BEHAVIORAL SCIENCE IN PEDIATRIC MEDICINE

NATHAN B. TALBOT, M.D.

Charles Wilder Professor of Pediatrics,
Harvard Medical School;
Chief, Children's Service, Burnham Division
for Children, Massachusetts General Hospital

JEROME KAGAN, Ph.D.

Professor of Human Development,
Department of Social Relations,
Harvard University

LEON EISENBERG, M.D.

Professor of Psychiatry,
Harvard Medical School;
Chief, Psychiatric Service,
Massachusetts General Hospital

1971 W. B. SAUNDERS COMPANY

PHILADELPHIA · LONDON · TORONTO

W. B. Saunders Company: West Washington Square
Philadelphia, Pa. 19105

12 Dyott Street
London, WC1A 1DB

1835 Yonge Street
Toronto 7, Ontario

Behavioral Science in Pediatric Medicine ISBN 0-7216-8750-4

Print No.: 9 8 7 6 5 4 3 2 1

CONTRIBUTORS

C. KEITH CONNERS, Ph.D.
Associate Professor of Psychology, Harvard Medical School. Psychologist, Massachusetts General Hospital, Boston, Massachusetts.

LEON EISENBERG, M.D.
Professor of Psychiatry, Harvard Medical School. Chief of Psychiatry, Massachusetts General Hospital, Boston, Massachusetts.

HOWARD D. FISHBEIN, Ph.D.
Associate Professor of Psychology, University of Cincinnati, Cincinnati, Ohio.

RONALD H. FORGUS, Ph.D.
Professor and Chairman, Psychology Department, Lake Forest College, Lake Forest, Illinois. Consulting Psychologist, Veterans Administration Hospital, Downey, Illinois.

BENSON E. GINSBURG, Ph.D.
Professor and Chairman, Department of Biobehavioral Sciences, The University of Connecticut, Storrs, Connecticut.

MARY C. HOWELL, M.D., Ph.D.
Chief, Family Evaluation Unit, Burnham Division for Children, Massachusetts General Hospital, Boston, Massachusetts. Instructor, Harvard Medical School, Cambridge, Massachusetts.

JEROME KAGAN, Ph.D.
Professor of Human Development, Department of Social Relations, Harvard University. Psychologist, Massachusetts General Hospital, Boston, Massachusetts.

ROSS A. McFARLAND, Ph.D., Sc.D. (Hon.)
Guggenheim Professor of Aerospace Health and Safety, Harvard University School of Public Health, Boston, Massachusetts.

ALLAN F. MIRSKY, Ph.D.
Professor of Psychiatry (Neuropsychology) and Neurology, Boston University School of Medicine, Boston, Massachusetts.

ROLAND C. MOORE, Ph.D.
Research Associate in Occupational Safety, Harvard University School of Public Health, Boston, Massachusetts.

NATHAN B. TALBOT, M.D.
Charles Wilder Professor of Pediatrics, Harvard Medical School. Chief, Children's Service, Burnham Division for Children, Massachusetts General Hospital, Boston, Massachusetts.

SHELDON H. WHITE, Ph.D.
Roy E. Larsen Professor of Educational Psychology, Harvard Graduate School of Education, Cambridge, Massachusetts.

REGINA M. YANDO, Ph.D.
Associate Professor, Clinical Psychology and Public Practice Program, Harvard University. Director, Psychological Training, Eunice Kennedy Shriver Center, Waltham, Massachusetts.

PREFACE

Current clinical experience with pediatric patients indicates that behavioral and social disorders are no less important than major physical and biologic agents as causes of disease and disability among infants, children and adolescents. This is gradually being recognized by medical schools, which have heretofore invested over 90 per cent of their curricular time, research resources and care facilities in the biophysical components of medicine. Therefore, many medical professionals have had limited opportunity to become familiar with the ways in which social conditions and personal behaviors may act singly or in combination with biophysical agents either to nourish and strengthen human beings or to injure and disable them. This poses a major challenge because the knowledge and skills of the behavioral sciences are now needed for solving contemporary health problems just as the natural sciences are essential for developing means to control diseases due primarily to organic pathogens.

The present volume comprises one of a number of current efforts by physicians and behavioral scientists to join together to meet this challenge through exchange of information and joint workmanship. This book is designed specifically for students and practitioners of pediatric medicine and allied health professions.

The first chapter presents a broad survey of the subject, viewed clinically. The next six chapters are concerned with basic considerations of certain phenomena clinically encountered by experts in specific fields of behavioral science. Thus, Chapter 2 is concerned with relations between behavior and mental function on the one hand and with the structural and functional state of the brain on the other. It brings into focus the fact that behavior is of neurofunctional origin, mediated by certain sets of brain cells subject to intrinsic biophysical and extrinsic sensory influences. Chapter 3 describes the elements of perception as a basic biosocial phenomenon and shows how this is related to information processing, learning, memory, thinking and behavioral adaptation to the environment. The authors of Chapter 4 have taken a fresh look at the processes of children's learning with a view to enabling members of the health care professions to deal with this subject in a realistically knowledgeable manner. Chapter 5 indicates how genetic and environmental factors can combine in various ways to produce behavioral phenotypes during the developmental period. In Chapter 6, the principles underlying assessment of intelligence and personality are detailed, with emphasis on their relation to clinical diagnosis and prognosis. Chapter 7 describes in considerable depth those components of the psychosocial system that have a bearing on the personality development of children particularly during their first decade. Chapter 8 deals with accidents, which now comprise a leading cause of death and disability among pediatric patients. Chapter 9 concerns psychopharmacology, which also is a subject of high importance because of its therapeutic implications and its relation to drug intoxication. Though some topics such as social anthropology are not considered *per se*, an effort has been made to include them where possible within the various chapters.

In discussing these subjects the authors have striven both to emphasize material bearing on clinical diagnosis or therapy and to present it in a way that the reader will gain critical insight and perspective on the subject at hand. Those who become actively interested in this field will undoubtedly want to pursue these subjects in greater depth. To facilitate this, references have been selected to open avenues for further reading as well as to provide detailed documentation on specific points. Particular effort has also been given to indexing this volume in a way that the reader can easily locate material of particular interest and discern the pertinence of the information represented by the basic behavioral sciences to practical clinical problems.

It is a pleasure to express here our sincere appreciation to Mr. John Dusseau, Vice President, and to Miss Pamela Herr, copy editor, of the W. B. Saunders Company for the splendid cooperation and patient support given us throughout the preparation of this book.

Nathan B. Talbot
Jerome Kagan
Leon Eisenberg

CONTENTS

1 SOCIAL AND BEHAVIORAL CAUSES AND CONSEQUENCES OF DISEASE AMONG CHILDREN

Nathan B. Talbot, and
Mary C. Howell

I. INTRODUCTION

> Man himself is now bringing about vast and rapid changes in his environment and is, thereby, producing an effect in which it is the environment created by him, rather than the environment of nature, that exerts a dominant influence upon his future evolutionary history—the transformation that is taking place is a shift from mainly physical diseases to social illness.
>
> *Salk, J. (1965)*

> It must be remembered that evidence is never complete, that knowledge of truth is always partial and that to seek certainty is to await eternity.
>
> *Bowlby, J. (1951)*

A. Essentiality of "Psychosocial Supplies"

Health and happiness as well as disease and disability derive not only from man's bodily constitution and the physical environment in which he lives, but also from his psychologic and behavioral interactions with the people who in his family, neighborhood and state comprise his social world.[1] To thrive, human beings must draw upon certain "psychosocial supplies," such as attention, affection, approval and control. Without an appropriate balance of these supplies, the individual may suffer from forms of "psychosocial malnutrition" which can produce results as disastrous to his health as is physical malnutrition induced by dietary imbalances. The way that biologic and physical factors can combine with social, psychologic and behavioral

[1] King, S. (1963); Talbot, N. B. (1968).

factors to cause—and also to correct—disorders of health is exemplified by the three following case abstracts.

CASE 1. MARKED DWARFISM SECONDARY TO PSYCHOSOCIAL MALNUTRITION[2]

This girl came to the Massachusetts General Hospital for diagnostic evaluation of dwarfism comparable to that seen in children with such organic conditions as primary hypopituitarism, hypothyroidism, dyschondroplasia, Cushing's syndrome and vitamin D resistant rickets. Although the problem involved biologic changes, it proved, in her case, to be the result of many interrelated psychosocial, psychophysiologic, behavioral and social-legal factors. Her response to treatment designed to overcome the social causes resulted in rates of gain and catch-up in growth that were of major proportions.

At a chronologic age of $7\frac{1}{4}$ years, this girl had a height age of 4 years and a weight age of $2\frac{1}{2}$ years. A detailed search for possible endocrine, metabolic or other organic causes of her dwarfism failed to yield any explanation other than the possibility that her failure to grow was in some way related to the fact that she was considerably underweight for her height. Metabolic balance studies were performed to determine whether or not she could gain and grow (as measured by nitrogen and mineral balances) if her caloric intake were raised to supermaintenance levels. The test results strongly suggested that the cause of her stunted growth at the biologic level was inadequate caloric intake (hypocaloricism).

However, it soon became clear that this was only part of the total web of causation, since the hypocaloricism was due to failure to eat (a behavioral phenomenon) because of lack of appetite (a psychophysiologic phenomenon). It was further noted that this anorexia might well be explained by the fact that this child was at risk of being separated from her foster mother, who was her only substantial source of affectionate attention and care. The child had been placed with this foster mother after the Division of Child Guardianship had removed her from the home of her grossly neglectful biologic parents (a psychosocial phenomenon). Now the parents were threatening to take her away. The foster mother, who had become fond of the child, wanted to stabilize the situation by adopting her. The responsible legal authorities, however, were reluctant to allow this because the child was abnormally small and therefore "a poor adoption risk" (a social-legal phenomenon). (See Fig. 1–1.)

In reviewing this situation it was clear that one had a wide choice of targets for therapeutic action. Theoretically, these included the possibility of giving the child growth hormone or of force feeding her in some manner. Likewise, she could have been given some pharmacologic agent to stimulate her appetite or to alleviate the anxiety on which her anorexia seemed to be based. Psychotherapy might

[2] Talbot, N. B., et al. (1947).

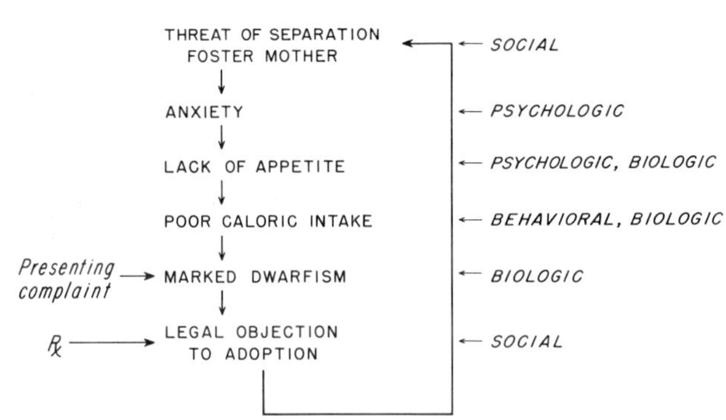

Figure 1–1 Case illustrative of the manner in which social, psychologic, behavioral and biologic factors can combine to cause dwarfism in a child. For details see Case 1 in the text. (*From* Talbot, N. B., et al., 1947, p. 25.)

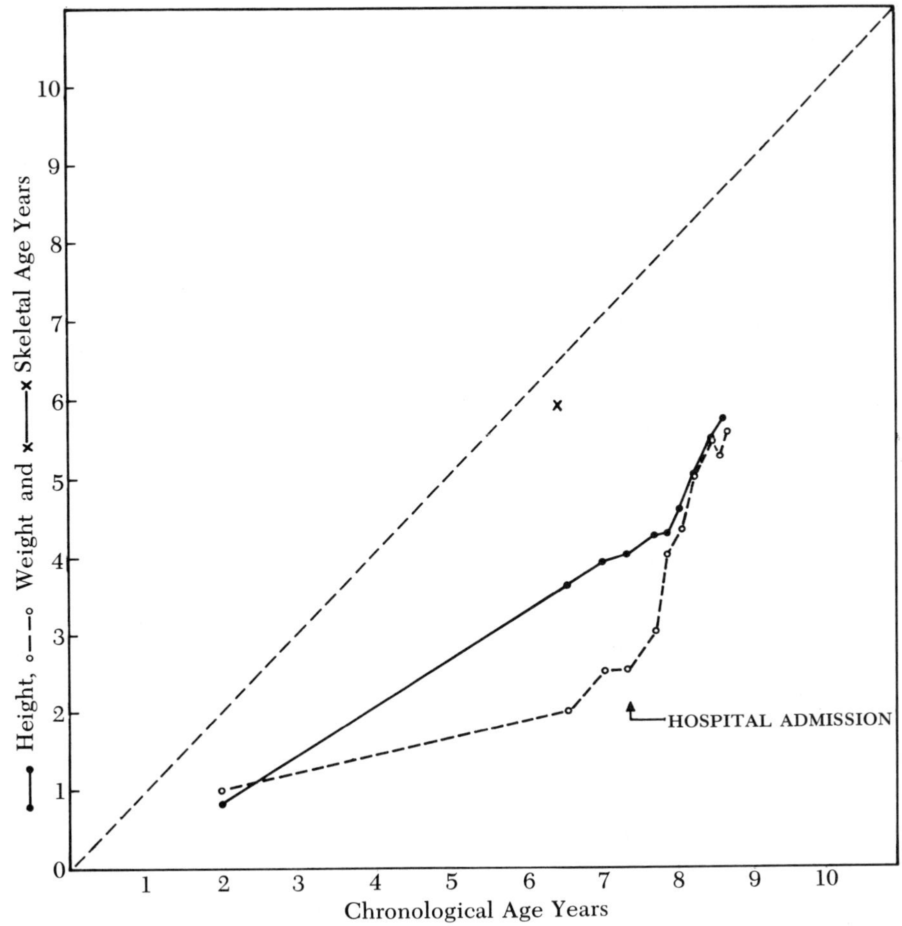

Figure 1–2 Effect of hospitalization and subsequent stabilization of the social environment on rates of gain in weight and growth in height of the patient of Figure 1–1.

have been recommended for similar purposes. However, from the overall biosocial medical point of view it appeared that the most logical way to deal with this problem was to try to persuade the legal authorities to permit the foster mother to adopt the child.

Happily, when the findings were presented to the guardianship authorities, they agreed to permit adoption proceedings. This action was accomplished shortly after the child's period of hospital studies. The results are shown in Figure 1–2. The child showed striking increases, first in weight gain and shortly afterwards in height. These gains occurred in the absence of any special diets, medications, psychotherapy or other standard forms of medical treatment. Thus, this case illustrates the importance of taking psychologic and behavioral, as well as biologic, factors into account even in the diagnosis and management of problems that appear to be primarily biomedical.

CASE 2. RESPONSE OF A RETARDED, NEGLECTED BOY TO CONSTRUCTIVE PERSONAL ATTENTION

Although the second case is in many respects similar to the first, it is characterized by retardation in cognitive and behavioral development as well as in physical development. Again, therapeutic provision of needed psychosocial supplies resulted in marked gains.

On admission to the Massachusetts General Hospital, this 21 month old boy corresponded in height to the average 6 month old, and in weight to the average 3 month old. In addition to being markedly dwarfed and underweight for his height, he had a bilateral partial cleft lip and considerable loss of vision due to cataracts, glaucoma, and congenitally cloudy corneas of both eyes. He tended to lie apathetic and inactive in his bed. He spoke no words and gave the impression of being grossly retarded in mental development. His history indicated that he had had a poor appetite; he had been eating poorly and had gained but one-half pound during the preceding nine months. He had been subject to repeated respiratory infections and gastrointestinal upsets.

For some time previously it had been noted that the child's mother was unconcerned about his difficulties and was preoccupied and overburdened with her many other problems. These included gallbladder disease, for which she could not afford an operation, heavy debts incurred as a result of the patient's multiple illnesses, low income and the need to work outside the home because her husband had lost his job. She had remarked that she felt better at work, where she was too busy to think, than at home. The mother had assumed that her husband could care for the baby while she worked, but observed that the child "would not eat for his father." Nonetheless, she planned to continue working even if her husband got a job.

Diagnostic studies failed to disclose any clearly observable organic cause of the child's small size, retarded mental and motor development and apathetic behavior. He was therefore transferred to the Children's Metabolic Unit to determine whether or not his stunting was due, as in Case 1, to hypocaloricism.

In this unit he came under the care of a nurse of friendly, gentle and happy disposition, who gave him several hours of almost undivided motherly attention each day. His responses to this affectionate care and general stimulation are portrayed in the sketches of Figure 1–3. As can be seen, he rapidly emerged from

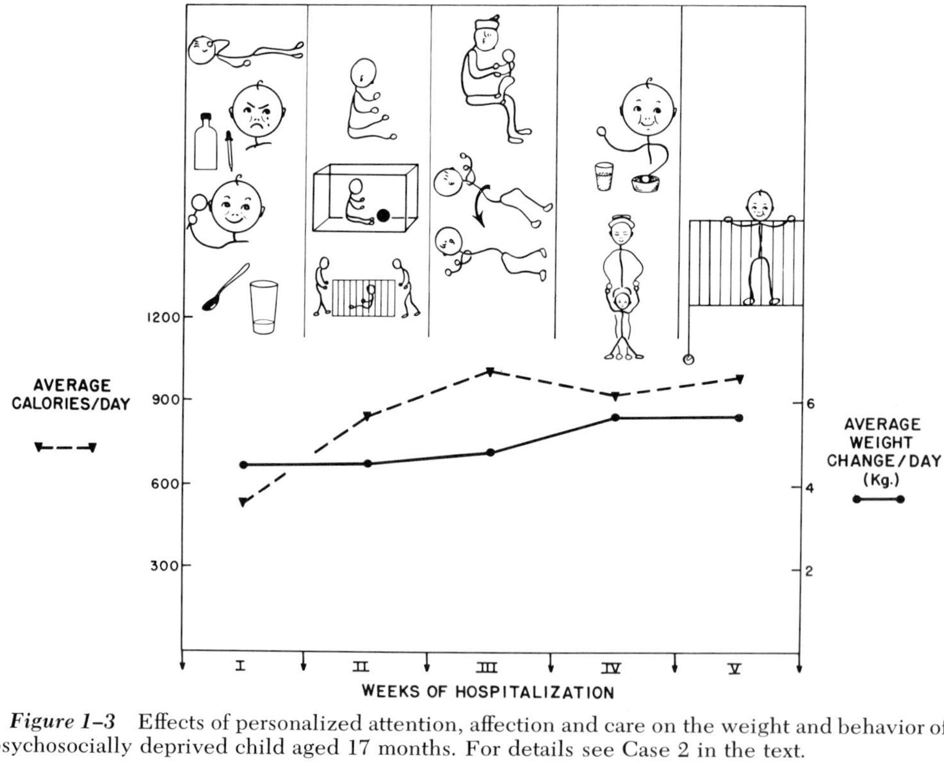

Figure 1–3 Effects of personalized attention, affection and care on the weight and behavior of a psychosocially deprived child aged 17 months. For details see Case 2 in the text.

his apathetic state to become an active, smiling, responsive, appealing youngster with evidence of normal capacity for neuromotor function and mentation. In addition, he was soon eating eagerly and beginning to gain weight.

His mother was pleased with these evidences of progress and promise for the future, and was able to accept the thesis that her child had a real need for personal attention from her. She therefore made arrangements that enabled her both to attend to his needs for a significant period of time each day, and to earn some much needed money. Unfortunately, the child's tendency to gain weight was interrupted by more upper respiratory infections following his return home. He continued to gain at a moderate rate but failed to accelerate sufficiently to make up for his growth deficit; consequently, he remained of abnormally short stature. On the other hand, he continued to show remarkable mental and behavioral progress. As mentioned above, he had originally appeared to be a grossly retarded child. When he was 4 years old, he was judged by standard tests to have an IQ of 60. However, when he was reexamined by tests appropriate for use with blind children, he was found to have an IQ of at least 85, with indications that he should function within the normal range if provided with the type of perceptual stimuli needed by visually handicapped individuals. This prediction was subsequently substantiated both by his mode of living and by standard tests of mental function.

Case 3. Sick Role as an Important Variable in Selection of Treatment of Thyrotoxicosis

The third case illustrates some of the social and personal life role disabilities that physicians may impose—unintentionally and perhaps unnecessarily—on patients during the course of treatment. These disabilities may affect not only the patients but their families as well.

This 14 year old girl presented with typical physical and chemical manifestations of juvenile thyrotoxicosis. The disease was of moderate intensity (serum protein-bound iodine was 13.5 mcg. per 100 ml.) and was clearly in need of therapy.

Thyrotoxicosis can be controlled by one of three means: An antithyroid medication such as propylthiouracil may be given by mouth every eight hours "by the clock," usually for two or more years, on the approximately 50–50 chance that the disease will burn itself out during that time. Another method consists in surgical removal of most of the thyroid gland. The third involves destruction of thyroid gland cells by means of an orally administered therapeutic dose of radioactive iodine. The first of these methods has the potential advantage of avoiding surgery and radiation, but carries the disadvantage that someone has to remember to give (or take) a pill on a regular schedule for a long period of time with no assurance that this will result in a permanent remission, even after over two thousand doses have been taken. It also may result in prominent enlargement of the thyroid gland and a consequent need to remove it surgically. Surgical management of thyrotoxicosis usually results in permanent control of the disease, but carries the small risks incident to general anesthesia and accidental injury to the parathyroid glands or to the nerves that control the vocal cords. It also leaves a scar in the neck, a scar considered by some girls as a disfigurement, and by others as a valuable means of gaining sympathetic attention. In about one in three cases, surgery results in a lifelong need for thyroid hormone substitution therapy. This can be taken in the form of a pill any time in the day and does not pose much of a problem. Treatment with radioactive iodine is painless and usually brings the disease permanently under control within a few weeks. There is a theoretical disadvantage of possible predisposition to tumor of the thyroid gland, but actual instances are rare. As with surgically managed patients, about one in three of these patients needs thyroid hormone substitution therapy once a day.

Administration of antithyroid medication had long been considered by many physicians to be the most conservative approach. Consequently, the patient was placed initially on the antithyroid agent, propylthiouracil. Recognizing that this medication could result in undesirable intensification of parental oversight and control of the adolescent girl, we strongly suggested that she herself be made responsible for taking the pills on time.

However, her mother, like many other mothers, found it difficult to grant this much independence and responsibility and personally made sure that the doses were taken on time, morning, afternoon, and night. As a result, the mother's supervision of this girl was markedly intensified at a time in life when most children are growing away from parental control and parents are relieved of the need to watch closely over their children's activities. Moreover, the life activities not only of the patient but also of her mother and, indeed, the rest of the family, began to be governed by the medication schedule. The net result was that several members of the family experienced almost as much of a "sick role" life style as the patient herself, to the dismay of all concerned.

At about the time when this social problem was becoming so intense that we were seriously considering shifting to a form of therapy that would not result in sick role existence, a circumstance arose which made a change in therapy desirable for biologic as well as for social reasons. This was the development of a drug rash of such intensity as to necessitate discontinuation of the propylthiouracil. As an alternate, the patient was given a single dose of radioactive iodine by mouth. During the ensuing three weeks, while the iodine was acting on her thyroid cells, she was asked to avoid strenuous physical exercise—another form of medically imposed sick role. During the two years since that time, however, she has been free to live a normal life with no medical treatment or supervision other than biannual checkups for signs of thyroid hormone excess or insufficiency. The entire family was profoundly relieved by the medical decision to manage the thyrotoxicosis in a manner that did not interfere seriously with their usual life activities.

These children represent only three among many hundreds of pediatric patients studied at Massachusetts General Hospital during the past 25 years whose cases demonstrate the close interrelationship of biophysical and sociobehavioral factors in the causes and consequences of disease. Pediatricians and internists are generally well prepared to diagnose and manage the biophysical aspects of disease. However, many are not yet equally well equipped to deal with the social and behavioral components of commonplace medical and surgical problems.[3] They lack familiarity with the nature and the importance of certain stresses which interfere with development, injure health and promote disease. They also lack appreciation of certain psychosocial supplies—such as those identified in the cases just described—necessary to prevent or to overcome disease.

There has been a paucity of clinically applicable diagnostic criteria and terminologies which take into account all of the complex factors in disease. There also has been a lack of systematic means of integrating sociobehavioral and biophysical information into a comprehensive diagnosis and plan of management. This book is one part of an overall effort to overcome these deficits.

B. Psychosocial Malnutrition —General Considerations

Section I has presented case studies to illustrate the interrelationship of biophysical and psychosocial factors in disease. Section II considers the basic components of the biosocial complex in health and disease. Section II-A deals with the nature, origins and modes of transmission and reception of psychosocial supplies. Healthy function and development of the human organism are contingent on receipt of the necessary psychosocial supplies, just as they are on receipt of such physical supplies as adequate diet. In both cases, supplies must be sufficient to cover minimum requirements, but not so great as to exceed tolerance limits.

---

[3]Rose, J. (1960); Talbot, N. B. (1964, 1965, 1968); Richmond, J. (1969).

When the input of psychosocial supplies exceeds or falls short of human limits of adaptive competence, psychosocial malnutrition may result. Some of these contributing factors, discussed in Section II-B, include deprivation, when psychosocial supplies are inadequate; intoxication, when supplies are overabundant; and injury, when either deprivation or intoxication reaches poisonous levels. Personal sources of the different varieties of psychosocial supplies are considered in section II-C, and impersonal sources are considered in section II-D. The nature of behavioral and physical problems resulting from an imbalance of psychosocial supplies is outlined in sections II-E and II-F.

Most physicians subscribe to the ideas expressed by Peabody[4] in his classic treatise "The Care of the Patient." However, few attempts have been made to define these ideas in terms of life roles, even though this is central to management of patients in relation to their environment and to the formulation of significant indices of therapeutic success. In section II-G, therefore, the effects of disease, disability or deformity on a child's parents, siblings or others is explored, and Section II-H describes the characteristics of a sick role existence.

It is essential that pediatricians and allied child health caretakers be able to prevent or manage commonplace forms of psychosocial deprivation, intoxication and injury during the early phases of psychosocial malnutrition, when the child is still capable of healing himself. Section II-I suggests appropriate therapeutic strategies. This concept may be understood through comparison with current pediatric practice in relation to vitamin D therapy for rickets. If the pediatrician can begin treatment soon enough, he can provide a rachitic infant with enough crystalline vitamin D_2 to enable the child's body to cure itself and remain free from rickets for life—at a cost of less than five dollars. However, if the child is not treated in the early stages of his disease, changes occur which cannot be handled in this simple, self-corrective manner and which may be only partially reversible at any price. The disease may develop beyond the pediatrician's competence, and his services may have to be supplemented by the orthopedic specialist. Similarly, the pediatrician's failure to cope with behavioral pathology in its early stages may make participation of a mental health professional necessary at a later time.

[4]Peabody, F. (1930).

Section III of this chapter deals with some of the clinical aspects of the interrelationship between biophysical and sociobehavioral pathology. Section III-A discusses the importance of sociobehavioral factors in the diagnosis and management of pediatric patients. Section III-B deals with psychosocial deprivation and intoxication syndromes, and section III-C with the child abuse syndrome as one form of psychosocial injury. Section III-D presents the Clinical Summary Abstract form, developed by the Children's Service of the Massachusetts General Hospital as a means of coordinating biophysical and sociobehavioral information into a comprehensive diagnosis and plan of management. A representative list of references is included at the end of the chapter.

II. COMPONENTS OF THE BIOSOCIAL COMPLEX IN HEALTH AND DISEASE

To treat and prevent diseases of children effectively, the physician needs to recognize not only the biophysical factors, but also the various forms of psychosocial malnutrition that can undermine a child's health. Such questions as the following therefore become relevant. What psychosocial supplies are required to prevent such malnutrition? Where are the sources (actual and potential) of these supplies in the child's social world? What are the effects of their presence or absence on his physical being and personal behavior, and what are the specific ways these supplies can be used as vital therapeutic tools?

A. Nature, Origins and Modes of Transmission and Reception of Psychosocial Supplies

Love is something like the
clouds that were in the sky
before the sun came out—
you cannot touch the clouds,
you know, but you feel the
rain and know how glad the
flowers and the thirsty earth
are to have it after a hot day.
You cannot touch love either,
but you feel the sweetness
that it pours into everything.
Without love you would not be
happy or want to play.

Words "spoken" by Ann Mansfield Sullivan to Helen Keller. Keller, H. (1954)

In every human society, human infants are born helpless and relatively undeveloped, dependent upon adult nurture and adult transmission of the great body of culture—beliefs, practices, skills— which make it possible for any human group and for this human group in particular to function as human beings. A child who does not participate in this great body of tradition, whether because of defect, neglect, injury or disease, never becomes fully *human.*

Mead, M., and Wolfenstein, M. (1955)

The behavioral elements as well as the structural ones are vital aspects of our biologic heritage—a craving by each individual for response from his social environment is a craving as fundamental as that for food.

Eisenberg, L. (1968)

Organisms like to be disturbed and indeed they cannot live normally and fully if they are not.

Thompson, W., and Melzack, R. (1956)

Attempts to ensure feelings of security in children and to avoid stress have led to prescriptions of continuity, stability and homogeneity as essential ingredients of an environment for development and learning. If the world were a great deal simpler, if it smacked more of a psychological laboratory, perhaps one could agree. But the world is not such a laboratory. It is essential to have and to develop in children, resources for dealing with the unexpected, the accidental and the unusual. It may be that a degree of security for children can be ensured by minimizing the quantity and variety of stimulation and thus eliminate stress. But this ill prepares them for the complex, ever-changing world with which they must deal as adults.

Martin, W. (1965)

It has long been known that human beings have a fundamental need for certain supportive psychosocial supplies, just as they have need for air, food and other nutriments. It is also probable that progressive exposure to changes in social environment, the requirement of delayed gratification, and other forms of psychosocial stress are as

*Table 1-1 Examples of Interpersonally Transmitted Psychosocial Supplies**

Category of Supply	Modes of Expression
Being valued	Acceptance[3]
	Affection[4]
	Approval[5]
Being attended to	Attention[6]
	Care[7]
	Protection[8]
Being controlled	Limit setting[9]
	Guidance[10]

*The chief personal sources of these supplies should be sufficiently stable, continuous and consistent to give the child a reasonable degree of *certainty of the future.*[1] On the other hand, progressive exposure to tolerable degrees of change in social environment, delay in gratification and other forms of psychosocial stress are important to the development of psychologic coping capacity.[2]

[1]Davis, K. (1949); Eisenberg, L. (1965); Bakwin, H., and Bakwin, R., et al. (1966); Caldwell, B. (1967); Provence, S. (1967).

[2]Reiser, D. (1963); Martin, W. (1965).

[3]Lowenfeld, B. (1956); Glaser, H., et al. (1964).

[4]Davis, K. (1949); Bowlby, J. (1951); Lowenfeld, B. (1956); Sears, R., et al. (1957); Schaefer, E. (1959); Peiper, A. (1963); Skeels, H. (1966); Caldwell, B. (1967); Provence, S. (1967); Conners, K. (1970).

[5]Bakwin, H., and Bakwin, R., et al. (1966); Provence, S. (1967).

[6]Davis, K. (1949); Bowlby, J. (1951); Skeels, H. (1966); Eisenberg, L. (1968).

[7]Fried, R., and Mayer, M. (1948); Bowlby, J. (1951); Lowenfeld, B. (1956); Green, M., and Solnit, A. (1964); Bakwin, H., and Bakwin, R., et al. (1966).

[8]Lowenfeld, B. (1956); Lapouse, R., and Monk, M. (1959); Witmer, H., et al. (1962); Bakwin, H., and Bakwin, R., et al. (1966).

[9]Lowenfeld, B. (1956); Jaco, E. (Ed.) (1958); Schutz, W. (1958); Schaefer, E. (1959); Richmond. J. (1960); Green, M., and Solnit, A. (1964; Bakwin, H., and Bakwin, R., et al. (1966); Provence, S. (1967).

[10]Green, M., and Solnit, A. (1964); Shapiro, M. (1965); Bakwin, H., and Bakwin, R., et al. (1966); Provence, S. (1967).

important to the development of the individual's psychologic coping capacity as exposure to various physical stresses is to the development of bodily ability to deal with infections, toxins and heavy physical demands.[5]

[5]Reiser, D. (1963); Martin, W. (1963, 1965).

The fact that most material resources can be held in the hand and weighed and analyzed by physical means has made it relatively easy to recognize, characterize and measure them with scientific precision. Psychosocial supplies pose more of a problem because they comprise various forms of interpersonally transmitted information concerning such matters as being valued, being the object of attention, being controlled and being reasonably secure about continuing to receive these supplies in the future.[6] (See Table 1-1.) *It is the recipient who decides whether he is being valued, attended to, controlled and so forth.* The fact that this decision is not always made evident to outside observers by the behavior of the recipient (in this case the child) may at times pose difficulties for the clinical diagnostician.

However, interpersonally transmitted information stems from the central nervous system of a living being. It is mediated by motions, sounds and other physical phenomena, which in turn stimulate the sensory systems of the recipient. For instance, when a parent wishes to express approval to his child, he may do so by smiling at him, giving him a pat on the back, saying "well done" or communicating this information in some other culturally appropriate way. The fact that these interpersonal exchanges are mediated by observable sounds and actions makes them subject to indirect definition and analysis by trained observers in accordance with scientific principles.[7] Thus, it is possible to establish norms of interpersonal behavior with relation to such variables as culture, sex, age and social class. These norms

[6]Spitz, R. (1946); Glaser, K., and Eisenberg, L. (1956); Maas, H., and Engler, R. (1959); Rose, J. (1959); Elmer, E. (1960); Eisenberg, L. (1962); Fanshel, D., and Maas, H. (1962); Scott, J. (1962); Silver, H., and Finkelstein, M. (1967).

[7]Rheingold, H. (1960).

provide points of reference from which the psychosocial supply status of a given individual can be compared with that of others who are developing and functioning well in similar environments.

For centuries poets and artists have portrayed mothers as the main purveyors of loving care for infants and little children. This is not surprising. The biologic relationship between mother and child is as old as mankind; monogamy, with its implied continuing bond between father and offspring, is a late event in our history and has no similar natural foundation.[8] Even today there are large numbers of American families in which the fathers are absent and the child's mother is his only stable source of nurture. Ordinarily, in our culture the natural mother is interested in assuming this role and is able to do so.

With the development of independent mobility, children gradually acquire additional personal sources of psychosocial supplies—siblings and other relatives, playmates, schoolmates, neighbors, teachers and so forth. Consequently, the initially predominant role of the mother becomes diluted as the child grows up. The shift from maternal care to care by others may be gradual, as is usually the case in American families, or very abrupt, as is characteristic of many of the old world cultures wherein mothers give a great deal of personal attention to their offspring up to the time of weaning and then suddenly transfer their attention from their now 2 or 3 year old child to his newborn sibling.

Variations in Mode of Expressing Psychosocial Supplies. Although parents, older sisters, nurses, teachers and other child caretakers share a common role as sources of psychosocial supplies for young children, the ways they provide these supplies vary considerably according to their culture and social class. Studies of children reared in different parts of the world under a variety of social, economic and physical circumstances provide rich sources of information concerning this subject.[9] Moreover, they indicate that human beings have a capacity to adjust, within certain limits, to variations in modes of providing essential psychosocial supplies, just as they do to variations in the nature of the foodstuffs from which they derive their essential dietary nutriments.

Table 1–2 is illustrative of the fact that dependable comparisons between various child care practices can be obtained. In this instance the comparisons were accomplished by a time sampling of the frequency with which various behaviors occurred over eight-hour periods of direct observation.[10] The subjects were 10 infants 3 to 4 months of age, five of whom were living at home and five who were residents in an institution. As in a Dutch study of maternal caretaking practices,[11] this study showed wide differences in the frequency of exposure of home reared infants to such maternal activities as looking at the child's face, talking to him, playing with him, patting him or holding him. A still greater difference was noted, however, between the care received by the home reared infants and the attention given those in the institution. The same types of care were recorded, but scores calculated from these observations indicate that the home reared infants received care about 4.5 times as often as the institutionalized children.

---

[8]Mead, M. (1949); Peiper, A. (1963).

[9]Mead, M. (1949); Mead, M., and Wolfenstein, M. (1955); Whiting, B. (Ed.) (1963); Ainsworth, M., and Salten, D. (1967); Rebelsky, F. (1967); Brazelton, R., et al. (1969); Caudill, W., and Weinstein, H. (1969); Bronfenner, M. (1970); Whiting, J., and Whiting, B. (1971).

[10]Rheingold, H. (1960).

[11]Rebelsky, F. (1967); Rebelsky, F., and Abeles, G. (1969).

***Table 1–2 Means and Ranges of Maternal Care and Infant Activity*††**
N of Infants in Each Group = 5
N of Observations for Each Infant = 1280

Item	Home Mean	Home Range	Institution Mean	Institution Range
**Caretaking	475.2	347– 617	105.8	74– 144
** *N* of caretakers	1.4	1– 2	6.0	5– 8
** Looks at face†	140.2	109– 173	28.4	6– 36
** Talks	55.8	26– 105	7.8	0– 19
** Talks to infant	166.2	51– 310	17.0	12– 22
** Pats	26.2	9– 44	2.0	1– 4
Shows affection	3.6	0– 14	0.2‡	0– 1
* Plays	11.8	4– 25	0.8‡	0– 4
** Holds	285.4	196– 394	45.6	11– 70
** Diapers	37.4	27– 57	5.6	1– 10
Bathes	35.2	0– 103	8.8	6– 11
** Feeds	154.4	72– 198	28.6	4– 43
Dresses	11.2	0– 28	16.2	6– 31
** Adjusts position	6.8	0– 11	2.2	1– 4
Rocks	37.2	0– 138	2.2	0– 4
Other	14.2	8– 20	11.4	3– 18
Location of Infant				
In crib	787.0	667– 908	908.4	699–1081
** In arms	258.6	179– 391	46.2	8– 76
** Seated	0.0	...	260.0	128– 530
Bathinette	86.0	27– 139	41.2	19– 70
Other location	148.2	2– 327	24.2	0– 112
** Out of own room	304.4	153– 391	43.0	21– 77
N Adults in Room				
** 0	690.0	466– 899	263.0	178– 352
1	534.8	372– 814	464.4	416– 568
** 2	34.8	0– 136	246.0	182– 329
** 3+	20.0	0– 99	304.2	210– 361
N Adults within 6 Ft.				
** 0	755.5	652– 919	1062.6	1022–1093
** 1	492.2	361– 621	161.0	130– 213
* 2	12.8	0– 38	45.0	33– 68
3+	19.5	0– 78	11.4	5– 18
Infant Activities				
Awake	847.4	565–1081	928.6	647–1042
Vocalizes	54.2	22– 81	38.4	1– 76
Vocalizes to mother	9.6	1– 30	3.0	0– 5
Protests	14.4	5– 21	20.6	1– 59
Fusses	31.4	14– 46	43.6	19– 71
Cries	23.6	2– 64	14.8	0– 47
Finger in mouth	103.8	0– 312	69.0	10– 111
** Bottle in mouth	54.4	0– 146	298.8	170– 435
* Plays with toy	62.8	0– 168	18.2‡	0– 91
Plays with hand	8.4	2– 20	41.6	1– 117
* Plays with dress	0.0	...	8.4	2– 20
Bursts of activity	32.6	13– 78	46.0	18– 92

†Caretaking items not mutually exclusive.
‡Mean based on one case.
*Difference between groups significant at .05 level, two-tailed test.
**Difference between groups significant at .01 level, two-tailed test.
††*The following quotation from Dr. Rheingold's text is given to clarify the procedure used in obtaining the data recorded in the table.*

Procedure

The Checklist. On the basis of observation and trial (3) a checklist composed of 42 items was drawn up, 30 for mothering activities and 12 for infant activities (Table [1–2] gives the items). Of the 30 mothering items six recorded the location of *S* in his environment, four the number of people in his room, and four the number of people within six feet of him.

The remaining 16 items recorded activities more closely related to mothering. "Caretaking" was an all-inclusive item which was checked if at the moment of observation someone was doing something for *S* while in proximity to him. "*N* of caretakers" recorded the number of different caretakers who cared for *S* during the eight-hour period of observation. The last 14 items were sufficient to cover all the caretaking operations performed by people in caring for three-month-old infants at the level of analysis selected for study here. Although all items were defined in detail, the behaviors included in them need no comment, with a few exceptions. "Talks" was checked when the caretaker talked to anyone and not specifically to *S*; her speech could be thought of as providing auditory stimulation for the infant. "Plays" included both social play of caretaker and infant *and* caretaker's initiating infant's play with toys. The item "Other" had to be used very infrequently; it covered such caretaking activities as giving *S* vitamins and weighing him.

It should be noted that the caretaking activities were not considered as mutually exclusive. Rather, all the activities occurring at any moment of observation were checked; thus, a caretaker could be bathing the infant, looking at his face, and talking to him on the same observation.

Although the purpose of the study was to measure the caretakers' activities, a number of infant activities which served to delineate maternal care were also included.

Time of Observation. For each *S* a period of eight hours was sampled according to the following schedule: *O* looked at S for a full second and then recorded on the checklist what he was doing, if someone was caring for him, the nature of the caretaking act, where he was, and how many other people were in his environment. *O* could take as long as 14 seconds to complete the record, but in any case she did not look up again until the 15th second when she again observed *S* for a full second. In this fashion, four observations were made in each minute for a total of 10 minutes. After a break of five minutes another sample of 10 minutes was observed. Thus, the first 10 minutes of each quarter hour were sampled for four consecutive hours, that is, from 9 A.M. to 1 P.M. on one day and from 1 P.M. to 5 P.M. on the next day, to make a total of eight hours. There were three *Os* in all, but only a pair for each infant, one observing the first four hours, and the other, the second four.

Observers' Behavior. The *Os* endeavored to put the mothers and the attendants at their ease by being friendly and by conspicuously making the infant the focus of observation. The *O*, for example, stayed in the room with *S*, whether he was asleep or awake, and continued to make observations. The readiness with which *Os* were accepted was reassuring, as was the extent to which people went about the business of caring for *S* *as though* they were not being observed. Mothers, on questioning subsequent to the period of observation, said that *O*'s presence inhibited only their more "foolish" behavior with the infant, e.g., using nonsense syllables, singing, etc. The effect of *O*'s presence will be raised again in the Discussion.

Scoring. The score was the frequency of occurrence of each item over the eight-hour period for each subject. From these scores a mean score for each item was derived for each group of five *S*s.

Since 40 observations were made during each 10-minute period, the total number of observations for the eight-hour period was 1280. Dividing the mean scores by 1280 could give percentages of occurrence; and, since the observations were systematically distributed throughout time, the mean score could also be translated into hours and minutes.

Observer-Agreement. To check the reliability of the observations, *Os* made independent simultaneous observations during 64 10-minute periods. Thirty-five of the periods occurred before the study began, the rest at intermediate points as the study progressed, in order to insure continuing agreement. The observations were made on seven *S*s, four in the institution and three in homes, none of whom were subjects in the study.

The amount of observer-agreement for each item was calculated by two different methods. In the first, a percentage of agreement was obtained by dividing the number of agreements by the combined number of agreements and disagreements. Here an agreement was a tally identical in both records; that is, both *Os* agreed not only in *identifying* the item but also in the *timing* of the item; agreement on the absence of an activity was *not* counted as an agreement. The median percentage of agreement for all items was 89.8 (range 16.7 to 100.0). As one might expect, there was some tendency for *Os* to agree more often on frequently occurring items. (The rank-order correlation between percentage of agreement and frequency of items was .71 $p < .01$).

In the second method, observer-agreement was calculated by correlating the frequencies obtained for each item. The median of the product-moment correlations was .97 (range .35 to 1.00).

On the basis of these findings the method was judged to have sufficient observer-agreement to warrant a measure of confidence in the results obtained by its use.

(*From* Rheingold, H. L.: The measurement of maternal care. *Child Develop.*, *31*:566–569, 1960. Courtesy The Society for Research in Child Development, Inc.)

Cultural Differences in Child Rearing. Many observers have reported interesting intercultural differences in the ways infants and children are provided with care, affection and control. Take, for example, the matter of maternal attention and care. In Nyansongo, Kenya, East African mothers carry their infants on their backs, or keep their babies close by but under the immediate care of someone else by day and sleep with them in their arms at night.[12] These babies are almost never left alone up to the time they are weaned, between 2 and 3 years of age. During this interval they are offered the breast without delay at the slightest indication of disquietude, hunger or discomfort. However, even though mother-child contact is close and nearly constant, it is unusual for these mothers to look at or fondle their offspring. Much the same kind of maternal care practices have been observed among families in Taira, Okinawa; in Tarong, an Ilocos Barrio in the Phillipines; and among the Mixtecans in Mexico.[13]

By contrast, in Khalapur, India, mothers have their infants sleep with them at night, but during the daytime when not in need of food or immediate attention, the babies are placed in cots, which are covered completely with quilts or sheets as protection against insects and envious glances.[14]

In Holland, Dutch mothers have their infants sleep in canopied beds in separate, unheated rooms, the doors to which are kept closed.[15] Because the mother also keeps the door to the room in which she is living closed, she is not always able to hear the baby cry. This practice is in keeping with the Dutch attitude that crying is a normal part of infantile behavior, is good for the lungs and is not, therefore, always something to stop. Although most of the Dutch mothers who were studied breast fed their offspring, they did so in accordance with their doctor's prescription for limited periods of time at three to four hour intervals.

Considerable differences in caretaker expressions of affection have been recorded. For instance, Nyansongo[16] and Zinacanteco[17] mothers rarely kiss, hug, coo or give other overt evidence of affection. By contrast, in Tarong, the infant is proffered much nurture by his mother and, indeed, by anyone and everyone in the community up to the time of weaning. Explicit expressions of affection have comprised a relatively small component of the normal mother-infant interactions observed among American, Dutch and Japanese families.[18]

Wide differences in respect to control, setting limits, discipline and allied matters have also been observed. In a number of the Old World cultures it is believed that infants are helpless creatures incapable of knowing, understanding or learning until they reach a certain age, usually the age of weaning. The thought is that they gain awareness and reason much as they cut their teeth and mature physically. Accordingly, such babies are treated indulgently with very little training during

---

[12]LeVine, R., and LeVine, B. (1963).

[13]Maretski, T., and Maretski, H. (1963); Nydegger, W., and Nydegger, C. (1963); Romney, K., and Romney, R. (1963).

[14]Minturn, L., and Hitchcock, T. (1963).

[15]Rebelsky, F., and Abeles, G. (1969).

[16]LeVine, R., and LeVine B. (1963).

[17]Brazelton, T., et al. (1969).

[18]Rheingold, H. (1960); Rebelsky, F. (1967); Rebelsky, F., and Abeles, G. (1969); Caudill, W., and Weinstein, H. (1969).

their first two to three years of life. For these children the day of change to a more responsible existence is a day of rude awakening. This is often marked by abrupt weaning, a shift from sleeping with parents to sleeping alone or with siblings and exposure to sometimes harsh discipline for transgressions of societal standards relating to personal conduct in elimination, obedience and aggressive behavior. As might be expected, this abrupt change often is markedly disturbing to the child, who may have tantrums and behave in a whining, obstinate and miserable manner during his adaptation to these new realities. New Englanders, by contrast, are described as having the attitude that parents and other adults can and should have an important influence on the development of their child from early on. They see themselves as being in a better position than the child to foresee the end product of development. It is therefore their duty to help the infant to realize the good aspects of his potential and to curb the bad.[19]

Cultural Values and Child Behavior. The ideals of parents in various societies may differ considerably. For instance, parents in many parts of the world consider the "ideal" infant to be one who cries little, eats well, needs no entertainment and goes happily to all adults. As the boy reaches preschool age it is hoped that he will be aggressive in defending himself, but not otherwise; will train easily in respect to eating, toilet and bedtime habits; will not be spoiled or shy or show off; and will get along well with his peers. On the other hand, in the Crow Indian culture, the child is encouraged to rebel against authority and to defy authoritarian demands, even from his own

[19]Whiting, B. (Ed.) (1963).

*Table 1–3 Percentage of Children in Each Culture Reported or Observed Performing the Listed Tasks**

Tasks	Percentage of Children					
	Nyansongo	Juxtla-huaca	Tarong	Taira	Khalapur	Orchard Town
Collecting firewood	44	27	58	13	13	*
Fetching water	75	64	20	18	29	*
Collecting fodder	0	5	13	8	17	*
Cleaning and sweeping	31	41	59	59	33	92
Preparing food	19	5	42	0	4	0
Harvesting vegetables	25	14	36	0	9	0
Grinding grain	38	9	8	0	0	*
Cooking	31	5	29	0	0	4
Gardening	75	14	13	13	4	*
Tending fowl	0	9	29	25	*	13
Tending household animals	0	23	33	21	13	*
Tethering	0	9	29	0	0	*
Herding	50	5	37	4	33	*

†*From* Whiting, J., and Whiting, B. (1971).
*Indicates that the task is not relevant for this culture.

*Table 1–4 Distribution of Children in Each Culture, Based on Their Scores on the Egoism-Altruism Scale**

SCORE	NYANSONGO	JUXTLA-HUACA	TARONG	TAIRA	KHALAPUR	ORCHARD TOWN
40						
+36–40					xxx	xx
+31–35					xx	xx
+26–30					xxxx	xxx
+21–25				xx	xx	xxxx
+16–20		x		xx	xxx	xxx
+11–15		x		xxx	x	xxxx
+6–10	x		xx	xxxxxx	xx	xxxx
+1–5		xx	xxxx	xxx	xx	x
0		xx	x	xxx		
−1–5		xxxx	xx	xx	xxx	x
−6–10	x	xx	xxxxxxx	x		
−11–15	xxxx	xxxxxx	xx	xx		
−16–20	xx		x			
−21–25	x	x	xx			
−26–30	xxx		xx			
−31–35	xxx	x	x			
−36–40		x				
−40	x	x				
Percentage of children more egoistic than altruistic	7	18	21	67	79	96

*The scores were computed by subtracting a child's score on the macro-altruism (the sum of *offers help, offers support* and *suggests reponsibility*) from his score on macro-egoism (the sum of *seeks help, seek attention* and *seeks dominance*). Each x indicates a child. (*From* Whiting, J., and Whiting, B., 1971).

parents. In the overall American culture this behavior might be interpreted as a lack of control, but among the Crows it is considered evidence that the child is learning to be a "man."[20]

Cultural values can have profound effects on the behavior of children, as illustrated by Whiting's observations on the altruistic-egoistic dimension of the behavior of 134, three to ten year old children reared in six different cultures.[21] (See Tables 1–3 and 1–4.) In the less complex societies of Tarong, Juxtlahuaca and Nyansongo, all family heads are subsistence farmers, and settlement patterns are composed primarily of dwellings with few if any specialized buildings. These communities depend primarily on an indigenous political system in which authority is localized and which has no class or caste system or indigenous priesthood. In these societies children, beginning at a very early age, are functioning members of the economy, and their assistance is expected and valued in performing such essential tasks as carrying wood and water, preparing and cooking food, gardening, caring for animals and looking after younger siblings, particularly infants. *Children reared under these circumstances behave in a predominantly altruistic (rather than egoistic) manner.* This judgment was based on the frequency with which children were observed helping others carry out a task, giving food or some desired object to another, cuddling, commiserating or otherwise providing emotional support to someone or acting in

[20]Benedict, R. (1949).
[21]Whiting, J. (1971).

a responsible way for the benefit of others (as when an older child attended a younger sibling).

By contrast, in Orchard Town, Khalapur and Taira, an appreciable number of family heads make their living at some occupation other than subsistence farming. In these communities the settlement pattern is complex, the political system is centralized. There is a class or caste system and a fulltime organized priesthood, and the children are assigned relatively few tasks clearly related to the welfare of the family. *Children reared under these circumstances behave in a predominantly egoistic manner.* They tend to seek help by crying, pleading, demanding, wheedling, whining or politely requesting help; they tend to seek attention by showing off, boasting, clowning or shouting or by direct requests such as "look at me," "see what I have done," and they tend to seek dominance by arrogantly issuing commands for purposes of self-interest more often than they offer help, support or responsible care.

Inborn Characteristics as a Factor in Child Behavior. Almost from the day of birth children exhibit observable differences in their threshholds of responsiveness, intensity of responses, activity levels, rhythmicity in sleeping, feeding adaptability, general moods and so forth. Sometimes these differences reflect transient results of such factors as prepartum medication to the mother and are therefore evident only during the neonatal period. Other differences are intrinsic and may persist and be discernible year after year.

The particular nature of each child, of course, influences the effects given sets of caretaking tactics have on his behavior.[22] These differences in the nature of the child may also have a bearing on the manner in which his parents and others deal with him. It is one thing to care for a child who is friendly, adaptable and positively responsive; it is another matter to cope with a child who is unfriendly, withdrawing, resistant to change or negatively responsive toward efforts to care for him. While it may be relatively easy to rear the former type of child, it takes an exceptionally loving and durable parent to continue to proffer affectionate care and guidance to the latter type and to avoid developing hostile, destructive attitudes and practices toward him. Yet this may be crucial to the evolution of the child as a healthy and effective person. Conversely, it may be difficult for a child to respond warmly and positively to a mother whose approach is cold, disapproving or harsh. Parent-child interrelationships are reciprocal and must, at least to a minimal extent, be mutually satisfactory to be constructive. Most children are adaptable rather than unadaptable, and positive rather than negative in mood.[23] This probably explains why so many children seem able to tolerate the wide differences in child rearing practices observed between cultures and from time to time within the same culture. These historic swings are interestingly reflected in articles on child training practices published in the *Ladies' Home Journal, Woman's Home Companion* and *Good Housekeeping* dating from 1890.[24] For instance, modes of infant discipline have varied from the "be tough with them, feed on schedule and let them cry it out" doctrine to a highly permissive, loosely scheduled "it is reasonable to feed a baby when he is hungry" approach. In 1890 writers were advising the use of rewards as a method of

[22]Brazelton, T. (1962); Kagan, J., and Moss, H. (1962); Thomas, A., et al. (1964); Brazelton, T., and Robey, J. (1965); Escalona, S, (1968); Thomas, A., et al. (1968).

[23]Thomas, A., et al. (1964).

[24]Stendler, C. (1950).

discipline, but 10 years later they were recommending that discipline be implemented by punishment. For some years physical manifestations of affection were discouraged in the belief that stimulation of any sort would lead to precocity in the older child and dullness in the man. Twenty years later a few daring writers protested, saying that "perhaps the greatest upheaval in nursery law is that which has been disciplining the young mother to hear her child's crying and make no response whatsoever. . . . It is good for some children to be allowed the privilege of crying unmolested, but there are some children who are definitely more or less seriously injured by this kind of neglect. . . . Perhaps it might be better for many young mothers if they had never heard of such a thing."[25] Many and more recent observers have noted that while children have considerable capacity to adapt successfully to variations in psychosocial environment, they cannot endure prolonged exposure to blatant degrees of psychosocial deprivation, stress or injury without residual scars.[26]

Need for Relativistic Approach to Evaluation of Psychosocial Input and Behavior. Evaluation of a child's psychosocial input and behavioral status must be approached relativistically.[27] One must consider not only the child's age, sex, temperament and other general characteristics, but also the local cultural ideals, customs and requirements. It is not necessary for the psychosocial supplies of children to conform to absolute standards, but it is essential that children receive from someone supplies of affection, care and control in amounts sufficient to prevent psychosocial deprivation, yet not so great to produce psychosocial intoxication. Though these limits have so far not been defined in absolute quantitative terms, it is clear that the range of human adaptability is broad enough to permit children to develop and function in a healthy manner under a wide variety of child rearing circumstances.

Recognition of Limits in Capacity to Adapt to Environmental Variations. As has been observed in respect to biologic homeostatic phenomena,[28] exposure to rates of input which exceed the range of physiologic tolerance always produces an abnormal deviation in some bodily function or structure. Serial observations of the function or structure may be used to determine whether the rate of biologic input of a substance is within the healthy range. The same appears to be true with regard to psychosocial input and certain bodily functions including, particularly, personal behavior. It is generally safe to conclude that when a child's behavior is normal and happy, his psychosocial input is within his range of physiologic tolerance. Conversely, when a child shows grossly prominent and frequent malbehavior, the possibility arises that there is some type of psychosocial deprivation, intoxication or stress.

If it is suspected that the child's problems are due to a socially pathological environment, as illustrated by Cases 1 and 2, valuable information may be obtained by observing the child's response to improvement of his environment. Disappearance of the behavioral manifestations is tentative evidence that the behavioral and functional disorders were in some way related to the environmental pathology. Continued favorable progress under normal environmental circumstances would tend to

[25]Stendler, C. (1950).

[26]Spitz, R. (1946 and 1946b); Davis K. (1947); Lowenfeld, B. (1956); Rose, J. (1959); Scott, J. (1962); Skeels, H. (1966); Eisenberg, L. (1968)

[27]Kagan, J. (1967).

[28]Talbot, N. B., et al. (1959).

support this tentative conclusion as would the observation that the manifestations of malbehavior or malfunction recurred when the child was returned to the original, presumably pathogenic environment. (See Figure 1–9.)

If malbehavior persists even after environmental circumstances have improved, two possibilities must be considered. One is the presence of organic causes of functional abnormality, such as brain damage, metabolic disorders or drug effects. The other is that prolonged psychosocial malnutrition may have so altered the child's capacity to respond that correction of his environment cannot bring about favorable changes in his behavior even when the initial cause was, indeed, environmental and not organic.

Environmental experiences, including child rearing practices, have many recognizable effects on the attitudes and behavior of children. However, except in cases of gross deprivation, it has thus far been as difficult to determine the exact extent to which the ordinary social experiences of childhood shape the ultimate characteristics of the fully developed individual as it has been to discern exact relationships between dietary intake during childhood and the ultimate bodily condition of the individual adult It is clear, however, that interpersonally transmitted supplies of affection, attention, control and related factors serve the essential function of sustaining the vitality of the psychologic system of human beings (and many other species),[29] and of enabling them to function and develop in accordance with intrinsic tendencies and in relation to extrinsic experiences. Psychosocial supplies deserve to be considered along with other key variables in searches for the causes and consequences of disease and disability among patients of all ages.

B. Varieties of Psychosocial Deprivation, Intoxication and Injury

The human being has considerable capacity for recovery: there is a drive toward health and harmony in development that is part of human nature. We must remember, however, that there is such a thing as too much stress, too much deprivation, and the infant's ability to adapt to stress or to recover from deprivation or hurt can be overtaxed.

Provence, S. (1967)

Has psychologic malnutrition taken the place of rickets and scurvy in contemporary pediatric practice?

Talbot, N. B. (1963)

Human beings have a considerable capacity to process and adapt to variations in input of psychologic supplies and stresses without becoming seriously disturbed. However, this capacity does have boundaries beyond which one cannot go for prolonged periods without developing signs of deficiency on the one hand or of intoxication on the other. The terms psychosocial deprivation, intoxication and injury are used to represent these pathogenic situations.

As indicated in Table 1–5, there are as many varieties of psychosocial deprivation and intoxication as there are types of psychosocial supplies (See also Table 1–1). *Acceptance* connotes a positive response to an individual even when certain facets of his personality or behavior are annoying. The mother of an active toddler says, "I can hardly keep up with him, but I get a bang out of

---

[29]Lorenz, K. (1957); Harlow, H. (1961, 1963); Foss, B. (Ed.) (1961, 1963, 1965).

*Table 1–5 Varieties of Psychosocial Deprivation, Intoxication and Injury**

Psychosocial Intoxication	Psychosocial Deprivation	Psychosocial Injury
Acceptance, excess of	Acceptance, lack of	Rejection[2]
Affection, excess of	Affection, lack of	Hostility[3]
Approval, excess of	Approval, lack of	Disparagement[4]
Attention, excess of	Attention, lack of	
Care, excess of	Care, lack of	
Protection, excess of	Protection, lack of	Abuse[5]
Control, excess of	Control, lack of	Indulgence[6]
Guidance, excess of	Guidance, lack of	

*Some of the conditions represented by these diagnostic terms have also been represented in the literature by such other familiar words and phrases as *smothered with affection, maternal overprotectiveness, overattentiveness, overcontrol, neglect* and *overpermissiveness.*[6]

[1]Levy, D. (1943); Spitz, R. A. (1946 a, b); Davis, K. (1947); Fried, R., and Mayer, M. (1948); Glaser, K., and Eisenberg, L. (1956); Lowenfeld, B. (1956); Solomon, P., et al. (1957); Rose, J. (1959); Eisenberg, L. (1962); Scott, J. (1962); Blodgett, R. (1963); Hollowell, J., and Gartner, L. (1965); Bakwin, H., and Bakwin, R. (1966); Eisenberg, L. (1968).

[2]Glaser, K., and Eisenberg, L. (1956); Lowenfeld, B. (1956); Jaco, E. (Ed.) (1958); Schaefer, E. (1959); Schutz, W. (1958); Eisenberg, L. (1962); Witmer, H., et al. (1962); Bakwin, H., and Bakwin, R. (1966); Krieger, I., and Sargent, D. (1967); Silver, H., and Finkelstein, M. (1967).

[3]Lowenfeld, B. (1956); Schaefer, E. (1959); Clarke, A., and Clarke, A. (1960).

[4]Jaco, E. (Ed) (1958); Kearsley, R., et al. (1962); Bakwin, H., and Bakwin, R. (1966); Mayer, J. (1966); Provence, S. (1967).

[5]Milowe, I., and Lourie, R. (1964); Caffey, J. (1965); Eisenberg, L. (1965); Silver, H., and Finkelstein, M. (1967).

[6]Levy, D. (1943); Schaefer, E. (1959); Schutz, W. (1958); Kearsley, R., et al., (1962); Green, M., and Solnit, A. (1964); Shapiro, M. (1965); Bakwin, H., and Bakwin, R. (1966).

seeing him explore and investigate everything." However, there can be too much of a good thing. An excess of acceptance is experienced by a child whose parent never allows himself an expression of irritation at the child's presence or behavior. The child may thus fail to learn that acceptance is usually variable and not wholly predictable. A lack of acceptance, on the other hand, is experienced by the child whose parent fails to communicate that the child remains acceptable as a person regardless of the quality of his behavior at any given moment. Lacking this assurance the child may fail to attain a conviction of his own worth as a person.

Affection, similarly, may be supplied by the parent in excessive or deficient amounts. Supportive affection is shown in small spontaneous ways—the pat on the shoulder in passing, the warm goodnight hug. Intoxication with an excess of affection, or "smothering," occurs when a parent indulges in exaggerated verbal or physical manifestations of fondness for the child, or singles out one child in the family for special attention. Deprivation is experienced by the child whose parent never communicates warmth or affection, even if he feels it, and maintains a cool, aloof attitude.

Approval is akin to acceptance but connotes a reaction to a specific behavior. On the way home from the doctor's office the mother of a 3 year old, tells him, "I was proud of you today—you were a good boy," or the father of a teenaged daughter comments that she is becoming a very good cook. An excess of approval occurs when the child is praised for nearly everything he does and is given no guidelines for assessing his own behavior in socially realistic terms. A lack of approval is experienced by a child whose parent punishes poor performance but fails to reward or comment upon good behavior.

Attention connotes not only providing the necessary protections and sanctions for a child but also being generally aware of him, his activities, his development and significant variations in his behavior. Excessive attention may take the form of anxious watchfulness, which allows the child no opportunity for autonomous development, whereas lack of attention occurs when the parent is indifferent or too preoccupied to keep track of the child's development, needs and interests.

Care refers to specific responses to the needs of the child—giving him his bottle or helping with shampoos. An excess occurs when a parent provides care with undue vigor or promptness, giving the child no opportunity to become independent in self-care. A lack of care, or neglect, occurs when a parent ignores the child's need or fails to respond appropriately. The consequences for the child vary with the degree of neglect, and with the age of the child. A grossly neglected infant cannot survive, while an older child can learn to get along after a fashion on his own or can seek care from other sources.

Protection, taking precautions against harm or injury to the child, becomes excessive when the parent anticipates all risks and forestalls all dangers. The child is thus denied an opportunity to develop his capacity to cope with the ordinary risks of life. Lack of protection occurs when a parent fails to take reasonable precautions for the child's safety and thus subjects him to dangers he may be unable to cope with.

Control is the exercise of restraint or direction over another. Reasonable degrees of control give the child leeway to function in accordance with his own tastes and inclinations and to learn self-control. Such control is compatible with respect for the child as an individual having personal tastes, desires and inclinations. An excess of control, experienced by the child whose parents require absolute conformity to certain behavioral standards which may or may not be within the child's developmental capacity, gives the child no opportunity to test his capacity to monitor his own behavior or to "be himself." Permissiveness or lack of control leaves a child with no set of personal or social standards by which to measure his own behavior and no means of learning the techniques of behavioral control.

Similarly, *guidance* helps to train and shape the child's behavior. Guidance becomes excessive when the child simply learns fixed rules of behavior and is given no opportunity to work out solutions for himself. A lack of guidance is experienced by the child whose parent fails to supply appropriate models of behavior or appropriate reinforcements for good or bad behavior in the form of reward or punishment.

Some children are deprived of all essential psychosocial supplies (pan deprivation) as a result of isolation or neglect. In all vertebrates studied, this usually results in markedly deviant behavior.[30] In other children, psychosocial injury may be induced by a single focus deficiency of a psychosocial supply, such as lack of control, or by an excess of a particular supply, such as overprotection.

Between these two extremes, varieties of deprivation and intoxication can occur in many combinations. The child who suffers from a general lack of care often also receives little attention, protection, guidance, control or approval. However, a child may receive an excess supply of acceptance and affection from a parent who treats

[30]Lorenz, K. (1957); Clarke, A., and Clarke, A. (1960); Harlow, H. (1961, 1963); Harlow, H., and Harlow, M. (1965); Skeels, H. (1966); Eisenberg, L. (1968).

him like a plaything but who fails to give him the physical care he needs. Or a child may receive meticulous care from a parent whose attitudes convey no real acceptance, affection or approval.

A child may suffer from two extremes of the same parental attitude. An ambivalent parent may alternate between smothering the child with an excess of affection and coldly shoving him aside. Or the parent may vacillate between total lack of guidance and control, and rigid insistence on the child's conformity to certain behavioral standards.

These varieties of psychosocial deprivation and intoxication also may result from such psychosocial injurers as rejection, hostility, disparagement, abuse or indulgence (See Table 1–5). The child suffers from rejection when the attitude of the parent reflects contempt, dislike and the opinion that the child is worthless or unsatisfactory. Hostility is a more active form of injury characterized by overt expressions of ill will, loathing or revulsion, whereas disparagement implies a tendency to belittle and underrate. Both physical abuse, such as beating or burning, and verbal abuse, characterized by comments that hurt and damage the child, are forms of psychosocial injury. These categories of injuries, of course, overlap, since disparagement and physical or verbal abuse are usually expressions of rejections and hostility. At the opposite end of the injury scale is indulgence, in which the parent caters to the child's every whim and fails to set appropriate behavioral standards and controls.

The relationships between psychosocial deprivation or intoxication, and psychosocial injury are intricate. A diagnosis of rejection, for example, is compatible with a lack of acceptance but not ordinarily with an excess of acceptance. However, it is possible for an ambivalent parent to alternate between showing excessive and intoxicating amounts of affection and injuring the child through overt expressions of hostility.[31] The excessively protective parent may suddenly injure the child with uncontrolled attacks of verbal or physical abuse.

Because it is still necessary to rely largely on gross observation of social situations and interpersonal behavior in evaluating the input of various social supplies and stresses a child receives, it is advisable to restrict application of these diagnoses to situations that are clear-cut enough to leave little doubt of their validity. It also is essential that information sufficient to indicate to others the basis for the diagnosis be appended to the diagnostic report. Many major advances in medical diagnosis and care have been initiated by the application of a given principle before refined means of measurement were available.

C. Personal Sources of Psychosocial Deprivation, Intoxication and Injury

The personal sources of childhood psychosocial malnutrition, stress and injury are apt to be those persons from whom they ordinarily derive their psychologic supplies (See Section II-A). The following paragraphs discuss some of the reasons, listed in Table 1–6, why parents and others behave in a stressful or harmful rather than in a nurturing way toward a child.

Lack of awareness of the child's psychosocial needs (Table 1–6A) at various ages accounts for some instances of psychosocial malnutrition. Parents are likely to use their own upbringing as a model for rearing their progeny. This may be adequate if they themselves were fortunately

[31]Witmer, H., et al. (1962).

*Table 1–6 Some Personal Sources of Psychosocial Deprivation and Injury Among Children**

SOURCE	CAUSE
A. LACK OF AWARENESS OF CHILD'S PSYCHOSOCIAL NEEDS	1. One's own inappropriate experiences[1] 2. Cultural prejudices or cultural isolation[2] 3. Lack of knowledge of characteristic psychosocial needs of children (see Section B in text p. 18) 4. Special characteristics of child
B. PERSONAL DISLIKE OF CHILD	1. Conception not wanted[3] 2. General or age-specific dislike of nurturing role[4] 3. Failure of child to fulfill parent's needs for child rearing satisfaction Because child is mentally retarded, malformed, "ugly," cripped, sickly, malbehaving and so forth[5] Because child does not live up to expections in scholastic performance, athletic prowess, social success and so forth[6] Because child does not gratify adult by (e.g.) reciprocating affection[7]
C. ANXIOUS OR GRIEVING PARENT[8]	1. Child sickly, failing to thrive or physically or functionally handicapped 2. Child has fatal disease
D. ABSENCE OF PARENT[9]	1. Death 2. Desertion or unmarried parent 3. Divorce 4. Involuntary separation due to military service, imprisonment and so forth

*During the years of development children usually derive their psychosocial supplies and stresses initially from their parents but eventually also from a wide variety of others (e.g., siblings, relatives, neighbors, teachers, schoolmates and playmates) with whom the child has significant contact. These persons may be sources of inappropriate social supplies for essentially the same reasons as those listed above for parents.

[1]Eisenberg, L. (1962); Kempe, C., et al. (1962); Leonard, M., et al. (1966); Silver, H., and Finkelstein, M. (1967).

[2]Eisenberg, L. (1968).

[3]Bowlby, J. (1951); Kempe, C., et al. (1962); Fontana, V., et al. (1963); Leonard, M., et al. (1966); Simons, B., et al. (1966).

[4]Lidz, T. (1949); Witmer, H., et al. (1962); Milowe, I., and Lourie, R. (1964).

[5]Lowenfeld, B. (1956); Clarke, A., and Clarke, A. (1960); Kempe, C., et al. (1962); Blodgett, F. (1963); Bakwin, H., and Bakwin, R. (1966); Powell, G., et al. (1967).

[6]Bakwin, H., and Bakwin, R. (1966); Mayer, J. (1966).

[7]Leonard, M., et al. (1966); Escalona, S. (1968); Thomas, A., et al. (1968).

[8]Keller, H. (1954); Richmond, J., and Waisman, H. (1955); Lis, E., et al. (1956); Browne, W., et al. (1960); Solnit, A. and Stark, M. (1961); Friedman, S. B., et al. (1963); Richardson, S. (1963); Agle, D. (1964); Glaser, H., et al. (1964): Talbot, N. B. (1964); Mattsson, A., and Gross, S. (1966); Howell, M. (1962).

[9]Reid, J. (1959); Caldwell, B. (1967); Powell, G., et al. (1967); Chilman, C. (1966); Coles, R. (1964).

Table 1–6 (Continued)

SOURCE	CAUSE
E. UNAVAILABILITY OF PARENT[9]	*1.* Conditions of employment *2.* Physical disability (i.e., hospitalized, bedridden, lack of mobility) *3.* Frequent voluntary absence due to marital discord, interest in job, community, social activities and so forth
F. PREOCCUPATION OF PARENT (i.e., psychologically unavailable though physically present) BECAUSE OF EXTRINSIC PROBLEMS OF LIVING[9]	*1.* Inadequate finances (poverty) *2.* Inadequate housing *3.* Inadequate employment *4.* Demands of other family members, such as elderly relative, disabled or retarded child or sick spouse *5.* Marital discord or tension
G. HANDICAPPED PARENT BECAUSE OF INTRINSIC PERSONAL PROBLEMS[10]	*1.* Personal social malnutrition such as lack of spouse, friends or extended family; or cultural isolation *2.* Immaturity; that is, when parents have poorly developed psychologic strengths (e.g., mothers of adolescent age) and are consequently unable to provide for the social needs of a dependent child *3.* Fatigue *4.* Sick role *5.* Mental subnormality, or sensory defects such as blindness, deafness or mutism *6.* Behavioral disorders Socially deviant behavior, including asocial and antisocial behavior and psychopathy Depression Anxiety Schizophrenia or schizoid behavior Addiction to abuse of alcohol or drugs Chronic anger *7.* Low self-esteem
H. DISCONTINUOUS SOURCE OF CARE[11]	*1.* Multiple placements in foster homes *2.* Placement in impersonal child care institution

[10]Bowlby, J. (1951); Rose, J. (1959); Elmer, E. (1960); Fanshel, D., and Maas, H. (1962); Eisenberg, L. (1962); Kempe, C., et al. (1962); Bain, K. (1963); Blodgett, F. (1963); Fontana, V., et al. (1963); McHenry, T., et al. (1963); Eisenberg, L. (1965); Hollowell, J., and Gardner, L. (1965); Leonard, M., et al. (1966); Simons, B., et al. (1966); Mayer, J. (1966); Powell, G., et al. (1967); Silver, H., and Finkelstein, M. (1967).

[11]Spitz, R. (1946 a, b); Glaser, K., and Eisenberg, L. (1956); Mass, H., and Engler, R. (1959); Rose, J. (1959); Elmer, E. (1960); Eisenberg, L. (1962); Fanshel, D., and Maas, (1962); Scott, J. (1962); Silver, H., and Finkelstein, M. (1967).

born to wise and caring parents. On the other hand, if they were raised under conditions of major psychosocial deprivation and trauma (i.e., lacked affectionate care, guidance or discipline, or perhaps were exposed to overt rejection, hostility or abuse) the chances are great that they will bring up their own children in a correspondingly pathogenic manner.[32] Parents are also subject to the sometimes deleterious influence of current cultural swings in regard to child rearing attitudes and practices.

Personal aversion or dislike for a child (Table 1–6 B) is another noteworthy cause of psychosocial malnutrition or injury. This may have its origin in the fact that conception of the child was not planned, not wanted or occurred at an inconvenient time.[33] In other instances the aversion may stem from parental uneasiness in managing children of a particular age. Some mothers enjoy caring for infants but are irritated by the incessant wanderings and curiosity of the toddler or by the rebellious independence of the older child or adolescent.[34]

Children who are mentally retarded, malformed, ugly, crippled, sickly or simply temperamentally "difficult" may be perceived as a burden by their parents. It is not unusual for such children to be treated in a punitive, irritable, hostile or rejecting manner.[35] The same may be true of physically healthy youngsters who cry incessantly, who soil themselves past the usual age of toilet training or who are stubborn, disobedient, hostile or otherwise a source of harassment and embarrassment rather than of pleasure and pride. Parental hostility and rejection may be concealed under a cloak of overprotection.[36] Older children who fail to satisfy their parents' sometimes unrealistic and unreasonable expections regarding scholastic honors, athletic prowess, social successes and so forth, also are at risk of experiencing hypercritical, overcontrolling and rejecting attitudes and practices.[37] A child living at home under the care of a hostile or rejecting parent may suffer psychosocial stress and injury as intense as that experienced by children living away from home under highly pathogenic institutional or foster placement circumstances.[38]

Parental anxiety about the health of a sick child may be a common source of psychosocial malnutrition (Table 1–6 C). This is apt to take the form of "smothering" care: overprotectiveness, overcontrol, excessive permissiveness, lack of control or indulgence.[39] In blind or otherwise seriously handicapped children, parents can become so preoccupied with the handicap that they forget the patient is primarily a child and needs the same love, discipline and social experiences that healthy children do.[40]

These reactions of parents vary with the nature of the child's condi-

---

[32]Kempe, C., et al. (1962); Milowe, I., and Lourie, R. (1964); Leonard, M., et al. (1966); Simons, B., et al. (1966); Silver, H., and Finkelstein, M. (1967).

[33]Bowlby, J. (1951); Kempe, C., et al. (1962); Fontana, V., et al. (1963); Leonard, M., et al. (1966); Simons, B., et al. (1966).

[34]Lidz, T. (1949); Witmer, H., et al. (1962); Milowe, I., and Lourie, R. (1964).

[35]Lowenfeld, B. (1956); Schaefer, E. (1959); Clarke, A., and Clarke, A. (1960); Kempe, C. et al. (1962); Blodgett, F. (1963); Bakwin, H., and Bakwin, R. (1966); Powell, G., et al. (1967). See also Section G, p. 36, concerning the effects on parents and others of having a disabled child in the family.

[36]Bakwin, H., and Bakwin, R. (1966).

[37]Bakwin, H., and Bakwin, R. (1966); Mayer, J. (1966).

[38]Leonard, M., et al. (1966).

[39]Richmond, J., and Waisman, H. (1955); Lis, E., et al. (1956); Browne, W., et al. (1960); Solnit, A., and Stark, M. (1961); Tisza, V. (1962); Friedman, S., et al. (1963 b); Richardson, S. (1963); Agle, D. (1964); Glaser, H., et al. (1964); Talbot, N. B. (1964); Bakwin, H., and Bakwin, R. (1966); Mattsson, A., and Gross, S. (1966); Howell, M. (1962).

[40]Lowenfeld, B. (1956).

tion. For example, mothers of children with life threatening renal disease may set lower goals with respect to obedience than do mothers of children with non-life-threatening allergies.[41] As one mother of a nephrotic child said, "As long as we have him I probably will do just about what he wants." In a study of pediatric patients with heart disease it was found, with only one exception, that all the mothers admitted that they treated these children differently, particularly in respect to physical punishment.[42] Some were afraid that spanking would precipitate an acute cardiac episode and perhaps even lead to early death. "If he hadn't been sick as much as he was, I would have clamped down on him a little more and he wouldn't be quite as spoiled as he is." On the other hand, this reaction is not universal, for as another mother remarked, "It does hurt me to take the belt to him, but he gets his beltings right along with Mary. He gets corrected and spanked and punished. I just close my eyes and give him two good swats and tell him to hush. I know if I don't punish him, I am going to have a spoiled brat on my hands."

Some parents of children with enduring maladies such as diabetes mellitus feel compelled to "beat the disease.[43] The net result is perfectionistic overcontrol of such intensity that the child's personality is crushed.

Parents who learn that a son or daughter has an imminently fatal disease, such as leukemia, frequently react to the intense anxiety generated by this grievous news by treating the child in a permissive, indulgent and overprotective manner.[44] This may result in, among other things, an unnecessary sick role existence. (See Section H, p. 39.)

Parental absence, unavailability, preoccupation with extrinsic problems of living and *handicap* because of intrinsic personal problems (Table 1–6 D through G) comprise some of the easily discernible explanations for psychosocial deprivation among children.[45] Absence may be involuntary as a result of death, military service, imprisonment or hospitalization; or voluntary, as with certain parents who have an overriding interest in job, community or social activities. However, the mother's involvement in a job or other outside activity does not necessarily result in the child's being psychosocially deprived for many mothers manage to provide enough personal attention to meet their children's basic needs while holding a job outside of the home. In essence, success here is contingent on the parent's being potentially available psychologically and physically, even when physically absent. Under these circumstances, parents who are away from home some of the time may do a better job of rearing the child than do parents who are physically present but psychologically unavailable because of boredom or restlessness.

Preoccupation with such extrinsic problems of living as poverty, inadequate employment, heavy family demands or marital tension likewise can result in failure to provide children with the necessary psychosocial attention. The same can be true of parents who lack psychosocial support from spouse, relatives or congenial friends. Likewise, fatigue and illness can so deplete a mother or

[41]Howell, M. (1962).

[42]Glaser, H., et al. (1964).

[43]Bruch, H. (1949).

[44]Keller, H. (1954); Bozeman, M., et al. (1955); Tisza, V. (1962); Friedman, S., et al. (1963 b); Agle, D. (1964); Mattsson, A., and Gross, S. (1966); Bergman, A., and Schulte, C. (1967); Rothenberg, M. (1967).

[45]Bowlby, J. (1951); Rose, J. (1959); Clarke, A., and Clarke, A. (1960); Elmer, E. (1960); Fanshel, D., and Maas, H. (1962); Kempe, H., et al. (1962); Bain, K. (1963); Blodgett, F. (1963); Fontana, V., et al. (1963); Eisenberg, L. (1965); Hollowell, J., et al. (1965); Leonard, M., et al. (1966); Mayer, J. (1966); Simons, B., et al. (1966); Powell, G., et al. (1967); Silver, H., and Finkelstein, M. (1967).

father that the ability to give to others is drained dry. The "immature" adolescent who becomes a mother before she has matured to the point where she herself no longer has a large need for mothering comprises a variant of this phenomenon.

Children living under the care of sociobehaviorally deviant parents are liable to both deprivation and abusive injury. The same is true of those being reared by people exhibiting any of the other forms of behavioral disorder listed under G-6 of Table 1–6.

Children are apt to suffer psychosocial deprivation or stress when they *lack* a *consistent* continuing *source of "parental" care* (Table 1–6 H). This is particularly true among children placed in a series of foster homes or located in busy, impersonal child care institutions.[46]

D. Material and Impersonal Sources of Psychologic Supplies, Stresses, and Injuries

> Narcotics can be abused, severely so, by people whose pain comes not from physical illness, but is surely as real and unpleasant—we refer to those brutalized by and trapped in the ghettoes of our cities. In those ghettoes great numbers of people, mostly black, suffer, and suffer, and suffer. Existing social and medical services have not been able to cope with the rage and the pain of the human beings trapped there. Narcotics offer one route of escape, and awful and ravaging route—a pathway of despair followed when personal and social pain becomes unbearable, and relief otherwise unobtainable.
>
> *Brenner, J., et al. (1970)*

[46]Spitz, R. (1946 a); Glaser, K., and Eisenberg, L. (1956); Maas, H., and Engler, R. (1959); Rose, J. (1959); Elmer, E. (1960); Eisenberg, L. (1962); Fanshel, D., and Maas, H. (1962); Scott, J. (1962); Silver, H., and Finkelstein, M. (1967).

> She was a handsome woman, tall and straight, with long, pure-white hair braided neatly on top of her head and large dark eyes set in a light-tan face. She was a bit stout, but it was a hard, muscular kind of heaviness collected slowly over the years rather than the fat of gluttony. "I'm supposed to lose some of my weight, but I can't do without my grits, and I can't give this child ice cream without taking just a little for myself. Tessie and I eat grits before going through these mobs, and we eat ice cream after we come home from them."
>
> *Coles, R. (1964)*

Human beings derive some psychologic supplies and stresses directly from material, or from essentially impersonal institutional and corporate sources as well as from the personal sources already described. For instance, good food, attractive clothing, comfortable housing and enough money to live decently may contribute to a person's sense of well being. Some people also derive positive input from living in an attractive and untroubled environment; from having access to satisfactory educational, job and recreatinal opportunities, and from being healthy and of attractive appearance. This is not to say that these impersonal resources are an adequate substitute for the human relationships which normally comprise the fundamental source of man's essential psychologic supplies. But people who lack these vital resources sometimes seek to compensate through material means, at times to their additional disadvantage. Typical of this are the people who try to compensate for lack of personal approval, acceptance or affection by means of food and as a result become unattractively obese.[47]

The history of mankind is also replete with examples of the many ways in which natural environmental

[47]Mayer, J. (1966, 1968).

Table 1–7 Some Material and Impersonal Sources of Psychologic Stress or Injury

Lack of material necessities (e.g., food, clothing, housing, money)
Threatening natural phenomena (e.g., extreme climatic conditions, floods, epidemics, volcanic eruptions)
Group violence (e.g., wars, riots, insurrections, terrorism)
Societal defamation of minority groups by majority groups (on the basis of race, color, creed)
Political upheavals
Governmental edict regarding taxes, civil rights, military draft status, jail sentence
Lack or loss of physical attractiveness or competence as a result of inborn or acquired defects in body form or function
Lack of job opportunities due to economic depression

occurrences such as floods, fires, epidemic diseases and famines can give rise to severe psychologic stress (See Table 1–7). The same may be said of such social phenomena as poverty, societal prejudices, political upheavals, governmental decisions on civil rights, draft status, imprisonment and taxes.[48]

E. Behavioral Problems Resulting from Psychosocial Malnutrition

A recurring behavioral characteristic is identified as being a problem when for one or more of the reasons listed in Table 1–8 a child:

(a) is not well adapted to his reference group (e.g., family or community) in respect to temperament, social behavior, personal habits or stereotyped behavior.

(b) is experiencing extreme emotional distress with loss of ability to work, play or love.

(c) is incapacitated in regard to learning and solving problems.

(d) is psychotic.

Most of these problem behaviors are distinguished from healthy behavior more by their frequency, intensity and duration in relation to the child's age, sex and surrounding circumstances than by absolute qualitative differences. For example, urinary and fecal incontinence is normal for an infant but not for an older child or adult. Similarly, young children in our society are expected to be somewhat dependent, but an extreme degree of dependency is maladaptive. A physically aggressive or abusive boy may be a hero on one city block but be labeled antisocial in a culturally different neighborhood. Moreover, certain behaviors may represent a temporary response to psychosocial stress or injury of momentarily high intensity just as fever is a temporary response to infection. This type of response is exemplified by small children who behave in a whining, obstinate manner during the days immediately following abrupt weaning from the breast (see p. 14). Likewise, in older children and adults behaviors indicative of grief or depression are commonly seen during the days or weeks immediately following the loss of a highly valued person through death or other causes.[49]

The behavioral problems listed in Table 1–8 are conditions usually encountered in pediatric practice. Those listed under *temperament* (Table 1–8 A) have to do with the intrinsic nature of the individual. They represent problem behavior when they differ from the norm in marked degree. Any normal child is active, but the hyperactive child is one who is constantly engaged in motion—running, fidgeting, swaying to and fro—and unable to remain quiet for any length of time. The hypoactive

[48]Coles, M. R. (1963, 1964); Haggstrom, W. (1964); Chilman, C. (1966); Dentsch, M. (1967); Brenner, J. H., et al. (1970).

[49]Lindemann, E. (1944).

*Table 1–8 Commonly Encountered Types of Childhood Behavioral Problems**

Areas in Which Behavioral Problems Occur	Behavioral Trait and Problem Characteristics
A. Temperament[1]	Physical activity[2] hyperactive hypoactive Responsiveness (mood)[3] apathetic excitable Adaptability[4] withdrawing slowly adapting Perceptual distractibility
B. Social Behavior	Asocial behavior[5] isolating shy Aggressiveness[6] toward others: manipulative verbally abusive physically abusive (cruel) violently assaultive (e.g., injuring, homicidal) toward self: reckless self-punishing suicidal Oppositional behavior[7] disobedient negativistic passive-aggressive Dependency[8] excessively conforming excessively dependent Antisocial behavior[9] lacking in conscience destructive dishonest truancy running away from home sexual nonconformity drug abuse Lack of empathy Inappropriate sex role behavior
C. Habit Disturbances[10]	Eating hyperphagia anorexia Drinking polydipsia Elimination constipation encopresis Sleeping insomnia day-night reversal Self-manipulation hair pulling auto-eroticism

Table 1–8 (Continued)

AREAS IN WHICH BEHAVIORAL PROBLEMS OCCUR	BEHAVIORAL TRAIT AND PROBLEM CHARACTERISTICS
	Speech stuttering lisping Disease related behaviors blindisms Addictive behavior
D. STEREOTYPED BEHAVIOR[11]	Compulsive Obsessive Phobic Perfectionistic
E. EMOTIONAL STATUS[12]	Anxious Depressed Chronic anger Low self-esteem
F. LEARNING[13]	Mental subnormality Academic achievement underachieving overachieving Specific learning disabilities (including disturbances in perception)
G. PSYCHOTIC BEHAVIOR[14]	Autism Hallucinations Delusions

*This list covers categorically most of the conditions encountered in the care of pediatric patients.

[1]Thomas, A., et al. (1968).

[2]Bakwin, H., and Bakwin, R. (1966).

[3]Eisenberg, L. (1962); Witmer, H., et al. (1962); Peiper, A. (1963); Fontana, V., et al. (1963); Bakwin, H., and Bakwin, R. (1966); Silver, H., and Finkelstein, M. (1967).

[4]Glaser, K., and Eisenberg, L. (1956); Bakwin, H., and Bakwin, R. (1966); Mayer, J. (1966); Silver, H., and Finkelstein, M. (1967).

[5]Eisenberg, L. (1965); Mayer, J. (1966); Bakwin, H., and Bakwin, R. (1966); Powell, G., et al. (1967).

[6]Lowenfeld, B. (1956); Lapouse, R., and Monk, M. (1959); Eisenberg, L. (1962); Agle, D. (1964); Bakwin, H., and Bakwin, R. (1966); Mattsson, A., and Gross, S. (1966); Powell, G., et al. (1967); Silver, H., and Finkelstein, M. (1967).

[7]Sommers, V. (1944); Lowenfeld, B. (1956); Lapouse, R., and Monk, M. (1959); Kempe, C., et al. (1962); Silver, H., and Finkelstein, M. (1967); Kenniston, K. (1970).

[8]Lapouse, R., and Monk, M. (1959); Richardson, S. (1963); Agle, D. (1964); Bakwin, H., and Bakwin, R. (1966).

[9]Bruch, H. (1949); Rose, J. (1959); Richmond, J. (1960); Eisenberg, L. (1962); Bain, K. (1963); Bakwin, H., and Bakwin, R. (1966); Krieger, I., and Sargent, D. (1967); Silver, H., and Finkelstein, M. (1967).

[10]Arnold, S. (1958).

[11]Glaser, K., and Eisenberg, L. (1956); Browne, W., et al. (1960); Clarke, A., and Clarke, A. (1960); Eisenberg, L. (1962); Kempe, C., et al. (1962); Caldwell, B., and Drachman, R. (1964); Bakwin, H., and Bakwin, R. (1966); Leonard, M., et al. (1966); Elmer, E., and Gregg, G. (1967); Powell, G., et al. (1967); Silver, H., and Finkelstein, M. (1967); Arnold, S. (1958).

[12]Bruch, H. (1949); Bowlby, J. (1951); Richmond, J. (1960); Bakwin, H., and Bakwin, R. (1966); Elmer, E., and Gregg, G. (1967).

[13]Clarke, A., and Clarke, A. (1960); Eisenberg, L. (1962); Eisenberg, L. (1965); Eisenberg, L. (1968).

[14]Creak, M. (1968).

child is sluggish, physically quiet and inactive; he tends to lie or sit still rather than move around.

Responsiveness, another aspect of temperament, constitutes problem behavior when the child's mood swings too far in one direction. He may be apathetic and show little or no outward sign of emotional response, or he may become overexcited and show intense emotionality.

Adaptability is commonly considered a desirable trait, but this, too, can reach problem dimensions. The child who withdraws from new situations or shows fear of any unfamiliar experience is adapting, but in an unhealthy way. The child who clings to old response patterns in adjusting to new situations is adapting, but slowly and with difficulty.

Normal children show a lively interest in all that goes on around them, but the child who tries to attend to every perceptual stimulus at the same time may be so distractible that he cannot focus productively on anything.

During the early weeks of life, many traits of temperament appear to be inborn. With passage of time, some of these may persist while others may be modified by life experience.[50]

The *social behaviors* listed in Table 1–8 B also emphasize the qualitative and quantitative nature of behavior. Everyone likes to be alone at times, but the child who is painfully shy and exhibits distrust and fear of people, or the one who avoids social contact and isolates himself as completely as possible manifests asocial behavior to a problem degree.

In our culture, the healthy individual is considered to be one sufficiently aggressive to "stand up for himself," "hold his own" or "get ahead." Aggressiveness becomes problem behavior when the individual is manipulative, verbally or physically abusive or assaultive toward others. The asthmatic child who manipulates her family by threatening to have an attack is showing aggressive problem behavior. The child who systematically demolishes the ego of his peers or his parents by vicious verbal abuse, or the bully who is impelled to grind every new child on the block into the sidewalk or pour kerosene on the cat and set it afire is showing problem behavior. So, too, are parents who abuse their children physically or undermine them by constant reminders that they are "bad all the way through" or "so stupid I can't stand to be in the same room with you."

Aggressiveness as a problem behavior may also be directed against onself. The accident-prone child who is forever breaking an arm in a reckless plunge down a steep hillside or who repeatedly injures himself in a variety of ways may be deliberately or subconsciously punishing himself. The child who attempts or accomplishes suicide—an astonishingly frequent phenomenon in our society—may be directing his aggression either against himself or against his parents.

Oppositional behavior can be considered a milder form of aggression. All normal children are disobedient at times and refuse to respond positively to reasonable requests. But the child who is consistently defiant and disobedient, the child who automatically says, "No!" to every request or command and the child who simply sits passively dawdling no matter what his mother says are carrying their opposition beyond the normal behavioral range. So is the child who is so clinging, so conforming and so dependent that he remains infantile long after such behavior is appropriate to his age level. Every child wants to be babied sometimes, but if he consistently abdicates his

[50]Thomas, A., et al. (1968).

responsibility to develop as an individual, possible causes—both biophysical and psychosocial—need to be explored.

Specifically antisocial behavior may take numerous forms. The child may be dishonest or destructive. He may become a chronic truant from school or engage in forms of sexual behavior unacceptable to his family or society. Or he may behave as if he "has no conscience," showing no evidence of internal control, no inhibitions about wrongdoing, and no remorse over past deeds.

Insensitivity or lack of empathy may represent an abnormal shutdown of the child's ability to recognize and respond to the needs of others and to modify his behavior accordingly. He may be described as selfish, uncooperative and inconsiderate.

The final form of social problem behavior listed in Table 1–6 B is inappropriate sex role behavior. Appropriate sex roles are different at different stages of life and in different cultures, and are subject to change even within the same culture. The sex role behavior of a child must therefore be viewed within the total social context, and be considered problem behavior when it deviates markedly from currently acceptable social norms, which may differ from those current when his parents were of similar age.

Habit disturbances (Table 1–8 C) frequently encountered in pediatric practice include excessive appetite or lack of appetite, excessive intake of fluids, abnormal elimination patterns such as chronic constipation and disturbances of sleep such as insomnia or day-night reversal. Behaviors often perceived by parents as "nervousness" may include such self-manipulations as hair pulling and masturbation, or speech disorders such as stuttering or lisping. Some problem behaviors are directly related to specific diseases, such as "blindisms" developed by visually handicapped children who lack the confidence to function normally.

The "drug habit" or addiction—a physiologic or psychologic dependence on alcohol, a drug or an inhalant—may cause alterations in the addict's behavior which affect other people to an even greater degree than they affect the addict himself. The alcoholic who beats his wife and children, the young heroin addict who kills the owner of the local grocery to get money to support his habit, or the young boy or girl who loses interest in his school work and becomes sullen and difficult to manage at school and at home after he becomes addicted to drugs or glue sniffing is manifesting behavioral problems which have far-reaching biosocial implications.

Stereotyped behavior (Table 1–8 D) represents a form of adaptation to psychosocial stress. It is therefore more reactive than temperamental in nature. It may take many forms ranging from the compulsive insistence of a tense child that every item on his toy shelf be exactly in its assigned spot, to obessive preoccupation with one persistent idea or desire. The child may develop ritual patterns of behavior to release tension or to ward off unreasoned phobias or anxieties which are out of proportion to any real threat to his safety or well-being. Or the child may place perfectionistic demands upon himself and others in an attempt to surround himself with a protective cocoon of predictable behavior and environmental regularity.

Emotional mood swings (Table 1–8 E) of moderate degree are experienced by everyone and are normal life phenomena. They become serious problems when they interfere with the capacity of an individual to carry on his normal life role and to relate in a warmly meaningful way to others. Most children are mildly disturbed over the prospect of the absence of a parent. If the child "comes all unglued" with nameless terror every time his mother steps out of sight, the sources of his anxiety need to be found. If he is chronically depressed or chronically angry, it may be very important to identify both biophysical and psychosocial factors which may be contributing to his emotional state. If he consistently undervalues his own capabilities and holds himself in low esteem, both his attitudes and those of the meaningful people in his world deserve close examination.

Learning disabilities (Table 1–8 F) are included in this taxonomy of behavioral problems because they may result from psychosocial deprivation as well as from organic disorders of the central nervous system, dietary insufficiencies or metabolic disorders. Lack of linguistic facility or lack of problem solving competence severe enough to prevent a child from coping with the ordinary demands of living may represent deficient mental capacity, but they may also represent correctible manifestations of psychosocial deprivation. Even a child who registers a very low IQ score on formal tests may be brought up to a normal level of functioning by environmental changes if his retardation has been psychosocial in origin, as indicated in Case 2 (p. 3). Academic achievement is often a poor indication of true intellectual potential. A 12 year old boy with an IQ of 120 may receive failing grades in school if he is bored, emotionally disturbed or reacting to any of a host of possible causes of psychosocial deprivation. The overachiever, on the other hand, may press himself almost beyond endurance to surpass the levels of achievement that might reasonably be expected of him. This is in the American tradition of the self-made man who achieves success through hard work, but it is a significant problem when it triggers medical or behavioral disorders.

When children of normal or high intelligence have specific learning disabilities in reading, writing or number usage, discovering the causes may be akin to putting a jigsaw puzzle together. A host of biophysical and psychosocial variables may have to be considered before the key piece of the diagnostic picture can be found.

Although *psychoses* (Table 1–8 G) are rarely encountered in pediatric practice, they occur frequently enough to merit inclusion in this listing. Autism is the most commonly recognized form of childhood psychosis.[51] It is characterized by extreme withdrawal, self-absorption, inaccessibility to interpersonal communication and the inability to form relationships with other persons. Hallucination—perception of external objects that do not exist—and delusions—irrational beliefs maintained in spite of perceptual and rational evidence which refutes their validity—are rarely seen in psychoses of young children. They may, however, be seen in adolescents, especially those who are taking hallucinogenic drugs.

Behavioral Clusters—Easy *versus* Difficult Children. Behavioral manifestations encountered in individual pediatric patients are apt to coexist as clusters of partially related variables.[52] An interesting example of this is provided by Thomas, Chess and Birch, who suggest that preschool age children can be classified as "easy" or "difficult" according to their dispositions (i.e., happy *versus* unhappy), habits (regularity *versus* irregularity of biologic functions), adaptability (approach *versus* withdrawal, and fast *versus* slow adjustment) and responsiveness or intensity of reaction (Table 1–9). They further indicate that the designation "difficult child" (aptly colabelled "mother-killer") is not necessarily synonymous with a diagnosis of a

[51] Creak, M. (1968).

[52] Kearsley, R., et al. (1962); Pavenstedt, E. (1967); Thomas, A., et al. (1968).

***Table 1–9 Temperamental Characteristics of "Easy"* versus *"Difficult" Children**[*]

CHARACTERISTICS	"EASY" TEMPERAMENT	"DIFFICULT" TEMPERAMENT
Overall mood	happy, smiling, positive	unhappy, crying, negative
Regularity of biologic functions	regular	irregular
Reaction to new situations	approach	withdraw
Rate of adaptation to new situations	rapid	slow
Intensity of reactions	mild or moderate	marked
PER CENT WHO DEVELOP BEHAVIORAL PROBLEMS	"small per cent"	70
PER CENT OF BEHAVIORAL PROBLEM CHILDREN HAVING TEMPERAMENT	23[**]	23

*Reprinted by permission of New York University Press from *Temperament and Behavior Disorders in Children* by Alexander Thomas, Stella Chess and Herbert Birch, copyright © 1968 by New York University.

**Note that the 10 cases of behavioral problem children with easy temperament is a small per cent of the total number of easy temperament children. But note, too, that the per cent of behavioral problem children with easy temperament is the same as that for behavioral problem children with difficult temperament. This seeming discrepancy occurs because the total number of easy temperament children in the sample was very much greater than the total number of difficult temperament children in the sample.

major behavioral disorder. Likewise, the designation "easy child" does not rule out the possibility that a child may develop a serious behavioral disorder, sometimes as a by-product of his very easiness. On the other hand, *it is probably true that difficult children are much more likely than are easy ones to develop major behavioral difficulties if for no other reason than that they are by definition hard to persuade, hard to please and generally a source of stress and worry to parents and others.* Case studies indicate that this type of child behavior is sometimes conducive to psychosocial deprivation or intoxication engendered by unfriendly, disapproving and punitive attitudes on the part of parents. These parental attitudes in response to the child's behavior may, in turn, cause intensification and fixation of the child's behavioral disturbances. However, other cases are cited which show that when parents can manage to deal in a moderately supportive way with such children, in some instances at least the child will outgrow his behavioral difficulties and become a healthy and effective person.

These observations, viewed in conjunction with those set forth under Sections III A, B and C (pp. 57 ff.), support the thesis that persons experiencing major degrees of psychosocial malnutrition are very likely to exhibit one or more of the behavioral disorders listed here. Though present findings suggest that certain types of psychosocial experience are apt to result in certain forms of malbehavior, clear descriptions of these relationships must await the gathering of more extensive, particularized information. Systematic recording of the malbehaviors encountered in pediatric practice, in association with various environmental and intrinsic circumstances should provide valuable information concerning this subject.

F. Direct and Indirect Effects of Psychosocial Stimuli on Bodily Functions

These reasons made his mouth to water.

Butler, S. (1600–1680)
Part I, Canto III
Line 277

In his treatise on ways in which emotion can effect the digestive tract,

Alvarez[53] points out that it has been recognized from time immemorial that the thought or smell of a luscious morsel will make the mouth water. Even primitive man could observe for himself that the salivary glands prepare for the approaching feast in response to psychic stimuli. More than a hundred years ago scientifically curious men extended these observations, by means of a gastric fistula, to lower segments of the digestive tract of dogs. Again they found that the mere sight of food would cause the gastric juices to flow.[54] Partly as an outgrowth of such observations, many have proposed that a variety of physical ailments are psychosomatic in origin. Although it is probably true that this is the case in certain situations, in many instances the relationships between psychologic events and somatic changes have not been tightly defined and are therefore of doubtful validity.

Cannon[55] was among the first to approach this problem in a scientifically controlled manner and to demonstrate how the organism may mediate psychosomatic reactions. He was able to demonstrate that the body responds to fear and other emotionally distressing situations through its sympathetic nervous system by secreting the hormonal agent epinephrine into the blood stream. This in turn prompts dilatation of the pupils, acceleration of the pulse, contraction of peripheral blood vessels, mobilization of glucose as a source of energy and other bodily changes, all of which appear to be designed to improve the ability to protect oneself from physical danger, if need be, by fighting, running or other forms of physical action.

In more recent times it has been demonstrated that even the normal newborn human responds autonomically, as evidenced by changes in heart rate and other variables, to sensory stimuli such as that provided by white sound of known composition (i.e., 20 to 20,000 cycles per second) and controlled density. All newborns respond to a stimulus intensity of 70 decibels, but some respond to less.[56] Similarly, increases in heart rates have been noted in older children who were witnessing an exciting movie under standardized circumstances. The greatest effect was in response to a story with which the children could really identify.[57]

In subsequent years others have discovered that the output of adrenocortical hormones also increases under conditions of emotional stress.[58] Hill, for example, measured the urinary 17-hydroxycorticosteroid output of varsity crewmen as they took part on different days in practice runs, time-trial runs and formal races. The values obtained indicated that adrenocortical activity was significantly higher on days when they were racing or undergoing time-trial runs than when they were simply practicing or not rowing at all. The level of physical activity was approximately the same on all rowing days, but the values were much lower on nonrowing days. The investigators concluded that emotional stress is probably much more potent than physical activity in effecting increased adrenocortical activity.

In line with this, elevations in adrenocortical activity have been observed in the absence of increased physical strain in students undergoing oral examinations[59] and in parents experiencing the distress of

[53]Alvarez, W. (1929).

[54]Bidder, F., et al. (1852) quoted by Alverez, W. (1929).

[55]Cannon, W. (1915).

[56]Steinschneider, A., et al. (1966).

[57]Lipton, E., et al. (1965).

[58]Thorn, G., et al. (1953); Hill, S., et al. (1956); Venning, E., et al. (1957); Friedman, S., et al. (1963); Hamburg, D. (1959, 1967).

[59]Venning, E., et al. (1957).

having one of their children admitted to the hospital for the first time with a life threatening, neoplastic disease.[60] It thus appears that emotional strain by itself is capable of inducing increased adrenocortical activity.

This thesis is supported by extensive studies[61] of mechanisms by which the organism mediates adrenocortical responses to stressful psychologic stimuli. It has been found that the response is initiated when an individual perceives an environmental situation to be emotionally threatening. This perception may either be in anticipation or in consequence of an event. Once initiated in the cerebral cortex, the response is mediated by a series of reactions involving the secretion of a corticotropin-releasing factor by cells in the hypothalamus, the secretion of adrenocorticotropic hormone by the adenohypophysis and, finally, the secretion of corticosteroids by the adrenal cortices. Whether and how these actions help the organism to deal with psychologic stress is not altogether clear. However, this information is of major significance in illustrating that bodily changes of psychologic origin can occur, and can be defined, measured and controlled in accordance with scientific principles. As already mentioned few such changes are as well understood as those just described.

For example, it has long been suspected that psychosocial stress may have something to do with the pathogenesis of clinical thyrotoxicosis. However, extensive efforts to demonstrate a dependable relationship between psychosocial events and thyroid function have not as yet yielded compelling evidence.[62] Likewise, it has often been suggested that other bodily maladies such as cardiac arrhythmias, eczema, asthma, acne, peptic ulcer, ulcerative colitis, amenorrhea, colic and abdominal pain, hypertension and even death may on occasion be at least partly of psychogenic origin.[63] Scientifically controlled observations in support of these possibilities is still lacking or at best tentative.

This paucity of evidence concerning psychosomatic mechanisms places major limitations on the application of psychosomatic principles to clinical diagnosis and therapy. This is not altogether surprising, considering that most practicing physicians and scientific investigators have tended to concentrate their attention *either* on the somatic *or* on the psychosocial aspects of health and disease. Yet, as Peabody pointed out 40 years ago in his essays *Doctor and Patient:*

> The proper interpretation of symptoms involves not only a comprehension of the (organic) causes of symptoms but also of the person in whom the symptoms arise. Every experienced physician knows that when one of his patients complains of a pain in the stomach it is probably a very trivial matter and when another makes apparently the same complaint it is probably a very serious matter. It all depends on the type of patient, and the better the physician knows his patient the better he will be able to decide on the proper treatment. Skilled physicians, gifted with peculiar insight in to human nature, can often estimate a personality with remarkable accuracy in a few minutes or even seconds, but in general the more the doctor knows of his patient's background the greater advantage he has in handling the case. This is the great advantage which

[60]Friedman, S., et al. (1963 a).

[61]Hamburg, D., and Lunde, D. T. (1967).

[62]Lidz, T. (1949); Jaco, E. (Ed.) (1958); Hamburg, D., and Lunde, D. (1967).

[63]Alvarez, W. (1929); Peabody, F. W. (1930); Spitz, R. (1946a); Reifenstein, E. (1946); Mac Keith, R., and O'Neill, D. (1951); Porter, R. W. et al., (1958); Engel, G. (1959); Richmond, J. (1962); Peiper, A. (1963); Apley, J. (1964); Mathis, J. (1964); Lipton, E. et al. (1965); Matsumoto, S. et al. (1965); Purcell, K. (1969); Bakwin, H., and Bakwin, R. (1966); Brooks, F. (1966); Steinschneider, A., et al. (1966); Coddington, R. (1968); Wolff, H., and Goodell, H. (1968); Engel, G. (1969).

the general practitioner has always possessed and still possesses. He knows the patient from childhood up—his physical health, the nervous and mental strain to which he has been subjected, the conditions of his social, business and domestic life, and, even more than this, he may have the same detailed knowledge of the patient's parents and of the circumstances of their life. *Now all this information, which is difficult to obtain except as a result of years of intimacy, has an infinitely important bearing on the question of health and disease. Not to have it is an enormous loss, and the loss falls, or course, primarily on the patient.* He is the one who suffers. The only person who can really gather together this fundamental knowledge of his patients is the general practitioner.

In the trend toward specialism the pendulum is swinging too far, and it is the duty of medical educators and leaders to indicate to their students the importance of general practice and the high professional attainments that are necessary for success in it.[64]

Today, the need for this approach to the maintenance of health and the diagnosis and management of disease is greater than ever. Today, however, it is necessary to go beyond the general practitioner pictured by Peabody to develop a modernized and highly sophisticated variety of primary physician generalist. These physicians must be equipped by training and experience to deal systematically and efficiently with the biosocial intermix of causes and consequences of disease, disability and health. It is hoped that present gaps in knowledge can be closed by showing that a given type of somatic change regularly occurs following exposure to psychosocial stress under specified environmental and biologic circumstances, and by defining the mechanism through which these changes are mediated. Information gathered under the leadership of well-informed representatives of this new breed of generalist should yield many clues to potentially significant relationships among social, environmental and intrinsic behavioral and organic phenomena. When pursued by means of scientifically controlled research techniques, these clues should lead to further substantial gains in the understanding of human health and disease.

G. Effects on Parents, Siblings and Others of Deformity, Disease or Disability in a Child

Long before social science could be identified as a discipline, physicians and others recognized that the presence of disease can have far-reaching effects not only on the patient but also on the lives of his family and others.[65] History provides no more compelling illustration of this than Massie's masterful account of the fateful effects of illness in the Tsarevitch, Alexis.[66] Born to the Tsar and Tsaritza, Nicholas and Alexandra, during what turned out to be the last years of Imperial Russia, Alexis had inherited hemophilia from his great grandmother, Queen Victoria. At birth he began to bleed from his navel, an occurrence that struck despair in the hearts of his parents. The historically crucial moments came a few years later when Alexis was recovering from a fall in a boat. The Empress, worried about her small son's being confined to the house, decided to take him for a drive. Not long after they started bounding and hostling over the rough country roads Alexis began to wince and complain of pain in his leg and abdomen. His mother ordered the driver to turn about and return home with all possible haste. Every time

[64]Peabody, F. W.: Doctor and Patient: Papers on the Relationship of the Physician to Men and Institutions. New York, The MacMillan Company, 1930, pp. 24–25.

[65]Castiglioni, A. (1947); Rosen, G. (1963); Arnold, M., et al. (1958).

[66]Massie, R. K. (1967).

the carriage jolted, young Alexis turned pale and cried out in pain, and by the time they reached home he was almost unconscious.

In terror, Alexandra telegraphed for medical help. One by one the doctors arrived, but to no avail, for the blood continued to flow. Day and night the boy's screams pierced the air and he became more and more desperately sick. When it appeared that the end was approaching, official announcements were made of the grave illness of the heir to the throne. Finally a night came when the boy's condition was so low that he was given the last sacraments with the expectation that he would be dead by morning.

It was on this night, when it seemed that doctors were powerless and that they were at the end of hope, that Alexandra called on the "Holy Man" Rasputin, begging him to pray for the life of her son. Rasputin cabled back from Siberia, "God has seen your tears and heard your prayers. Do not grieve, the Little One will not die. Do not allow the doctors to bother him too much." Even though no immediate improvement in Alexis' condition was noted, and the beneficial effects of Rasputin's advice on the outcome are hard to assess, the effect of his reassurance on Alexandra was profound. By the next morning she was smiling and said, "I am not a bit anxious myself now.... During the night I received a telegram from Father Gregory [Rasputin] and he has reassured me completely." The bleeding stopped a day later.

To quote Massie directly, "Whatever the cause, everyone—doctors, court officials, grand duchesses, people who believed in Rasputin and those who hated him—recognized that a remarkably eerie coincidence had occurred. Only to one person was the mystery not a mystery. In her own mind, Alexandra understood clearly what had happened. To her it seemed quite natural: after the best doctors in Russia had failed, after her own hours of prayer had gone unanswered, her plea to Rasputin had brought the intervention of God and a miracle had taken place. From that time, Alexandra was unshakably convinced that her son's life lay in Rasputin's hands. From this belief enormous consequences were to flow."

At the center of these consequences was what Alexis' tutor Gulliard termed "the phenomenon of Rasputin," who through this episode gained enormous influence over Alexandra and hence over the government of Russia in the critical days which led to the disintegration of the dynasty and eventually to the Russian Revolution.

This is an unusually dramatic example of the impact of a child's illness on the lives and attitudes of other people, but every disease or disability has consequences beyond its direct effects on the patient. (See Table 1–10.) Many studies have shown that pregnancy is normally a period of hopeful expectation. To have pregnancy culminate in the birth of a malformed infant is therefore profoundly disappointing and may be catastrophic to the parents.[67] In instances when the child is severely deformed or handicapped mentally or physically, the parents know they have to give up their aspirations and hopes for an offspring of whom they can be proud. They realize also that they are trapped in a situation where they may have to provide their child with extra and special care for an indefinite period, perhaps a lifetime.

As one author aptly put it, "What happens to parents following the birth of an abnormal baby is a nightmare."[68] This distress often is com-

---

[67]Solnit, A., and Stark, M. (1961); Tisza, V. (1962); Tisza, V., and Gumpertz, E. (1962); Bergmen, A., and Schulte, C. (1967).

[68]Parmelee, A. (1962).

Table 1–10 Possible Effects of a Malformed, Sick, Disabled or Dying Child on Parents and Siblings

Parental disappointment, shame or guilt over malformed or handicapped child
Parental resentment and anger over burden, or sublimation thereof in constructive actions
Parental anxiety leading to overprotective, overrestrictive, overindulgent care, with problems secondary thereto
Overconcentration of attention on sick child with resultant underattention to needs of other members of the family, fatigue, depression, family impoverishment
Distortion of normal family life in respect to where to live, what to do and so forth
Sibling resentment of patient as recipient of special and favored attention; also, shame due to having abnormal sibling
Sibling vulnerability in respect to parental transference of overprotective attitudes and practices to them after patient dies
Grief and depression in anticipation of experiencing fatal or disastrous outcome

pounded by personal shame and guilt at having produced an abnormal child.[69] In instances where the disease is acquired rather than inherited, parents are apt to blame themselves on the basis that they could and should have prevented it by being more alert, by handling the child differently, and so forth.

The reactions of parents to the news that their child has a fatal disease such as leukemia also follow somewhat predictable patterns. Among these is a deep dismay regarding the child's loss of opportunities for self-fulfillment, and personal sorrow at the inevitability of the forthcoming separation. A few become totally overwhelmed, disorganized and unable to work for a period of time.[70] While the *threat of loss* exists, some try to deny the situation by screening out reality or by making compulsive efforts to reverse it (as by shopping around among diagnostic and therapeutic agencies).[71] Some also begin to mourn in anticipation of the loss of the child; this may involve some degree of emotional detachment from the dying child and increased involvement with other children on the hospital ward even when their own child is critically ill.[72]

Parental child-caring practices in respect to malformed, disabled and dying children also tend to conform to predictable patterns. Those who bitterly resent being burdened with a defective child may treat him in a neglectful, rejecting manner with resultant psychosocial deprivation.[73] Other parents may focus their hostility and anger on the medical profession, or sublimate it by organizing or becoming active in associations of parents having children with conditions such as mental retardation, cerebral palsy, nephrosis or cystic fibrosis.[74]

Green et al.[75] have pointed out that the anxieties occasioned by caring for a dying child engender parental attitudes and practices which may cause severe behavioral problems either in the patient himself, if he unexpectedly survives, or, by displacement, in a brother or sister if he does not.

Among the most common (and perhaps most damaging) responses of parents to the anxiety and dismay at having a handicapped or dying child

[69]Bozeman, M., et al. (1955); Lis, E., et al. (1956); Browne, W., et al. (1960); Solnit, A., and Stark, M. (1961); Tisza, V. (1962); Tisza, V., and Gumpertz, E. (1962); Friedman, S., et al. (1963 b); MacKeith, R. (1964); Mattsson, A., and Gross, S. (1966); Berman, A., and Schulte, C. (1967).

[70]Bergman, A., and Schulte, C. (1967).

[71]Bozeman, M., et al. (1955); Tisza, V. (1962); Green, M., and Solnit, A. (1964); Mattsson, A., and Gross, S. (1966).

[72]Tisza, V. (1962); Tisza, V., and Gumpertz, E. (1962); Bergman, A., and Schulte, C. (1967).

[73]Lis, E., et al. (1956); Howell, M. (1962); Friedman, S., et al. (1963 b); MacKeith, R. (1964).

[74]Bozeman, M., et al. (1955); Tisza, V. (1962); Friedman, S., et al. (1963 b); MacKeith, R. (1964).

[75]Green, M., and Solnit, A. (1964.

are tendencies to overprotect the child from ordinary small risks, to over-restrict physical activities, to withhold discipline and to overindulge whims.[76] The damaging effects of these forms of psychosocial malnutrition may be compounded by marital discord over the proper way to treat, protect and discipline the child. It is not unusual for parents to go further than this and in effect make the patient the central figure around whom the whole family revolves. The mother becomes heavily preoccupied with preparing the diet, supervising the medication, curtailing the child's activities and handling the child's own emotional reactions to the limitations and deprivation imposed on him as a result of his illness. (See also Section H, p. 39.)[77]

Such focus on the child inevitably results in distortions of normal patterns of living such as evenings out, vacations and other family social activities. For example, the parents of one diabetic child reported that they had not spent a single evening or weekend away from home during the five years following the onset of her condition. In another instance a family moved to Alaska to get away from the embarrassment and stress of raising a sexually precocious 7 year old boy in a Boston suburb. The brothers and sisters of the patient (and sometimes the father) are likely to resent any and all extreme forms of special or favored treatment for a sick sibling, especially if this results in marked reduction of attention to their own needs and interests.[78] The family life style then becomes "child specific," and behaviors regarding psychosocial supplies become governed by the "sick child."

H. Characteristics of Sick Role Existence Among Children

> I wish I knew what you mean about being sick. Sometimes I've felt so bad I could curl up and die, but had to go on because the kids had to be taken care of and because we didn't have the money to spend for the doctor. How could I be sick? How do you know when you're sick anyway? Some people can go to bed anytime with anything, but most of us can't be sick even when we need to be.
>
> *Koos, E. (1954)*

> Being sick is a cultural phenomenon in itself and may or may not accompany clinically definable ill health. One may instance cases in which clinically very serious ill health—schizophrenia or epilepsy, to name only two—is evaluated culturally as an enviable state. Thus the limitations of a culture may make its participants simply oblivious to a given kind of ill health. . . . It may seem too much to assert that a man is as sick as he feels, but there is considerable evidence to support such a statement.
>
> *Maclachlan, J. (1958)*

During the years following the introduction of biologic science to medicine a half century ago, it was natural and appropriate that attention be concentrated on saving lives, on physical restoration and on the maximization of bodily function. The gains yielded by this approach are now handsomely reflected in the relatively low infant and child mortality rates in the United States and other countries.[79] In the United

---

[76]Broene, W., et al. (1960); Howell, M. (1962); Tisza, V. (1962); Richardson, S. (1963); Friedman, S., et al. (1963 b); Agle, D. (1964); Glaser, H., et al. (1964); MacKeith, R. (1964); Mattsson, A., and Gross, S. (1966).

[77]Solnit, A., and Stark, M. (1961); Tisza, V. (1962); Friedman, S., et al. (1963 b); Bergman, A., and Schulte, C. (1967).

[78]Bozeman, M., et al. (1955); Friedman, S., et al. (1963 b); Mattsson, A., and Gross, S. (1966); Bergman, A., and Schulte, C. (1967).

[79]Harper, P. (1962); Wallace, H. (1962); Shiffer, C., and Hunt, E. (1963).

States, more than 97 per cent of all live-born babies and more than 99 per cent of all fullterm infants now survive to adult age with an average life expectancy in excess of 70 years. Corresponding reductions have been achieved in physically crippling disorders. Many of the complaints and concerns expressed by patients a few decades ago have disappeared, and opportunities have emerged for the health care professions to foster levels of wellness never before possible. However, detractions from personal well-being remain. The lives of many patients are marred by their assumption of "sick role" behavior which may or may not be necessary.[80]

Parsons[81] defines role as the organized participation of an individual in a social system such as a family or a neighborhood. An individual's role is expressed in the performance of a number of different tasks which have some function in relation to his role or his personality. Somatic health is the state of optimal capacity for effective performance of valued tasks, whereas psychologic health signifies capacity for performance of valued roles. The term sick role applies when a person becomes unable to perform normally expected tasks or roles. Generally, it is assumed that the ill person cannot overcome this incapacity by a process of decision making alone but that some kind of therapeutic process, spontaneous or aided, is necessary for recovery.

Table 1–11 shows a number of the factors in sick role behavior that detract from personal well-being. Some have been discussed previously, and others are self-evident. Some, however, need additional comment.

Certain individuals with a visible handicap are apt to be given a rela-

[80]Bergman, A., and Schulte, C. (1967).
[81]Parsons, T. (1951, 1958).

Table 1–11 Some Characteristics of "Sick Role" Existence Among Children

A. Psychosocial Deprivation, Intoxication or Injury*
Rejection or lack of acceptance (devalued status)
Hostility or lack of affection
Excess control or lack of freedom
Indulgence or lack of control
"Smothering" or excess attention
Excess protection
Abuse
B. Restrictions in Ordinary Life Experiences
Interpersonal communication (as in blindness, deafness, cleft palate)
Mobility and opportunities for physical explorations and social contacts
Self-care
Activity level
Education (e.g., being able to go to school)
Plans for career, marriage and so forth
C. Experiences Typical to Illness
Diet (e.g., increased, restricted, measured, special)
Medication (e.g., scheduling, unpleasant tastes, discomfort)
Physical therapy (e.g., postural drainage, excercises, braces, mist tent, surgery)
Pain (e.g., injections, dressings)
D. Behavioral Problems
Characteristics of temperament
hyperactivity
hypoactivity
withdrawal
Psychosis
Social behavior
asocial behavior (isolation, shyness)
aggression (especially manipulation, self-punishment)
oppositional behavior (disobedience, negativism, passive aggression)
dependency
Emotional behavior
anxiety
depression
Stereotyped behavior (especially compulsiveness)
Suicide
Addiction
Habit disturbances

*See also Tables 1–6 and 1–10.

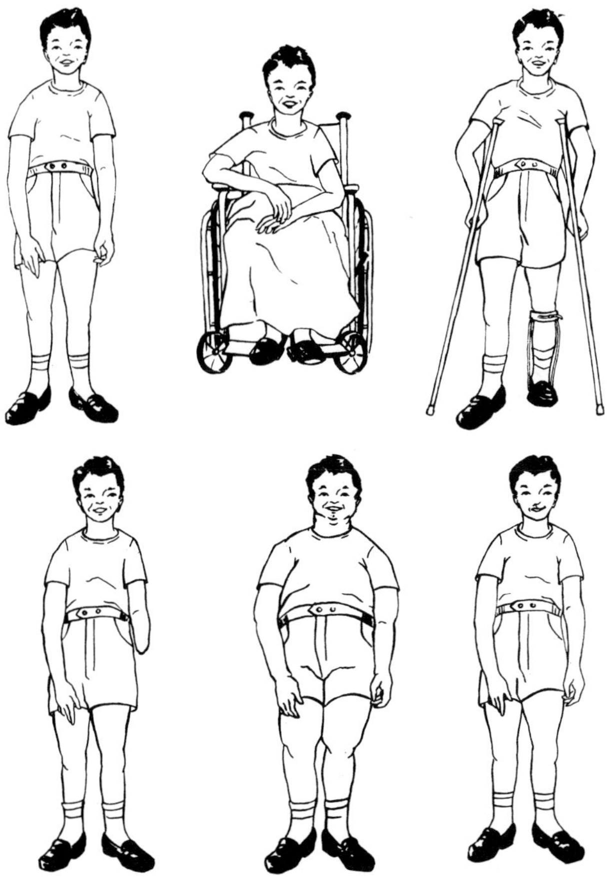

Figure 1–4 Figures used in studies of attitudes of various groups of children and adults toward children with visible physical handicaps. The same individual is depicted variably (*top, left to right*) as normal, as unable to walk, on crutches for disabled leg, (*bottom, left to right*) with amputated left arm, as obese and with harelip. (*From* Richardson, S., et al., 1961.)

tively low status by other persons.[82] Richardson has studied this phenomenon systematically and has determined that when children and their parents are asked to give a preferential ranking to a standard set of pictures of children who differ only in respect to the presence or absence of visible disabilities (Figure 1–4), they indicate choices with a high degree of uniformity. The nonhandicapped child is liked most, followed by the child with leg brace and crutches, the child in the wheel chair, the child with amputation of the left hand, the child with slight facial disfigurement (harelip) and, lastly, the obese child. Thus, a person with a visible handicap may have one strike against him irrespective of any functional disability or competence he may have. The same appears to be true with regard to invisible maladies such as diabetes, hemophilia and cardiac disease if others are aware of the disorder.[82]

Helen Keller's life history is instructive when considering restrictions in ordinary experience in gen-

[82]Fischer, A., and Dolger, H. (1946); Bruch, H. (1949); Abel, T. (1952); Davis, F. (1961); Richardson, S., et al. (1961); Richardson, S. (1963); Swift, C., et al. (1967).

eral (Table 1–11 B), and in interpersonal communications in particular. Anyone who has read the story of her life or seen *The Mircle Worker* on stage or screen will have an acute appreciation of the impact on a child of blindness, deafness and the inability to communicate verbally. The notes and letters of Anne M. Sullivan also give valuable information on the necessity (for healthy human behavior and cognitive development) of providing the child, through one channel or another, with love, discipline and constructive cognitive stimuli.[83] (See also Section I, p. 44.)

Restrictions in mobility consequent to blindness, cerebral palsy or other conditions are important when they curtail exploration of the physical world and restrict opportunity for developing social contacts.[84] Some handicapped children spend hours with almost nothing to do simply because play and work objects are beyond reach. Thus, dependence on care given by others can be an important component of this type of sick role.

Limitations of physical activity such as bed rest, restriction to wheelchair or house or even minor restrictions in outdoor work and play activities can also comprise significant components of sick role existence. In the past, many parents and physicians considered bed rest an important adjunct to the treatment of respiratory infections, rheumatic fever, rheumatoid arthritis, tuberculosis, nephritis and a wide variety of other childhood illnesses.[85] Over the years students of these conditions have challenged this concept, and some have concluded that this form of sick role limitation not only may be unnecessary and psychosocially detrimental, but also may be less beneficial in overcoming the physical complaint than is a more liberal regimen.[86] Moreover, Bass demonstrated that subjects 6 to 13 years of age who had been hospitalized for a variety of chronic physical diseases were no less active during days of bed rest than when allowed full activity around the ward. Children can be as lively in bed as out, but under most circumstances they limit their activity to levels that conform to their current condition and even get into bed spontaneously when they feel ill enough.

Riseborough, in working with scoliotic children, has concluded that these patients do as well or better physically, and much better psychologically, if allowed unlimited activity during the long postoperative period when they are incased in a cast, than if subjected to a regimen of prolonged bed rest.[87] Similarly, Agle, and Mattsson and Gross have observed that hemophiliacs are no more likely to bleed when they are encouraged to be fully active than when they are restricted.[88]

The patient represented in Figure 1–5 illustrates two additional points. One is that absence from school can comprise a large component of sick role existence for children. The other is that the attitude of caretakers can be an important factor in determining whether a person lives a "well" or a "sick" role. This child developed asthma at an early age. Though the astma was mild, his mother perceived him to be in need of protection from the ordinary rigors of school. As a result he was kept out of school for one-third of the school year. In con-

[83]Keller, H. (and Sullivan, A.) (1954).

[84]MacKeith, R. (1964); Barker, R., and Wright, H. (1955).

[85]Bass, H., and Schulman, J. (1967).

[86]Capps, R., and Barker, M. (1947); Beaumont, G. (1954); Chalmers, J. (1955); Gibson, J. (1956); Joseph, M., and Polane, P. (1958); McCrory, W., et al. (1958); Browne, W., et al. (1960); Wynn-Williams, N., and Shaw, J. (1960); Feinstein, A. (1962).

[87]Riseborough, E. (1967).

[88]Agle, D. (1964); Mattsson, A., and Gross, S. (1966).

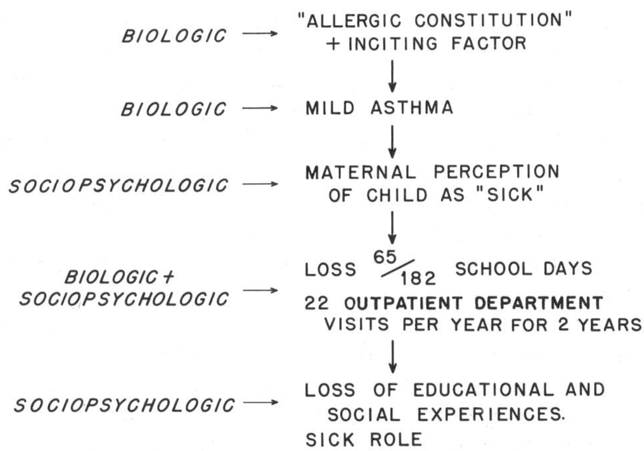

Figure 1–5 Example of the importance of perception of disease in determining whether patients with biologic handicaps live a well or a sick role. (*From* Talbot, N. B., 1968.)

sequence of this and the fact that he was taken to the doctor over 20 times a year, he was as seriously disabled in respect to his educational and social experiences as if he had had a major limitation in respiratory function from, for instance, cystic fibrosis.

Limitations in capacity to plan for education, career, marriage and other healthy, mature activities begin to loom large as the invalid child approaches the time in adolescence when he would normally grow out of a state of dependency and perhaps get a job, marry and think about developing a family of his own. MacKeith,[89] in writing on this subject, emphasizes the crucial importance of encouraging basic healthy activities in the handicapped as well as in the healthy young individual.

The list of experiences characteristic of illness (Table 1–11 C) includes such familiar items as diet, medications, treatments, surgery, pain and so forth. The manner in which these experiences can influence a patient's daily life has been illustrated by the thyrotoxic patient (Case 3, p. 5) mentioned in the introduction to this chapter. The two principles represented by this case apply to all patients requiring medical attention for any length of time: *first,* treatment schedules can be socially and behaviorally disabling, even when they are organically beneficial; *second,* decisions concerning the optimum balance between the dual desiderata of satisfactory body function and a rewarding way of life are one of the chief responsibilities of the primary physician.

Most of the sick role behavioral problems in Table 1–11 D have been discussed in relation to the psychosocial effects of being malformed or disabled (Table 1–11 A) and to the behavioral responses to psychosocial malnutrition and injury (Table 1–8). Some of these behavioral problems, such as hypoactivity, withdrawal and dependency, may reflect a tendency to use sickness as an excuse to escape from the stresses of ordinary existence,[90] or to use the malady as a weapon for manipulating others and getting one's own way (i.e., "If you hit me, I'll bleed," or "If you punish me, I'll tell the doctor.")[91] Oppositional behavior may be one of the few

---

[89]MacKeith, R. (1964).

[90]Parsons, T. (1958); King, S. (1962, 1963); Knutson, A. (1965).

[91]Browne, W., et al. (1960).

ways bed ridden or seriously disabled children have to protect themselves against a powerfully dominant and controlling environment.

Sick and disabled children, like their adult counterparts, may be anxious and depressed about alarming realities such as difficulty in breathing, bleeding, threat of separation from loved ones, a gloomy outlook regarding cure or relief of symptoms, or, in some instances, survival. The concept of death as a reality to which they may be subject grows gradually and is usually well established by the age of puberty.[92] Prior to that time children have only a partial understanding and awareness of this phenomenon. In children under 3 to 4 years of age, concern is apt to center around separation from parents on whom they depend for care. Preschool children are curious about burials and about the characteristics of dead animals and flowers, and they may fear the loss of love and attention which occurs as a result of death. Death begins to be personified between 5 and 9 years of age, after children have had sufficient experience to comprehend the difference between dying and going away, between death and absence.

Suicidal behavior is by no means a rarity among children who are suffering profoundly from physical pain, bodily disfigurement, social isolation or rejection, traumatic dressings, multiple anesthesias and so forth.

Psychotic behavior as a manifestation of sick role is rare except in cases of marked brain damage or under conditions of intoxication with hallucinogenic or psychopathogenic drugs. Drug addiction also is unusual but is a risk in children given addicting medications over prolonged periods.

Habit disturbances are common. They often reflect a tendency to regress more childish or infantile behavior when illness results in intense psychologic stress.

The variables discussed in this section are central to "the care of the patient" as a person. Though attention has been focused largely on factors that detract from healthy and happy living, the intended implication is that it is well within the purview and competence of members of the health care professions to upgrade the quality of living of their patients by reducing these detractions to the lowest level compatible with a reasonable life span. Patients all too frequently experience sick role phenomena *unnecessarily*. Some of this may be of parent or even patient origin; but some—and perhaps most—are either instilled by the physician or can be prevented or corrected by him. (See Case 3, p. 5.)

I. Therapeutic Strategies

> Solving problems of disease is not the same thing as creating health. . . . This task demands a kind of wisdom and vision which transcends specialized knowledge of remedies and treatments and which apprehends in all their complexities and subleties the relation between living things and their total environment.
>
> *Dubos, R. (1959)*

> All scientific work is incomplete—whether it be observational or experimental. All scientific work is liable to be upset or modified by advancing knowledge. That does not confer upon us a freedom to ignore the knowledge that we already have, or to postpone the action that it appears to demand at a given time.
>
> *Hill, A. (1965)*

[92]Leventhal, H. (1965); Bergman, A., and Schulte, C. (1967); Green, M., and Solnit, A. (1964).

General Considerations. When protected against undue stress and provided with adequate psychosocial supplies, children have an intrinsic capacity to heal themselves of disturbances caused by psychosocial malnutrition. Appropriate therapy can help them take advantage of this capacity.

The particular nature and origin of the patient's psychosocial deprivation, intoxication or injury determine what therapeutic strategy will be most effective. The patient must be provided with essential supplies at rates that fall between the minimum requirements and the maximum tolerance levels of his own homeostatic, adaptive ranges. Fortunately, the ranges of adaptive competence normally are broad, and considerable variations in the quality and quantity of social supplies can be tolerated.

For example, the successful results obtained by placing socially starved babies in the hands of institutionalized retardates suggest that infants can make gains even when the purveyors of affection and attention are not intellectually well endowed.[93] On the other hand, the caretakers do have to be persons who can love and be interested in their charges.[94] The requirement holds for children's biologic parents as well as for parent substitutes. This fact has led a number of authors to recommend when there is lack of harmony between mother and child, or that the child be removed from his home and placed in a more nurturing environment when there is a vicious kind of parent-child interaction as seen in some cases of neglect, abuse or marked temperamental misfit.[95] Under all circumstances, it is preferable that persons tending children be knowledgeable about the child's needs.[96] It is desirable, too, that the child's care be provided consistently by one or, at most, two persons.[97]

Quantitatively speaking, it has been observed that in institutions where infants have developed gross evidence of social deprivation the ratio of caretaker to charges has been on the order of one nurse to more than five infants.[98] Under these thinly staffed circumstances the nurses were able to take care of the physical needs of the babies but had little time to attend to them in a personal way. In nicely arranged experiments, Goldfarb found that supplementing this impersonal care by means of a mothering person who spent one hour a day five days a week cuddling, playing with, talking to and otherwise giving individual and personal attention to an infant resulted in the elimination of most manifestations of psychosocial malnutrition, and in rapid developmental gains.[99]

Looking at the opposite end of the scale, it is safe to assume that a ratio of one mother to one child is compatible with enough attentiveness and affection. However, the upper limits of human tolerance for this psychosocial nutriment can be overreached by an overanxious parent who practically never lets a child out of her sight, has him sleep in the same room with her and in general devotes most of her social energies to this one individual.[100] The result, for the child, may be psychosocial intoxication.

---

[93]Skeels, H. (1966); Caldwell, B. (1967).

[94]Provence, S. (1967).

[95]Bowlby, J. (1951); Glaser, K., and Eisenberg, L. (1956); Rose, J. (1959); Clarke, A., and Clarke, A. (1960); Witmer, H., et al. (1962); Bain, K. (1963); Peiper, A. (1963); Silver, H., and Finkelstein, M. (1967).

[96]Engel, G. (1959).

[97]Glaser, K., and Eisenberg, L. (1956); Clarke, A., and Clarke, A. (1960); Fanshel, D., and Maas, H. S. (1962); Witmer, H., et al. (1962); Leonard, R., et al. (1966); Powell, G., et al. (1967).

[98]Spitz, R. (1945); Yarrow, L. (1961); Witmer, H., et al. (1962); Skeels, H. (1966).

[99]Goldfarb, W. (1945).

[100]Bowlby, J. (1951); Lapouse, R., and Monk, M. (1959); Green, M., and Solnit, A. (1964); Bakwin, H., and Bakwin, R. (1966).

Under such circumstances, as with the opposite situation of deprivation, relatively small changes in maternal practices may be sufficient to restore the intensity of attention to tolerable levels. However, the risk of recurrence is less if the level of input is comfortably distant from pathogenic levels.

As mentioned earlier, a normally endowed infant may be able to attain a completely healthy status if psychosocial deficiencies and excesses are corrected before the child reaches the age of one to one and half years.[101] Depending on their duration and intensity, longer periods of psychosocial malnutrition can result in irreversible changes.[102] This is not to say, however, that a deprived individual's capacity to respond favorably to an enrichment program becomes nil by the end of childhood. In any given case the surest way to assess a child's capacity for recovery is to give him a therapeutic trial of assured, adequate psychosocial nutrition.[103] As exemplified by Cases 1 and 2 (pp. 2 ff.) and by many other patients reported in the literature, the capacity for favorable response on the part of markedly deprived infants and children can become clearly and strikingly manifest within two to four weeks.[104]

Failure to respond favorably may indicate that the therapeutic arrangements were inadequate. It is often difficult for the physician to be sure what kind of care children receive when they live in an uncontrolled environment (as at home). Failure also may be due to the presence of neurologic, metabolic or other primarily physical disease, which may have the effect of reducing the child's homeostatic responsiveness.

Specific Therapeutic Strategies. Therapeutic efforts to overcome psychosocial deprivation, intoxication or injury in accordance with the principles just outlined may take several forms. As in the management of biologic problems, the chances of success are greatest when treatment is directed as closely as possible toward primary causative factors (see Tables 1–5, 1–6 and 1–7). Depending, therefore, on etiologic relationships, one or more of a variety of approaches may be indicated. Included among these are (a) instruction of the child's principal caretakers, (b) fulfillment of the parents' social and material requirements, (c) supplementation of parental care taking, (d) provision of a substitute parent or parents, (e) medical or surgical correction of a primary disorder in the child and (f) modification of the attitudes and practices of other important persons and institutions.

PARENTAL EDUCATION. Many normal parents and other adults simply do not realize that infants and children have basic needs for attention, control, acceptance and affection as well for the obvious physical necessities (See Table 1–6 A).[105] Some of these people may read books on child rearing by Spock, Ginott, Fraiberg, Holt and Brazelton[106] and consequently learn enough about the principles of psychosocial nutrition in relation to human behavior and development to be able to meet the needs of children. On the other hand, it has been repeatedly observed by students of the therapeutic

---

[101]Goldfarb, W. (1945); Witmer, H., et al. (1962); Caldwell, B., and Drachman, R. (1964); Bakwin, H., and Bakwin, R. (1966).

[102]Bowlby, J. (1951); Bakwin, H., and Bakwin, R. (1966).

[103]Davis, K. (1947); Hollowell, J., and Gardner, L. (1965); Bakwin, H., and Bakwin, R. (1966); Chilman, C. (1966).

[104]Talbot, N. B., et al. (1947); Fried, R., and Mayer, M. (1948); Glaser, K., and Eisenberg, L. (1956); Elmer, E. (1960); Peiper, A. (1963); Powell, G., et al. (1967); Eisenberg, L. (1968).

[105]Reid, J. H. (1959); Samora, J., et al. (1962).

[106]Spock, B. (1958); Fraiberg, S. (1959); Holt, J. (1967); Ginott, H. (1969); Brazelton, T. (1970).

process that patients and parents are much more likely to absorb instruction and respond to advice if it is personally given by an accepted and respected member of a health care profession.[107] Moreover, it may be necessary to translate the principles of psychosocial nutrition into terms that are meaningful to parents of different cultural, educational and experiential backgrounds. This is especially true in the case of parents brought up under socially deprived or injurious circumstances.

When the child has a chronic illness or an enduring physical or mental handicap, it may be necessary to call the parents' attention to the dangers inherent in expecting more from the child than can realistically be expected (see Table 1–6, B-3). Parents may also need to be alerted to the damage they may do by being overattentive or overprotective,[108] overanxious,[109] overindulgent[110] or overcontrolling[111] or by failing to provide the child with adequate allotments of control,[112] approval[113] and acceptance.

In presenting information on these subjects to parents, it is well to remember that fear-arousing strategies are not very likely to motivate persons to change their ways.[114] On the other hand, the strategy of generating opinion and stimulating action through the news media, social gatherings and other semipublic channels are effective ways of influencing individual members of society.[115]

There needs to be a nationwide effort to explore and evaluate means of increasing the public's understanding of the impact of adult attitudes and practices on child health. Widespread dissemination of information concerning children's needs, tolerances and responses among high school students and through parent-teacher associations could be one effective yet inexpensive way of reducing the high incidence of psychosocial malnutrition among children. However, this effort must extend beyond the school and other neighborhood educational and social institutions. An effort should be made to educate individuals such as writers, publishers of magazines and other popular forms of literature, performers and creators of television programs and movies, so that they, in turn, will use their influence to spread this knowledge. The results of the *Sesame Street* television program and studies on attitude formation have shown that such media can be an effective positive force.

FULFILLMENT OF PARENTAL SOCIAL AND PHYSICAL REQUIREMENTS. In situations where a child's parents are failing to provide for his essential needs because they themselves are starved for social supplies, sick, poverty stricken, jobless or otherwise overburdened with problems with which they cannot cope, one of the best ways to meet the child's needs may be to help the parents. Viewed broadly, this may involve major changes in societal value systems and arrangements.[116]

Fortunately, however, in many instances much can be accomplished on an individual family basis. Social

[107]Senn, M. (1948); Korsch, B. (1956); Solnit, A., and Stark, M. (1961); Tisza, V. (1962); Bakwin, H., and Bakwin, R. (1966).

[108]Lowenfeld, B. (1956); Rose, J. (1959); Browne, W., et al. (1960); Witmer, H., et al. (1962); Fontana, V., et al. (1963); Friedman, S., et al. (1963); Agle, D. (1964); Glaser, H., et al. (1964); Green, M., and Solnit, A. (1964).

[109]Bruch, H. (1949); Green, M., and Solnit, A. (1964).

[110]Friedman, S., et al. (1963); Green, M., and Solnit, A. (1964).

[111]Bowlby, J. (1951); Green, M., and Solnit, A. (1964).

[112]Green, M., and Solnit, A. (1964); Caffey, J. (1965); Bakwin, H., and Bakwin, R. (1966).

[113]Bakwin, H., and Bakwin, R. (1966); Mayer, J. (1966).

[114]Janis, I., and Feshbach, S. (1953).

[115]Glasser, M. (1958).

[116]Coles, R. (1964); Chilman, C. (1966).

Table 1–12 Approximate Costs Per Person Per Year in 1969–1970 of Various Forms (A) of Parent Supplementation and Substitution Arrangements and (B) of Correctional and Supportive Care for Youth and Adults

A. FORMS OF PARENT SUPPLEMENTATION AND SUBSTITUTION	COST		
	MINIMUM*	ACCEPTABLE	DESIRABLE
Foster Day Care (generally for children under 3)[1]	$1423	$2032	$2372
Group Day Care (generally for children 3 to 5)[1]	$1245	$1862	$2320
Before and After School and Summer Care (generally for children 6 to 13)[1]	$ 310	$ 653	$ 653
Live-in Foster Home (exclusive of medical bills, clothing, and extra care if necessary)[2]			
Birth to 10 years		$ 936	
Ten years and older		$1144	
Private Day School (for school-age children)[3]			
Girls		$ 800 to $1625	
Boys		$ 885 to $1750	
Private Boarding School			
Girls		$3100 to $3700	
Boys		$2700 to $3300	

B. FORMS OF CORRECTIONAL, SPECIAL TRAINING, MENTAL HEALTH AND WELFARE CARE	COST
Bureau of Special Education[4]	
Nonresidential school	$2500 to $3300
Residental school	$7500 to $8700
Youth Service Training School[5]	$2000 to $5000
Department of Mental Health[6]	
As outpatient	$1825 to $8212
As inpatient	$4380 to $14,600
State Correction Institution[7]	$4109 to $9433
County Correction Institution	$2471 to $9375
Training School	$2000 to $5000

Table 1–12 (Continued)

B. FORMS OF CORRECTIONAL, SPECIAL TRAINING, MENTAL HEALTH AND WELFARE CARE	COST
Department of Public Welfare[8]	
Maintenance cost for persons 18 to 65 years old, living alone (exclusive of rental exceptions, medical costs, special diet and other special needs if necessary)	$2000
Aid for families with dependent children. Allowance per family of 1 adult and 3 children under 7 years old ($165 additional for each child 7 to 12 years; $240 additional for each child 13 to 20 years)	$2972

*"Minimum" is defined as the level essential to maintaining the health and safety of the child, but with relatively little attention to his developmental needs. "Acceptable" is defined to include a basic program of developmental activities as well as provision of minimum custodial care. "Desirable" is defined to include the full range of generalized and specialized activities suitable to individual development. Most experts feel that the disadvantages to children of a "minimum" level program far outweigh the advantages of having the mother work.

[1]Standards and Costs of Day Care (1969). See also Family Health Services, Department of Public Health, Commonwealth of Massachusetts, which is paying at "Desirable" rates.

[2]Chamberlin, J., Office of Commissioner of Research and Planning, Department of Public Welfare, Commonwealth of Massachusetts, 600 Washington Street, Boston, Massachusetts.

[3]*Tuition Fees 1970–1971.* National Association of Independent Schools, 4 Liberty Square, Boston, Massachusetts, 02109. These costs vary with the age of the child, being lowest in the first grade and highest for grades 9 to 12; this age factor accounts for most of the range shown in the table. In addition, however, there are geographic differences; the costs are lowest in the southeastern and southern states and highest in the New England and the Middle Atlantic states.

[4]Peterson, E., Bureau of Special Education, Department of Education, Commonwealth of Massachusetts, 182 Tremont Street, Boston, Massachusetts.

[5]McLaughlin, M., Youth Service Division, Commonwealth of Massachusetts, 14 Somerset Street, Boston, Massachusetts.

[6]Dermody, W., Division of Settlement and Support, Department of Mental Health, Commonwealth of Massachusetts, 190 Portland Street, Boston, Massachusetts.

[7]Division of Research, Correction Department, Commonwealth of Massachusetts, 100 Cambridge Street, Boston, Massachusetts.

[8]Chamberlin, J., Office of Commissioner of Research and Planning, Department of Public Welfare, Commonwealth of Massachusetts, 1970. Family Health Service, 600 Washington Street, Boston, Massachusetts.

service agencies and workers have traditionally played a major role in solving problems at this level. For optimal gains from efforts directed at this level, it is almost essential that the pediatrician join forces with his internist and social service colleagues in a family oriented, closely coordinated effort. Correction of a child's psychosocial malnutrition may involve providing a socially isolated mother with a culturally congenial source of friendship, training a father for a job that will enable him to be a self-respecting breadwinner or helping a mother to get medical treatment so that she feels physically well enough to attend to the needs of her family.

SUPPLEMENTATION OF PARENTAL CARETAKING. Though supplementation of parental caretaking is included here among other therapeutic strategies, it could also be considered a normal and perhaps even essential component of the child rearing matrix. In the animal world, for instance, when a bottle-nosed dolphin gives birth to a calf, other adult females instinctively help the mother by keeping her offspring afloat until she can take care of his needs or until he can fend for himself.[117] Adult female elephants likewise remain close to a pregnant member of the herd, protecting and supporting her until she and her progeny are able to take care of themselves. In earlier generations, grandparents, aunts, sisters, neighbors, old family friends and, in some instances, household help were readily available to support young mothers in the performance of their child rearing responsibilities. These resources, however, have all but disappeared as a result of the transition from a relatively stable, well-rooted way of life to the highly mobile, rootless existence that isolates today's young couples from these traditional sources of help. The widespread use of high school and college students as "baby-sitters" indicates that these couples need supplementary help. Unfortunately, this "baby-sitter" mode of supplementation is apt to be characterized by inconstancy of personnel, many of whom have had little or no training or experience in child caretaking and no more than a transient interest in their charges.

The significance of this subject is underscored by the fact that in the United States as of March, 1967, there were 27.5 million working women 16 years of age and over. Of these women, 10.6 million were mothers with children under 18 years of age. About 2.2 million of these working mothers had children under 3 years of age, 1.9 million had children 3 to 5 years of age (with none under 3) and almost 6.5 million had children 6 to 17 years of age (with none under 6).[118] The fact that the number of working mothers with preschool children increased from 2.9 million in 1960 to 4.2 million in 1969 indicates that this phenomenon is growing rapidly, and it is estimated that the proportion of working mothers with children living at home will rise to 60 to 70 per cent during the 1970's as compared to 42 per cent in 1960 and only 10 per cent in 1940.[119]

In recognition of these startling realities, many have come to believe that supplementary help should now be made available on a community-wide basis in the form of professionally staffed day care centers, nursery school enrichment programs and professionally coordinated physician-parent-teacher cooperative schemes.[120] In Table 1–12 the approximate monetary cost of parent

[117]Raphail, D. (1970).

[118]Low, S., and Spindler, P. (1968); Chenoweth, A. (1970).

[119]Bray, T. (1970).

[120]Bower, E. M. (1963); Pines, M. (1966); Caldwell, B. (1967); Eisenberg, L. (1968); Chenoweth, A. (1970); Bray, T. (1970).

supplementation and substitution services for needy children are listed along with current data concerning the expense to society of caring for children who grow up to be mentally subnormal, delinquent or otherwise socially disabled as a consequence of psychosocial malnutrition or other causes. Even at an average price of $2000 per year for 15 years (total $30,000), the expense of providing for an individual child who is at high risk of maldevelopment as a consequence of inadequate parental care appears small relative to charges for managing a mentally handicapped child ($2500 to $8700 per year), educating a youth out of delinquent behavior or housing him in a correctional institution ($2000 to $9000 per year) or carrying a person as a dependent adult for approximately 50 years (total about $100,000). However, pressure for providing care away from home for large numbers of children could easily overtax the supplies and energies of qualified day caretakers to the point where many children would become at risk of deprivation or injury as a result of inadequate parent-substitution arrangements. Already there are signs that this may be happening as a result of insufficient training, inadequate pay and lack of appreciation of the importance to child health and development of human as well as physical factors. Indeed, day care specialists of the Office of Child Development of the U.S. Department of Health, Education and Welfare are now warning that the disadvantages to children of "minimum" (i.e., inadequate) day care, parent-substitute programs far outweigh the advantages of having the mother work.[121]

It is hoped that the public in general and the child health professional in particular will choose to give this matter the close attention it deserves. Moreover, if we are to avoid major errors in corporate child caretaking practices, some of this attention should take the form of research designed to define optimal social nurture in terms of the qualifications of caretakers, the ratio of caretakers to children, the need for interpersonal compatibility and the content of the nurturing relationship.[122]

As has been demonstrated many times, parental supplementation of appropriate quality can be remarkably effective and valuable. It would be hard to find a more striking example of this than that provided by the role of Anne Sullivan in the early development of Helen Keller,[123] Helen's parents supplied her with an abundance of love and solicitude but were quite incapable of providing her with a means of communication or with the firm discipline she needed. Anne Sullivan's success in fulfilling these specific needs earned her the love and appreciation of her remarkable subject, as well as the title of "Miracle Worker" from an admiring world of onlookers. The miracle was not only that Anne Sullivan succeeded in reaching through the perceptual deficits preventing Helen from communicating and leading her to behave in a widely uncontrolled and extremely disruptive manner, but also especially that Miss Sullivan had the sense to appreciate the child's specific needs and potentials and the strength to persevere until these were fulfilled.

Some 50 years ago F. B. Talbot[124]

---

[121]Day Care Specialists, Office of Child Development, (1969).

[122]Spitz, R. (1945); Engel, G. (1959); Rose, J. (1959); Yarrow, L. (1961); Witmer, H., et al. (1962); Peiper, A. (1963); Willoughby, J., and Haggerty, R. (1964); Eisenberg, L. (1965); Leonard, M., et al. (1966); Skeels, H. (1966); Caldwell, B. (1967); Werner, E., et al. (1968).

[123]Keller, H. (1954).

[124]Talbot, F. B., quoted in Glaser, K., and Eisenberg, L. (1956).

observed a form of maternal supplementation in the Children's Wards in Düsseldorf. He noted that there was always an "Old Anna" wandering around the ward with a baby on her hip. On inquiry, he was told that whenever medical care failed to make a malnourished child thrive, the child was handed over for loving and mothering to old Anna "who never failed"! We are thus reminded that relatively unstructured supplementation may be effective under certain circumstances. At the same time, as we move into more professional methods of supplementary mothering, it should be remembered that physicians may be able to cover, by prescription, specifically identified psychosocial needs of individual child patients.

PARENT SUBSTITUTION. It has been observed many times that it is not essential to the mothering role that the mothering person be the child's biologic parent.[125] Nevertheless, most members of the health care professions are reluctant to recommend parent substitution as a means of overcoming psychosocial malnutrition among basically normal children (a) unless the child is at high risk of severe deprivation or injury because his mother or father (particularly the former) treats him in a grossly neglectful, rejecting, hostile or abusive manner and (b) unless the likelihood of overcoming the problems within a reasonable period of time by any of the means already described is very slight, thereby making unacceptable the risks of leaving the child with his parents. This latter condition is most likely to obtain where the biologic mother is unavailable, delinquent, mentally retarded, totally uninterested in caring for the child or otherwise ill suited to the mothering role.

These criteria may be open to easement when a child is unable to function as a member of a family in a personal sense because of mental retardation or other grossly handicapping conditions, or when, as in intractable asthma, there are indications that a physical malady may be due in considerable part to deep-seated psychologic stresses of familial origin.[126]

In attempting to establish a satisfactory substitute parent-child relationship, there are a number of points that deserve thoughtful consideration. One is that the person who is to assume the role of surrogate parent be temperamentally compatible with the child and be interested and able to provide the personal attention, affection and guidance that all children need.[127] The substitute parent should like the appearance of the child and be pleased by his behavior. In older children this attraction between parent-to-be and child should be mutual. Because there is a limit to the amount of personal attention that any mothering person can give to her children, it is well to make sure also that the potential substitute mother is not already at the outer limit of her capabilities in this regard.[128]

Another requisite to success is that the ties between the child and his natural parents[129] be interrupted to such an extent that the child and his new parent are able to develop a warm, secure and meaningful relationship (see Case 1, p. 2).

[125] Glaser, K., and Eisenberg, L. (1956); Clarke, A., and Clarke, A. (1960); Witmer, H., et al. (1962).

[126] Bakwin, H., and Bakwin, R. (1966); Purcell, K., et al. (1969).

[127] Glaser, K., and Eisenberg, L. (1956); Rose, J. (1959); Clarke, A., and Clarke, A. (1960); Fanshel, D., and Maas, H. (1962); Witmer, H., et al. (1962); Bain, K. (1963); Peiper, A. (1963); Chapter by Gerard, H. in Leiderman, P., and Shapiro, D. (Eds.) (1964); Eisenberg, L. (1965); Provence, S. (1967); Silver, H., and Finkelstein, M. (1967).

[128] Witmer, H., et al. (1962).

[129] Glaser, K., and Eisenberg, L. (1965); Rose, J. (1959); Clarke, A., and Clarke, A. (1960); Eisenberg, L. (1962); Bain, K. (1963); Silver, H., and Finkelstein, M. (1967).

The child's age at the time of placement is an additional important factor. Transfer to another parent seems to be well tolerated by infants before the time they begin to distinguish the faces of their principal caretakers—before 4 months of age. Thereafter, infants pass through a period of one to two years during which they recognize their principal mothering person but are as yet unable to understand much spoken language. Consequently, it is difficult during this period to explain to a child why his care has been transferred from one person to another. The result may be intense separation anxiety and identity confusion.[130] The same may be true for older children unless the reasons for transfer are understood and accepted by the child.

This leads to consideration of some of the hard realities about child placement in this country. The magnitude of the problem is reflected in national statistics indicating that there were approximately 268,000 children in foster care in the late 1950's. Of these, 44,000 were in preadoptive homes, while the remainder were in institutions or foster family homes. Figures for 1960 indicate that approximately 260,000 children had been placed away from their natural homes because of neglect and deprivation. Of these, 28 per cent were in institutions and 72 per cent in foster homes.[131]

Though it is difficult for an institution to function as a source of mothering, it has been repeatedly observed that it can serve this purpose well (as evidenced by striking gains in the physical and behavioral status of children) when a serious effort is made to provide the children with "parental" care.[132] The same is potentially true with respect to foster home placement.[133] Unfortunately, however, foster home placements are often transient in nature. This may make little difference when foster or institutional placement is temporary and a means of affording a family the opportunity to regain stability and competence.[134] The same may be true of halfway houses for teenagers. Under circumstances requiring longer placement, however, it leaves the child in limbo, often with dire results.

Eisenberg's studies of foster children who were referred to a psychiatric clinic[135] showed that 40 per cent of these children had been placed in foster care before they were 4 years old, and 70 per cent before they were 10 years old. All under 10 years of age had been committed as neglected, dependent children. Thirty per cent of the 10 to 15 year old group had been judged delinquent. More than half of the total group had had three or more placements, more than one third had had four or more placements and one fifth of the children had had five or more placements. Of children in foster care for two years or more, 60 per cent had had three or more placements, and 50 per cent had had four or more placements. Goldfarb[136] reported behavioral differences between children in continuous placement and those who were moved one or more times. Only one member of a group of 40 children who had been in

[130] Fanshel, D., and Maas, H. (1962). See also Chapter 4.

[131] Reid, J. (1959); Fanshel, D., and Maas, H. (1962).

[132] Talbot, N. B., et al. (1947); Davis, K. (1947); Fried, R., and Mayer, M. (1948); Witmer, H., et al. (1962); Hollowell, J., and Gardner, L. (1965); Talbot, N. B. (1965); Powell, G., et al. (1967).

[133] Glaser, K., and Eisenberg, L. (1956); Eisenberg, L. (1962); Fanshel, D., and Maas, H. (1962); Witmer, H., et al. (1962); Fontana, V., et al. (1963); Eisenberg, L. (1965); Silver, H., and Finkelstein, M. (1967); Eisenberg, L. (1968).

[134] Hollowell, J., and Gardner, L. (1965).

[135] Eisenberg, L. (1962).

[136] Goldfarb, W. (1947).

continuous foster placement had to be removed from a foster home because of behavioral difficulties. By contrast, in another group of 40 who had originally been placed in an institution and subsequently transferred to foster home care, replacement because of unacceptable behavior became necessary in 12 cases, and seven of these had to be replaced at least twice.[137]

These realities, coupled with the fact that there probably will never be enough permanent, private adoption opportunities to meet the need of "lost" children for a stable home environment, have led Eisenberg[138] to propose that serious consideration be given to cultivating professionally staffed group homes. As with the day care centers mentioned in the preceding paragraphs on parent supplementation, this appears to be worthy of vigorous attention. Again, participation by physicians and other professionals concerned with child care is very much needed, because there are still people in positions of authority who remain unconvinced that it is necessary to provide destitute children with anything more than a house to live in, clothes to wear, food to eat, a school to go to and perhaps a place to play. They must be helped to understand that children need a real sense of belonging, of being wanted and useful and accepted by one or more responsible people.[139]

The response of deprived infants and children to adequate substitute parenting is apt to be good if a stable placement in a family (i.e., adoption) is accomplished before the child is 1 year old,[140] and favorable results may be had in children up to 18 months of age.[141] The response of children who have suffered deprivation beginning at older ages is so heavily contingent on preceding circumstances that it is very difficult to make any general predictions as to outcome. However, it is usually worthwhile to carry out the diagnostic therapeutic stratagem of observing how the child responds to substitute parenting of known quality under reasonably well-controlled conditions.

The costs of parent substitution arrangements are indicated in Table 1–12.

CORRECTION AND CONTROL OF CHILD'S PRIMARY PHYSICAL DISORDERS. There are times when the child's psychosocial malnutrition represents a parental reaction to the reality that the child has a disabling, expensive, unattractive or unpleasant physical problem. Some problems, such as blindness, severe mental retardation, dyschondroplasia and osteogenesis imperfecta may be beyond correction by current medical methodology. Others, however, such as harelip, cleft palate, lop ears, squint, exstrophy of the bladder, sexual malformations, failure to mature (as in gonadal dysgenesis), excessively tall stature in girls, excessively short stature (due to hypopituitarism or hypothyroidism) and obesity secondary to Cushing's syndrome or to infantile overfeeding, may be amenable to medical or surgical correction.[142] Such correction benefits both the child and his parents.

CASE 4. ORGANIC DISEASE MISTAKENLY ASSUMED TO BE PSYCHOGENIC

A specific example of a physical, correctable problem was provided by a girl of 6 years who presented with the chief complaint of fecal soiling in association with a tendency to chronic constipation. Because the child's problems were thought to be behavioral rather than organic in origin, she had had psycho-

---

[137]Goldfarb, W. (1947); Glaser, K., and Eisenberg, L. (1956).
[138]Eisenberg, L. (1968).
[139]Reid, J. (1959).
[140]Eisenberg, L. (1968).
[141]Witmer, H., et al. (1962).
[142]Richardson, S. (1963); Crawford, J., and Haessler, J. (1967); Barnett, H. L. (1968).

therapy over a period of two years. The parents were so distressed by the messy clothes and malodor incident to the soiling, and by all of the problems these created, that they had become intensely disapproving and strongly directive toward their daughter. However, examination disclosed that the child's difficulties were actually caused by a relatively minor congenital abnormality in the rectal region. This abnormality consisted chiefly of forward displacement of the anal opening with the formation of a thin shelf of tissue in the area where the anal opening normally is located. As a result of this the child could not move her bowels normally, nor could she prevent fecal leakage.

Surgical correction of this malformation and subsequent administration of a mild laxative for a few weeks totally eliminated her gastrointestinal difficulties. As the parents became aware of the fact that they now had a functionally normal child who had not "willfully" caused her previous trouble, their attitude toward her became spontaneously accepting and approving. Eventually all signs of pathology disappeared in parents and child alike.

Striking degrees of improvement in attitudes, behavior and parent-child relationships have been observed following surgical removal of diseased bowel in children with ulcerative colitis. In these cases the restitution of a general sense of well-being and release from special diets, multiple medications, fatigue, the need for proximity to a bathroom and other sick role manifestations often outweigh by a generous margin the nuisance of having to live with an ileostomy. This treatment often results also in spontaneous disappearance of the intense maternal protectiveness and directiveness frequently present as a component of the childhood ulcerative colitis syndrome.[143]

PHYSICIAN STRATEGIES IN RELATION TO PATIENTS AND COMMUNITIES. A number of variables must be kept in mind in implementing the various therapeutic strategies that have just been discussed. Most of these center about a number of obvious realities. For instance, it is one thing to order that a patient do such-and-such when he is hospitalized and subject to the almost unlimited control of the doctors and nurses, and it is quite another to persuade him or his parents to follow medical recommendations while living independently at home. Controlled conditions can bring about obedience and conformity, but these superficial changes in behavior may not represent changes in inner attitudes. Induced behavior is apt to disappear when the force of authority is removed.[144]

This phenomenon has been documented by studies of differences between prescriptions and actual therapeutic practices.[145] For instance, in one group of patients who had been instructed to take a 10 day course of oral penicillin for control of infection while living at home, 83 per cent said that they had taken all the pills prescribed. However, counts of the number of pills remaining in the bottles disclosed that in actuality 50 per cent had stopped taking the medication by the third day, 71 per cent by the sixth day and 82 per cent by the ninth day. This was confirmed by urinary penicillin assays.[146] It follows that the patients' perception of what is important, and how well he follows orders as a result, is a factor of high importance to medical care practice.

The relationship between the patient and his physician can have an important bearing on this matter. Compliance is apt to be greatest if the physician is interested in and sensitive to the patients' personal com-

[143]Point, W., Personal communication, 1970.

[144]Leventhal, J. (1965).

[145]Berkowitz, N., et al. (1963); Haessler, H., and Crawford, J. (1966).

[146]Bergman, A., and Schulte, C. (1963).

plaints, problems and concerns rather than in only the scientifically intriguing aspects of the patient's malady.[147] The physician needs to be aware of the kinds of attitudes, fears and behaviors that are likely to prevail in patients and parents under certain circumstances. For example, in dealing with parents of a defective newborn, the physician needs to recognize that they may be experiencing sorrow as profound as that suffered by parents who learn that an older child has developed a fatal disease or acquired a seriously crippling handicap.[148]

Although the physician-patient relationship may have a much more important bearing on the patient's or parent's performance of prescribed plans than does their intellectual knowledge about the disease and its treatment, it is important to recognize that the patient's lack of health knowledge can be a potent barrier to effective medical care.[149]

Unrealistic choice of goals by either physician or patient also can predispose to almost certain therapeutic failure.[150] The recommendation that the obese child of equally obese parents be placed on a low calorie diet while other family members around the table eat heartily according to their appetites is an example of this all-too-common occurrence. Contrariwise, physicians must realize that it may be as much or more of a problem for parents to permit a child with heart disease, asthma or diabetes to participate in normal activities than it is for them to enforce restrictions.[151] One mother reported that she found herself "interrupting playtime, hiding the jump rope, driving her child to and from school, refusing swimming lessons and keeping the child off that horse just one more month."

It is evident in all that has been said in prior pages that human competence and life satisfaction are functions of the total environment. As Eldredge comments in *Taming Megalopolis*,[152] "In order to tame that sprawling beast, the metropolis fast becoming megalopolis, it is first necessary to understand his characteristics and have some idea of the sort of useful and handsome creature one would like. . . . All serious students of the urban scene by now agree that there are not going to be any new and shining cities without new and shining people in some as yet not entirely clear reciprocal relationship. . . . And the people must eat and have shelter which spells out the truism that space, social and economic planning are parts of a trinity—and cannot be worshipped separately with any anticipation of reward. . . . And finally, altered space/time relations can conceivably foster new types of human society and settlements in the future with shapes and social structure as yet unglimpsed."

Although it is beyond the scope of most members of the health care profession to be engaged directly in this complex, multifaceted task of "taming megalopolis," they can contribute significantly to the design thereof. Specifically, it falls within their purview to provide urban planners with information concerning the kinds of biosocial supplies and opportunities the community must be able to offer to its constituents if malnutrition of body and mind is to be avoided and if life is to be a rewarding experience.

---

[147]Korsch, B. M. (1956); Parmelee, A. (1962); Green, M., and Solnit, A. (1964); Bergman, A., and Schulte, C. (1967).

[148]Parmelee, A. (1962); Green, M., and Solnit, A. (1964); Bergman, A., and Schulte, C. (1967).

[149]Clausen, J., et al. (1954); Samora, J., et al. (1962); Williams, T., et al. (1967).

[150]Tisza, V. (1962); Davis, M., and Eichhorn, R. (1963).

[151]Glaser, H., et al. (1964).

[152]Eldredge, H. W. (1967).

III. CLINICAL ASPECTS OF THE INTERRELATIONSHIP BETWEEN BIOPHYSICAL AND SOCIOBEHAVIORAL PATHOLOGY

A. Importance of Social and Behavioral Factors to the Diagnosis and Management of Pediatric Patients

Recorded frequency rates for various conditions vary greatly according to the strictness of diagnostic criteria and the thoroughness of the research procedures employed. To obtain some information concerning the latter factor, systematic observations have been made at Massachusetts General Hospital on a group of 28 randomly selected Children's Service patients with enduring maladies of various sorts.[153] The following sampling procedure was used: Every fourth week an aggregate list of all the child patients coming to the Ambulatory Clinics of the hospital was prepared. From this list, every tenth patient was selected. The first patient chosen in each sample was determined by reference to a random number table. The study sample was then obtained by subjecting this primary sample to secondary criteria. These were that the child be under 14 years of age, live within six miles of the hospital, be a "service" as contrasted to a "private" patient and have a condition which needed continuous medical attention for at least one year but which was not likely to be lethal within the next five years. Since 75 per cent of the clinic population of Massachusetts General Hospital lived within a six mile radius of the hospital the study may be considered representative of the Ambulatory Clinic population.

Thirty-one patients were selected by this procedure. It was possible to develop a reasonably complete picture in 28 of these patients. In two instances the family refused to cooperate, and one patient died unexpectedly before comprehensive evaluation was initiated. In each of the 28 cases, as an initial step, the clinic record was analyzed for its content of information concerning the child's physical, cognitive and behavioral status and the nature of the biologic and social factors that had caused his problem. Next, irrespective of the chief complaint, the child was re-evaluated to obtain a comprehensive picture. This evaluation was done by a team comprised of a senior staff pediatrician, a social worker and clinical psychologists. The social worker collected information by making at least one home visit (except in two instances where parents refused), by interviewing the mother, by screening through the Social Service Index and other agencies having knowledge of the family and by contacting the patient's school. The clinical psychologist tested the intelligence of each patient of school age, using the Wechsler Intelligence Scale and, as indicated, the Figure Copying, Gilmore Oral Reading (Form B), Eye-Hand-Foot Dominance, Graham-Kendall, House-Tree-Person, Reversed Figure or Stanford-Binet tests. Psychologic evaluation by means of TAT, Rorschach and Draw-A-Person tests also was performed by a senior staff psychologist.

As Table 1–13 indicates, the children of this study came largely from families of low economic status, limited educational experience and limited functional competence. The father was absent from the home in half the cases. Four-fifths of the families had had multiple prior contacts with community agencies. However, only three fell into the poverty category.

[153]Talbot, N. B., et al. (1966). This work was supported by U.S. Children's Bureau Grant No. H-103.

Half of the children were boys and half were girls. They ranged in age from 1.5 to 14 years. Table 1–14 itemizes the effects of the biosocial evaluation on the diagnostic status. The diagnoses represented in their clinical records prior to the study indicated that of the 28 patients subsequently studied completely, 26 (92 per cent) had one or more physical disorders, seven (25 per cent) showed signs of retarded motor or mental development and seven (25 per cent) presented one or more of the behavioral disorders listed in Table 1–6. The physical disorders were varied and included five instances of organic neurologic disease; five of asthma; four of allergic rhinitis; two each of renal disorder, respiratory tract infections, stunted growth and idiopathic abdominal pain; and one each of scars secondary to burn injury, shortening of one leg secondary to poliomyelitis, obesity, purpura, congenital cataracts and enuresis without evidence of organic cause. The behavioral diagnoses included two instances of being antisocial and one each of being asocial, of hyperactivity, of sexual promiscuity; of suicidal gesture and of immaturity.

The right hand column of Table 1–14 shows that the comprehensive work-up resulted in new physical diagnoses in six (21 per cent) patients, and in the deletion of prior physical diagnoses in two (7 per cent) patients. It also led to the addition of behavioral and social diagnoses in 18 (64 per cent) children and in the deletion of these in three (11 per cent) children. In two patients the diagnosis deleted was "mental retardation."

The overall effects of these changes on the ultimate diagnostic picture are indicated in Table 1–15. Whereas it appeared prior to the study that almost two thirds of the children were suffering only from physical problems, at the close of the study the indications were that in reality most had a combination of physical, social and behavioral disorders. Included among these were 16 instances of inadequate or inappropriate parental care incident to paternal absence, to maternal depression, decompensation, inadequacy or the like, or to antisocial paternal behavior. Among the pediatric diagnoses there were

Table 1–13 Family Characteristics of the Massachusetts General Hospital Random Sample Comprehensive Child Evaluation Study

COMPOSITION	Father absent in 14 (50 per cent) families. Psychotic mother living at home while receiving weekly shock treatments in one (3.5 per cent) family.
EDUCATIONAL STATUS	Average maternal education: 10.3 years Average paternal education: 10.2 years (data not available in 10 cases).
FINANCIAL STATUS	Average income: $4319. 40 per cent of families relying on Aid to Families with Dependent Children.
FUNCTIONAL COMPETENCE	21 per cent fitted the general description of "multiproblem family" and were disorganized with respect to their ability to utilize medical care facilities. 82 per cent of the families had prior contact with community agencies. The average number of agency contacts per family was 6.7 (range: 0 to 27). Multiple agency contacts were greatest in those families with the least parental educational achievement.

*Table 1–14 Effects of Systematic Biosocial Evaluation on the Apparent Diagnostic Status of 28 of 31 Randomly Selected Ambulatory Child Patients with Enduring Maladies of Various Sorts**

Case	Sex	Age (Years)	Diagnoses Recorded Before Study	Duration of Condition (Years)	Diagnoses Added (+) or Subtracted (–) Through Systematic Study
1	M	5.5	Mental retardation	5.5	Mental retardation (–)
			Asocial behavior	2	Asocial behavior (–)
					Specific learning disability (+)
					Poverty (+)
					Hyperactive behavior (+)
2	F	9	Asthma	1.25	Lack of parental care (+)
					Asocial behavior (+)
3	M	2.5	Hydrocephalus	2	
			Motor retardation	2	
			Poverty	2	
4	F	2	Dietary malnutrition	2	Malabsorption (–)
			Stunted growth	2	Motor retardation (–)
			Malabsorption	1	Immature behavior (–)
			Motor retardation	2	Maternal Decompensation (+)
			Immature behavior		Lack of maternal care (+)
5	M	7	Father deserted		
			Mother inadequate		
			Lack of maternal care	7	
			Mental retardation	7	
			Hyperactive behavior	2	
6	F	10.5	Allergic rhinitis	0.5	Father divorced (+)
					Mother self-preoccupied (+)
					Lack of maternal care (+)
					Unnecessary sick role re school absences (+)
					Asocial behavior (+)
7	F	14	Anorexia nervosa	1	Anorexia nervosa (–)
			Suicide gesture (drug ingestion)		Father separated (+)
8	M	13	Chronic bronchitis	12	Asthma (+)
					Excessive maternal possessiveness (+)
					Excessive paternal disapproval (+)
					Asocial behavior (+)
					Unnecessary sick role re limited physical activities (+)
9	F	10	Scarring and contractures post third degree burn	8	
10	M	7	Enuresis	7	Father divorced (+)
			Asthma	2	Mother depressed (+)
					Lack of maternal

**From* Talbot, N. B., et al. (1966).

Table 1–14 Effects of Systematic Biosocial Evaluation on the Apparent Diagnostic Status of 28 of 31 Randomly Selected Ambulatory Child Patients with Enduring Maladies of Various Sorts (Continued)*

Case	Sex	Age (Years)	Diagnoses Recorded Before Study	Duration of Condition (Years)	Diagnoses Added (+) or Subtracted (–) Through Systematic Study
					attention (+) Asocial behavior (+) Unnecessary sick role re school absences (+)
11	F	13	Allergic rhinitis	10	Father divorced (+) Father antisocial re molest wife, daughter (+) Unnecessary sick role re school absences (+)
12	M	5	Nephrosis	2.5	Father deserted (+) Father antisocial (+) Father inappropriate role model (+) Lack parental discipline (+) Unnecessary sick role re special diet (+) Antisocial behavior re firesetting (+) Asocial behavior (+)
13	M	13	Allergic rhinitis and conjunctivitis	8	
14	M	1.5	Recurrent pneumonitis	1.33	
15	M	11	Father divorced Congenital cataracts Allergic rhinitis Antisocial behavior re lying, stealing	11 11 9	Unnecessary sick role re limited physical activities (+)
16	F	6	Petechiae (idiopathic)	1	Parents not married (+) Mother not interested in child (+) Lack of maternal care (+) Hyperactive behavior (+)
17	F	8	Abdominal pains (cause not known)	1	Father deserting intermittently (+) Lack of parental care (+) Obsessive behavior (+)
18	F	14	Abdominal pains (cause not known)	3	Father deserted (+) Mother inadequate (+) Lack of parental care (+) Truant behavior (+) Trichomonal vaginitis (+)
19	F	2	Mental retardation	0.75	Father separated (+) Mother decompensated (+) Lack of maternal care (+) Self-aggressive behavior (hit self) (+)

Table 1–14 (Continued)

Case	Sex	Age (Years)	Diagnoses Recorded Before Study	Duration of Condition (Years)	Diagnoses Added (+) or Subtracted (−) Through Systematic Study
20	F	3.5	Father dead Obesity	3.5 1	
21	M	7	Asthma Chronic otitis media	4 4	Father separated (+)
22	F	5.5	Seizure disorder Right hemiparesis (postictal, clearing)	0.25 0.25	Abstract reasoning disability (+)
23	M	10	Father deserted Mother depressed Lack of maternal care Dietary malnutrition Stunted growth Mental retardation ("borderline" I.Q.)	10 10 10 10 10 2	Antisocial behavior re stealing (+)
24	M	11.5	Mental retardation (abnormal EEG, I.Q. 76)	11.5	Father deserted (+) Inadequate mother (+) Lack of maternal care (+) Antisocial behavior (+)
25	M	13	No family (born out of wedlock) No caring parent Mental retardation (abnormal EEG, "borderline" I.Q.) Antisocial behavior re stealing	13 13 5 1	
26	M	13	Short right leg (due to old poliomyelitis)	9	Excess parental disapproval, discipline (+) Habit disturbance re head banging (+) Scholastic underachievement (+)
27	M	9	Nephritis, familial	6	
28	M	12.5	Asthma Otitis media, chronic	4	Perceptual cognitive defect (+)
29	F	1	Nephrocalcinosis Death, cause unknown		Case not available for comprehensive study
30	F	6	Precocious puberty	0.5	Case not available for comprehensive study
31	M	13	Seizure disorder	0.5	Case not available for comprehensive study

Table 1–15 Summary of Effects of Systematic Biosocial Evaluations on the Diagnostic Status of Patients of Table 1–14

	PHYSICAL PROBLEMS ALONE (PER CENT CASES)	SOCIOBEHAVIORAL PROBLEMS ALONE (PER CENT CASES)	PHYSICAL PLUS SOCIOBEHAVIORAL PROBLEMS (PER CENT CASES)
Before Study	64	4	32
After Study	22	7	71

six instances of apparently unnecessary sick role, five each of asocial and antisocial behavior, three of hyperactivity, two of specific learning disability, two of self-directed aggression and one each of scholastic underachieving, obsessiveness, sexual promiscuity, truancy and habit disturbance.

In the 16 cases where there were indications of psychosocial deprivation or intoxication of parental origin, behavioral disorders were evident in 15 and dietary malnutrition and stunted growth in the remaining one (case 4). Conversely, in 14 of the 16 children with behavioral disorders there were coexistent indications of

*Table 1–16 Frequency of Occurrence of Physical, Cognitive and Sociobehavioral Problems Among Children**

GROUP	TYPE OF PROBLEM (PER CENT CASES)		
	PHYSICAL	COGNITIVE	SOCIOBEHAVIORAL
A. Survey of random sample of 32 MGH child outpatients with chronic diseases[1]			
1. Precomprehensive diagnostic survey	96	25	32
2. Postcomprehensive diagnostic survey†	93	32	78
B. Survey of 349 Chelsea grade school children[2]			
1. Through routine school examination	9	0	0
2. Through MGH comprehensive diagnostic survey†	36	15	21
C. Survey of nonrandomly selected MGH child inpatients[3]	100	14	36
D. USA child population through independent agencies, national statistics and other sources[4]	7	3	10

*Data are approximate and expressed as per cent of the group studied. The diagnoses for groups A, B and C were concurrent and the result of simultaneous examinations of individual children. The diagnoses for group D were obtained on separate groups of children and hence cannot be considered coexistent for any particular child or group of children.

†Signifies that the corresponding results were obtained by means of a systematic biosocially comprehensive examination of the same children.

[1]See Tables 1–13 and 1–14.

[2]Connelly, J., et al. (1966).

[3]Peebles, T. (1967).

[4]Rowntree, L., et al. (1945); Masland, R. et al. (1958); Eisenberg, L. (1962); Harper, P. (1962); The President's Panel on Mental Retardation (1962); Wallace, H. (1962); Howels, J. (1963); Shiffer, C., and Hunt, E. (1963); Silver, G. (1963); Caplan, G. (1964); Lesser, A. (1964); Miller, L. (1964); Glaser, K., and Clemmens, R. (1965); Werner, E., et al. (1971).

psychosocial deprivation or intoxication. In the two cases where specific indications of deprivation were lacking, it was noted that the father was absent because of separation or divorce. Of the seven children with retarded motor or mental development, five had evidence of organic disease; three of these, plus two others who did not have any specific evidences of primary neurologic disease, lacked adequate mothering.

Review of the etiologic relationships revealed by all available data suggests that biologic factors had initiated the problem in 19 (68 per cent) of the cases and that social factors, either singly or in combination with biologic factors, had done so in nine (32 per cent) of the cases. This underscores the importance of the pediatrician, and of physical health as a key to the early identification of psychosocial and behavioral problems.

The impression gained from the foregoing random sample that the causes and consequences of many of the more serious problems of child patients are comprised of a mixture of physical, social and behavioral problems is reinforced by the observations carried out by Connelly and his associates on 349 Chelsea School Children (Table 1–16B), and by Peebles in a month long survey of the diagnostic characteristics of every child admitted to two pediatric inpatient floors of the Children's Service of the Massachusetts General Hospital (Table 1–16C).[154] Though comparable data are not available for the population at large, it is interesting to relate the above data to presently available national statistics and individual impressions concerning rates of occurrence, respectively, of physical, cognitive and behavioral problems among children (Table 1–16D). These data may be more nearly comparable to those in parts A-1 and B-1 of the table, which represent the types of problems identified during routine school examinations and prior to comprehensive diagnostic survey, than they are to parts A-2 and B-2, which represent problems recognized after comprehensive diagnosis.

[154]Connelly, J. P. (1966); Peebles, T. (1967).

B. Psychosocial Deprivation and Intoxication Syndromes

Many diagnostic terms have been used to represent situations in which children suffer from the forms of psychosocial deficiency or excess listed in Table 1–5. A number of these terms with corresponding references to their authors are set forth below.

Criminal Neglect—Silver, K., and Kempe, C. (1959).

Deprivation—Clarke, A., and Clarke, A. (1960); Eisenberg, L. (1965).

Deprivation Dwarfism—Silver, H., and Kempe, C. (1967).

Disadvantaged Infants—Richmond, J., and Caldwell, B. (1966).

Disturbed Family Environment—Hollowell, J., and Gardner, L. (1965).

Emotional Deprivation—Powell, G. F., et al. (1967).

Environmental Handicap—Dennis, W., and Najarian, R. (1957).

Hospitalism—Spitz, R. A. (1945, 1946a, 1946b); Coleman, R. W., and Provence, S. (1957).

Loneliness (in Infants)—Bakwin, H. (1942).

Maternal Deprivation—Glaser, K., and Eisenberg, L. (1956); Yarrow, L. (1961); Patton, R., and Gardner, L. (1962); Witmer, H., et al. (1962); Blodgett, F. (1963); Patton, R., and Gardner, L. (1963); Whitten, C., et al. (1969).

Maternal Overprotection—Levy, D. (1943).

Pathogenic Parental Attitudes—Tamkin, A. (1964).

Psychologic Deprivation—Goldfarb, W. (1945).

Psychologic Privation—Goldfarb, W. (1945).

Psychosocial Malnutrition—Talbot, N. B. (1963).
Sensory Deprivation—Solomon, P., et al. (1957); Krieger, I., and Sargent, D. (1967).
Social Isolation—Davis, K. (1947).

The closely allied subject of *child abuse* has also been labeled in various ways.

Abused Child—Reinhart, J., and Elmer, E. (1964); Elmer, E., and Gregg, G. (1967); Gil, D. (1970).
Battered Child—Kempe, C., et al. (1962); Harper, F. (1963); Milowe, I., and Lourie, R. (1964).
Maltreatment Syndrome—Fontana, V., et al. (1963).
Child Abuse—DeFrancis, V. (1963); Simons, B., et al. (1966).
Physical Abuse—Silver, H., and Kempe, C. (1959); Bain, K. (1963).
Slaughter of the Innocents—Adelson, L. (1961).

These titles remind us that the origins, modes of mediation, quality, duration, intensity and behavioral and bodily manifestations of deprivation and abuse among children vary considerably from case to case and family to family. This is emphasized because we hope that by alerting physicians and others to the existence of this syndrome complex, we may also promote close scrutiny of specific causes and consequences of psychosocial malnutrition in individual patients. This, together with development of individualized therapeutic and preventive strategies, should greatly enhance the capacity of the health care professions to deal effectively with these important and widespread problems.

Manifestations of Deprivation and Intoxication Syndromes. The following case summary is illustrative of the many problems of diagnosis and management which may be encountered in dealing with these patients.

CASE 5. RETARDATION AND MALNUTRITION DUE TO PSYCHOSOCIAL DEPRIVATION

This 5 year and 10 month old boy was referred to the Massachusetts General Hospital by a member of the Visiting Nurse Association who had by chance seen him during her visit to his mother, who was awaiting the delivery of her eighth child. The child was the height of a 3½ year old and the weight of a 2⅓ year old. His skin was rough and scaly, and scabs covered his entire body. His eyes were inflamed. There were bruises and abrasions on his head and body. His mother reported that these had been caused by bumping into the stove. He had a pigeon breast deformity of the chest and signs of pulmonary infection. He was emaciated in appearance, and his abdomen was distended. (See Fig. 1–6A.)

The Visiting Nurse Association had been following this family for two years and had the impression that the mother was a capable person who gave her children good care. However, on the latest visit the nurse had been shocked by the condition of the apartment, this boy's obviously sick appearance and behavior and the mother's attitude of unconcern toward him, which contrasted sharply with her warm and loving attitude toward her other children. When the seriousness of his condition was pointed out, she agreed to let the nurse arrange hospitalization for him.

The boy was the next to the oldest of seven children. His father, a 55 year old Negro, was a furniture mover. His mother, who was white, was 33 years old and a high school graduate, and appeared to be intelligent and interested in her children. She talked easily and well, and gave a story of family harmony, good diet and excellent care for the patient. She indicated, however, that she was puzzled by changes in his weight and behavior and could not explain them. Until about a year previously, she said, he had been in good health and spirits. Then he began to wet his bed and soil his underwear. He became sullen and withdrawn and had on occasion kicked his mother. His appetite was so ravenous that his mother had to keep the pantry locked, and he would eat catfood, newspapers, wood and garbage as well as food. Nevertheless, in six months his weight had dropped from 55 pounds to 25 pounds.

A review of the boy's past history indicated that he had suffered first and second degree burns over his back, chest and armpits which required hospitalization when he was a year and a half old. He

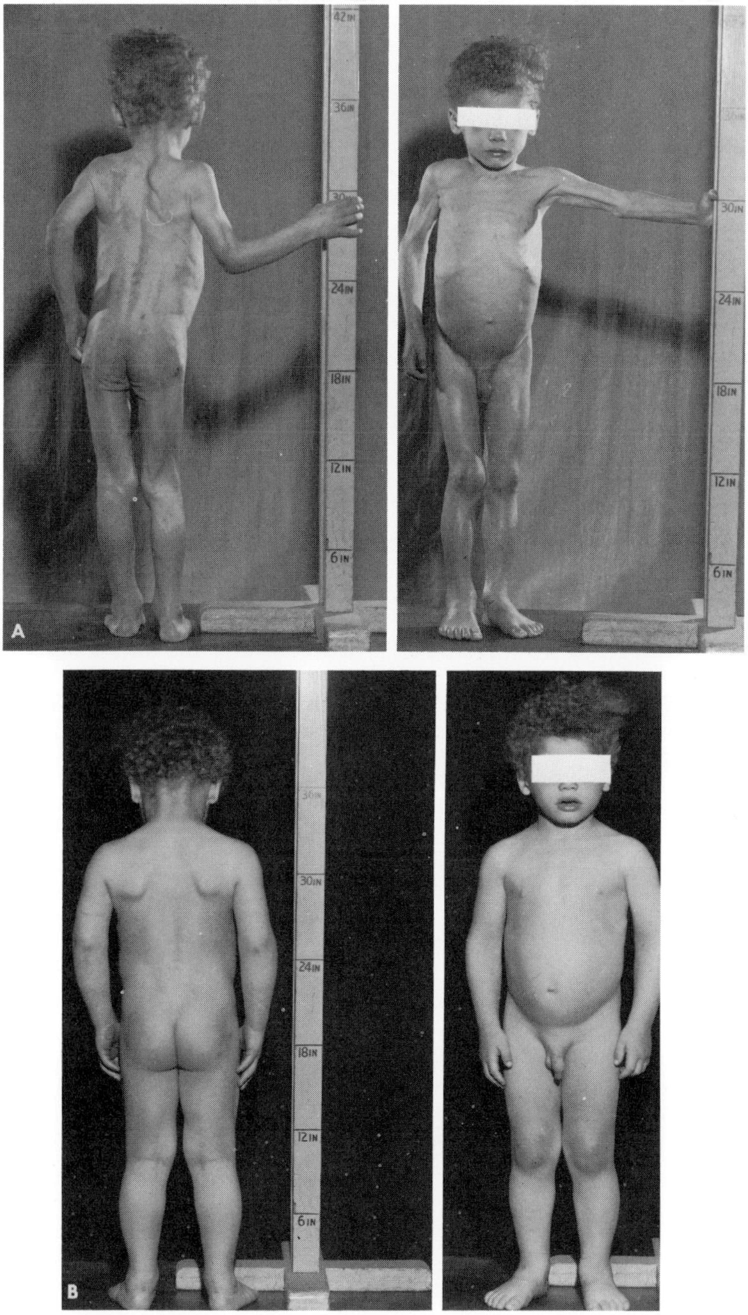

Figure 1–6 Appearance of patient described in Case 5 (A) on admission to hospital and (B) after five weeks in the hospital.

was again admitted to a hospital at the age of 2 for treatment of an infected traumatic injury to his jaw.

When admitted to Massachusetts General Hospital, the boy behaved in a markedly withdrawn manner. His speech appeared to be grossly retarded. Intelligence tests revealed an overall mental age score of 3 years and 5 months, which gave him an IQ of 50. On the basis of these findings, a primary working diagnosis of gross physical, mental and psychosocial retardation with severe nutritional deficiency was made, and studies were begun to determine the cause. Attention was directed almost entirely to organic diseases such as congenital syphilis, tuberculosis, malignancy, hypermetabolism and cystic fibrosis. The test results showed few abnormalities and no clear organic disease.

Meanwhile, on a standard diet with supplementary vitamins, despite many interruptions for diagnostic studies, the boy began to gain weight at a phenomenal rate almost immediately following admission (see Fig. 1–7). The reason was obvious: he spent most of his waking hours for three weeks stuffing food into his mouth. By the end of five weeks, he had gained 17 pounds, was normal weight for his height, and appeared well nourished (see Fig. 1–6B). After a month in a convalescent home he was readmitted to the hospital for further studies. He had grown more than an inch. He was an active, vigorous child with no physical abnormalities other than a slight heart murmur. He was friendly and cooperative and spoke clearly. Retesting with Stanford-Binet Form M indicated an overall mental age of 4 years and 3 months, a gain of 10 months in 2 months time. His IQ was 71.

Despite these observations, some members of the physician staff found it difficult to believe that abnormalities of the magnitude he had shown could be due primarily to psychosocial deprivation. Unfortunately, the ultimate outcome of this case is unknown, since the child moved with his family to a different city shortly after his return home.

This case is significant because it illustrates that the possibility of

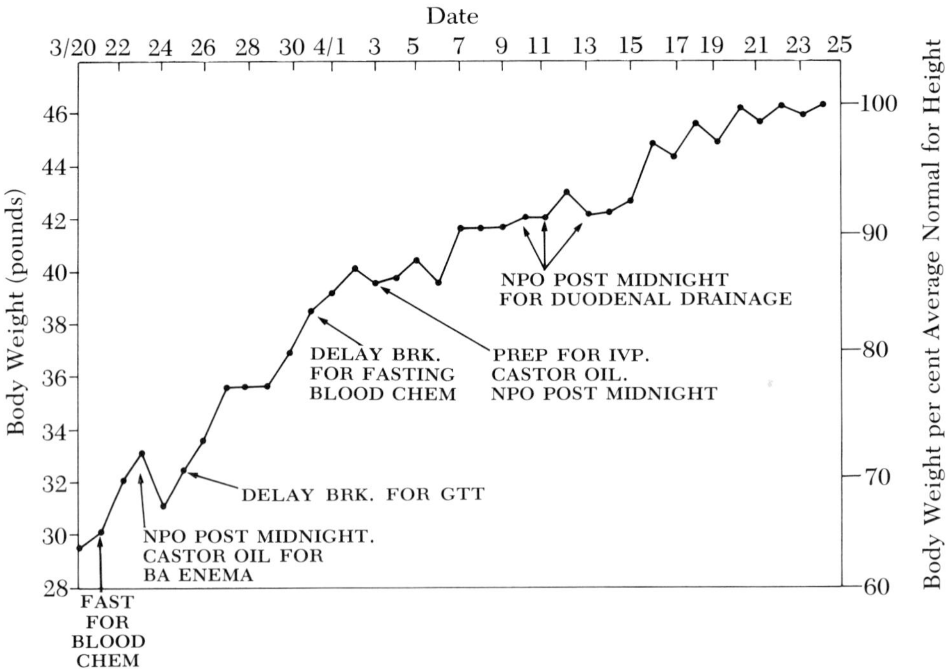

Figure 1–7 Weight gain observed during the first five weeks of hospitalization of the patient described in Case 5. The meaning of the abbreviations is as follows: NPO – nothing by mouth, BA – barium, GTT – glucose tolerance test, IVP – intravenous pyelogram for defining kidney tract architecture.

dietary and psychosocial deprivation must be kept in mind when children show significant retardation of bodily growth and maturation, even if the child's parents appear to be intelligent and caring. Failure to recognize this can result in the performance of many unnecessary diagnostic tests and perhaps in delay in correcting the real causes of the child's problems.

As Case 5 demonstrates, the syndrome of psychosocial deprivation or intoxication is really a family disorder. No level of society is exempt.[155] Pathology is usually evident in one or both parents (or parent substitutes) as well as in the child. The problems encountered at the parental level are made up of the various difficulties listed earlier in Table 1–6. Among the most frequent are adverse childhood rearing experiences on the part of one or both parents, disturbed marital relations, broken home, illegitimacy, unwanted child, maternal decompensation, depression or ambivalence (with respect to the child as an individual or to the mothering role), paternal unemployment, alcoholism, institutional or foster home placement, overcrowding and poverty.[156] Though poverty is a relatively frequent concomitant, the psychosocial deprivation and intoxication syndrome occurs among the well-to-do and highly educated as well as the financially and educationally disadvantaged.

As a result of such parental disturbances, children may suffer from any of a variety of forms of psychosocial deprivation or injury. Most commonly they miss the warmly intimate care and attention provided by a competent mothering person.[157] In consequence of this, they lack many of the sensory, social and emotional stimuli required for the healthy development and function of the human organisms. These psychosocial deficiencies may be compounded by frank expressions of rejection.[158] They also may be the indirect consequence of isolating practices incidental to parental overprotection.[159] In some instances the psychosocial supply disturbances have been accompanied by physical privations such as underfeeding,[160] locking a child in the attic for prolonged periods or keeping him tied to a chair.[161] More traumatic forms of abuse and battery are considered separately later in the text (p. 76). In all cases, noxious parental attitudes and practices may be concealed under a camouflage of apparent overconcern or overprotection.[162]

Vulnerability to deprivation is greatest during the early years of life when infants and children are most heavily dependent upon parents (or parent substitutes) as caretakers and as providers of essential sensory and psychosocial stimuli. The effects of deprivation on such children may be manifest in a variety of behavioral, intellectual, motor and physical disorders. Though almost all of the behavioral problems listed in Table 1–8 have been encountered in deprived children, certain ones stand out as prominent features of a marked degree of generalized psychosocial deprivation. For example, these pa-

---

[155] Patton, R., and Gardner, L. (1962).

[156] Talbot, N. B., et al. (1947); Clarke, A., and Clarke, A. (1960); Yarrow, L. (1961); Patton, R., and Gardner, L. (1962); Witmer, H., et al. (1962); Davis, M., and Eichhorn, R. (1963); Eisenberg, L. (1965); Chilman, C. (1966); Leonard, M., et al. (1966); Powell, G., et al. (1967); Silver, H., and Finkelstein, M. (1967).

[157] Bakwin, H. (1942); Goldfarb, W. (1945a, b); Bowlby, J. (1951); Clarke, A., and Clarke, A. (1960); Patton, R., and Gardner, L. (1962); Witmer, H., et al. (1962); Sours, J. (1963); Silver, H., and Finkelstein, M. (1967); Hirsch, J. (Ed.) (1968).

[158] Goldfarb, W. (1964a,b); Patton, R., and Gardner, L. (1962); Witmer, H., et al. (1962); Silver, H., and Finkelstein, M. (1967).

[159] Witmer, H., et al. (1962); Blodgett, F. (1963).

[160] Leonard, M., et al. (1966).

[161] Davis, K. (1947); Clarke, A., and Clarke, A. (1960).

[162] Witmer, H., et al. (1962).

tients often have an unhappy, anxious appearance.[163] Infants who have been severely deprived may be apathetic, generally unresponsive to social stimuli and lacking in cuddlesomeness.[164] Infants 7 to 21 months of age who have been deprived of sensory stimuli may assume a posture similar to that seen normally only in infants less than 4 or 5 months of age. This posture is evident whether the child is supine, sitting, standing or being held. The arms are in a state of tonic immobility for prolonged periods of time with the elbow flexed 90 degrees or more. The humerus is abducted and usually outwardly rotated. The hands are pronated and positioned at a variable distance from the side of the head, or they come to rest on top of the head.[165] Such infants may show little or no dismay at being separated from their parents and may give no indication of discriminating between familiar persons and strangers.

Some infants are hypertonic, irritable, difficult to comfort, cry a great deal and sleep only fitfully; others are depressed, relatively immobile, slow of action and generally listless. As they grow older and become more independent they are apt to become demanding, negativistic, distrustful and aggressively hostile toward their parents. Still later, problems in respect to school performance, running away, stealing and the like are common.[166] Tendencies to asocial behavior, habit disturbances (including encopresis) and self-directed aggressive behavior have also been observed.

In the very young, neuromotor development in respect to reaching out, sitting unsupported, standing without aid, pulling himself up, walking alone and so forth may be so retarded as to raise serious questions about the possibility of brain damage.[167] Concern about this possibility has in many instances been intensified by the fact that many of these children display limitations in vocalization, inarticulateness and retardation in language development.[168] The same is true with respect to their apparent intellectual development, which, as evaluated by standard psychologic testing procedures, may be indicative of mental retardation in general,[169] and of defects in time and space concepts and in capacity for abstract thinking in particular.[170]

Stunting of growth is common and may be of a degree comparable to that observed in children with hypothyroidism, hypopituitarism or Cushing's syndrome (Fig. 1–8A and Table 1–17).[171] Most of these children are not only markedly undersized for their age but are also either proportionately or actually underweight

[163]Bakwin, H. (1942); Goldfarb, W. (1945); Bowlby, J. (1951); Leonard, M., et al. (1966); Whitten, C., et al. (1969).

[164]Bakwin, H. (1942); Bowlby, J. (1951); Coleman, R., and Provence, S. (1957); Patton, R., and Gardner, L. (1962); Witmer, H., et al. (1962); Eisenberg, L. (1965); Leonard, M., et al. (1966); Krieger, I., and Sargent, D. (1967); Powell, G., et al. (1967); Silver, H., and Finkelstein, M. (1967); Whitten, C., et al. (1969).

[165]Krieger, I., and Sargent, D. (1967).

[166]Bakwin, H. (1942); Goldfarb, W. (1945a,b); Bowlby, J. (1951); Patton, R., and Gardner, L. (1962); Witmer, J., et al. (1962); Willoughby, J., and Haggerty, R. (1964); Eisenberg, L. (1965); Leonard, M., et al. (1966); Krieger, I., and Sargent, D. (1967); Silver, H., et al. (1967).

[167]Davis, K. (1949); Patton, R., and Gardner, L. (1962); Witmer, H., et al. (1962); Blodgett, F. (1963); Leonard, M., et al. (1966); Whitten, C., et al. (1969).

[168]Bakwin, H. (1942); Goldfarb, W. (1945a,b); Bowlby, J. (1951); Clarke, A., and Clarke, A. (1960); Witmer, H., et al. (1962); Blodgett, F. (1963); Eisenberg, L. (1965); Leonard, M., et al. (1966).

[169]Goldfarb, W. (1945a,b); Patton, R., and Gardner, L. (1962); Witmer, H., et al. (1962); Eisenberg, L. (1965); Krieger, I., and Sargent, D. (1967); Powell, G., et al. (1967); Whitten, C., et al. (1969).

[170]Glaser, K., and Eisenberg, L. (1956).

[171]Talbot, N. B., et al. (1947); Bowlby, J. (1951); Talbot, N. B., et al. (1952); Coleman, R., and Provence, S. (1957); Patton, R., and Gardner, L. (1962); Blodgett, F. (1963); Leonard, M., et al. (1966); Krieger, I., and Sargent, D. (1967); Silver, H., et al. (1967); Talbot, N. B. (1968); Whitten, C., et al. (1969).

for their height (Fig. 1–8B). Some are emaciated in appearance (Fig. 1–6A). However, many simply look thin, having sparse stores of subcutaneous fat and thinly developed musculature. Protuberant abdomen is occasionally observed.[172]

These children are apt to have a history of feeding difficulties and sometimes of other disturbances of gastrointestinal function.[173] Some have large appetites and tend to steal food, eat out of garbage cans, gorge and vomit or ruminate. Some have a tendency to drink a great deal, including, at times, drinking out of toilet bowls. On the other hand, many others have a history of anorexia and inadequate nutritional intake particularly with respect to calories. Bowel habits may vary from constipation to frequent stools. In some the stools are foul smelling, as in steatorrhea.[174]

POSSIBLE CAUSES OF STUNTED GROWTH. These observations have led to much discussion of the role of inborn errors *versus* psychosomatic, nutritional and other factors in causing stunted growth in these children. In 1947 evidence was presented which suggested that the stunting of growth was a function of hypocaloricism due either to unavailability of sufficient food or to anorexia.[175] This thesis was supported by metabolic balance data which showed in a typical case that growth (as measured by nitrogen balance) changed from negligible to strongly positive as caloric balance was increased from submaintenance through equilibrium to strongly positive levels.

In order to determine whether the stunting of growth observed in such children was due directly to caloric insufficiency or to some effect of psychosocial deprivation on the child's growth control mechanisms, one group of investigators made arrangements designed to find out whether children with this condition would grow at a significantly accelerated rate if fed an ample diet under home conditions which were kept unchanged insofar as their apparently pathogenic psychosocial characteristics were concerned.[176] To accomplish this they arranged to have a trained observer present at feeding times at home, thereby obtaining an on-the-spot record of the child's actual dietary intake. They found that *when the food intake was held at satisfactory levels,* these children gained and grew at "catch up" rates similar to those observed in such patients when they were extricated from abnormal home environments and placed in more adequate ones. Notwithstanding the possibility that the mere presence of an observer in the household of these home-managed patients resulted in changes in maternal perception, attitudes and practices as well as increases in the child's food intake, it is probably true that the gains in growth rate observed in these patients were similar in nature to those recorded in Figures 1–2 and 1–7.

Though it would thus appear that inadequate caloric intake may be a major and perhaps the chief reason why so many psychosocially deprived children tend toward stunted growth, it could be a mistake to discard prematurely the possibility that the failure to grow and gain may in certain instances be mediated by other, more direct "psychosomatic" mechanisms. For instance, some of these psycho-

[172]Blodgett, F., (1963); Leonard, M., et al. (1966).

[173]Bakwin, H. (1942); Talbot, N. B., et al. (1947); Patton, R., and Gardner, L. (1962); Eisenberg, L. (1965); Leonard, M., et al. (1966); Krieger, I., and Sargent, D. (1967); Powell, G., et al. (1967); Silver, H., et al. (1967).

[174]Bakwin, H. (1942); Bowlby, J. (1951); Leonard, M., et al. (1966); Powell, G., et al. (1967).

[175]Talbot, N. B., et al. (1947).

[176]Whitten, C., et al. (1969).

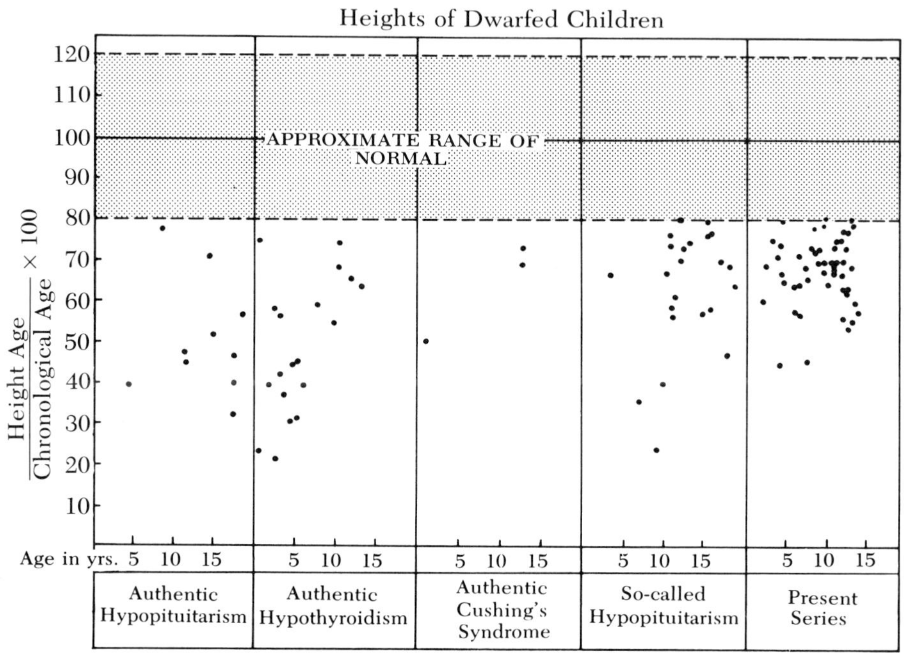

Figure 1–8 A, Heights of dwarfed children. The height age of a child is found by determining the average age of normal children of the same height and sex. Note the consistent tendency to dwarfism in patients with authentic hypopituitarism. Similar degrees of dwarfism may be observed in children with hypothyroidism, Cushing's syndrome and so-called hypopituitarism (i.e., the diagnosis was presumptive) and in children suffering from caloric undernutrition (indicated by the term Present Series).

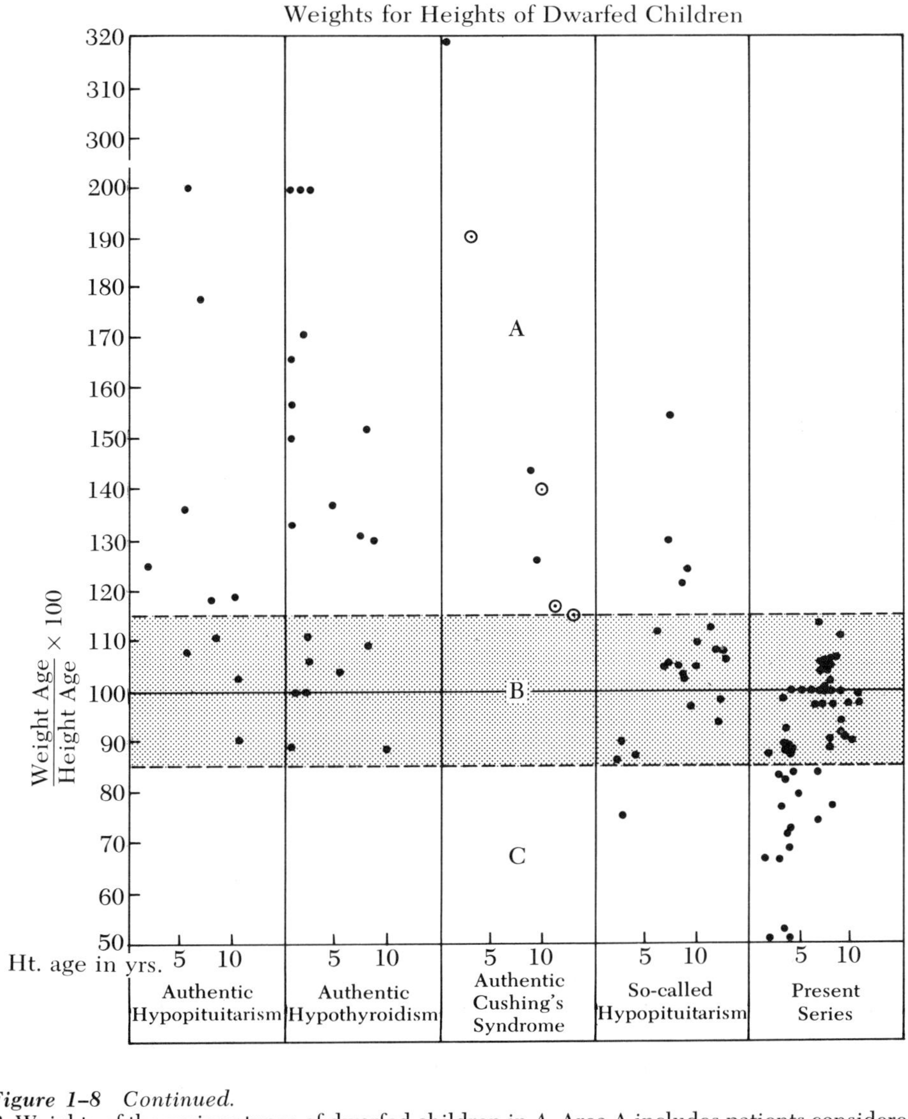

Figure 1–8 *Continued.*

B, Weights of the various types of dwarfed children in *A*. Area A includes patients considered to be overweight for their height. Area B includes patients whose weight is within normal limits. Area C includes patients who are underweight for height.

Studies by Dr. Lindemann on 21 of the thin dwarfs (i.e., Present Series group) indicated that in 34 per cent of the cases the child was being rejected by his parents; in 19 per cent there were evidences of mental subnormality; and in 14 per cent each, respectively, the children were members of impoverished families, the mother was delinquent (or otherwise incapacitated) and the child's behavior was indicative of chronic grief. In the remaining 5 per cent of cases no social or behavioral pathology was found. This was in contrast to the observations carried out simultaneously upon seven well-nourished dwarfs, 43 per cent of whom were apparently free of sociobehavioral problems. However, there were evidences of maternal delinquency in 45 per cent and of chronic grief in 14 per cent of these patients. (*From* Talbot, N. B., Sobel, E., Burke, B., Lindemann, E., and Kaufman, S., 1947, p. 783.)

*Table 1–17 Growth Measurements of Psychosocially Deprived Infants and Children**

Author	Sex	Actual Age	Height Age	Weight Age	Weight for Height Age (per cent)	Height (cm.)	Weight (kg.)
Coleman and Provence (1957)	M	17 mo.	Birth	5 mo.		46	7.8
	F	9 mo.	6 mo.	3 mo.		67	6.5
Patton and Gardner (1962)	F	15 mo.	3 mo.	1 mo.		58	4.4
	F	36 mo.	12 mo.	4 mo.		73	7.0
	F	14 mo.	9 mo.	1 mo.		69	4.5
	M	78 mo.	42 mo.	24 mo.		100	12.9
	M	22 mo.	8 mo.	3 mo.		68	6.0
	M	18 mo.	9 mo.	5 mo.		70	7.7
Blodgett (1963)	M	5 yr.	2.6 yr.	1.7 yr.		92	12.5
Leonard et al. (1966)	F	10 wk.	2 mo.	1 mo.		57	
	M	10 wk.	3 mo.	1 mo.		59	
	M	10 wk.	1 mo.	Birth		52	
	F	15 wk.	Birth	Birth		50	
	M	15 wk.	1 mo.	Birth		52	
	M	19 wk.	7 mo.	3 mo.		67	
	M	7 mo.	6 mo.	3 mo.		66	
	F	7 mo.	6 mo.	3 mo.		66	
	F	7 mo.	5 mo.	3 mo.		62	
	F	10 mo.	11 mo.	7 mo.		74	
	M	23 mo.	12 mo.	6 mo.		75	
	M	26 mo.	22 mo.	15 mo.		85	
	M	27 mo.	12 mo.	9 mo.		75	
Powell et al. (1967)	M	3.3 yr.	1.8 yr.		+15		
	M	3.8 yr.	2.0 yr.		−19		
	M	3.9 yr.	1.2 yr.		−20		
	M	3.9 yr.	2.6 yr.		0		
	M	4.4 yr.	2.0 yr.		0		
	F	5.1 yr.	2.8 yr.		+2		

*Age values in months represented to nearest whole number.

Table 1–17 Continued

AUTHOR	SEX	ACTUAL AGE	HEIGHT AGE	WEIGHT AGE	WEIGHT FOR HEIGHT AGE (PER CENT)	HEIGHT (CM.)	WEIGHT (KG.)
	M	5.1 yr.	2.0 yr.		−13		
	M	5.3 yr.	3.5 yr.		−18		
	M	5.8 yr.	3.0 yr.		−23		
	M	6.9 yr.	3.5 yr.		− 6		
	F	7.2 yr.	4.0 yr.		0		
	M	7.8 yr.	4.5 yr.		+ 7		
	M	11.5 yr.	5.3 yr.		+ 6		
Silver and Finkelstein (1967)	M	56 mo.	18 mo.	15 mo.			
	F	56 mo.	18 mo.	14 mo.			
	M	16 yr.	9 yr.	8 yr.			
	F	84 mo.	20 mo.	20 mo.			
	F	47 mo.	16 mo.	14 mo.			
Whitten et al. (1969)	M	7 mo.	3 mo.	1 mo.			
	M	9 mo.	3 mo.	1 mo.			
	M	5 mo.	2 mo.	2 mo.			
	M	11 mo.	7 mo.	4 mo.			
	M	11 mo.	9 mo.	5 mo.			
	F	7 mo.	3 mo.	1 mo.			
	M	4 mo.	2 mo.	1 mo.			
	M	19 mo.	11 mo.	5 mo.			
	F	13 mo.	7 mo.	6 mo.			
	M	18 mo.	11 mo.	10 mo.			
	F	23 mo.	12 mo.	4 mo.			
	M	17 mo.	15 mo.	7 mo.			
	M	13 mo.	5 mo.	5 mo.			
	M	23 mo.	7 mo.	4 mo.			
	F	19 mo.	10 mo.	6 mo.			
	F	11 mo.	7 mo.	4 mo.			

socially deprived children are constantly on the go. Such physical activity results in increased caloric expenditures, a phenomenon that could predispose to negative caloric balance under conditions of average normal caloric intake. Psychosocial stress may give rise to marked alterations in the function of the gastrointestinal tract,[177] alterations which could result in a tendency toward maldigestion or malabsorption manifested by diarrhea or steatorrhea. Some infants with "deprivation dwarfism" have had stools suggestive of steatorrhea. Stress may give rise to markedly increased levels of cortisone output.[178] This hormone can markedly suppress growth.[179] In short, there may be substantial reasons why some of these children are scrawny and fail to thrive despite ravenous appetites.

Treatment of psychosocial deprivation is not likely to be very successful unless the underlying cause can be indentified and corrected in accordance with one or more of the tactics outlined in Section II-I (p. 44) of this chapter. However, as discussed in Chapter 9, the use of psychoactive drugs may be helpful in quieting a hyperactive child. Moreover, when they help to make the child less troublesome for a parent, they may serve indirectly to make the parent-child interrelationship more satisfactory and hence less pathogenic. The use of pituitary growth hormone and androgens as growth-promoting agents has been unsatisfactory in improving the ultimate stature of children with the deprivation dwarfism syndrome. Pituitary hormone is essentially ineffective in the presence of caloric undernutrition.[180] Androgens will cause a growth spurt, but they also artificially induce masculinization and acceleration of skeletal maturation, thereby shortening the growth period and stunting ultimate stature.[81] Forced feeding rarely results in a significantly increased caloric balance for any prolonged period of time. Moreover, it predisposes to parental overdirectiveness, which is one form of psychosocial intoxication.

Effect of Environmental Improvement. As has been illustrated, children who have suffered marked degrees of psychosocial deprivation, stress or intoxication can improve dramatically within a few weeks following correction of the environmental disorders, provided these disorders have not existed for a long period of time. Caution must always be used in concluding that a therapeutic move was the *cause* of an improvement in a patient's condition. However, in most instances there is little likelihood that a child with the deprivation syndrome will improve spontaneously and dramatically in the absence of a favorable change in his environment. Accordingly, the behavioral improvements that occur within a few days or weeks after the elimination of severe psychosocial deprivation or stress can reasonably be tentatively attributed to these environmental changes. If this is a real and significant relationship, it will tend to persist except when the psychosocial situation is allowed to revert back to the deprivation levels which prevailed originally. Under these circumstances, the child is likely to stop progressing abruptly and in some instances to retrogress in his behavioral and body weight status (Fig. 1–9). On the other hand, failure to respond to presumably improved psychosocial arrangements may signify that the child is either suffering from a primary organic disorder or has experienced an irreversible degree of damage from the originally

[177]Wolff, P. (1966).
[178]Hamburg, D. (1959).
[179]Blodgett, F., et al. (1956).
[180]Bode, H., Unpublished observations, 1970.
[181]Sobel, E., et al. (1956).

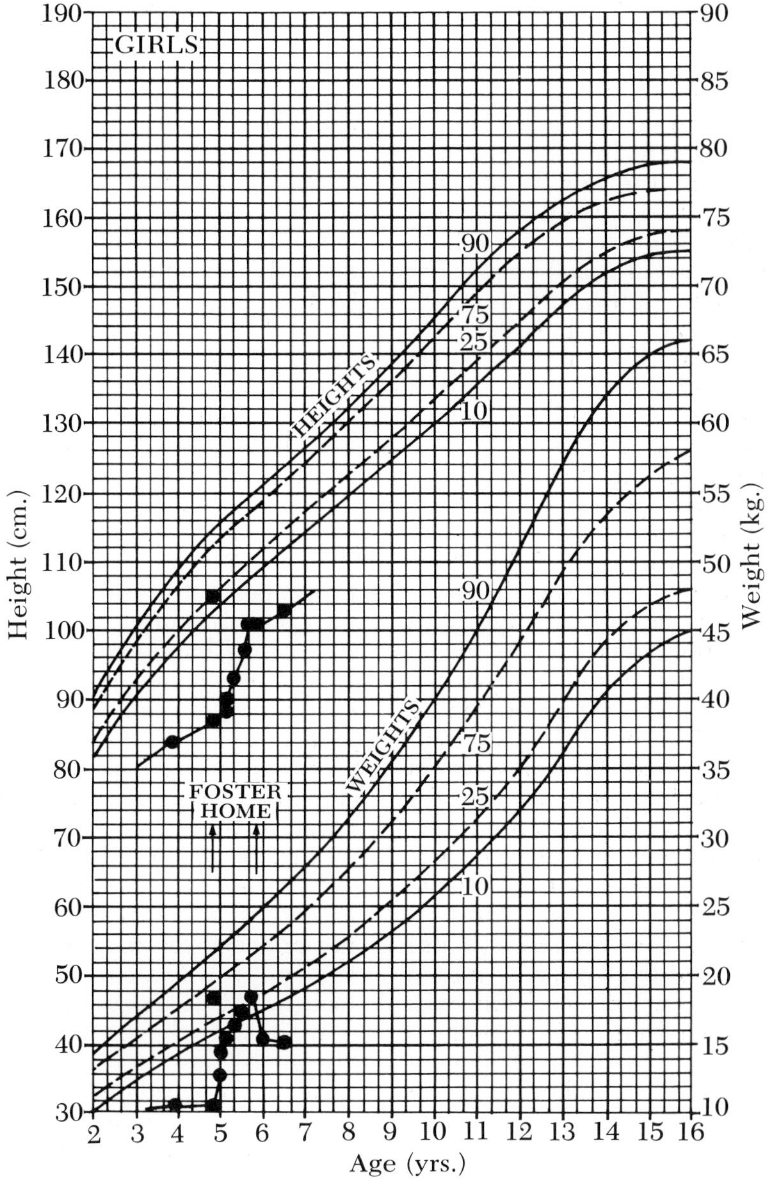

Figure 1–9 Effects, on rate of weight gain (and loss) and growth in height, of transferring a child suffering from psychosocial deprivation from her natural home to a foster home and back again. The black squares give the height and weight of a healthy twin. The curves coursing upward from left to right give the percentile distribution of values for normal children of corresponding age and sex.

simple primary psychosocial deprivation.

C. Child Abuse Syndrome

In many respects the child abuse syndrome is an extreme version of the psychosocial deprivation-intoxication syndrome outlined in the foregoing section. Attention to this problem rose sharply in the late 1950's and early 1960's when several investigators reported shockingly high incidences of severe physical or psychological, or both, abuse and injury to children brought to hospitals for treatment.[182] Within a few years every state had passed some form of legislation that required physicians to report cases of suspected abuse to local authorities but that protected physicians from legal suits resulting from such reports.[183]

In the background of child abuse cases, the incidence of social pathology at the familial level is high.[184] In some cases the roots can be traced back a generation to the fact that the parents themselves were beaten or battered as children. Less than half of one series of 313 children were on welfare, a finding which indicates that this condition is by no means restricted to the poor.[185] In two-thirds of the cases the parents of the patients were married. The proportion of those born out of wedlock (32 per cent) was considerably greater than that obtaining for New York City as a whole (12 per cent). The mothers were the abusers in about 30 per cent of the cases, and the fathers in about 20 per cent, with baby sitters, paramours, siblings and a few unknowns accounting for the remainder. In 60 per cent of the instances the child had experienced active abuse, and in 24 per cent the trauma was the accidental result of neglect. In the remaining 16 per cent the exact causes could not be pinned down.

It is often difficult to tell whether or not abuse has occurred. As in Case 5 (p. 64), parents may "explain away" current injuries by reporting the child has fallen or bumped into something. Or they may report prior hospitalizations of the child for extensive burns or traumatic injuries of various sorts which raise often unanswerable questions about how these injuries actually occurred. Accidents are the chief cause of death among children in the United States, accounting for approximately 14 deaths per 100,000 annually.[186] There is no way to know how many of these deaths may, in fact, be consequences of child abuse. (See also Chapter 8.)

Among married parents of abused children there has been a record of marital discord or separation in one of three cases, and of prior institutionalization in a mental hospital or penal institution or prior treatment of mental or social problems in one of six instances. Half the children's caretakers had psychologic counseling or social service help; nearly half this group was alcoholic or addicted to drugs. Insofar as parents are concerned, it is thought that frank psychosis is the single most common factor in precipitating a fatal degree of abuse.[187] There are on record seven instances where fathers attempted to or succeeded in wiping out entire families, and eight instances in which mothers killed a total of 10 children.

These findings are in keeping with those of others who have observed

---

[182]Silver, H., and Kempe, C. (1959); Kempe, C., et al. (1962).

[183]Reinhart, L., and Elmer, E. (1964); Gil, D. (1970).

[184]Silver, H., and Kempe, C. (1959); Adelson, L. (1961); Kempe, C., et al. (1962); Bain, K. (1963); De Francis, V. (1963); McHenry, T., et al. (1963); Milowe, I., and Lourie, R. (1964); Simons, B., et al. (1966); Elmer, E., and Gregg, G. (1967); Yankauer, A. (1967).

[185]Simons, B., et al. (1966).

[186]Fontana, V., et al. (1963).

[187]Adelson, L. (1961).

that the injurers are likely to be alcoholic, sexually promiscuous or unstable marriage partners, or to have criminal records.[188] Temperamentally they are apt to be immature, impulsive, self-centered, hypersensitive, quick to react and under poor self-control. In addition, the pregnancy may have been unwanted, having occurred before marriage, too soon after marriage or at an inconvenient time.

The problem of abuse can occur in children of any age, but it is most frequently recognized in children under three years.[189] Sometimes several children in the family are subjected to maltreatment, and sometimes one is singled out while the others are treated in a loving or overprotective manner. In certain instances the child himself may contribute to the etiology by being a source of tension and worry because he cries frequently, is stubborn, does not obey well, is subject to fecal soiling, tends to harass or goad his parents and so on.[190] In about 10 per cent of cases the child has had a severe prior disability, such as brain damage, disfiguring eye, orthopedic impairments or other deformities.[191]

The means employed to damage the child are many and varied. Among the more extreme cases, gunshot wounds, asphyxiation (by ligature around the neck, drowning, smothering, manual strangulation) and carbon monoxide and other forms of poisoning have been recorded.[192] Manual assault with the hand, the foot or an instrument also has occurred, as have stabbing, burning, sexual molestation and starvation. A number of children have died as a result of repeated beatings administered for disciplinary reasons. In other instances the injuries have been more nearly accidental in origin as in the case of a father who comes home inebriated and who under these circumstances decides to toss his child back and forth with a family friend as a form of play.

Considering the ease and frequency with which children are seized by the arms and legs, it is not surprising that injuries of the appendicular skeleton are the most common in this syndrome. Even when the major injuries involve the skull, spine, ribs and other organs, the extremities are usually involved also.[193] There are apt to be associated swellings, with or without local tenderness and discoloration of the skin, and limitation of motion of the injured part. The radiographic findings include typically metaphyseal infractions (i.e., chip fracture fragments are evident at the ends of the shafts of tubular bones) in association with new bone formation in the form of long traumatic involucra which cloak the shaft of the bone.[194] These involucra do not appear before the eighth to tenth day following the injury, a fact useful in dating the time of an injury and in recognizing the occurrence of recurrent traumatic episodes due to beatings or other causes.[195] Such evidence of multiple injuries in various stages of development and repair are common among these patients.

Other clinical manifestations include soft tissue swellings, skin bruises, poor skin hygiene, fever or leucocytosis or both (the former particularly following internal

---

[188]Kempe, C., et al. (1962).

[189]Kempe, C., et al. (1962); Fontana, V., et al., (1963); Simons, B., et al. (1966).

[190]Adelson, L. (1961); Kempe, C., et al. (1962).

[191]Simons, B., et al. (1966).

[192]Adelson, L. (1961); Kempe, C., et al. (1962); Caffey, J. (1965); Simons, B., et al. (1966).

[193]Bakwin, H. (1956); Kempe, C., et al. (1962); Caffey, J. (1965); Elmer, E., and Gregg, G. (1967).

[194]Caffey, J. (1946); Silverman, F. (1953); Caffey, J. (1957); Caffey, J. (1965).

[195]Caffey, J. (1965).

bleeding), convulsions (in instances of subdural hematoma or brain injury), hematuria (following trauma to the kidneys) and failure to thrive with signs of malnutrition.

Because parents and others frequently fail to tell about abuse and even about accidental injuries (the latter for fear of being criticized for negligence), it is important for health care professionals to be alert to the possibility that unusual or unexplained manifestations similar to those just outlined may be due to maltreatment. The need for this is underscored by the fact that some of these manifestations are compatible with other diagnoses such as hemorrhagic disease, leukemia, collagen disease, inflammation, scurvy, syphilis, infantile cortical hyperostosis, osteogenesis imperfecta and paraplegia with sensory defect. Under most circumstances the simplest way to discover whether findings are caused by trauma from abuse or by disease is to make a roentgenographic search of the skeleton for the characteristic radiologic changes caused by abuse.

Apart from the obvious necessity of attending to the child's physical injuries, major objectives of the treatment of these patients are the provision of an adequate source of essential psychosocial supplies and the prevention of further physical or psychologic injuries. The probability of accomplishing this while the child continues to live at home is apt to be small in seriously disturbed homes, particularly in cases where the trauma was inflicted during periods of uncontrollable rage.[196] Reported death rates among seriously abused children have run as high as 10 per cent, and permanent brain damage has been evident in as many as 15 of every 100 of these children.[197] It follows that it may be advisable and sometimes essential to move a child from his home to a safe and supportive environment when the child's natural caretakers are not likely to respond to other, less drastic therapeutic measures designed to improve the parent-child relationship and to protect the child from fatal injury. On the other hand, if a child can be considered safe from further assault and can be followed closely, such measures as provision of a homemaking helper, day care for an infant or psychotherapy for a parent may be appropriate. Juvenile and family courts and other social agencies in the community may be helpful in implementing therapeutic arrangements.[198]

The requirement that the physician report suspected cases of child abuse to appropriate authorities has several purposes. One is to keep him constantly aware of his responsibility to consider the possibility of abuse in suggestive cases. Another is to establish a network of protection for the child. Through his report, the physician may alert others in health care and social welfare positions to the possibility that a given child may be at risk of serious injuries of abusive origin.

D. The Clinical Summary Abstract—A Means of Coordinating Biophysical and Sociobehavioral Information into a Comprehensive Diagnosis and Plan of Management

Viewed as a whole, the data of the preceding three sections suggest that:

1. Sociobehavioral and physical disorders occur with approximately equal frequency among children today.

2. These two forms of disability are apt to coexist in patients with enduring forms of physical disease.

---

[196] Kempe, C., et al. (1962).

[197] Fontana, V., et al. (1963); Simons, B., et al. (1966); Gil, D. (1970).

[198] Fontana, V., et al. (1963).

3. Recognition of and management of the biosocial character of children's diseases is more likely to occur as systematic efforts are made to identify social and behavioral as well as physical and biologic causes and consequences of human disabilities.

A useful biosocial approach to clinical care demands that all pertinent diagnostic information and decisions concerning clinical management be easily accessible in the patient's record. The form represented in Figure 1–10 has been developed by the Children's Service of the Massachusetts General Hospital to make systematic recording of such information a regular component of patient care. The form occupies both sides of a single sheet of standard-sized clinical record paper. The diagnoses of the patient's physical, social, behavioral and cognitive status are recorded on the upper half of the front side. The etiologies for each of these conditions are recorded on the lower half. On the back there is space for explicit statement of the goals of therapy, of the variables to be used as indices of progress (i.e., therapeutic success or failure) and of the specifics of therapy (i.e., the name, dosage and timing of drugs or other forms of medical management; the nature and means of any social, educational or psychologic prescriptions; and the names of those who have been involved in, and who are to be responsible for the management of the patient).

The diagnostic terms representing information regarding biophysical factors correspond to those commonly used in medical texts; those used for recording social and behavioral findings are derived from the taxonomies given in this chapter. Though these listings are open to additions and modifications, they cover essentially all problems commonly recognized in caring for the pediatric patients at the Massachusetts General Hospital.

Experience with such record forms indicates that they do promote a comprehensive biosocial approach to diagnosis and treatment, and facilitate continuity and coordination in caretaking practices. They also enable physicians, consultants and allied health professionals who carry only brief or occasional responsibilities for the patient to understand the case without having to read detailed information spread out over many pages of the clinical record. The need for supplementary search for details may be largely eliminated by subtending to each diagnosis information indicating the findings on which it is based.

The important thing about this form is its intent and content, not the details of its design, which may be subject to modification to suit local conditions. Like the form developed by Weed, it recognizes that patients are apt to have multiple problems of diverse though perhaps related etiology.[199] One of its chief purposes is to stimulate primary physicians and their associates to select therapeutic goals designed to sustain a satisfactory way of life through avoidance of unnecessary sick role phenomena, to the fullest extent compatible with the control of physical difficulties.

ACKNOWLEDGMENTS

Many of the thoughts expressed in this chapter are based on work which was supported in part by grants in aid received from the Commonwealth Fund of New York, the United States Children's Bureau, the Godfrey Hyams Trust, the Massachusetts General Hospital General Research Support Grant and donations from Mr. George Harrison, the Ladies Visiting Committee of the Massachusetts General Hospital and other generous individuals.

[199]Korsch, B. (1956); Lapouse, R., and Monk, M. (1964); Weed, L. (1968).

CLINICAL SUMMARY ABSTRACT

Name: Case 1 Age: $7\frac{1}{4}$ Sex: F Unit No.__________

Admission or clinic visit date: Discharge date: Date prepared:

DIAGNOSES

Include and number serially all major physical, behavioral*, and social* disorders. Indicate essential supporting evidence for each diagnosis.

1. Dwarfism (ht.-41 in., ht. age-4 yrs.).
2. Underweight for height (wt.-30 lbs., wt. age-$2\frac{1}{2}$ yrs.).
3. Anorexic behavior.
4. Inadequate parents (child neglected).
5. Foster placement, temporary by Division Child Guardianship.

ETIOLOGIC FACTORS

Relate by number to above diagnoses.

1., 2. Caloric undernutrition due to undereating.
3. Apparently related to anxiety incident to threat of separation from foster mother.
4. Unknown.
5. Necessitated by condition of child.

GENERAL COMMENTS

The foster mother wishes to stabilize this child's relationship with her by adopting her. The legal authorities have been reluctant to allow this. Meanwhile the child's natural parents have been trying to take the child away from the foster mother.

Figure 1–10 Clinical Abstract Summary form developed by the Children's Service of the Massachusetts General Hospital. The information set forth here represents a summary of the findings presented in more detail in Case 1 at the beginning of this chapter.

GOALS OF THERAPY	INDICES OF FUTURE PROGRESS
1. Stabilize child's relationship with foster mother. 2. Eliminate signs of anxious behavior. 3. Restore child's rates of gain, growth, and development to satisfactory levels.	Permanent placement or equivalent. Height, weight, etc. measurements. Eating, learning, social, and other behavior.

THERAPEUTIC PLAN

Give specifics.

Social Service with physician back-up to discuss findings with Division Child Guardianship and other legal authorities, with the aim of convincing them that it is advisable to permit this foster mother to adopt this child.

PERSONS RESPONSIBLE FOR MANAGEMENT

Referring M.D. Name: Visiting Nurse Assoc. Tel. No. ______ Copy Sent ______

Address: ------------, Mass. Date Called ______

MGH Staff:

	Name	Discipline	Tel. No.	Copy Sent
Primary Physician*	Dr. D. B-----	Pediatrician		
Consultants	Dr. J. A-----	Endocrinologist		
	Dr. R. S-----	Psychiatrist		
	Miss D. H-----	Social Worker		

House Officer Signature ______ Senior Staff Physician Signature ______ Date ______

Figure 1–10. *Continued.*

We also wish to express our deep appreciation to Miss Mary Ann Van Beek, Mrs. Kathleen Mickiewicz and Mrs. Henrietta Jackman for their care and patience in gathering and cataloging reference material and in typing the many working revisions of this chapter. We are also grateful to Mrs. Leora Wood Wells for numerous valuable editorial suggestions concerning the wording of the text.

REFERENCES

Abel, T. M.: Facial disfigurement in psychological aspects of physical disability. *Rehabilitation Series, No. 210,* Washington, D.C., Office of Vocational Rehabilitation, 1952.

Adelson, L.: Slaughter of the innocents. *New Eng. J. Med., 264*:1345–1349, 1961.

Agle, D.: Psychiatric studies of patients with hemophilia and related states. *Arch. Intern. Med., 114*:76–82, 1964.

Ainsworth, M., and Salter, D.: *Infancy in Uganda. Infant Care and the Growth of Love.* Baltimore, The Johns Hopkins Press, 1967.

Alvarez, W. C.: Ways in which emotions can affect the digestive tract. *J.A.M.A., 92*:1231–1237, 1929.

Apley, J.: *The Child with Abdominal Pains.* Oxford, Blackwell Scientific Publications, Ltd., 1964.

Arnold, M. B., Talbot, N. B., and Cope, O.: Concerning the choice of therapy for hyperthyroidism. *Pediatrics, 21*:47–53, 1958.

Bain, K.: The physically abused child. *Pediatrics, 31*:895–898, 1963.

Bakwin, H.: Loneliness in infants. *Amer. J. Dis. Child., 63*:30–40, 1942.

Bakwin, H.: Multiple skeletal lesions in young children due to trauma. *J. Pediat., 49*:7–15, 1956.

Bakwin, H., and Bakwin, R. N.: *Clinical Management of Behavior Disorders in Children,* 3rd ed. Philadelphia, W. B. Saunders Company, 1966.

Barker, R. G., and Wright, H. F.: *Midwest and its Children—The Psychological Ecology of an American Town.* Evanston, Illinois, Row-Peterson and Company, 1955.

Barnett, H. L.: *Pediatrics,* 14th ed. New York, Appleton-Century-Crofts, 1968.

Bass, H. N., and Schulman, J. L.: Quantitative assessment of children's activity in and out of bed. *Amer. J. Dis. Child., 113*:242–244, 1967.

Beaumont, G. E.: Discussion: Use and abuse of rest as a therapeutic measure. *Proc. Roy. Soc. Med., 47*:177–182, 1954.

Benedict, R.: Continuities and discontinuities in cultural conditioning. *In* Benedict, R. (Ed.): *A Study of Interpersonal Relations.* New York, Hermitage Press, Inc., 1949.

Bergman, A. B., and Schulte, C., III: Care of the child with cancer. *Pediatrics, 40*:487–546, 1967.

Bergman, A. B., and Werner, R. J.: Failure of children to receive penicillin by mouth. *New Eng. J. Med., 268*:1334–1338, 1963.

Berkowitz, N. H., Malone, M. F., Klein, M. W., and Eaton, A.: Patient follow-through in the outpatient department. *Nurs. Res., 12*:16–22, 1963.

Birch, H. G., and Gussow, J. D.: *Disadvantaged Children: Health, Nutrition, and School Failure.* New York, Harcourt Brace Jovanovich, Inc., 1970.

Blodgett, F. M.: Growth retardation related to maternal deprivation. *In* Solnit, A. J., and Provence, S. A. (Eds.): *Modern Perspectives in Child Development.* New York, International Universities Press, 1963.

Blodgett, F. M., Burgin, L., Iezzoni, D., Gribetz, D., and Talbot, N. B.: Effects of prolonged cortisone therapy on the statural growth, skeletal maturation and metabolic status of children. *New Eng. J. Med., 254*: 636–641, 1956.

Bode, H.: Personal Communication, 1970.

Bower, E. M.: Primary prevention of mental and emotional disorders: A conceptual framework and action possibilities. *Amer. J. Orthopsychiat., 33*:832–848, 1963.

Bowlby, J.: Maternal care and mental health. *Monograph Series No. 2,* World Health Organization, 1951.

Bozeman, M. F., Orbach, C. E., and Sutherland, A.: Part I. Psychological impact of cancer and its treatment; Part II. The adaptation of mothers to the threatened loss of their children through leukemia. *Cancer, 8*:1–47, 1955.

Bray, T.: Day-care centers find favor as more women flock into work force. *Wall Street Journal,* Vol. 175, No. 70, April 10, 1970.

Brazelton, T. B.: Observations of the neonate. *J. Amer. Acad. Child Psychiat., 1*:38–58, 1962.

Brazelton, T. B.: *Infants and Mothers: Differences in Development.* New York, Delacorte Press, 1970.

Brazelton, T. B., and Robey, J. S.: Observations of neonatal behavior: The effect of perinatal variables, in particular that of maternal medication. *J. Amer. Acad. Child Psychiat., 4*:613–637, 1965.

Brazelton, T. B., Robey, J. S., and Collier, G. A.: Infant development in the Zinacenteco Indian of southern Mexico. *Pediatrics, 44*: 274–290, 1969.

Brenner, J. H., Coles, R., and Meagher, D.: *Drugs and Youth—Medical, Psychiatric and Legal Facts.* New York, Liveright, 1970.

Bronfenbrenner, M., with assistance of

Condry, J. C.: *Two Worlds of Children. U.S. and U.S.S.R.* New York, Russell Sage Foundation, 1970.
Brooks, F. B.: Central nervous system control of gastric secretion. *Texas Med., 62*:48–50, 1966.
Browne, W. J., Mally, M., and Kane, R. P.: Psychosocial aspects of hemophilia: A study of twenty-eight hemophilic children and their families. *Amer. J. Orthopsychiat., 30*: 730–740, 1960.
Bruch, H.: Physiologic and psychologic interrelationships in diabetes in children. *Psychosom. Med., 11*:200–210, 1949.
Caffey, J.: Multiple fractures in the long bones of infants suffering from chronic subdural hematoma. *Amer. J. Roentgen., 56*:163–173, 1946.
Caffey, J.: Some traumatic lesions in growing bones other than fractures and dislocations: Clinical and radiological features. *Brit. J. Radiol., 30*:225–238, 1957.
Caffey, J.: Significance of the history in the diagnosis of traumatic injury to children. *J. Pediat., 67*:1008–1014, 1965.
Caldwell, B. M.: What is the optimal learning environment for the young child? *Amer. J. Orthopsychiat., 37*:8–21, 1967.
Caldwell, B. M., and Drachman, Robert H.: Comparability of three methods of assessing the developmental level of young infants. *Pediatrics, 34*:51–57, 1964.
Cannon, W. B.: *Bodily Changes in Pain, Hunger, Fear and Rage.* New York, Appleton-Century-Crofts, 1915.
Caplan, G.: *Principles of Preventive Psychiatry.* New York, Basic Books, Inc., Publishers, 1964.
Capps, R. B., and Barker, M. H.: Management of infectious hepatitis. *Ann. Intern. Med., 26*:405–416, 1947.
Castiglioni, A.: *In* Krumghaar, E. B. (Ed.): *The History of Medicine.* New York, Alfred A. Knopf, Inc., 1947.
Caudill, W., and Weinstein, H.: Maternal care and infant behavior in Japan and America. *Psychiatry, 32*:12–47, 1969.
Chalmers, T. C., et al.: The treatment of acute infectious hepatitis. *J. Clin. Invest., 34*: 1163–1235, 1955.
Chenoweth, A.: Care of young children of working mothers. *The Woman Physician, 25*:166–169, 1970.
Chess, S.: Individuality in children, its importance to the pediatrician. *J. Pediat., 66*: 676–684, 1966.
Chilman, C. S.: *Growing Up Poor.* Social and Rehabilitation Service Publication No. 109, U. S. Department of Health, Education and Welfare, 1966.
Clarke, A. D. B., and Clarke, A. M.: Some recent advances in the study of early deprivation. *Child Psychology and Psychiatry, 1*: 26–36, 1960.
Clausen, J., Seidenfeld, M. A., and Deasy, L. C.: Parent attitudes toward participation of their children in polio vaccine trials. *Amer. J. Public Health, 44*:1526–1536, 1954.
Coddington, R. D.: Study of an infant with a gastric fistula and her normal twin. *Psychosom. Med., 30*:172–192, 1968.
Coleman, R. W., and Provence, S.: Environmental retardation (hospitalism) in infants living in families. *Pediatrics, 19*:285–292, 1957.
Coles, M. R.: Southern children under desegration. *Amer. J. Psychiat., 120*:332–344, 1963.
Coles, M. R.: *Children of Crises.* Boston, Little, Brown and Company, 1964.
Connelly, J. P., et al.: Survey of 349 Chelsea grade school children. Unpublished observations, 1966.
Conners, C. K.: Symptom patterns in hyperkinetic, neurotic and normal children. *Child Develop., 41*:667–682, 1970.
Crawford, J. D., and Haessler, H. A.: Obesity—A pediatric viewpoint. *Med. Times, 95*:1269–1280, 1967.
Creak, M.: Psychosis in childhood. *In* Miller, E. (Ed.): *Foundations of Child Psychiatry.* Oxford, Pergamon Press, 1968.
Davis, F.: Deviance disapproval: The management of strained interaction by the visibly handicapped. *Social Problems, 9*:120, 1961.
Davis, K.: Final note on a cause of extreme isolation. *Amer. J. Sociol., 52*:432–437, 1947.
Davis, M. S., and Eichhorn, R. L.: Compliance with medical regimens: A panel study. *J. Health Hum. Behav., 4*:240–249, 1963.
DeFrancis, V.: Child Abuse—*Preview of a Nationwide Survey.* Denver, The American Humane Association, Children's Division, 1963.
Dennis, W., and Najarian, P.: Infant development under environmental handicap. *Psychol. Monogr., 71*:1–12, 1957.
Densen, P. M., Ullman, D. B., Jones, E. W., and Vandow, J. E.: Childhood Characteristics as indicators of adult health status. *Public Health Rep., 85*:981–996, 1970.
Deutsch, M.: *The Disadvantaged Child.* New York, Basic Books, Inc., Publishers, 1967.
Deutsch, M., Katz, L., and Jensen, A.: *Social Class, Race and Psychological Development.* New York, Holt, Rinehart & Winston, Inc., 1968.
Dubos, R. J.: *Mirage of Health: Utopias, Progress and Biological Change* (World Perspectives, Vol. XXII), New York, Harper & Row, Publishers, 1959.
Eisenberg, L.: The sins of the fathers: Urban decay and social pathology. *Amer. J. Orthopsychiat., 32*:5–17, 1962.
Eisenberg, L.: Deprivation and foster care. *J. Amer. Acad. Child Psychiat., 4*:243–253, 1965.
Eisenberg, L.: The social development of

human intelligence. *The Harvard Medical Alumni Bulletin, 43*:2–8, 1968.

Eldredge, H. W.: *Taming Megalopolis.* New York, Anchor Books, 1967.

Elmer, E.: Failure to thrive: Role of the mother. *Pediatrics, 25*:717–725, 1960.

Elmer, E., and Gregg, G.: Developmental characteristics of abused children. *Pediatrics, 40*:596–602, 1967.

Engel, G. L.: Psychogenic pain and the pain-prone patient. *Amer. J. Med., 26*:899–918, 1959.

Engel, G. L.: Psychological factors in ulcerative colitis in man and gibbon. *Gastroenterology, 57*:362–365, 1969.

Escalona, S. K.: *The Roots of Individuality.* Chicago, Aldine Publishing Company, 1968.

Fanshel, D., and Maas, H. S.: Factoral dimensions of the characteristics of children in placement and their families. *Child Develop., 33*:123–144, 1962.

Feinstein, A. R.: Physical activity and rheumatic heart disease in asymptomatic patients. *J.A.M.A., 180*:1028–1031, 1962.

Fischer, A. E., Dolger, H., et al.: Behavior and psychologic problems of young diabetic patients. *Arch. Intern. Med., 78*:711–732, 1946.

Fontana, V., Donovan, D., and Wong, R.: The "maltreatment syndrome" in children. *New Eng. J. Med., 269*:1389–1394, 1963.

Foss, B. M. (Ed.): *Determinants of Infant Behavior.* London, Methuen & Co. Ltd., 1961, 1963, 1965.

Fraiberg, S. H.: *The Magic Years: Understanding and Handling the Problems of Early Childhood.* New York, Charles Scribner's Sons, 1959.

Fried, R., and Mayer, M. F.: Socio-emotional factors accounting for growth failure in children living in an institution. *J. Pediat., 33*: 444–456, 1948.

Friedman, S. B., Mason, J. W., and Hamburg, D. A.: Urinary 17-hydroxycorticosteroid levels in parents of children with neoplastic disease. *Psychosom. Med.,* 25:364–376, 1963a.)

Friedman, S. B., Chodoff, P., Mason, J. W., and Hamburg, D. A.: Behavioral observations of parents anticipating the death of a child. *Pediatrics, 32*:610–625, 1963b.

Garrard, S. D., and Richmond, J. B.: Psychogenic megacolon manifested by fecal soiling. *Pediatrics, 10*:474–481, 1952.

Gibson, J. P.: How much rest is necessary for children with fever? *J. Pediat., 49*:256–261, 1956.

Gil, D. G.: *Violence Against Children: Physical Abuse in the United States.* Cambridge, Massachusetts, Harvard University Press, 1970.

Ginott, H. G.: *Between Parent and Teenager.* New York, The Macmillan Company, 1969.

Glaser, H., Harrison, G. S., and Lynn, D. B.: Emotional implications of congenital heart disease in children. *Pediatrics, 33*:367–379, 1964.

Glaser, K., and Eisenberg, L.: Maternal deprivation. *Pediatrics, 18*:626–642, 1956.

Glaser, K., and Clemmens, R. L.: School failure. *Pediatrics, 35*:128–141, 1965.

Glasser, M. A.: A study of the public's acceptance of the Salk vaccine program. *Amer. J. Public Health, 48*:141–146, 1958.

Goldfarb, W.: Effects of psychological deprivation in infancy and subsequent stimulation. *Amer. J. Psychiat., 102*:18–33, 1945a.

Goldfarb, W.: Psychological privation in infancy and subsequent adjustment. *Amer. J. Orthopsychiat., 15*:247–255, 1945b.

Goldfarb, W.: Variations in adolescent adjustment of institutionally-reared children. *Amer. J. Orthopsychiat., 17*:449–457, 1947.

Green, M., and Solnit, A. J.: Reactions to the threatened loss of a child: A vulnerable child syndrome. *Pediatrics, 34*:58–66, 1964.

Haessler, H. A., and Crawford, J. D.: Lipolysis in homogenates of adipose tissue: An inhibitor found in fat from obese rats. *Science, 154*:909–910, 1966.

Haggstrom, W.: The power of the poor. *In* Riessman, F., Cohen, J., and Pearl, A. (eds.): *Mental Health of the Poor.* New York, The Free Press, 1964.

Hamburg, D. A.: Some issues in research on human behavior and adrenocortical function. *Psychosom. Med., 21*:387–388, 1959.

Hamburg, D. A.: Genetics of adrenocortical hormone metabolism in relation to psychological stress. *In* Hirsh, J. (Ed.): *Behavior and Genetic Analysis.* New York, McGraw-Hill Book Company, 1967.

Hamburg, D. A., and Lunde, D. T.: *Relation of Behavioral, Genetic, and Neuroendocrine Factors to Thryoid Function.* Chicago, Aldine Publishing Company, 1967.

Harlow, H. F.: The development of affectional patterns in infant monkeys. *In* Foss, B. M. (Ed.): *Determinants of Infant Behavior.* London, Methuen & Co. Ltd., 1961, pp. 51–74.

Harlow, H. F.: The maternal affectional system. *In* Foss, B. M., (Ed.): *Determinants of Infant Behavior II.* London, Methuen & Co. Ltd., 1963.

Harlow, H., and Harlow, M.: The effect of rearing conditions on behavior. *Int. J. Psychiat., 1*:43–51, 1965.

Harper, F. V.: The physician, the battered child, and the law. *Pediatrics, 31*:899–902, 1963.

Harper, P. A.: *Preventive Pediatrics.* New York, Appleton-Century-Crofts, 1962.

Hill, A. B.: The environment and disease: Association or causation. *Proc. Roy. Soc. Med., 58*:295–299, 1965.

Hill, S. R., Goetz, F. C., Fox, H. M., Murawsky, B. J., Krakauer, L. J., Reifenstein, R. W., Gray, S. J., Reddy, W. J., Hedberg, S. E.,

Marc, J. R., and Thorn, G. W.: Studies on adrenocortical and psychological response to stress in man. *Arch. Intern. Med.,* *97*:269–298, 1956.
Hirsch, J. (Ed.): *Behavior-Genetic Analysis.* New York, McGraw-Hill Book Company, 1968.
Hollowell, J. G., and Gardner, L. I.: Rumination and growth failure in male fraternal twin, association with disturbed family environment. *Pediatrics,* *36*:565–571, 1965.
Holt, J.: *How Children Learn.* New York, Pitman Publishing Corp., 1967.
Howell, M. C.: Some effects of chronic illness on children and their mothers. Unpublished Doctoral Dissertation, University of Minnesota, June, 1962.
Howels, J. G.: *Family Psychiatry.* Edinburgh, Oliver & Boyd, Ltd., 1963.
Jaco, E. G. (Ed.): *Patients, Physicians and Illness; Sourcebook in Behavioral Science and Medicine.* Glencoe, Illinois, The Free Press, 1958.
Janis, I. L., and Feshbach, S.: Effects of fear-arousing communications. *J. Abnom. & Soc. Psychol.,* *48*:78–92, 1953.
Joint Commission on Mental Health of Children: *Crisis in Child Mental Health: Challenge for the 1970's.* New York, Harper & Row, Publishers, 1970.
Joseph, M. C., and Polani, P. E.: The effect of rest on acute hemorrhagic nephritis in children. *Guy Hosp. Rep.,* *107*:500, 1958.
Jussor, R.: Psychosocial deprivation and personality development. *In* La Veck, G. (Ed.): *Perspectives on Human Deprivation: Biological, Psychological and Sociological.* National Institute of Child Health and Human Development, U.S. Dept. of Health, Education and Welfare, 1968.
Kagan, J.: On the need for relatavism. *Amer. Psychol.,* *22*:131–142, 1967.
Kagan, J., and Moss, H. A.: *Birth to Maturity: A Study in Psychological Development.* New York, John Wiley & Sons, Inc., 1962.
Kearsley, R., Snider, M., Richie, R., Crawford, J. D., and Talbot, N. B.: Study of relations between psychologic environment and child behavior. *Amer. J. Dis. Child.,* *104*:12–20, 1962.
Keller, H.: *The Story of My Life.* Garden City, New York, Doubleday & Company, Inc., 1905, 1954.
Kempe, C. H., Silverman, F., Steele, B. F., Droegemueller, W., and Silver, H. K.: The battered-child syndrome. *J.A.M.A.,* *181*:17–24, 1962.
Kenniston, K.: Youth and violence: The contexts of moral crisis. *In* Gustafson, J. M., et al.: *Moral Education: Five Lectures.* Cambridge, Massachusetts, Harvard University Press, 1970.
King, S.: *Perceptions of Illness and Medical Practice.* New York, Russell Sage Foundation, 1962.
King, S.: *In* Freeman, H. E., et al. (Eds.): *Some Psychological Factors in Illness: Handbook of Medical Sociology.* Englewood Cliffs, New Jersey, Prentice-Hall, Inc., 1963.
Knutson, A. L.: *The Individual, Society, and Health Behavior.* New York, Russell Sage Foundation, 1965.
Koos, E. L.: *Health in Regionville.* New York, Columbia University Press, 1954.
Korner, A. F., and Grebstein, R.: Individual differences at birth. Implications for mother-infant relationship and later development. *S. Amer. Acad. Child Psychiat.,* *6*:676–690, 1967.
Korsch, B. M.: Practical techniques of observing, interviewing and advising parents in pediatric practice as demonstrated in an attitude study project. *Pediatrics,* *18*:467–490, 1956.
Krieger, I., and Sargent, D. A.: A postural sign in the sensory deprivation syndrome in infants. *J. Pediat.,* *70*:332–339, 1967.
Lapouse, R.: Who is sick? *Amer. J. Orthopsychiat.,* *35*:138–144, 1965.
Lapouse, R., and Monk, M. A.: Fears and worries in a representative sample of children. *Amer. J. Orthopsychiat.,* *29*:803–818, 1959.
Lapouse, R., and Monk, M. A.: Behavior deviations in a representative sample of children: Variation by sex, age, race, social class and family size. *Amer. J. Orthopsychiat.,* *34*:436–446, 1964.
La Veck, G. D.: *Perspectives on Human Deprivation: Biological, Psychological and Sociological.* The National Institute of Child Health and Human Development, U.S. Dept. of Health, Education and Welfare, 1968.
Leiderman, P. H., and Shapiro, D. (Eds.): *Psychobiological Approaches to Social Behavior.* Stanford, California: Stanford University Press, 1964.
Leonard, M., Rhymes, J. P., and Solnit, A. J.: Failure to thrive in infants. *Amer. J. Dis. Child.,* *111*:600–612, 1966.
Lesser, A.: *Health of Children of School Age.* Welfare Administration, Children's Bureau, U.S. Department of Health, Education and Wefare, 1964.
Leventhal, H.: Fear communications in the acceptance of preventive health practices. *Bull. N. Y. Acad. Med.,* *41*:1144–1168, 1965.
LeVine, R. A., and LeVine, B. B.: Nyansongo: A Gusii Community in Kenya. *In* Whiting, B. B. (Ed.): *Six Cultures.* New York, John Wiley & Sons, Inc., 1963.
Levi-Strauss, C.: *The Savage Mind.* Chicago, University of Chicago Press, 1966.
Levy, D. M.: *Maternal Overprotection.* New York, Columbia University Press, 1943.
Lidz, T.: Emotional factors in the etiology of hyperthyroidism: The report of a preliminary survey. *Psychosom. Med.,* *11*:2–8, 1949.
Lindemann, E.: Symptomatology and manage-

ment of acute grief. *Amer. J. Psychiat., 101*: 141–148, 1944.

Lipton, E. L., Steinschneider, A., and Richmond, J. B.: The anatonomic system in early life. *New Eng. J. Med., 273*:147–153, 201–208, 1965.

Lis, E. F., Pruzansky, S., Koepp-Baker, H., and Kobes, H. R.: Cleft lip and cleft palate. *Pediat. Clin. N. Amer., 3*:995–1028, 1956.

Lorenz, K.: Companionship in bird life. *In* Schiller, C. H. (Ed.): *Instinctive Behavior.* New York, International Universities Press, 1957.

Low, S., and Spindler, P. G.: *Child Care Arrangements of Working Mothers in the United States.* Children's Bureau Publication No. 461, U.S. Department of Health, Education and Welfare, 1968.

Lowenfeld, B.: *Our Blind Children—Growing and Learning with Them.* Springfield, Illinois, Charles C Thomas, Publisher, 1956.

Maas, H. S., and Engler, R. E.: *Children In Need of Parents.* New York, Columbia University Press, 1959.

MacKeith, R.: The adolescent who has a handicap. *Medical World, 100*:296–302, 1964.

MacKeith, R., and O'Neill, D.: Abdominal pain in children. *Lancet, 2*:278–282, 1951.

Maretzki, T., and Maretzki, H.: Taira: An Okinawan village. *In* Whiting, B. B. (Ed.): *Six Cultures.* New York, John Wiley & Sons, Inc., 1963.

Martin, W. F.: Introduction: Relevance of research in child development to child welfare. *In* Norris, M., and Wallace, B. (Eds.): *The Known and Unknown in Child Welfare Research: An Appraisal.* New York, Child Welfare League of America, 1965.

Masland, R. L., Sarason, S. B., and Gladwin, T.: *Mental Subnormality: Biologic, Psychologic and Cultural Factors.* New York, Basic Books, Inc., Publishers, 1958.

Mason, W., and Sponholz, R.: Behavior of rhesus monkeys raised in isolation. *J. Psychiat. Res., 1*:299–306, 1963.

Massie, R. K.: *Nicholas and Alexandra.* New York, Atheneum Publishers, 1967.

Mathis, J. L.: A sophisticated version of voodoo death. *Psychosom. Med., 26*:104–107, 1964.

Matsumoto, S., Thoma, K., Kubo, H., Watanabe, M., Hosaka, H., and Utsuno, A.: Environmental menstrual disorders. *Gunma J. Med. Sci., 14*:1–15, 1965.

Mattsson, A., and Gross, S.: Social and behavioral studies on hemophilic children and their families. *J. Pediat., 68*:952–964, 1966.

Mayer, J.: Medical progress—Some aspects of the problem of regulation of food intake and obesity. *New Eng. J. Med., 274*:610–616, 722–731, 1966.

Mayer, J.: *Overweight: Causes, Cost and Control.* New Jersey, Prentice-Hall, Inc., 1968.

McCrory, W. W., Fleisher, D., and Sohn, W. B.: The course of acute nephritis in children allowed early resumption of normal physical activity. *Amer. J. Dis. Child., 96*:576–578, 1958.

McHenry, T., Girdany, B. R., and Elmer, E.: Unsuspected trauma with multiple skeletal injuries during infancy and childhood. *Pediatrics, 31*:903–908, 1963.

Mead, M.: *Male and Female.* New York, William Morrow & Co., Inc., 1949.

Mead, M., and Wolfenstein, M.: *Childhood in Contemporary Cultures.* Chicago, University of Chicago Press, 1955.

Miller, L. M.: *Dropouts: Selected References.* Superintendent of Documents Catalog No. F 85 220:20070, Washington, D.C., U. S. Government Printing Office, 1964.

Miller, N. E.: Physiologic and cultural determinants of behavior. *In The Scientific Endeavor.* New York, Rockefeller Institute Press, 1965.

Milowe, I. D., and Lourie, R. S.: The child's role in the battered child syndrome. *J. Pediat., 55*:1079–1081, 1964.

Minturn, L., and Hitchcock, J. T.: The Rajputs of Khalapur, India. *In* Whiting, B. B. (Ed.): *Six Cultures.* New York, John Wiley & Sons, Inc., 1963.

Nydegger, W. F., and Nydegger, C.: Tarong: An Ilocos Barrio in the Philippines. *In* Whiting, B. B. (Ed.): *Six Cultures.* New York, John Wiley & Sons, Inc., 1963.

Parmelee, A. H.: The doctor and the handicapped child. *Children, 9*:189–193, 1962.

Parsons, T.: *The Social System.* Glencoe, Illinois, The Free Press, 1951.

Parsons, T.: Definitions of health and illness in the light of American values and social structure. *In* Jaco, E. G. (Ed.): *Patients, Physicians and Illness.* Glencoe, Illinois, The Free Press, 1958.

Patton, R. G., and Gardner, L.: Influence of family environment on growth: The syndrome of "maternal deprivation." *Pediatrics, 30*:957–962, 1962.

Patton, R. G., and Gardner, L.: *Growth Failure in Maternal Deprivation.* Springfield, Illinois, Charles C Thomas, Publisher, 1963.

Pavenstedt, E.: The nursery school, day care centers and developmental studies. *J. Amer. Acad. Child Psychiat., 5*:349–359, 1966.

Pavenstedt, E.: The drifters. Children of disorganized families. *Int. Psychiat. Clinic, 4*:1–13, 33–44, 323–334, 1967.

Peabody, F. W.: *Doctor and Patient: Papers on the Relationship of the Physician to Men and Institutions.* New York, The Macmillan Company, 1930.

Peebles, T. P.: A biosocial survey of 146 consecutive admissions to the Massachusetts General Hospital Children's Service. Unpublished observations, 1967.

Peiper, A.: *In* Wortis, J. (Ed.): *International Behavior Series; Cerebral Function in Infancy and Childhood.* New York, Consultants Bureau Enterprises, Inc., 1963.

Pines, M.: *Revolution in Learning: The Years*

from Birth to Six. New York, Harper & Row, Publishers, 1966.

Porter, R. W., Brady, J. V., Conrad, D., Mason, J., Galambos, R., and Rioch, D.: Some experimental observations on gastrointestinal lesions in behaviorally conditioned monkeys. *Psychosom. Med., 20*:379–394, 1958.

Powell, G. F., Brasel, J. A., and Blizzard, R. M.: Emotional deprivation and growth retardation simulating idiopathic hypopituitarism. *New Eng. J. Med., 276*:1271–1278, 1967.

President's Panel on Mental Retardation. *National Action to Combat Mental Retardation.* Washington, D.C., U. S. Government Printing Office, 1962.

Provence, S.: *Guide for the Care of Infants in Groups.* New York, Child Welfare League of America, Inc., 1967.

Provence, S., and Lipton, R. C.: *Infants in Institutions.* New York, International Universities Press, 1967.

Psychopathological Disorders in Childhood: Theoretical Considerations and a Proposed Classification. Formulated by the Committee on Child Psychiatry. New York, Group for the Advancement of Psychiatry, Vol. VI, Report No. 62, June, 1966.

Purcell, K., Brady, K., Chai, H., Muser, J., Molk, C., Jordon, N., and Means, J.: The effect on asthma in children of experimental separation from the family. *Psychosom. Med., 31*:144–164, 1969.

Rakoff, A. E.: Psychogenic factors in anovulatory women. I. Hormonal patterns in women with ovarian dysfunctions of psychogenic origin. *Fertil. Steril., 13*:1–10, 1962.

Raphail, D.: When mothers need mothering. *New York Times Magazine,* February 8, 1970, p. 67.

Rebelsky, F.: Infancy in two cultures. *Nederlands Tijdschrift voor de Psychologie en haar Grensgebieden, 22*:379–385, 1967.

Rebelsky, F., and Abeles, G.: *Infancy in Holland and the United States.* Paper presented at the Society for Research in Child Development, April, 1969, Santa Monica, Calif.

Reid, J. H.: Action called for—Recommendations. *In* Mass, H. S., et al. (Eds.): *Children in Need of Parents.* New York, Columbia University Press, 1959.

Reifenstein, E. C., Jr.: Psychogenic or "hypothalamic" amenorrhea. *Med. Clin. N. Amer., 30*:1103–1114, 1946.

Reinhart, J. B., and Drash, A. L.: Psychosocial dwarfism: Environmentally induced recovery. *Psychosom. Med., 31*:165–172, 1969.

Reinhart, J. B., and Elmer, E.: The abused child: Mandatory reporting legislation. *J.A.M.A., 188*:108–112, 1964.

Reiser, D. E.: Psychosis of infancy and early childhood, as manifested by children with atypical development. *New Eng. J. Med., 269*:790–798, 844–849, 1963.

Rheingold, H. L.: The measurement of maternal care. *Child Develop., 31*:565–575, 1960.

Richardson, S. A.: Some social psychological consequences of handicapping. *Pediatrics, 32*:291–297, 1963.

Richardson, S. A., Boodman, N., Hastorf, A. H., and Dornbush, S. M.: Cultural uniformity in reaction to physical disabilities. *Amer. Sociol. Rev., 26*:241–247, 1961.

Richmond, J. B.: The pediatrician and the individual delinquent. *Pediatrics, 26*:126–131, 1960.

Richmond, J. B.: Discussion of juvenile paroxysmal supraventricular tachycardia: Psychosomatic and psychodynamic aspects. *J. Amer. Acad. Child Psychiat., 1*:265–268, 1962.

Richmond, J. B.: *Currents in American Medicine: A Developmental View of Medical Care and Education.* Cambridge, Massachusetts, Harvard University Press, 1969.

Richmond, J. B., and Caldwell, B.: The effectiveness of day-care program for disadvantaged infants and young children—Results after one year. *J. Pediat., 69*:885–886, 1966.

Richmond, J. B , and Waisman, H. A.: Psychologic aspects of management of children with malignant diseases. *Amer. J. Dis. Child., 89*:42–47, 1955.

Riseborough, E. J.: Current concepts: Treatment of scoliosis. *New Eng. J. Med., 276*: 1429–1431, 1967.

Robinson, D.: *When "Illness" is not Illness.* Presented at the Second International Conference on Social Science and Medicine, Aberdeen, Scotland, September, 1970.

Romney, K., and Romney, R.: The Mixtecans of Juxtlahuaca, Mexico. *In* Whiting, B. B., (Ed.): *Six Cultures.* New York, John Wiley & Sons, Inc., 1963.

Rose, J. A.: Delayed recognition of childhood emotional disorders. *Child Welfare, 38*:7–13, 1959.

Rose, J. A.: Commentaries: The dimensions of comprehensive pediatrics. *Pediatrics, 26*: 729–734, 1960.

Rosen, G.: *In* Freeman, H. E., et al. (Eds.): *The Evolution of Social Medicine: Handbook of Medical Sociology.* Englewood Cliffs, New Jersey, Prentice-Hall, Inc., 1963.

Rothenberg, M. B.: Reactions of those who treat children with cancer. *Pediatrics, 40*: 507–510, 1967.

Rowntree, L. G., et al.: Mental and personality disorders in Selective Service registrants. *J.A.M.A., 128*:1084–1087, 1945.

Salk, J.: From an address on the occasion of his receipt of the Congressional Award. *New York Times,* April 13, 1965.

Samora, J., Saunders, L., and Larson, R. F.: Knowledge about specific diseases in four selected samples. *J. Health Hum. Behav., 3*:176–185, 1962.

Schaefer, E. S.: A circumplex model for maternal behavior. *J. Abnorm. Soc. Psychol., 59*: 226–235, 1959.

Schneck, H. M.: Control by brain studied as way to curb body ills. *New York Times*, January 10, 1971, p. 1.

Schutz, W. C.: *A Three Dimensional Theory of Interpersonal Behavior.* New York, Holt, Rinehart & Winston, Inc., 1958.

Scott, J. P.: Critical periods in behavioral development. *Science, 138*:949–958, 1962.

Sears, R. R., Maccoby, E. E., and Levin, H.: *Patterns of Child Rearing.* Evanston, Illinois, Row-Peterson and Company, 1957.

Senn, M. J.: The psychotherapeutic role of the pediatrician. *Pediatrics, 2*:147–153, 1948.

Shapiro, J. I.: Teen-agers and venereal disease – The threat to our youth. *J.A.M.A., 194*: 147–149, 1965.

Shiffer, C. G., and Hunt, E. P.: *Illness Among Children.* Welfare Administration, Children's Bureau, U. S. Department of Health, Education and Welfare, 1963.

Silver, G. A.: *Family Medical Care.* Cambridge, Massachusetts, Harvard University Press, 1963.

Silver, H. K., and Finkelstein, M.: Deprivation dwarfism. *J. Pediat., 70*:317–324, 1967.

Silver, H. K., and Kempe, C. H.: The problem of parental criminal neglect and severe physical abuse of children. *Amer. J. Dis. Child., 98*:528, 1959.

Silverman, F. N.: The roentgen manifestations of unrecognized skeletal trauma in infants. *Amer. J. Roentgen., 69*:413–427, 1953.

Simons, B., Downs, E. F., Hurster, M. M., and Archer, M.: Child abuse – Epidemiologic study of medically reported cases. *New York J. Med., 66*:2783–2788, 1966.

Skeels, H. M.: Adult status of children with contrasting early life experiences: A follow-up study. *Monogr. Soc. Res. Child Develop., 31*:1–65, 1966.

Sobel, E., Raymond, C. S., Quinn, K. V., and Talbot, N. B.: The use of methyltestosterone to stimulate growth: Relative influence on skeletal maturation and linear growth. *J. Clin. Endocr., 16*:241–252, 1956.

Solnit, A. J., and Provence, S. A. (Eds.): *Modern Perspectives in Child Development.* New York, International Universities Press, 1963.

Solnit, A. J., and Stark, M. H.: Mourning and the birth of a defective child. *Psychoanal. Stud. Child, 16*:523–537, 1961.

Solomon, P., Leiderman, H., Mendelson, J., and Wexler, D.: Sensory deprivation: A review. *Amer. J. Psychiat., 114*:357–363, 1957.

Sommers, V. S.: *The Influence of Parental Attitudes and Social Environment on the Personality Development of the Adolescent Blind.* New York, American Foundation for the Blind, 1944.

Sours, J. A.: Narcolepsy and other disturbances in the sleep waking rhythm: A study of 115 cases with review of the literature. *J. Nerv. Ment. Dis., 137*:525–543, 1963.

Spitz, R. A.: Hospitalism: An inquiry into the genesis of psychiatric conditions in early childhood. *Psychoanal. Stud. Child, 1*:53–74, 1945.

Spitz, R. A.: Hospitalism: A follow-up on investigation described in Volume 1, 1945. *Psychoanal. Stud. Child, 2*:113–117, 1946(a).

Spitz, R. A.: Anaclitic depression: An inquiry into the genesis of psychiatric conditions in early childhood, II. *Psychoanal. Stud. Child, 2*:313–342, 1946(b).

Spock, B.: *Baby and Child Care.* New York, Pocket Books, 1958.

Standards and Costs of Day Care. Compiled by Day Care Specialists, Washington, D.C., Office of Child Development, U.S. Department of Health, Education and Welfare, 1969.

Starfield, B., and Borkowf, S.: Physicians' recognition of complaints made by patients about their children's health. *Pediatrics, 43*: 168–172, 1969.

Steinschneider, A., Lipton, E. L., and Richmond, J. B.: Auditory sensitivity of the infant: Effect on cardiac and motor responsivity. *Child Develop., 37*:233–252, 1966.

Stendler, C. B.: Psychologic aspects of pediatrics: Sixty years of child training practices. *J. Pediat., 36*:122–134, 1950.

Stine, O. C.: Content and method of health supervision by physicians in child health conferences in Baltimore, 1959. *Amer. J. Public Health, 52*:1858–1865, 1962.

Swift, C. R., Seidman, F., and Stein, H.: Adjustment problems in juvenile diabetics. *Psychosom. Med., 29*:555–571, 1967.

Talbot, N. B.: Has psychologic malnutrition taken the place of rickets and scurvy in contemporary pediatric practice? *Pediatrics, 31*:909–918, 1963.

Talbot, N. B.: Pediatrics redefined. *J. Pediat., 64*:464–468, 1964.

Talbot, N. B.: Pediatric frontiers in developmental medicine. *Amer. J. Dis. Child., 110*: 287–290, 1965.

Talbot, N. B.: Concerning the need for behavioral and social science in medicine. *In* Knowles, J. H. (Ed.): *Views of Medical Education and Medical Care.* Cambridge, Massachusetts, Harvard University Press, 1968.

Talbot, N. B., Richie, R. H., and Crawford, M. D.: *Metabolic Homeostasis.* Cambridge, Massachusetts, Harvard University Press, 1959.

Talbot, N. B., Robinson, J. C., Loescher, L., et al.: Development of plans for a long range action oriented comprehensive medical care study and training program for children with chronic disabilities. Report on Children's Bureau Grant H-103, July 1, 1966.

Talbot, N. B., Sobel, E. H., Burke, B. S.,

Lindemann, E., and Kaufman, S. B.: Dwarfism in healthy children: Its possible relation to emotional, nutritional and endocrine disturbances. *New Eng. J. Med.*, *236*:783–793, 1947.

Talbot, N. B., Sobel, E. H., McArthur, J. W., and Crawford, J. D.: *Functional Endocrinology from Birth Through Adolescence.* Cambridge, Massachusetts, Harvard University Press, 1952.

Tamkin, A. S.: Survey of pathogenic parental attitudes in parents of emotionally disturbed children. *Psychol. Rep.*, *15*:36, 1964.

Thomas, A., Chess, S., and Birch, H. G.: *Temperament and Behavior Disorders in Children.* New York, New York University Press, 1968.

Thomas, A., Chess, S., Birch, H. G., and Hertzig, M. E.: *Behavioral Individuality in Early Childhood.* New York, New York University Press, 1964.

Thompson, W. R., and Melzack, R.: Early environment. *Sci. Amer.*, *194*:38–42, 1956.

Thorn, G. W., Jenkins, D., and Laidlaw, J. C.: The adrenal response to stress in man. *Recent Progr. Hormone Res.*, *8*:171, 1953.

Tisza, V. B.: Management of the parents of the chronically ill child. *Amer. J. Orthopsychiat.*, *32*:53–59, 1962.

Tisza, V. B., and Gumpertz, E.: The parents' reaction to the birth and early care of children with cleft palate. *Pediatrics*, *30*:86–90, 1962.

Twaddle, A. C.: The concept of health status. Presented at the Second International Conference on Social Science and Medicine, Aberdeen, Scotland, September, 1970.

Venning, E. H., Dyrenfurth, I., and Beck, J. C.: Effect of anxiety upon aldosterone excretion in man. *J. Clin. Endocr.*, *17*:1005–1008, 1957.

Wallace, H. M.: *Health Services for Children.* Philadelphia, W. B. Saunders Company, 1962.

Weed, L. L.: Medical records that guide and teach. *New Eng. J. Med.*, *278*:593–600, 652–657, 1968.

Werner, E., et al.: Reproductive and environmental casualties: A report on the 10-year follow-up of the children of the Kauai pregnancy study. *Pediatrics*, *42*:112–127, 1968.

Werner, E., Bierman, J. M., and French, F. E.: *The Children of Kauai.* Honolulu, University of Hawaii Press, 1971.

White, M. S.: Social class, child rearing practices and child behavior. *Amer. Sociol. Rev.*, *22*:704–712, 1957.

Whiting, B. B. (Ed.): *Six Cultures: Studies in Child Rearing.* New York, John Wiley & Sons, Inc., 1963.

Whiting, J. W., Child, I. L., and Lambert, W. W.: *Field Guide for a Study of Socialization.* New York, John Wiley & Sons, Inc., 1966.

Whiting, J. W., and Whiting, B. B.: *Children of Six Cultures. Part I: Egoism and Altruism.* To be published 1971 or 1972.

Whitten, C. F., Pettit, M. G., and Fischhoff, J.: Evidence that growth failure from maternal deprivation is secondary to undereating. *J.A.M.A.*, *209*:1675–1681, 1969.

Williams, T., Martin, D. A., Hogan, M. D., Warkins, J. D., and Ellis, E. V.: The clinical picture of diabetic control, studied in four settings. *Amer. J. Public Health*, *57*:441–451, 1967.

Willoughby, J. A., and Haggerty, R. J.: A simple behavior questionnaire for preschool children. *Pediatrics*, *34*:798–806, 1964.

Witmer, H. L., Yarrow, L. J., Ainsworth, M. D., and Glaser, K.: *Maternal Deprivation.* New York, Child Welfare League of America, Inc., 1962.

Wolff, H. G., and Goodell, H.: *Stress and Disease.* Springfield, Illinois, Charles C Thomas, Publisher, 1968.

Wolff, P. H.: The causes, controls, and organization of behavior in the neonate. *Psychological Issues.* New York, International Universities Press, 1966, Vol. V, No. 1, Monograph 17.

Wynn-Williams, N., and Shaw, J. B.: Is cavity closure in pulmonary-tuberculosis influenced by bed rest? *Tuberculosis*, *41*:352–357, 1960.

Yankauer, A.: Mortality and morality. *Pediatrics*, *40*:547–549, 1967.

Yarrow, L. J.: Maternal deprivation: Toward an empirical and conceptual re-evaluation. *Psychol. Bull.*, *58*:459–490, 1961.

2 PHYSIOLOGICAL PSYCHOLOGY

Allan F. Mirsky

Physiological psychology may be defined as that area of specialization within behavioral science which is concerned with relating behavior and mental processes to the structure, function, and state of the central nervous system. Few would disagree with the premise that mental life, be it overt, or inferred and unobservable, is dependent upon the existence of an intact brain. Disagreements have arisen, however, as to whether efforts to explain thought in terms of central neural events are misdirected at this time. Some have argued forcefully that the role of the psychologist or behavioral scientist is to describe with precision the relation between environmental events and the responses emitted by the organism; study of the central nervous system should be reserved to the physiologist, anatomist or neurologist (Skinner, 1938). Nevertheless, many psychologists have disagreed with this point of view (for example, Hebb, 1949) and have devoted their efforts to understanding the way in which mental processes stem from and are dependent upon the nervous system. This chapter will review and attempt to summarize some of these efforts, and where possible will seek to integrate studies which highlight developmental issues or which contrast the effects of experimental procedures upon immature and mature animals.

The general organization of the chapter is as follows: It begins with a review of the anatomy of the central nervous system. This review emphasizes the structure, subdivisions, and vocabulary of special relevance for physiological psychological research. This is followed by a discussion of the techniques in use in this area of research, and then by a consideration of the substantive material of physiological psychology itself. For purposes of organization the latter is divided into three major areas: intellectual behavior, emotional behavior, and sleep and attentive behavior. Where possible—i.e., where the available data permit—relevant human and animal data which bear on the same issues are presented together.

THE ANATOMY OF THE CENTRAL NERVOUS SYSTEM

The brain of an adult human is shown in lateral view in Figure 2–1A. To highlight similarities and differences, Figure 2–1*B* shows a corresponding view of the brain of a rhesus macaque (*Macaca mulatta*) monkey. The brain of this animal has been selected for presentation because of the extensive use of macaques in neuropsychological research. The gross subdivisions of the brain are often referred to by names derived from embryological terminology: thus, the *telencephalon* or end brain includes the cerebral hemispheres, the olfactory bulbs and tract, the lateral ventricles and a nuclear mass known as the corpus striatum. The corpus striatum is in turn composed of the caudate nucleus, the putamen, the globus pallidus and the claustrum. These are best seen in the cross sectional views in Figure 2–2.

The major component of the telencephalon, both in terms of mass and importance, is the cerebral cortex. Aside from the subdivision according to lobes (frontal, parietal, temporal, occipital), the cortex is usefully subdivided in several other ways. A distinction may be drawn between the *primary sensory cortex* and the *motor cortex* on the one hand, in which the afferents and efferents linking the brain to the periphery are paramount, and *association cortex* on the other hand. The "association" or "intrinsic" cortex is believed to be concerned primarily with relating or elaborating intracortical events. In both man and monkey, the larger proportion of the cerebral mantle is association cortex. By far the greatest amount of research and the greatest degree of controversy have been concerned with assigning higher behavioral functions to the frontal association cortex, and to the parieto-temporo-preoccipital association cortex.

A far more elaborate scheme for subdividing cortical areas is based on the detailed study of the six cortical cell layers. By *cytoarchitectonics,* anatomists such as Brodmann, Campbell, von Economo, Bailey and von Bonin have subdivided the cortex into various regions. Differences of opinion exist as to how many distinctive and differentiable areas are in fact present. However, Brodmann and von Economo believe that one can identify 50-odd regions. It is not clear that all of these structurally different regions have independent functional roles, but this may simply be a matter of further research. Figure 2–3 presents a lateral and medial view of the human brain cortex according to the most popular system, that of Brodmann. The cortical areas referred to so far are described as *neocortex.* This phylogenetically newer cortex (also called *isocortex*) is distinguished from the older paleocortex (or allocortex) by the presence of six layers in the adult or embryonic brain. The layers may differ widely in development from area to area; in the primary visual receiving area (17 in Brodmann's terminology), layer 4, which is the main afferent layer, is particularly prominent. Although this is characteristic of sensory cortex generally, it is especially marked in area 17, so that this region is referred to as the striate cortex, and the striation is called the *stripe of Gennari* or the *stripe of Vicq d'Azyr.* In contrast, in the motor cortex (area 4 of Brodmann), layer 4 is much reduced in size and layer 5 (the pyramidal cell layer) is prominent. Paleocortex is found throughout the *rhinencephalon* (discussed later): for example, in the medial and ventral surfaces of the temporal lobe. A further subcategory of cortex, which seems to be a transitional form between neo- (iso-) and paleo- (allo-) cortex, is referred to as *mesocortex* or *juxta-allocortex.* This is also widely seen in rhinencephalic areas.

The *diencephalon* comprises the hypothalamus, the thalamus, and the associated structures of the "limbic system," including the amygdala, the hippocampus, the fornix, the mamillary bodies, the septum and the tracts which interconnect the several com-

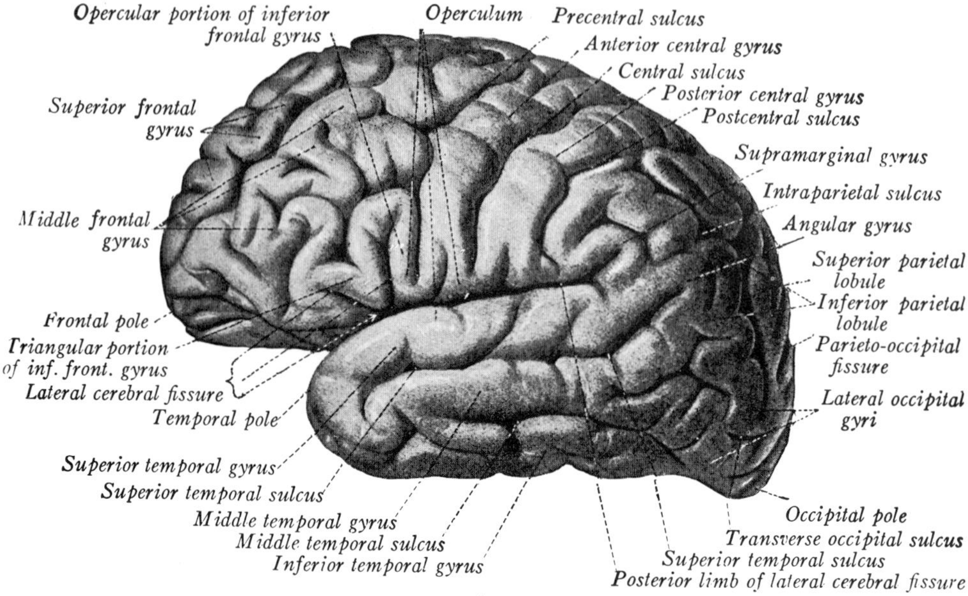

Figure 2–1 A, Lateral view of the left cerebral hemisphere of an adult human. (*From* Ranson, S. W., and Clark, S. L.: *The Anatomy of the Nervous System*, 10th ed. Philadelphia, W. B. Saunders Company, 1959, p. 55.)

ponents of the "limbic system." The term limbic system is an inference based on neurophysiological and behavioral evidence which suggests that some of the structures encompassed by the term are part of a functional entity. The use of the word limbic, however, is derived from Broca's use of the designation *limbic lobe* to describe the ring of structures that surround the midbrain and brain stem and appear to be homologous in a number of vertebrate species. The telencephalon and diencephalon collectively are often referred to as the forebrain.

The *mesencephalon* or midbrain is somewhat more difficult to delimit anatomically in the adult brain than are the preceding major divisions, but it may be said to include the superior and inferior colliculi and the tegmentum (the roof of the third ventricle). Caudal to the mesencephalon is the *metencephalon,* which comprises the pons, the cerebellum and most of the fourth ventricle. Finally, the *myelencephalon* is the term reserved for the medulla oblongata, the last "brain" area before the spinal cord. The majority of the cranial nerves (from part of the Vth or trigeminal through the XIIth or hypoglossal) either exit or enter the central nervous system through the medulla. The metencephalon and myelencephalon jointly comprise the *hindbrain.*

There are in common use several quasi-anatomical terms which are frequently a source of confusion. *Rhinencephalon* (literally nosebrain)

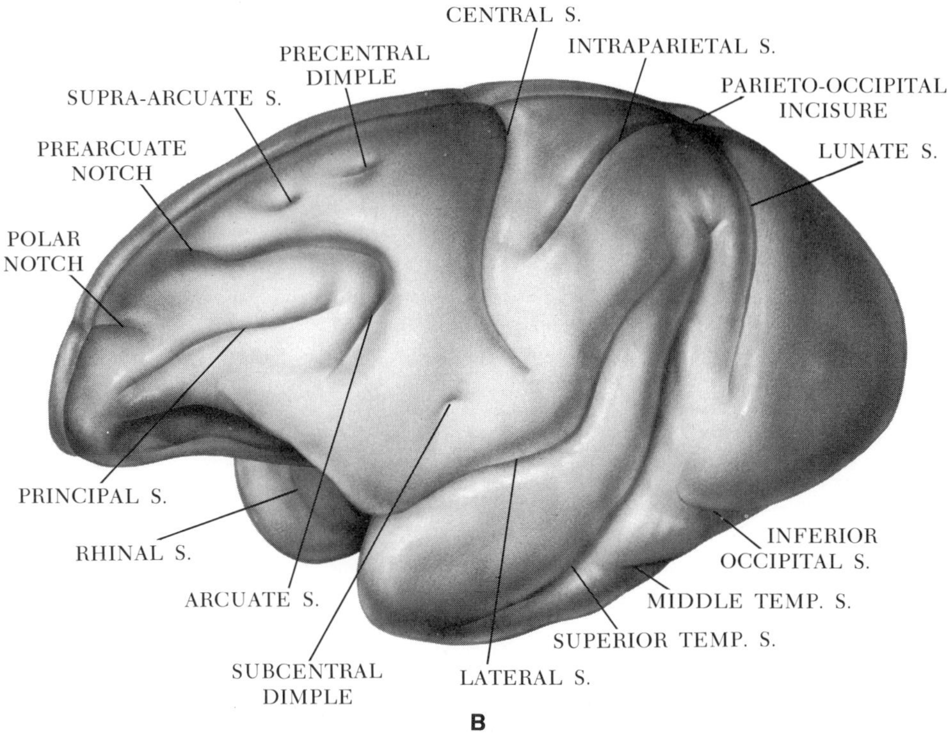

Figure 2–1 *Continued.*
B, Lateral view of the left cerebral hemisphere of a macaque monkey. The brain is tilted so that the anteromedial surface of the right temporal lobe is visible. Note, in comparison with *A*, the smaller number of gyri and sulci in the macaque brain and the greatly reduced extent of the prefrontal area. (Adapted from Krieg, W. S.: *Connections of the Frontal Cortex of the Monkey.* Springfield, Illinois, Charles C Thomas, Publisher, 1954, p. 5. Modified after J. Morgan.)

includes both telencephalic (olfactory bulbs, olfactory tract) and diencephalic (limbic system) structures and is a vestige of the belief held by anatomists that all of these structures formed a system concerned exclusively with the sense of smell. More current theory assigns the function of emotion, rather than exclusively smell, to this system.

Brain stem is used to refer to that area of the metencephalon and myelencephalon comprising the pons and medulla. The 'stem" referent is explained by some anatomists as though the entire encephalon were a lima bean within a pod attached to a stalk or stem. Breaking off the whole forebrain (the lima bean) would destroy the midbrain, since this is the junction twixt fore- and hindbrains. The stalk remaining would be the brain stem; the ring of structures or scar on the bean corresponding to the point of attachment to the stalk would be the limbic lobe.

Reticular formation is one of a number of terms that are more or less interchangeable; all of them refer to the same general concept but differ somewhat. Reticular formation refers generally to that area of the brain stem which comprises the polysynaptic nuclear and fiber mass dorsal to the pons and lateral and ventral to the

(Text continued on page 98)

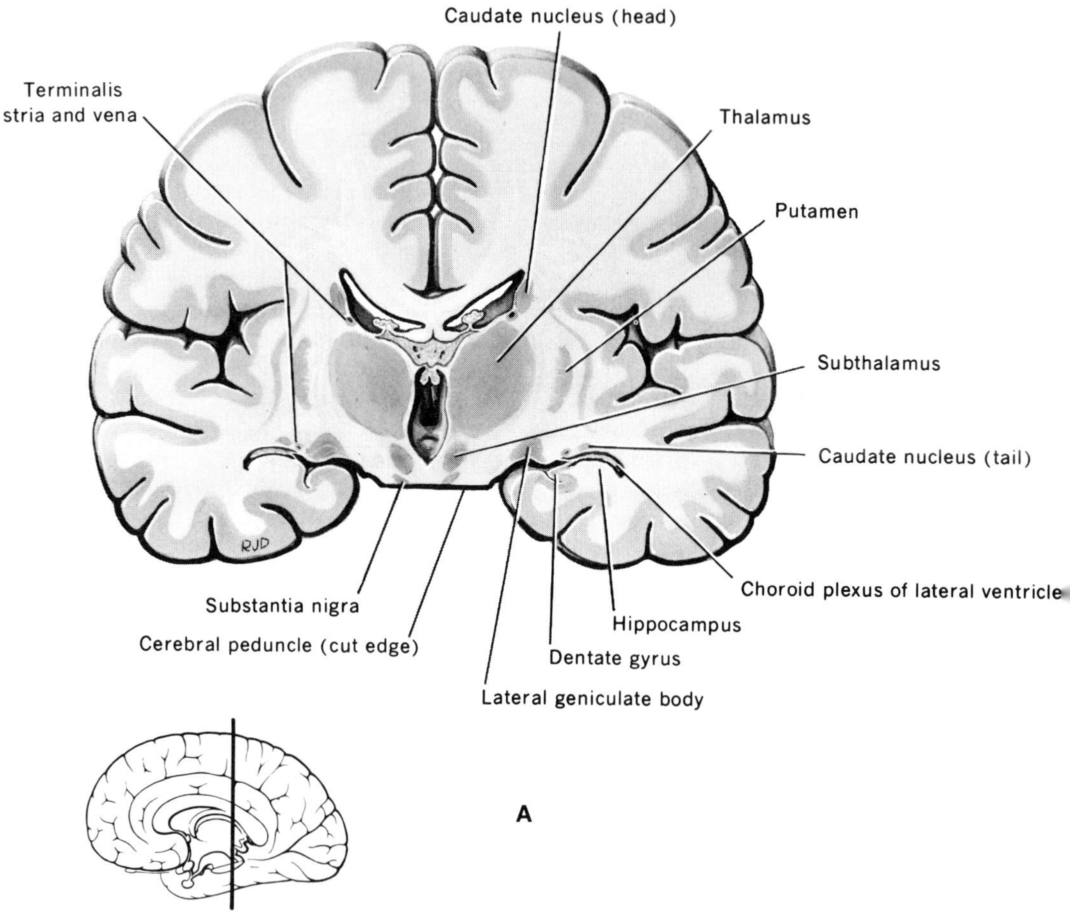

Figure 2–2 A, Cross sectional (coronal) view through the cerebrum at the level of the head of the caudate nucleus and the anterior limb of the internal capsule.

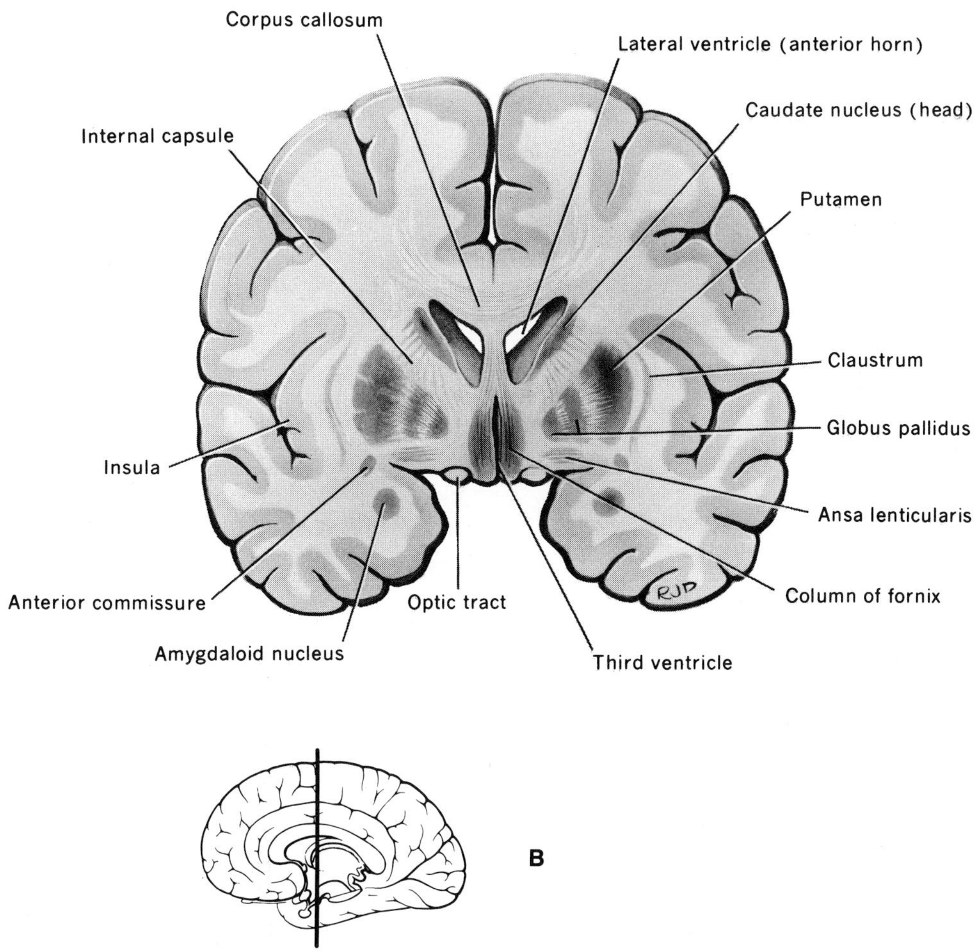

Figure 2–2 *Continued.*
B, Cross sectional (coronal) view through the cerebrum at the level of the globus pallidus and the genu of the internal capsule.

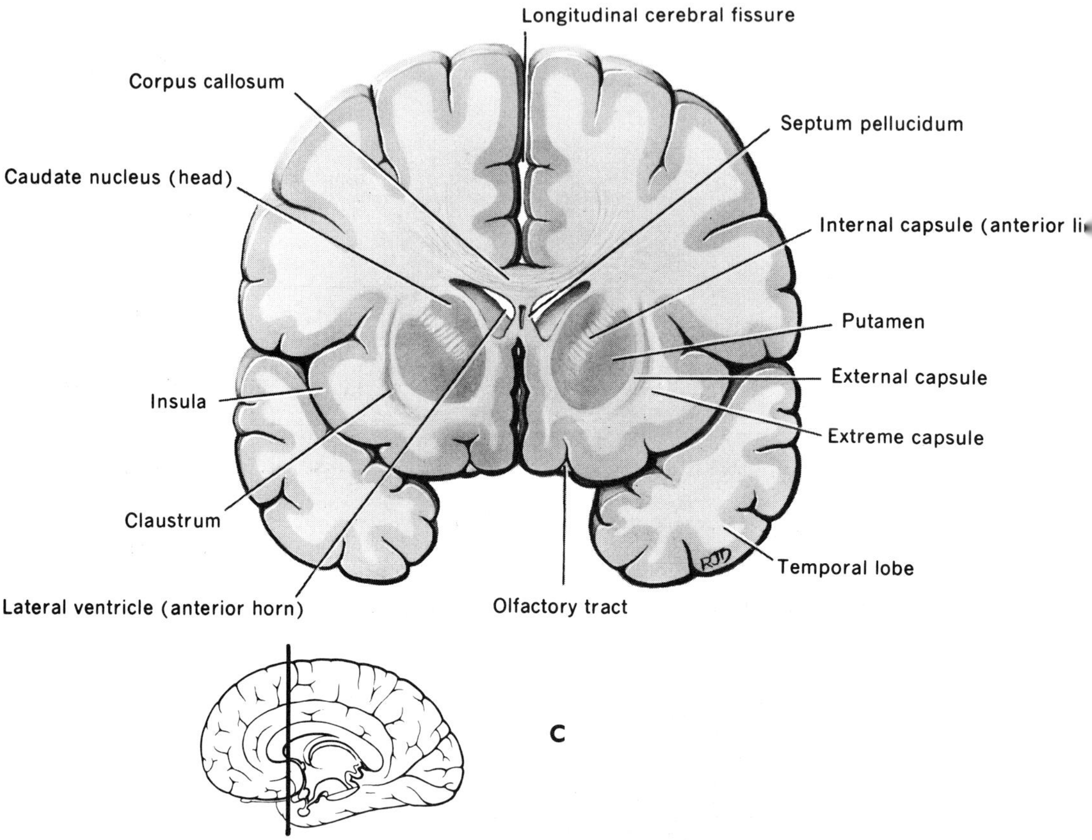

Figure 2–2 *Continued.*
C, Cross sectional (coronal) view through the cerebrum at the level of the thalamus and the anterior portion of the lateral geniculate body. (*From* Noback, C. R.: *The Human Nervous System.* New York, McGraw-Hill Book Company, 1967, pp. 15, 16 and 17.)

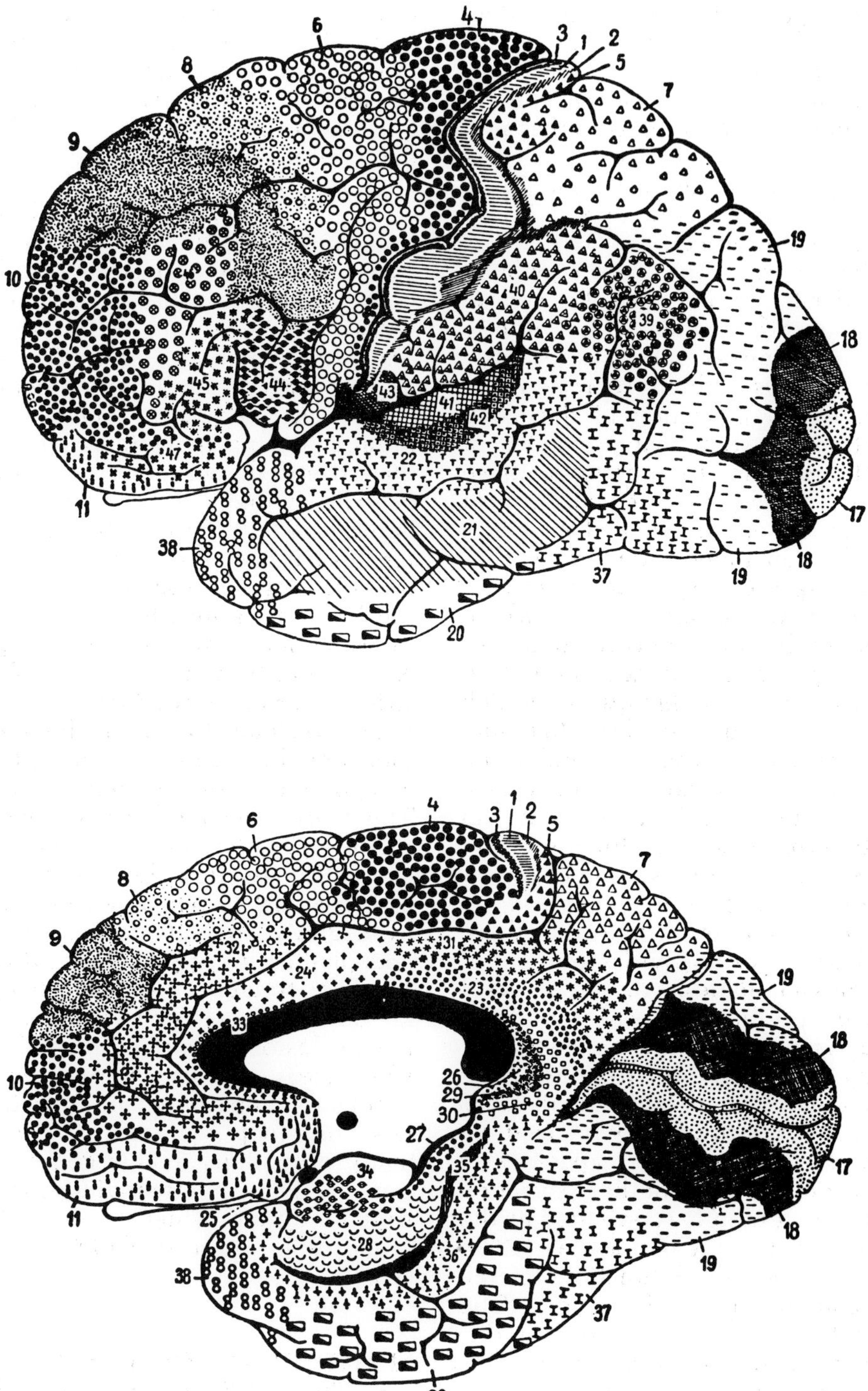

Figure 2–3 A, Lateral view of left human cerebral hemisphere, showing the cytoarchitectural areas of the cortex, as derived by Brodmann.

B, Medial view of right human cerebral hemisphere, showing Brodmann areas. (*From* Grossman, S. P., 1967, p. 121.)

central gray substance. *Brain stem reticular formation*, or *pontine reticular formation*, would be the more exact terminology. *Mesencephalic reticular formation* refers to that area within the tegmentum which is functionally continuous with the brain stem reticular formation. *Meso-diencephalic reticular formation* has as its referent the mesencephalic reticular formation, as well as those portions of the thalamus (the midline and intralaminar nuclei, the reticular nucleus) which represent the most rostral extension of the same functional system that originates in the brain stem. In contrast to these terms, which refer to anatomical locus, there are several that are somewhat less anatomic and more psychophysiologic; examples are *ascending reticular activating system* (which refers to the ultimate cortical goal or behavioral effect of activity within this system) *reticular system* (which has more of a functional cast to it than does reticular formation) and *reticular arousal system.* Other terms, which are combinations of an anatomical locus, a function and some reference to a system or organization, exist as well.

It is of interest to note that there has been a rostral-caudal gradient of neuropsychological research effort which has followed the rostral-caudal organization of the encephalon. Many studies in the latter part of the nineteenth century and early decades of the twentieth century focused exclusively on assigning capacities to the various regions of the association cortex. An example is provided by the classic study by Karl Lashley (1929) on the intellectual functions of the association cortex of the rat. (The contributions of this work are discussed subsequently.) Somewhat later, experimental interest turned to the role of areas of the thalamus and hypothalamus, and to other subcortical forebrain areas as well. The work of Anand and Brobeck (1951) on the hyperphagia produced by lesions in the medial hypothalamus in rats is illustrative of this period. The 1950's and 1960's have been marked by exploration of midbrain and brain stem function; the paper by Lindsley et al. (1949) on the impaired consciousness and EEG effects produced by lesions in the brain stem reticular formation is one of the studies which signals the beginning of the present era. Although studies of cortical and of subcortical forebrain functions have continued and increased in number during the middle years of the twentieth century, the rostral-caudal gradient has nevertheless been manifest. Part of the impetus for this has been the effort to describe the total vertical organization within the brain of various behaviors; thus, investigations which may have begun with describing the effects of restricted cortical resections have later been broadened to include the role of diencephalic and mesencephalic components of the "system" as well. The gradient also reflects, however, a rough parcellation of neuropsychological function: lesions in cortical areas are accompanied primarily by cognitive defects; lesions in diencephalic (and, particularly, limbic system) structures produce changes in emotional or drive-related behavior; lesions in midbrain and brain stem areas produce permanent or temporary impairment in consciousness or sleep patterns. There are many exceptions to this generalization, of course, but it provides a crude rule of thumb which is helpful in organizing neuropsychological research.

METHODS OF STUDYING THE CENTRAL NERVOUS SYSTEM

The oldest and most widely used method of determining whether a particular behavioral function is subserved by a given brain area is to remove that brain area and study the capacities of the surviving organism. Thus, after removing the posterior cerebral cortex of an armadillo, one might test the animal's capacity to perform a visual discrimination task based upon color cues. If the armadillo failed to learn that food was always behind the red door, as opposed to the green door, the conclusion might be that the posterior cerebral cortex is necessary for color discrimination in the armadillo. Although this conclusion might in fact be correct, it is erroneous on the basis of the experiment described. Several things are wrong with the conclusion, and it is instructive to discuss them in the context of methods in neuropsychological research. The experiment did not establish that a color discrimination is within the behavioral repertoire of a normal armadillo; prior information from other research, or careful preoperative study of the behavior in question and careful design of the study are necessary. This would include making certain that it was in fact the *hue* of the two stimulus patches that the animal was discriminating and not simply the *brightness* of the red *versus* the green door. Moreover, it is necessary to study more than a single animal, since the one chosen might have been a particularly stupid specimen. Instructive also would have been the tactic of teaching the animal two or more discrimination tasks, or a discrimination task and a simple maze habit. If the armadillo failed both tasks postoperatively, it would be difficult to establish a case for a specific association between the lesion in the posterior cerebral cortex and the deficit on color discrimination.

If one had established that performance of the color discrimination task did suffer as a result of the lesion, whereas other tasks were spared, there is still the possibility that the loss is somehow related to difficulty. If the color task were more taxing or demanding for the animal than the other tasks, it could still be argued that no specific association between discrimination of hue and posterior cortex existed; rather, there was simply an association between difficulty or effort and this cortical lesion.

The most powerful method for establishing an association is by the technique of *reverse* or *double dissociation.* To illustrate this in the present instance would require two (or more) lesions, two or more) tasks, and two groups of animals. Each group is trained to perform two tasks: a color discrimination and smell discrimination. One group is then subjected to a posterior cortical lesion, the other to an anterior cortical lesion. If the group with the posterior lesion is unimpaired on the smell task but deficient on the color task, and (contrariwise) if the group with the anterior lesion is unimpaired on the color task but deficient on the smell task, then one has established a specific task-lesion association. The difficulty dimension is rendered irrelevant by this experimental outcome.

To press further with this example, the question could then be raised as to what has been learned from this experiment. True, there is reason to believe that the posterior cortex is necessary for a color discrimination task. What is not clear is whether the behavioral loss reflects the blindness of the subject, or some higher order associative or cognitive weakness. Does the armadillo fail because he is blind or because the association between food and a specific hue is weakened? If the armadillo has simply forgotten this task, then perhaps he can be retrained. If retraining fails, then the assumption is strengthened that the function somehow resides in the posterior cortex and is now forever lost. If retraining

Table 2–1 Survey of Methods and Variables Encountered in Neuropsychological Research

INDEPENDENT VARIABLES	DEPENDENT VARIABLES
EXPERIMENTER-PRODUCED VARIABLES	BEHAVIORAL VARIABLES
Destructive lesions	Intelligence, problem solving capacity, memory
Surgical ablation or removal.	
Cutting connections or tracts.	Emotion, affect, drive
Suction.	
	Sensory, motor capacity
Destruction *in situ* without removal.	
Electrocoagulation, electrocautery (thermocautery).	Consciousness, sleep-wakefulness, attention
Irritative lesions: aluminum hydroxide cream, tungstic acid gel (to induce seizures).	PHYSIOLOGICAL VARIABLES Brain electrical activity
Ultrasonic energy.	EEG.
Radiation to exposed brain or via implanted materials.	Evoked potentials. Single neural elements. Slow, baseline (DC) effects.
Section of neuraxis.	
Cerveau isolé (midcollicular).	Hormonal, biochemical bodily constituents
Encéphale isolé (first cervical level).	
Midpontine pretrigeminal cut.	ANATOMICAL VARIABLES Tracing of pathways, connections
Nondestructive (reversible) agents	
Electrical stimulation	Nuclear areas; cell density, size, conformation
Specific brain area: direct, remote, self-stimulation.	Brain weight: thickness
Electroconvulsive shock.	
	Ultramicroanatomy
Drugs: depressants, stimulants, tranquilizers, transmitters, convulsants, memory enhancers or disrupters, hormones; administered systemically or directly into brain.	
Spreading depression.	
Cooling: whole brain, local.	
Environmental effects: work, sleep loss, oxygen loss.	
Environmental deprivation or enrichment: sensory, experimential (*N.B.*, may be irreversible).	
NATURALLY OCCURRING VARIABLES	
Epilepsy	
Brain injury: traumatic wounds, tumors, vascular accidents	
Mental retardation	
Schizophrenia, autism, other psychoses	
IATROGENIC VARIABLES	
Psychosurgery: frontal lobe, temporal lobe	
Neurosurgical therapy of epilepsy, Parkinson's disease	

succeeds, then the speculation is that other brain areas have come to assume the function. The factors involved in the recovery of a function which has been lost following a brain lesion are of considerable importance. This question is discussed at some length later in the chapter, but it has special relevance for pediatrics; the effects of destruction of apparently equivalent areas of brain tissue may differ depending upon the age of the organism at the time of the insult.

The discussion thus far has evolved from a consideration of the effects of a destructive lesion. The methods of producing a destructive lesion are numerous, and some of them are summarized in Table 2–1. Many of the individual entries in the table are discussed in connection with specific topics in the text; for the present, we will only touch on the major outlines of the table. The *independent variables* refer to a manipulation, operation or circumstance, either produced by the researcher or studied by him, the consequences of which are investigated. Clearly, such variables as epilepsy and mental retardation are not the result of the experimenter's action and are consequently classified as *naturally occurring variables.* The difference between *experimenter-produced variables* and what is here called *iatrogenic variables* lies not in method but in intent. That is, the several neurosurgical approaches to mental disease, epilepsy and degenerative diseases such as parkinsonism may employ the same tissue destruction techniques used in experimental animals. However, in the course of producing a desired therapeutic outcome it is often difficult to spare intact brain substance, and in removing a brain tumor the surgeon may destroy healthy tissue in order to facilitate removal of the tumor. The consequences for behavior may be grave but unavoidable.

Other means of destroying brain tissue will be discussed only briefly. Electrocoagulation (as well as other techniques) is usually used in conjunction with the stereotaxic method as developed by Horsley and Clarke (1908). By this method, various subcortical areas have been mapped in terms of three spatial coordinates (anteroposterior, lateral, vertical) which are located with reference to certain landmarks on the skull. Each subcortical area may be specified with respect to these coordinates; these in turn can serve to locate an electrode which may be positioned in this structure either temporarily or permanently. The purpose may be to record from depth locations, to stimulate or to produce a destructive lesion by the passage of sufficient amounts of electrical energy. This technique reduces the damage to brain tissue overlaying the structures of interest, since the tissue loss due to the electrode wires or shaft is usually far less than that consequent to direct surgical approach. Using stereotaxic methods, tissue may be destroyed by chemical means (e.g., aluminum hydroxide; Kopeloff, et al., 1950) or by ultrasonic energy (Lele, 1962). The latter method avoids the damage produced by the electrode, but is technologically difficult and expensive.

An alternative approach to the destructive lesion involves the use of *nondestructive* (*reversible*) *agents.* With this method there is hopefully only a temporary disruption or disturbance of the function of some brain area. The use of electrical stimulation or drugs provides the most common example of such techniques, although the precise effect such agents have on the brain may be difficult to specify. Sometimes it is clear that electrical "stimulation" may resemble ablation. Depending upon the amount of electrical energy delivered and the parameters of stimulation (pulse width, amplitude, frequency) employed, a lesion may in fact be produced by stimulation. In order to guard against the possibility of accidental or unintended damage, Lilly (1961) has proposed the use of a special pulse form (i.e., an integrated biphasic square wave) for brain research.

An example of research in which stimulation and ablation has similar effects is provided by the study of Rosvold and Delgado (1956), in which electrical stimulation of the caudate nucleus via implanted electrodes produced an impairment of delayed alternation behavior similar to that seen following electrolytic lesions in the caudate nucleus (Battig et al., 1960). On the other hand, the effect of stimulation of the ventromedial hypothalamus of the rat,—i.e., the suppression of eating (Larsson, 1954)—is opposite in action to the effect of lesions in this area—i.e., enhancement of eating (Anand et al., 1955). Stimulation in this instance appears to augment or intensify the normal function subserved by a particular brain region. Other questions arise in interpreting stimulation effects: Is the effect due to the deposition of metallic ions from the electrode? Does stimulation produce a small localized seizure? Of what relevance for normal functioning of neurons is the massive current (as contrasted with "physiological" levels) that is usually applied in this work? What about spread of current to adjacent brain regions? Is the effect restricted to the structure in which the electrode is embedded, or is the effect due to remote stimulation of other areas connected anatomically to the one in question? Many of these ambiguities can be resolved by appropriately designed studies. However, despite these questions, stimulation remains a popular technique in brain research. A special case of stimulation is the method of self-stimulation, in which the experimental subject is permitted to deliver the electrical energy to his own brain. This method, pioneered by Olds and Milner (1954) and explored extensively by Olds, Lilly, Valenstein, and their colleagues, has led to the concept of reward *versus* punishment "systems" within the brain. Experimental animals will perform responses repeatedly to deliver stimulation via electrodes located in "reward" areas, on the other hand they will learn behavioral sequences to avoid stimulation of "punishment" areas. Further discussion of this technique may be found in the section *Drive and Emotional Behavior.*

Electroconvulsive shock (ECS) will be noted briefly. By this method, a convulsion is produced by the passage of current through electrodes positioned on the head. Earlier research (Rosvold, 1949; Stone, 1946) stemmed from an interest in the neural mechanisms which underlie the recovery from psychiatric disease that may follow use of ECS. Recent interest results from the disruptive effect that ECS is believed to have upon the temporary neural circuits which are presumably set up during the process of short-term memory.

The vast literature concerning the effects of drugs upon brain activity (Toman, 1963), is testimonial to the usefulness of pharmacological agents as methods of altering behavior, as well as to the effort to understand how central neural events are altered by drugs. Some of the phenomena studied have included memory (McGaugh and Petrinovich, 1965), learning (Burns et al., 1967), the performance of various problem solving tasks (Bakay Pragay et al., 1969), attention (Mirsky and Kornetsky, 1968), feeding (Grossman, 1960), drinking (Grossman, 1960) and sexual behavior (Michael, 1965). Drugs in solution or in crystalline form may be administered directly into the brain via cannula (Grossman, 1964), or they may be injected into various cerebral arteries (Rothballer et al., 1961). These two methods are designed to restrict the action of the drug to certain localized areas. Drugs may also be administered systemically (orally, intravenously, intramuscularly). In neuropsychological research, the interpretation of the results of systemic administration of drugs depends heavily upon inferences from the results of direct neuropharmacological study of the compounds. Research of this type, based as it is upon inferences, often suffers from lack of precision with respect to the neural variables which may be involved. However, combining this research with other methods (stimulation, ablation, recording) may fortify it. Furthermore, often one wishes to learn specifically about the effects of systemic administration, since this is the route most frequently used clinically.

Spreading depression has been used extensively in neuropsychological research by Bures and Buresova (1960). Typically, the method involves the direct irrigation of brain surface with a small amount of potassium chloride solution. As described by Leão (1944), originally a wave of negatively polarized activity sweeps over the cortical surface, stopping only when the boundaries of a sulcus are reached. Succeeding waves of negativity recur, depending upon the amount of potassium ions present. During this time, all electrical activity in the affected area ceases, and the behavioral effects of this temporary deafferentation may be studied. Spreading depression is used most effectively with smooth-brained (lissencephalic) animals such as rodents; the absence of sulci allows the temporary inhibition or depression of neural activity to spread unhindered over an entire cerebral hemisphere.

Local cooling of restricted brain areas is accomplished by means of appropriately designed miniature coils or grids through which a coolant flows (Byck and Dirlik, 1963). Activity in the brain area in question is temporarily inhibited; brain temperature may be monitored through thermisters embedded in the cooling device. Whole-body cooling is used to reduce the temperature and neural activity of the entire brain. Experimental hypothermia has been initiated in this way to induce hibernation behavior in small rodents.

Research involving environmental manipulation has resulted either from practical, applied concerns or from more basic theoretical interests. Thus, scientists employed by the military have been concerned with the effects on brain function (usually, as monitored by the EEG) of reduced oxygen (as encountered in high altitude conditions), increased carbon dioxide (as encountered in prolonged submersion in submarines), jet-engine noise, prolonged work, or sleep deprivation.

In the 1950's there was considerable interest in the behavioral and EEG effects of restriction or reduction of sensory input, with the period of isolation ranging up to several days.

Research on oxygen deprivation, particularly during the perinatal period, has focused on the neurological and behavioral effects of neonatal asphyxia in monkeys (Windle, 1964). Also from a theoretical point of view, research has been conducted on the effects of deprivation of sensory experience or manipulative experience, or both (Held and Hein, 1958), on the later development of sensory, motor or problem solving capacity (Melzack, 1962). Restriction of visual input may result in irreversible retinal damage (Riesen, 1961), so that the effects of these restrictions may be permanent. The effects upon dogs of complete social isolation during development have been investigated neuropsychologically by Melzack (1962). Environmental deprivation, and its opposite, environmental enrichment, have been studied extensively in rats by Krech et al. (1962). Marked changes in brain weight (Krech et al., 1966) have been observed, dependent upon the conditions of rearing used with the subjects.

Behavioral variables, under *dependent variables* in Table 2–1, summarizes the essential material of the chapter; consequently, extended discussion of it is deferred to the appropriate sections. The following general comments seem in order, however, to integrate the *behavioral* and *physiological variables.* The last decade or so has seen a vast increase in the number of studies which combine behavioral and physiological measurements in the same subject, and some experiments have used the two types of measures simultaneously. This is in contrast to earlier types of research in which the effects of a lesion or of some reversible agent were measured on behavior. Such behavior may have been acquired before the experimental manipulation; alternatively, the behavior may be observed during the process of acquisition, as modified by the central neural intervention. Although this type of research has been enormously productive of information, it is essentially static and does not yield information about the neuropsychological *processes* or functions *underlying* the maintenance (or disruption) of behavior. Functions, mechanisms, and systems must be inferred and pieced together, borrowing heavily in some cases from neurophysiological studies of the same brain areas. This observation has somewhat less force in respect to studies with reversible agents. Often, the processes underlying a behavior may be inferred from the nature of the impairment observed. Understanding is hampered, however, by incomplete knowledge of the processes by which reversible agents exert their effects. Furthermore, there is a risk of error inherent in borrowing information from physiological studies in order to infer processes which can not be observed directly in static types of investigation. Most classic neurophysiological preparations are heavily anesthetized or have had some radical insult to the central nervous system (see discussion of cerveau isolé and encéphale isolé, p. 139) in order to facilitate recording. Because of the conditions of measurement, such research may provide only the barest outline of the complex processes occurring in a conscious, behaving animal. Although the static approach will undoubtedly continue to be productive, the type of information yielded by the more functional approach offers the promise of illuminating the dynamic state of the brain as behavioral events take place.

In this more recent kind of research, as illustrated by John and Killam (1959), Adey et al. (1960), and Olds et al. (1969), behavioral- and electrophysiological-dependent variable measurements are made simultaneously. The electrophysiological variables have ranged from single neural units, to evoked potentials, to computer aided analysis of the EEG background activity. This type of study has led to insights as to how discrimination behavior develops and is maintained; how the focus of neural activity gradually narrows or shifts during the mastery of a problem solving task and, thus, how the system necessary for the maintenance of a bit of behavior differs depending upon the point in time at which the behavior is sampled.

LEARNING AND INTELLECTUAL BEHAVIOR

This section deals primarily with studies that have been conducted on the functions of association cortices of the frontal, temporal and parietal lobe. The bulk of neuropsychological research has involved these brain regions which together form the great mass of association cortex or "intrinsic cortex" (Pribram, 1958) of the primate brain.

Guiding Principles

The approach of researchers to the neuropsychology of intellectual behaviors reflects their view of the general organization of the brain with respect to behavior. Traditionally, there have been two views: the holistic view, derived from or influenced by the Gestalt school of psychology, and the connectionistic view, which stems from reflex-oriented physiology and more recently from the impact of computer technology and the general influence of the cybernetic "revolution." According to the first view, the brain is conceived of as totally involved in the acquisition or execution of any skilled behavior; consequently, damage anywhere in the nervous system is regarded as detrimental to all behaviors, and experiments aimed at specifying the locus of specific behavioral functions are believed to be unproductive. According to the connectionistic view, the brain is regarded as a series of complexly organized reflexes or systems with quite separate functions or capacities residing within them or mediated by them. But these two approaches are not new; they are the conceptual descendants of theories of the brain that were prevalent in the eighteenth and nineteenth centuries. Flourens (1824) represented the view that intelligence is a function of the brain as a whole; in contrast was the view of Gall and Spurzheim (1810–1819), the fathers of phrenology, who maintained that specific human abilities and propensities were strictly localized in the brain and could be evaluated by examining the conformation of the head.

Exponents of the holistic view in the twentieth century have been few in number, but they have had enormous impact, particularly in that area of clinical psychology dealing with the identification and diagnosis of brain damage. Two persons in particular stand out: Kurt Goldstein and Wolfgang Köhler. Goldstein was a neurologist who derived his "organismic" theory from observations of brain-injured veterans of World War I. According to this theory (Goldstein, 1951), all humans are capable of approaching the world on either an abstract or a concrete level. The characteristics of the abstract attitude included the following abilities: to assume and to shift a mental set voluntarily; to keep in mind, simultaneously, various aspects of a situation; to grasp the essentials of a given whole or to break it down to its components; to generalize, abstract, plan ahead, to entertain the merely possible. The concrete attitude was defined as the absence of these qualities; to be stimulus bound, to be governed by and unable to escape from the characteristics of the immediate situation. Broadly speaking, the adoption of the concrete attitude by brain-injured persons was seen as a defensive maneuver. It represented an attempt to avoid facing the realization that one's basic means of dealing with the environment, one's uniquely human problem solving equipment (i.e., the capacity to assume the abstract attitude) is defective. To confront this would lead to a "catastrophic situation" (in Freudian terms, to be overwhelmed by anxiety) which is intolerable. Consequently, the assumption of the concrete attitude would avoid this confrontation. This was an inevitable sequela of brain damage; Goldstein believed that impairment of the abstract attitude could follow damage anywhere in the brain, although it was most likely to occur after frontal lobe damage. Goldstein and Scheerer

(1941) developed a battery of tests which are still widely used to measure qualitative changes in the abstract attitude. Some of the results of studies employing these tests are discussed later.

Köhler, the other major figure representing the holistic approach, is famous for his contributions to the Gestalt school of psychology (Köhler, 1947), a body of theory which stressed the wholeness or unity of perceptual events and which was, in part, a reaction against the prevailing physiological approach to mental life in the early twentieth century. According to this latter view, as represented in the writings of Pavlov (1960) and Sherrington (1947), complex behaviors were built up out of smaller sensorimotor units or reflexes such as those observed in the peripheral nervous system. Against this, the Gestaltists argued that, for example, a circle was perceived directly as a circle and not as a mosaic of individual perceptions of individual arcs. The brain organization which forms the basis of such unitary perceptions must therefore have the appropriate characteristics: the perception of a circle must somehow be represented on the field of the cortical surface as a series of excitations that in some fashion corresponds to a circle. Köhler suggested the term *psychophysical isomorphism* to call attention to the parallel between the psychological experience and the physical representation of it in the brain; he suggested that differential concentrations of hydrogen ions (H^+) on the cortex might provide the mechanism for the physical representation of perceptions.

The switchboard, connectionistic, localization-of-function tradition in neuropsychology is by far the more prevalent one and has guided or shaped the vast majority of research on the brain. Pavlov (1960) suggested that "analyzers" for different behavioral functions were located in different brain areas, thus providing one impetus for parcellation of behaviors in the nervous system. Also, the whole anatomical and neurological traditions of the nineteenth century—the cytoarchitectonic maps of the cortex prepared by Brodmann and others, the writings and studies of influential neurologists such as Broca (1888), Jackson (1931) and others—led almost inexorably to the belief that specific regions of the brain had responsibility for specific functions.

An example of a theoretical approach to cerebral organization based on the switchboard-connectionistic hypothesis was provided in the writings of Hebb (1949). Influenced strongly by the detailed anatomical drawings of cortical cells of Lorente de Nó (1943) Hebb, dealing primarily with perception, proposed that the basic unit of cerebral structure was the "cell assembly." This was defined as a contiguous group of two or more cells or systems of cells that become "associated" by virtue of being repeatedly active at the same time. The implication of this association is that activity in one cell facilitates activity in the other. Groups of cell assemblies are gradually built up into "phase sequences," which form the basis of the learned neuropsychological organization underlying behavioral events. Hebb's cell assembly notion (presented here in barest outline) was later amended and modified by Peter Milner (1957) to take account of some of the more recent facts of neurophysiology. Basically, Milner's modification added the notion of inhibitory cells, suggested that the cell assembly be confined to the cortex and incorporated some of the facts about the subcortical nonspecific arousal system. Generally, his modification consisted in reduction of the theoretical possibility that all brain cells become associated into one giant assembly which fires convulsively every time some excitation impinges upon the central nervous system.

A computer-oriented approach to brain organization was provided by McCulloch and Pitts (1943), who drew the analogy between a neuron and the primary unit of information of a computer, the bivalent binary digit or bit. Assuming that a neuron can be in either of two states (i.e., firing or not firing) they provide an explanation of how a relatively small number of neural units can economically represent a large number of "states." According to the principles upon which digital computers are assembled, the number 2 to the exponent of the number of units involved represents the number of different states to which a given number of units may correspond. Thus, three units (2^3) can represent 8 states, five units (2^5) can represent 32 states and so forth. If the brain has 10^{10} neurons, then it is possible to represent $2^{10^{10}}$ states at any one time, a number sufficiently large to account for the complexity and subtlety of behavior. McCulloch and Pitts showed how "formal neural networks," built up on these principles (with the additional assumption of certain principles concerning threshold, excitation and inhibition), could model any given function so long as it was defined logically and unambiguously. Research based broadly on these outlines, modeling various aspects of brain function (including the phenomena of the EEG), and employing digital computers has been conducted by Farley and Clarke (1954).

A more recent, more behavioral-oriented computer analogy to brain functions has been provided by Miller et al. (1960).

Standing somewhere between the two antipodal views of the operation of the brain (i.e., the connectionistic and the holistic) is the position offered at one point by Lashley (1951). He suggested that the fundamental aspect of brain integration was not provided by an aggregate of isolated reflex units but was rather to be understood in terms of patterns of excitation over large areas of cortical surface. Lashley drew the analogy between the brain surface and the surface of a pond: as pebbles are dropped into the pond from different locations, concentric waves overspread the pond, overlapping and intersecting in patterns of increasing complexity. In contrast to Köhler's approach, which might account for this in terms of a spreading electrical field in a fluid medium, Lashley's view was more structural. He assumed that the "waves" of excitation were represented by the coordinated, sequential action of the dense network of cortical cells of short axons. It should be noted that neither Köhler's view nor Lashley's view has withstood experimental test. Neither short circuiting cortical electrical fields by gold foil strips (Lashley et al., 1951) nor multiple surgical interruption of short-axon transmission (Sperry et al., 1955) produces substantial impairment of visual discrimination behavior in cats.

The various theories of cerebral integration that have been briefly noted here are still influential in that they condition the way that experiments on learning and memory are conducted and the kinds of variables and interpretations that come into play. A clear example of the relationships among theory, experiment and interpretation is provided in the work of Lashley himself, in a study which is still of considerable heuristic value notwithstanding the fact that it is over 40 years old. Although he was not the first to perform experimental lesions in animals and to study the effects of these lesions on problem solving behavior, Lashley may be credited with founding the tradition of modern neuropsychological research. In 1929 he published *Brain Mechanisms and Intelligence,* which was the account of a systematic and detailed effort to relate intellectual functions to the cerebral cortex in rats. Lashley used a series of problem solving tasks, including three mazes of differing degrees of complexity. His definition of "intelligence" in the rat was thus provided by measures of the animal's performance (speed, errors, trials to a given criterion of mastery) in several situations. In this work, studies were made of the effects of cortical lesions, which were produced by thermocautery, on both acquisition and retention of the tasks; from 1.5 percent through 82 percent of the brain surface was destroyed. Lashley sought to correlate the amount and locus of damage with the extent of behavioral deficit produced by the lesions. The basic conclusions reached by Lashley were these: (1) The greater the difficulty in initial learning of a task, the more it was affected by a given lesion (and the more predictable the relation between lesion size and deficit). (2) The larger the lesion, the greater the behavioral deficit observed. (3) The locus of the lesion appeared to be relatively unimportant compared with the amount of tissue destroyed. To Lashley, three principles in particular seemed to capture the essence of these results: (1) *vicarious functioning,* which means that one brain region apparently can assume the role of behavior ordinarily subserved by another area; (2) the corollary of this, *equipotentiality,* which states that brain areas are equally capable of assuming different behavioral functions; and (3) *mass action,* which means that it is the mass of remaining brain tissue rather than its locus which is critical for the preservation of intellectual behavior.

The results of this study underlie a part of Lashley's later holistic approach to cerebral organization. The impact of the findings has been enormous, and the principles just listed have guided much research and generated considerable controversy over the interpretation of experimental data. The study itself has been criticized on a number of methodological grounds, including the relability of the mazes used, and subsequent research has often failed to confirm the principles of equipotentiality and mass action. Thus, for example, Lansdell (1953), using the Hebb and Williams (1946) "closed field" intelligence test for rats, found that posterior cortical lesions were more detrimental than anterior lesions. The closed field test presents the rat with a series of different maze problems, one each day, and measures the level of performance achieved over the series rather than the number of trials to a specific, fixed criterion on a single task. It is argued that this is more formally similar to the way intelligence is measured in man and hence a more appropriate translation of the concept of intelligence for studies with the rat.

If the principles of equipotentiality and mass action are suspect as far as the rat is concerned, there is serious doubt as to their validity (at least as originally enunciated by Lashley) in the monkey and higher primates. Research on intellectual functions in monkeys has not been preoccupied with global concerns such as intelligence but has focused on specific functions and their cerebral loci. The cortical area which has received the greatest amount of experimental attention (and this applies to man as well) is that region of the frontal lobes which lies anterior to the motor and premotor areas (i.e., areas 9, 10, 11 and 44, which are rostral to areas 4 and 6 in Brodmann's notation; see Fig. 2–3). As is evident in Figure 2–1, there is a striking difference between the relative size of this "prefrontal" area in man and in monkey, which has suggested to some theorists (e.g., Halstead) that this is the portion of the brain responsible for the enormous intellectual superiority of man over his nearest phylogentic neighbors (i.e., the infrahuman primates).

Studies of Frontal Lobe Functions in Monkeys

Research on the intellectual functions of the frontal lobe in monkeys and chimpanzees was initiated in the 1930's by Jacobsen, Fulton, Nissen and others (Jacobsen and Nissen, 1937). A persistent finding is that bilateral removal of the prefrontal lobes results in permanent loss of the ability to perform either delayed alternation or delayed response tasks. In the delayed alteration task, the monkey is trained to alternate between two food cups (in which the bait is concealed until the cup is overturned); in delayed response, the animal is allowed to see the cup baited, but a delay is interposed between the baiting and the time when a response is permitted. Subsequent studies have established additional facts about this deficit: it will follow lesions which are restricted to the dorsolateral as opposed to the ventromedial portions of the prefrontal areas (Pribram et al., 1952); the principal sulcus of the frontal lobe is especially critical for this function (Mishkin, 1957), although lesions in the more posterior arcuate area and in the orbital surface may produce moderate losses of function; and subcortical lesions in the caudate nucleus or the corpus callosum may produce behavioral deficits similar to those of the prefrontal lesion (Battig et al., 1962). Other research has clearly established that the orbital surface of the frontal lobes (Brodmann areas 10, 11 and 12) subserves a different behavioral role than the dorsolateral surface, a role which may be more closely related to the suppression of strong response tendencies or to the failure of habituation to occur (Butter et al., 1963; Mishkin et al., 1962). This raises the issue of how the celebrated delayed alternation–delayed response deficit itself is to be interpreted. First, it should be noted that some lesions which impair delayed alternation may spare delayed response (e.g., the caudate lesion), so that the two tasks may depend upon separable, although overlapping, neuropsychological organizations. Some recent data by Goldman et al. (1969) also bear this out. Over the course of the years, however, both behaviors have been viewed as measuring such factors as attention, short-term memory and postural-spatial orientation capacity, or the capacity to maintain a set or orientation to respond. The contribution of hyperactivity (continuous circling is a common sequela of frontal lobe damage) has also been mentioned as a possible cause of the defect. Mishkin (1964) has summarized much of this thinking. A great deal of the work of Mishkin, Pribram, Rosvold and others has been aimed at providing evidence for one or another of these hypotheses. No single explanation seems to capture all of the facts; however, those which invoke such factors as "perseveration of central sets" (Mishkin, 1964) are particularly attractive, since they resemble explanations of the behavioral losses following frontal lobe damage in man. A complication arises in that the perseveration hypothesis has been advanced to account for the orbital rather than the dorsolateral effect on behavior. In any case, the possible relations to the human studies will be discussed subsequently. First, however, there are two other issues which should be mentioned: (1) In terms of the distinction made earlier between "static," and "dynamic" or "functional" approaches to the brain, the majority of studies discussed in this section have been of the static (ablation) variety. It is of interest to note that the dynamic approach has been tried, at least, and that the results seem to dovetail with the lesion studies. Weiskrantz et al. (1962), Stamm (1964) and others have shown that electrical stimulation of the prefrontal cortex (but not other cortical areas) can produce a severe but reversible defect on the two delay tasks. This kind of result suggests that the nature of the electrical activity over this cortical region is clearly related in some fashion to the behavioral function. A recent study by Abplanalp (1969) has shown that there are EEG changes over the frontal cortex during the acquisition of delayed alternation which differ from the changes seen during the learning of visual discrimination tasks. Further studies along these lines may help to illuminate the nature of the function and may aid in selection among the several alternative hypotheses that have been proposed to account for the defect. (2) The other issue concerns the role of developmental factors in the manifestation of the deficit.

Research on the recoverability of function following damage to frontal lobe tissue was initiated by Margaret Kennard in the 1930's. She published three studies of monkeys (1936, 1938, 1942) in which the age of the animal at the time of surgery and the extent of the damage were explored. No behavioral tasks were investigated; instead, the research focused on motor functioning following ablations of motor and premotor frontal cortex. Early lesions (prior to three weeks of age) produced no deficit; later lesions were accompanied by motor deficits which diminished over time so long as the lesion was made earlier than about seven months of age. Lesions made after this time produced permanent spasticity and other motor disabilities. Although lesions which were extended to include frontal association or parietal cortex increased the disability, destruction of the tissue alone was not accompanied by motor losses. Other studies of early effects of lesions are summarized by Kling and Tucker (1967). More recent research has focused on recoverability of delayed response deficits following lesions in frontal association cortex (and related areas), and much of this work is described in Harlow et al. (1968) and in Kling and Tucker (1967). Removal of prefrontal association cortex up to about 150 days of age may have no effect on delayed response learning (Harlow et al., 1964), whereas lesions made at one year of age or later produce the deficit seen in animals receiving lesions in adulthood. If a lesion made in an animal prior to 50 days of age includes both prefrontal cortex and portions of the caudate nucleus, then no recovery of function may be seen when the animal is tested at one year of age (Kling and Tucker, 1967). However, this combined cortical-subcortical lesion so debilitates the animal (including the production of seizures) that the interpretation is somewhat clouded.

Clearly, a promising start has been made in this area of research. Factors (discussed by the authors just mentioned) which complicate any generalization of the present findings include: (1) the normal time in the animal's development that the behavior under study may be acquired and (2) the possibility of subsequent defects appearing in the later life of the animal. Nevertheless, it seems reasonable to state that the skilled visuomotor behavior such as that required by the delayed alternation habit must be dependent upon a complex, vertically (if not horizontally) organized neural system; this system may involve telencephalic, diencephalic and lower levels of the brain. What may be happening in the young animal with lesion is that other cortical or subcortical way stations of the system may assume the role usually fulfilled by the dorsolateral frontal cortex. The possibility exists, therefore, that Lashley's principles of equipotentiality or vicarious functioning may apply to the monkey, but only up to certain levels of maturation. Whether the maturation at issue is that of brain cells or of brain organization (as suggested previously) is not clear at this time.

Studies of Frontal Lobe Functions in Man

Research on frontal lobe function, and brain function generally, in man is beset with a number of technical difficulties that are not encountered in animal studies. From an anatomical point of view, it is frequently impossible to specify the precise locus of the lesion in persons who have had brain wounds or surgical removal of tumors. Although the surgeon's notes describing the extent of damage may be careful and complete, the remote effects of tumors (e.g., compression effects upon other proximal structures) or of interruption of the vascular supply to the brain may be difficult to specify until an autopsy and histological verification can be performed. Further, even in patients who come to surgery for removal of an epileptogenic focus and in whom the lesion may be diagrammed with considerable exactness (Penfield and Jasper, 1954), it is often unclear whether other parts of the brain are not also pathologically involved because of the continuing, longterm presence of the epileptogenic process). Then too, in studies such as these it is virtually impossible to find two or more patients with closely similar damage or removals. Nevertheless, Brenda Milner of the Montreal Neurological Institute has made extensive and careful use of these subjects, as provided by the surgery conducted by Drs. Penfield, Rasmussen and Feindel. A unique subject population has been studied by a group of investigators working at the New York University–Bellevue Medical Center. Several years after World War II, Hans-Lukas Teuber and associates began to accumulate a series of veterans who had sustained brain wounds and who were sufficiently recovered to be able to participate in psychological testing. Later, the series was augmented by brain-injured veterans of the Korean War, and it eventually included more than 200 men. For controls, a population of over 100 men who had had penetrating injuries to one or more peripheral nerves were also studied. For more than 10 years this group of subjects was investigated extensively by Teuber and a group of neuropsychologists including Sidney Weinstein, Josephine Semmes and Lila Ghent. Also affiliated with this group in one or more specific investigations were Stanley Battersby, Morris Bender and Mortimer Mishkin. Studies were conducted on a wide variety of functions, including various measures of intellectual capacity (some of which have been referred to in the section *Frontal Lobe Functions*), sensory (visual, tactile, somesthetic) functions and motor capacity. Not only were studies of individual sensory, motor or intellectual abilities conducted on this population, but comparisons were made among the results of different studies so that the congruences possibly existing among the data could also be described. This coordinated, sustained and productive investigative effort is probably without parallel in the area of human neuropsychology. The advantage that it provided, in addition to the opportunity to see congruences, was that it represented a population of subjects who were essentially normal before their injury, and in whom such complications as epilepsy, the problematical remote effects of tumors or cerebral vascular accidents and the existence of severe behavior pathology (as in schizophrenia) were absent. The disadvantage that the population presented was that the locus and extent of injury were often imprecise or not well known, and could often only be estimated from the extent of the

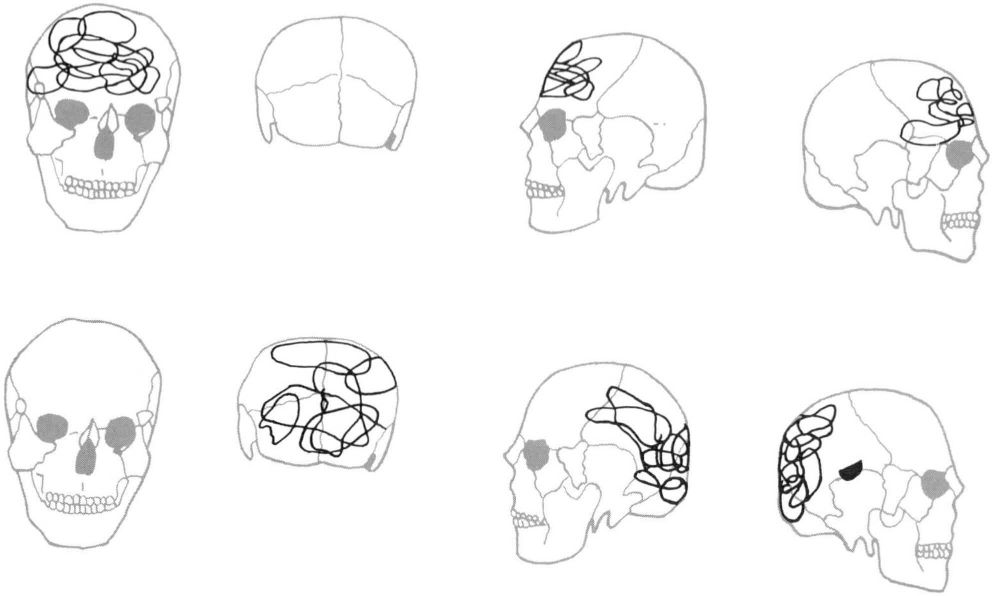

Figure 2–4 Composite diagrams showing outlines of skull defects in 20 men with anterior (frontal) missile wounds of the brain, and in 20 men with posterior (parieto-occipital) missile wounds of the brain. Anterior wounds appear at the top, posterior wounds at bottom. (*From* Teuber, H. L., and Mishkin, M.: *J. Psychol.*, 38:164, 1954.)

bony defect (actually, only the point of entrance of the missile) on the skull (see Fig. 2–4). In contrast with the careful description and measurement (and often, photography) of the surgical lesion as obtained by Milner in her cases from the Montreal Neurological Institute, the Teuber group often had only a terse description of the wound and the extent of the damage as dictated by a miliary surgeon under the exigencies of near-battlefield conditions. A further disadvantage was that with the exception of certain routine military screening instruments, no preinjury test information was available on this subject population.

Despite these drawbacks, the population has proved to be a useful one to study. The most successful studies, possibly, from a neuroanatomical point of view have involved the planned removal of identical brain areas from a group of psychotic patients (described, for example, in Mettler, 1949) in whom evidence of overt brain damage was absent.

These studies often suffer from built-in ineradicable weaknesses from the point of view of the design of the behavioral investigation. Studies of clear or relatively precise neurosurgical removals are invariably conducted on subjects in whom the essential normality or intactness of the brain is in serious doubt (i.e., psychotic or epileptic persons). Consequently, preoperative measures of behavior are often of doubtful validity insofar as their generalizability to normal persons is concerned. Persons with a normal history who have suffered traumatic brain wounds have almost never had any careful preoperative behavioral evaluation; the occasion for such evaluation never arose. Although records of school attainment, scholastic rank and the like are of some value, they cannot substitute for standardized, objective tests. The single, partial exception to this rule is provided by war veterans who have sustained brain injuries such as those from missile wounds. All men inducted into the service were administered quasipsychometric tests to aid in their military assignments, tests such as the Army General Classification Test (AGCT) or the Armed Forces Qualification Test (AFQT). The availability of the premorbid data has allowed some inferences to be drawn about the effect of brain injury on intelligence (of the I.Q. variety), and this is discussed later in the text. In view of these factors, the results of human studies must be considered with some caution; the issues of consistency and duplication of the finding, selection of the patient subjects, the nature of the brain insult and the existence of carefully selected brain lesion and nonlesion controls all have to be weighed carefully in the evaluation of findings.

In considering the effects of frontal lobe damage in man, the issue of effects on personality or character traits has almost invariably been intermixed with effects on intellectual functions. The largest single source of subjects with frontal lobe damage has been psychiatric patients who have had removals of prefrontal cortex for relief of their psychotic symptoms (usually, violent, assaultive or destructive behavior). Clearly, an effect on *emotional* or social behavior was intended, and any subsequent intellectual defect, if any, was regarded as an unfortunate if inevitable side effect.

As illustrative material this discussion will use three representative bodies of work on the prefrontal lobes, since a complete review of the studies in this area is beyond the scope of this chapter. The studies revolve around the work of Halstead, Goldstein and Brenda Milner. Halstead (1947) published a widely influential experimental study of the effects of frontal and more posterior lesions in man. His basic position was that the frontal lobes were the seat of "biological intelligence," which he was careful to differentiate from psychometric (the I.Q. variety) intelligence. Influenced in part by Goldstein's views on abstract *versus* concrete behavior, Halstead maintained that four factors comprised his brand of intelligence: abstraction, power, modality and a factor more or less equivalent to memory. These factors were derived from a battery of tests requiring simple psychomotor and visuomotor skills. They comprised such items as measurement of critical flicker fusion frequency, or CFF (that frequency at which a flickering source of light ceases to flicker and appears steady), performance on a form board (fit the square block in the square hole, the round one in the round hole and so forth) as well as other manipulative and discriminative tasks. Halstead claimed that his patients with frontal lobe damage performed more poorly on this battery than did patients with posterior cerebral damage and hence showed impairment of "biological intelligence." Although no attempt has been made to replicate Halstead's work in its entirety, studies have been conducted using specific portions of his battery; e.g., CFF and the form board (Teuber and Weinstein, 1954; Teuber et al., 1951; Mettler, 1949). None of these studies was able to confirm his results. In fact, when patients with posterior lesions were studied, they generally either were as impaired as those with frontal lesions or showed even more impairment. This suggests either that the damage to the frontal lobe patients in Halstead's study was not confined to the frontal lobes or that factors other than locus of injury contributed to the results he obtained. The animal data, together with the human data of the Teuber group, suggest that invasion of visual pathways (which is likely to accompany posterior temporal or occipital damage) is responsible for CFF deficit; the relation to frontal lobe damage, if any, remains obscure, and the concept of "biological intelligence" is somewhat shaken by this result.

Nevertheless, the notion of a complex multitest battery as a means of diagnosing and classifying brain injury still has considerable currency (Reitan, 1964) although not used precisely in the way that Halstead intended.

The approach of Goldstein has already been described. In collaboration with a number of other workers (Goldstein and Scheerer, 1941), he developed a battery of tests for use in the diagnosis brain injury. All the tests, he believed, reflected impairment of the abstract attitude. These included tests of sorting, categorizing objects, color matching, design construction, and measures of the capacity to shift. Since impairment of the abstract attitude was particularly likely to follow frontal lobe damage, it was natural that several of his tests were selected to assess the effects of selective partial ablations in the prefrontal cortex in man. During the late 1940's and 1950's, following the clinical reports provided by Egas Moniz (1936) and Freeman and Watts (1942), a number of fairly systematic investigations of the effect of prefrontal lobotomy were launched. The relationship between human and animal studies deserves comment here. Moniz was prompted to attempt prefrontal ablation on the basis of a paper by Fulton and Jacobsen (1935) reporting the effect of this procedure in two chimpanzees named Becky and Lucy. The study was actually concerned with some aspect of the delayed alternation deficit. Fulton described the calming effect that the surgery had upon Becky, who had been a somewhat difficult and intractable performer preoperatively. Egas Moniz suggested that this procedure might be of use in ameliorating the assaultive, destructive behavior seen in some psychiatric patients, and shortly thereafter reported the favorable outcome of this operation in a small series of patients (Moniz, 1936). Freeman and Watts (1942) did an extensive series in the United States with favorable results and may be said to have launched the lobotomy era. During this time, tens of thousands of patients with a variety of diagnoses were subjected to this psychosurgery (as it was called), in which various parts of the forebrain were severed, ablated, coagulated, undercut, bombarded with ultrasound and otherwise damaged. This era ended in 1956 when phenothiazine (e.g., chlorpromazine) medication was introduced and proved equally effective in controlling psychotic behavior; it also had the virtue of returning the responsibility of treatment from the neurosurgeon to the psychiatrist. Leaving aside the question of the longterm success of psychosurgical procedures, this period did provide an opportunity for some extensive research on frontal lobe function in man. The Columbia-Greystone studies (Mettler, 1949), in which some of Goldstein's tests were used, were among the most elaborate studies done. Patients not undergoing surgery were used as controls, and there were several preoperative as well as a number of postoperative tests on all subjects. The tests relevant to the present discussion included a color-form sorting test, originally developed by Weigl, which measured the capacity to shift from sorting geometric forms on the dimension of color, to sorting geometric forms according to another dimension. Also of interest was the Porteus Maze Test (Porteus and Peters, 1947), which indexed the capacity to plan ahead, at least with respect to the moves necessary for solving a series of pencil-and-paper mazes. Other tasks in various ways measured the ability to maintain a set. Of particular relevance, in view of the animal studies, was an effort to use a version of the delayed response task to assess frontal lobe damage. The pattern of results on these tests was similar to that seen on many of the psychologi-

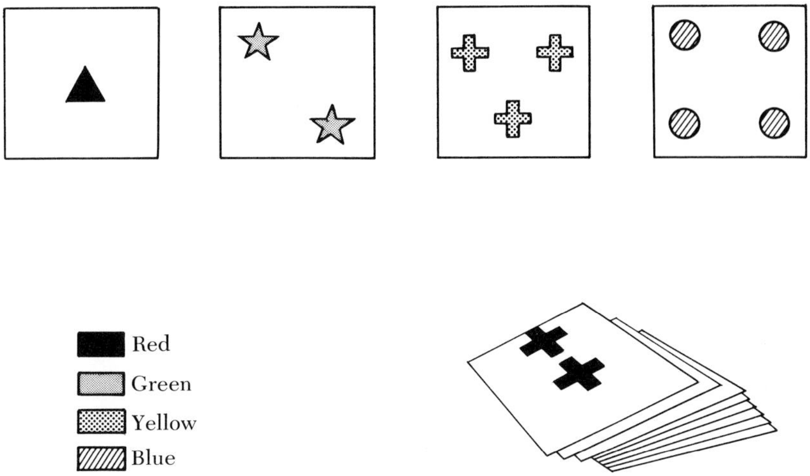

Figure 2–5 The Wisconsin Card Sorting Test, showing the material as presented to the subject. (*From* Milner, B. *In* Warren, J. M., and Akert, K. (Eds.): *The Frontal Granular Cortex and Behavior.* New York, McGraw-Hill Book Company, 1964, p. 315.)

cal procedures: postoperatively there was either no consistent effect or a small but significant drop in performance which disappeared on subsequent testing. In a second study, Mettler (1952, p. 315) concluded that "all changes resulting from the surgery used in this project were nonspecific and transitory."

The results of these studies are in contrast with one reported by Brenda Milner (1963), in which epileptic patients were subject to surgical removal of frontal cortex containing a focus of epileptogenic activity. Milner used a more complex version of the Weigl test—the Wisconsin Card Sorting Test—developed by Grant and Berg (1948) to provide a quantitative index of sorting and shifting behavior. The test is depicted in Figure 2–5, which is reprinted from Milner's study, as is the following description of the method:

[The figure] shows the test material as it appears to the patient. In front of him are four stimulus cards, differing in color, form, and number: one red triangle, two green stars, three yellow crosses, and four blue circles. He is given a pack of 128 response cards which vary along these same dimensions of color, form, and number; thus, in the example shown in the figure, the two red crosses on the response card correspond to Stimulus Card 1 in color, Stimulus Card 3 in form, and Stimulus Card 2 in number. The patient is then instructed to place each response card in front of one or other of the stimulus cards, wherever he thinks it should go, and is told that the experimenter will then inform him whether he is "right" or "wrong." He is told to make what use he can of this information and to try to get as many cards "right" as he can. No other cues are given. A noncorrection technique is used throughout.

The patient is arbitrarily required to sort first to color, all other responses being called "wrong;" then, once he has achieved ten consecutive correct responses to color, the required sorting principle shifts to form without warning, and color responses are therefore "wrong." After ten consecutive correct responses to form, the principle shifts to number, and then back to color once more. This procedure continues until the subject has successfully completed six sorting categories (color, form, number, color, form, number), or until all 128 cards have been placed. To succeed requires a readiness to abandon one method of approach when it ceases to work and also perhaps some interest in solving the problem.

This task was chosen because it provided some objective and quantitative measures of sorting behavior. In addition to yielding total error scores, this technique yields separate measures for perseverative and nonperseverative errors and for the number of sorting categories achieved. A perseverative response is defined as one which would have been correct on the immediately preceding stage of the test, or, in the first stage, as a continued response in terms of the patient's initial preference. All other errors are nonperseverative.[1]

Milner compared patients having dorsolateral frontal excisions with patients having temporal, parietal and other lesions. All excisions were done for relief of epilepsy. Some patients were tested both pre- and postoperatively, whereas others were examined postoperatively only. The results indicated a clear inferiority of the dorsolateral frontal group, both in number of perseverative errors and in number of categories sorted. The deficit was seen even in preoperative testing and was markedly accentuated in the postoperative testing.

This result is one of the clearest obtained in studies of frontal lobe function in man and suggests that the capacity to maintain a set, to shift set and to sort objects on the basis of different categories (all characteristics of the abstract attitude described by Goldstein) may be dependent upon the dorsolateral frontal cortex in man. Furthermore, this result bears a resemblance to the hypothesis regarding difficulty in overcoming perseverative tendencies (Brush et al., 1961; Mishkin et al., 1962), which has been invoked to account for effects of frontal lobe removals in monkeys. There may be, therefore, similar kinds of factors involved in the deficit seen in frontal lobe damage in differing species of primates, although the same *task*—i.e., delayed response—may not be appropriate to demonstrate it in both man and monkey. There is some evidence to suggest that the chimpanzee, which falls between man and monkey in brain development and complexity, will show initial postoperative deficit on delayed response tasks after dorsolateral frontal cortex removals; however, with repeated testing the chimpanzee may recover his preoperative performance (Rosvold et al., 1961). A result of this kind has never been reported in the monkey. The failure to see sorting- and set-related deficits in the psychotic patient who has had a frontal lobe operation, as described in the Greystone studies, may be due to characteristics of the specific tasks used. Other problems in the interpretation in these studies arise from the fact that the appearance of a defect may have been obscured by recovery from psychosis (with the attendant amelioration of behavior), or that the schizophrenic process may already involve so much functional (if not structural) damage to frontal lobe tissue that the effect of subsequent psychosurgical ablations may not be discernible. A review by Mirsky (1969) discusses some of the evidence of brain damage in schizophrenia.

Studies of Temporal Lobe Functions in Monkeys

An important stimulus for the investigation of the intellectual functions of the temporal lobes in monkeys was provided by the classic study of Klüver and Bucy (1939), in which the bizarre effects of bilateral temporal lobectomy were described. One of the symptoms noted (the syndrome is discussed more fully in the section *Drive and Emotional Behavior*) was that of "psychic blindness": the animals behaved as though they could not discriminate among familiar objects (i.e., food *versus* nonfood, monkey *versus* other animals, animate *versus* inanimate

[1]Milner, B.: Effects of different brain lesions on card sorting. *Arch. Neurol.*, 9:91, 1963.

objects and so forth). Although Klüver (1965) was skeptical of attempts to subdivide either the temporal lobe lesion or the behavioral syndrome, efforts have nevertheless proceeded along these lines. Studies by Chow (1951), Mishkin and Pribram (1954) and Mishkin (1954) have established that visual discrimination defects follow lesions restricted to the inferior, ventral surface of the temporal cortex. The hippocampus and the superior surface of the temporal lobe do not seem to be involved in the performance of these tasks. An interesting feature of the deficit is that it appears to be more pronounced, both in initial learning and in postoperative retention, in pattern discriminations (e.g., $\triangle$ *versus* ∇, or $\Diamond$ *versus* $\equiv$) than in color or brightness discriminations. The latter discriminations are learned with fewer trials, and the finding is reminiscent of Lashley's results with the study involving easy and difficult mazes and rats with brain lesions. It is important to note that the inferotemporal lesion does not render the monkey "blind." Losses in visual acuity do follow lesions in the striate cortex (area 17) but not those in the inferotemporal region. Further, the striate lesion is without marked effect on visual discrimination performance (Wilson and Mishkin, 1959). Efforts to implicate subcortical structures as part of the system necessary for visual discrimination behavior (as in the case of the caudate nucleus in the frontal cortical delayed response loss) have thus far proved unsuccessful. Lesions in the pulvinar (Chow, 1950) and in the superior colliculus (Mishkin, 1966) have not yielded defects in discrimination. These results, as well as certain anatomical considerations, have led Mishkin to conclude that the role of the inferotemporal cortex in visually guided behavior is to be understood via a relay through the prestriate cortex and thence to the striate (visual) cortex of area 17. Some of the neuropsychological anatomical studies lending confirmation to this hypothesis are described by Mishkin.

Studies of Temporal Lobe Functions in Man

The question immediately arises as to whether or not temporal lobe lesions in man are accompanied by loss in visual discrimination ability identical to that seen in the monkey. As might be anticipated, there is no direct evidence of a strictly comparable loss in man; there is, however, evidence suggesting that a loss in higher order visual cognitive processing ability occurs following temporal lobe damage in man. Bilateral temporal lobe removals or lesions, which are necessary to produce the deficit in monkeys, are very rare in man. Surgeons are extremely reluctant to remove both temporal lobes for relief of epilepsy, even though the EEG and clinical signs may indicate the presence of independent bilateral temporal lobe foci. This is in contrast to psychosurgery in which bifrontal removals were the rule. Furthermore, the likelihood of survival with a traumatic wound which involves both temporal lobes is virtually nil, since the missile or other object would also be likely to damage the deep midline subcortical structures necessary for consciousness and for vital functions such as respiration.

Another complication is the fact that the two cerebral hemispheres in man are quite asymmetric in function. It has been known since the time of Broca that speech is usually mediated by the frontotemporal regions of the left or dominant hemisphere. What has in fact been shown is that there are higher order visual deficits following unilateral lesions in man, and they appear to be most pronounced following right temporal lobe damage. Milner (1958) has shown that such lesions are likely to produce impairment of a task measuring the ability to perceive incongruous features in a series of cartoon-like drawings. In this task, the McGill Picture Anomalies Test, the patient is required to recognize that a picture of a goldfish bowl contains a bird, or that a sketch of a chimpanzee cage (complete with chimpanzee) shows a picture hanging on the wall. Other visual deficits have been described following right temporal lobe excisions in man (Lansdell, 1968; Kimura, 1963). There also is evidence for behavioral deficits following left temporal lobe excision, and several of these have been described by Milner. Patients with such lesions have deficits on tasks requiring the memorization and subsequent recall of verbal materials (Milner, 1963). Although such deficits can be demonstrated in patients who are not aphasic (at least as measured by standard tests), there may be some relationship between this impairment and the language losses subsequent to left hemisphere damage.

A study by Dorff et al. (1965) of patients who have had temporal lobe removal provides some evidence that both temporal lobes may be involved in visual function—evidence that

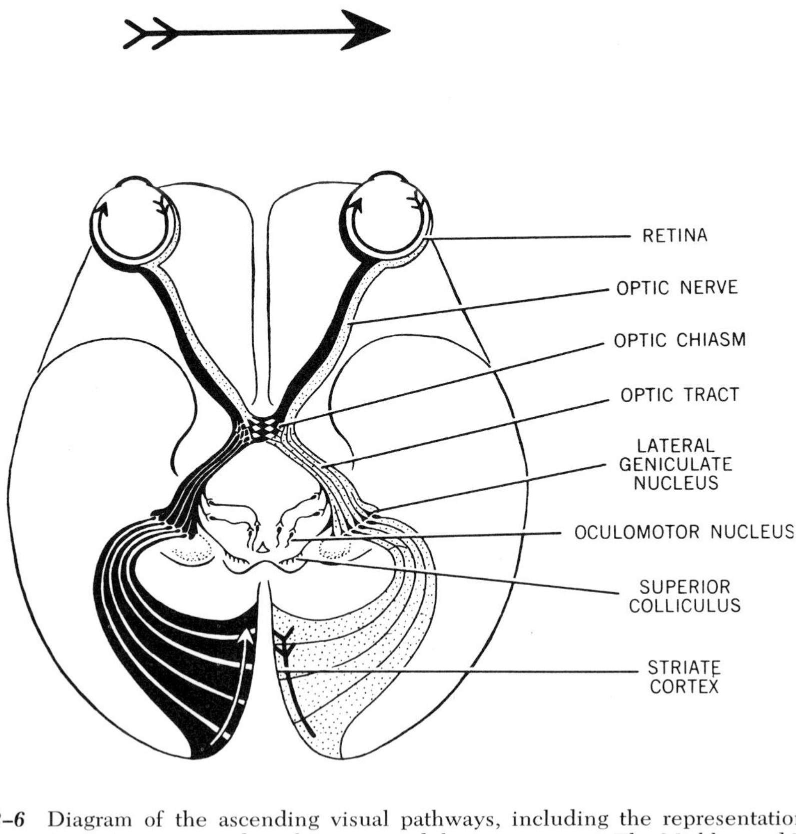

Figure 2–6 Diagram of the ascending visual pathways, including the representation of an object in space (*arrow*) as projected on the retina and the striate cortex. The Mishkin and Forgays (1952) and Heron (1957) findings indicate that words or letters presented at or near the point of the arrow (right visual field) will usually be perceived with more accuracy than material presented at or near the tail of the arrow (left visual field). That portion of the visual pathway represented as black is therefore more efficient in verbal recognition than is the portion represented as stippled. (*From* Polyak, S.: *The Vertebrate Visual System.* Chicago, The University of Chicago Press, 1957, p. 289.)

blurs somewhat the distinction just mentioned. This work was based on earlier reports by Mishkin and Forgays (1952) and Heron (1957), which showed that in normal persons, verbal material presented tachistoscopically to either visual field separately or to both fields simultaneously would generally be recognized better in the right field. This suggests, incidentally, that normally the *left* hemisphere is involved in visual functions, at least insofar as the processing of some kinds of verbal material is concerned. This relationship is depicted schematically in Figure 2–6. The presence of this asymmetry provided normative baselines with which to evaluate lesion effects. Dorff found that the ability to recognize simple nonverbal material (geometric forms) was equal in the two fields, but that the capacity for letter recognition was impaired by removal of both the left and the right temporal lobes. The effect was generally greater in the field contralateral to the removal. One condition of the study yielded results similar to those reported by Milner (1958) and Kimura (1963): when letters were presented simultaneously in both

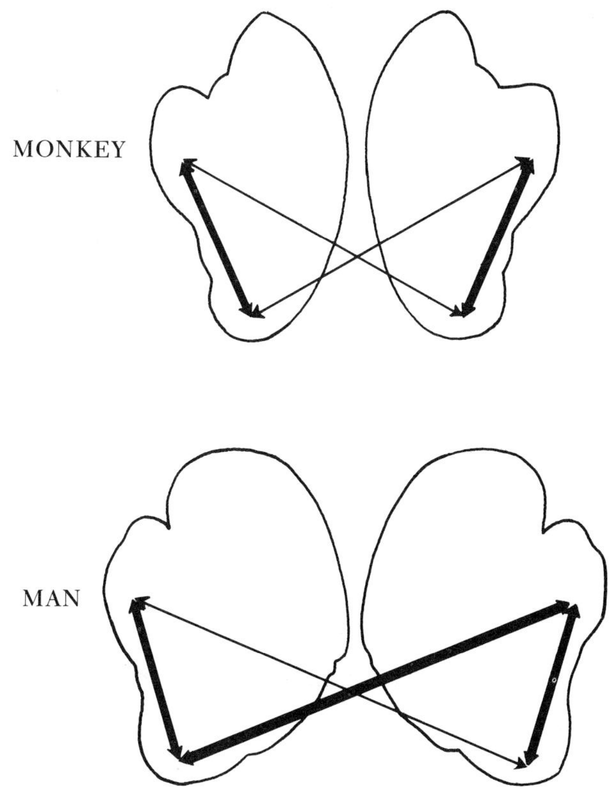

Figure 2–7 Hypothetical striate-inferotemporal connections in monkey and man, showing the postulated asymmetry in the strength of connections in man. Those interhemispheric connections between the right temporal cortex and the left striate cortex are presumed to be stronger than those between the left temporal cortex and the right striate cortex. The homologous connections in the monkey are considered to be symmetric. This suggestion would account for (a) the lack of effect on visually guided behavior produced by unilateral lesions in the monkey and (b) the deficit on visually guided behavior produced by right temporal lobe lesions in man. (*From* Mishkin, M. *In* Mountcastle, V. P. (Ed.): *Interhemispheric Relations and Cerebral Dominance.* Baltimore, The Johns Hopkins Press, 1962, p. 104.)

fields, the patients with left temporal lobe removals were impaired only in the right field, whereas the patients with right temporal lobe removals were significantly impaired in both fields. Mishkin (1966) has speculated that this means that the right temporal lobe interacts with the visual systems of both hemispheres (possibly because of stronger intrahemispheric and callosal connections), thereby facilitating recognition in both fields; by contrast, the left temporal lobe interacts mainly with the visual system of the left hemisphere (see Fig. 2–7). This theory lends some unity to the several findings concerning the role of the right temporal lobe in visually guided behavior.

The parcellation of function which has been described (i.e., verbal defects follow left temporal lobe damage, nonverbal and visual defects follow right temporal lobe damage) does not exhaust the intellectual functions of the temporal lobes. Prompted in part by the studies of Neff (1961), which showed that complex auditory (including tonal patterns) discrimination in cats may be impaired by temporal lesions whereas simple frequency or pattern discriminations are undisturbed, Milner (1962) reported the effects of temporal lobectomy on various measures derived from the Seashore Measures of Musical Talents. As before, asymmetries in the effect of the lesion were described: removals of the right temporal lobe impaired judgment of tonal pattern or quality, whereas simpler discriminations were less affected. Left temporal lesions either were without effect or produced smaller effects. The use of a different technique, derived from Broadbent's study (1954) of information processing in the auditory system, yielded results completely opposite to those just described. Digits were presented simultaneously to the two ears, according to a systematic design, and the subject was allowed to report them in any order. The performance in patients with left temporal epilepsy was significantly worse than that of patients with right temporal epilepsy (who were unimpaired), and this difference was enhanced by surgical ablation of the affected lobe. In regard to recognition in the two ears separately, in both groups there was loss following the removal, but it affected only the contralateral ear. This result emphasizes the greater effectiveness of the contralateral auditory pathway in this function. Obviously, the loss was much larger in the patients with left temporal defects than in those with right temporal defect. Another finding, which Kimura (1961) has also shown to apply to normal persons, is that efficiency of recognition is always greater in the right ear than in the left ear. This is reminiscent of the results of the studies with tachistoscopically presented verbal material. Together, the several findings (using the tachistoscopic material and the Broadbent test) suggest that man's left temporal region has a special role in the processing of verbal material, whether it be presented in the visual or in the auditory mode. In contrast, other kinds of discriminative abilities (e.g., visual, tonal pattern and quality) are more dependent upon the integrity of the right temporal lobe. An interesting anatomical finding which may relate to this difference has recently been reported by Geschwind and Levitsky (1968). In a series of 100 human brains, they found that in 65 specimens the upper surface of the left temporal lobe in the region of the planum temporale was uniformly larger than the corresponding surface of the right temporal lobe. It was larger on the right in only 11 cases. The reason for this structural asymmetry is unknown, but the fact of its existence provides a basic neurobiological understructure upon which the functional asymmetries in man (i.e., preponderant localization of speech on the left) are built.

Studies of Parietal Lobe Functions

Investigations of the parieto-preoccipital area of the parieto-temporo-preoccipital region of the association cortex (reviewed by Chow and Hutt, 1953) have suggested that the parieto-preoccipital area might be differentiated from the inferotemporal area in the monkey: whereas the inferotemporal area plays a role in vision, the parieto-preoccipital regions may be more concerned with somesthesis. Although investigation of this area in recent years has not been as extensive as that of other association cortices, the results that have been obtained bear out this differentiation. H. Pribram and Barry (1956) contrasted parieto-preoccipital lesions with those of the inferotemporal cortex. Animals with the inferotemporal lesion were impaired in visual pattern discrimination performance, but not in tactile-somesthetic discrimination of shapes or weights. Monkeys with parieto-preoccipital lesions, on the other hand, performed without difficulty on the visual task but showed some impairment in the retention of preoperatively learned tactile tasks. The deficit was greatly enhanced in the capacity for postoperative acquisition of a length discrimination. A very extensive program of testing somatosensory functions in brain-injured war veterans was reported by Semmes et al. (1960). Although the population of subjects tested was not restricted to those with parietal or parieto-preoccipital lesions, the results of that study have particular relevance for this group of patients. A large number of brain-injured subjects, together with control subjects having peripheral damage, were measured in pressure sensitivity threshold, two-point discrimination threshold, point localization and sense of passive movement. All tests were conducted on each hand separately. The results suggested that there was a focus of these sensorimotor functions in the parietal region of the left hemisphere, since defects in the tasks were seen in the right hand of those with such injuries. The effect of lesions elsewhere in the left hemisphere was much less pronounced. In contrast, lesions in the right parietal region were not more likely to be associated with defects in these somatosensory procedures than were lesions in other areas of the right hemisphere. The greater diffuseness of organization of the right as compared with the left hemisphere in regard to these measures of primary somatic sensation calls to mind the hemispheric differences for visual and auditory tasks discussed in the section *Temporal Lobe Functions*.

However, when more complex, cognitive tasks dependent on somesthetic function were studied (i.e., three-dimensional size discrimination and blindfold performance on a two-dimensional form board), the results suggested that the right hemisphere rather than the left hemisphere has a greater focalization of somatosensory function. Patients with either left or right parietal lesions made more errors than did patients with lesions thought to spare this region; in addition, the performance of patients with right parietal damage was inferior to the performance of those with left parietal damage. A similar finding was seen in speed of finger oscillation.

But a further complication is added to the question of cerebral localization and cerebral dominance of somatosensory function: a number of tasks are equally impaired after lesions of either parietal area; these include measures of the tendency to overestimate the intensity of two successive tactile stimuli, roughness discrimination and tacile discriminations of various types. The several studies just discussed are summarized by Weinstein (1964).

Dissociability of Functions

A thread runs through this discussion of frontal, temporal and parietal lobe functions: specific higher order cognitive capacities are localized in distinct areas of the brain. Researchers in human neuropsychology have always aimed at or have at least been influenced by the model of double, triple or even multiple dissociations of function seen in studies involving monkeys. Thus, dorsolateral frontal cortical lesions produce delayed alternation deficit but not visual discrimination loss or somesthetic discrimination loss; similar exclusive associations exist between inferotemporal cortical resections and visual discrimination loss, and between parieto-preoccipital lesions and somesthetic impairment. Although a case can be made for some kind of parallel parcellation in man (prefrontal cortex—losses in shift and set capacity; temporal lobes—losses in verbal and visual processing ability; parietal lobes—losses in somatosensory capacity) the situation is far more complex. There is strong evidence for hemispheric differences, a phenomenon not clearly seen in monkeys; further, there is evidence for a reversal of the importance of the hemispheres, depending on a seemingly trivial change in the method of testing or in task parameters within the same modality (be it vision, audition or touch). Two interpretations come to mind: One is that the human brain is just simply a vastly complicated organ and that the seemingly obscure or confusing organization of higher mental processes is based upon a host of anatomical, developmental and experiential factors that have not yet been understood or even identified. Another interpretation is that the brain is not as complexly organized as the studies discussed previously suggest, but that the pathological processes in the brains of those heretofore studied are themselves obscuring the simpler relations between brain and behavior. That is, shifting dominance within modalities (and possibly between them) may not reflect normal processes so much as the effects of long-standing epilepsy or undetectable, remote effects of missile-induced lesions or even of psychosis. And these effects represent compensatory processes, which tell more about how a damaged brain copes with the environment than about how the intact brain operates. The two interpretations may not be completely incompatible; in any event, the whole problem is the stuff of human neuropsychology. One additional note: since the majority of the data presented in this section are based upon lesion studies (as are the experiments using monkeys) they are open to all the criticisms of lesion studies. It is hoped that dynamic approaches, which reveal more of the activity of the intact brain, may be fruitfully employed in studies of human cognitive functioning.

The Cerebral Localization of Intelligence

As was seen in the discussion of the research on frontal lobe function in man, the question of whether "intelligence" (at least as measured by I.Q. tests) is impaired by brain damage is rather controversial, and all of the arguments which have appeared in print will not be reviewed here. However, it should be noted that many scientists feel that it is less useful to talk about "intelligence" than about specific cognitive and sensorimotor abilities. In the Greystone studies (Mettler, 1949, 1952), it was found that frontal lobe removals caused no permanent effect on I.Q., beyond a slight postoperative drop in score. Rowe (1937) has reported a case of a person who was subjected to a nearly complete hemispherectomy and who still had an I.Q. of 115. Other reports of preserved intellectual capacity following cerebral insult have been published. Despite these reports, the bulk of clinical evidence strongly suggests that I.Q. is impaired by brain damage, and that hemispheric differences exist as well. Milner (1962), Doehring et al. (1961) and others have reported on separate series of cases in which the Wechsler-Bellevue verbal I.Q. was impaired by left hemisphere (in particular, left temporal in Milner's study) pathology. This effect was seen in the absence of aphasia. Performance I.Q. on the Wechsler-Bellevue test, on the other hand, was more impaired by right hemisphere involvement, although this correlation was probably not as robust as that for verbal I.Q. and left hemisphere involvement. In Milner's cases, the differential lowering of I.Q. was seen to be an accompaniment of the lateralized epileptogenic focus itself and was simply enhanced by later surgical removals. These data seem to accord well with the data discussed earlier concerning the localization of verbal-memorization skills in the left hemisphere and of visual-spatial skills (as are required in the performance I.Q. subtests) in the right hemisphere. There have been only two studies in which data from intact normal persons were obtained prior to cerebral insult. In both cases, these were based on wounded war veterans whose premorbid AGCT (U. S. War Department, Adjutant General's Office, 1945) scores were available. Ross (1958) administered a brief verbal intelligence test to a series of brain-injured soldiers in order to match their general intellectual level with that of a group of control subjects who had not sustained brain injury. The question arose as to whether the groups would still be matched on the basis of AGCT scores, comparing the premorbid values of the brain-injured group with those obtained at an earlier time from the controls. The results indicate that the brain-damaged group prior to injury was significantly superior to the controls on the AGCT. To the extent that the brief intelligence test and the AGCT are comparable (and Ross provides evidence that they are), this result suggests that the brain damage had impaired the intelligence of the injured group and made them comparable to a group to which they otherwise would have been superior. Weinstein and Teuber (1957) reported a similar result with more specificity as to lesion effect. About ten years after injuries were sustained, a number of the veteran population that they had studied extensively were again given the AGCT. Those cases who had wounds of the left parietotemporal region showed a loss of AGCT score; other patients did not. It is not clear whether there is any discrepancy between the two results, since Ross does not specify the contribution of locus of specific injuries to the score differences he obtained. There is in any case clear agreement between Weinstein and Teuber's finding and the results of studies by Milner and others on verbal I.Q. losses following left temporal lobe removals; the AGCT is primarily a test of verbal intelligence.

A tentative integration of these results which seems to fit reasonably well with the material in prior sections is that the functions comprising the verbal I.Q. may be dependent upon the integrity of the left temporal lobe rather than the frontal lobe. Performance I.Q. is less well established in terms of cerebral localization, perhaps, but evidence strongly suggests a dependence upon the right hemisphere and possibly the right temporal region. The intellectual functions mediated by the frontal lobes appear to be too subtle to be measured by I.Q. tests, which show only a transient effect of frontal lobe damage.

Memory

Within the past 10 years, research on cerebral factors in memory has been concerned largely with biochemical factors rather than with anatomical ones. There are, nevertheless, a number of studies related to the localization of memory within the cerebrum, and these will be described. Some definitions should be introduced at this juncture. The term *amnesia* refers to the loss of memory for events occurring within a specified period; in *retrograde amnesia* the loss is for events occurring prior to a given point in time; for example, prior to a traumatic blow to the head. In *anterograde amnesia* the loss covers events occurring after a given point in time. Retrograde amnesia, to a greater or lesser extent, is a commonly observed consequence of head injury. Recent research has also suggested that a distinction should be drawn between the processes occurring in "short-term" as opposed to "longterm" memory consolidation or storage. Some of these studies are discussed subsequently.

The studies which have been conducted on cerebral localization of memory processes are chiefly the work of Brenda Milner (summarized in Milner, 1966), and they strongly implicate the role of structures within the temporal lobe. In some of the work described earlier, patients were required to remember either verbal or visual material for a short span of time. Those with left temporal lobe damage were deficient in the recall of verbal material, whereas those with right temporal lobe damage had impaired ability to recall the nonverbal material. But subsequent studies have suggested that it may not be temporal cortex *per se* so much as damage to the hippocampus, a diencephalic structure lying in the medial portion of the temporal lobe. Striking evidence for this was provided in a series of patients in whom there was severe and marked anterograde amnesia after surgery (Scoville and Milner, 1957). These patients had been subjected to bilateral medial temporal lobectomy, either for psychosurgical reasons or for relief of epilepsy. One of these, case H.M., is described as follows:

> The patient was drowsy for the first few postoperative days but then, as he became more alert, a severe memory impairment was apparent. He could no longer recognize the hospital staff, apart from Dr. Scoville himself, whom he had known for many years; he did not remember and could not relearn the way to the bathroom, and he seemed to retain nothing of the day-to-day happenings in the hospital. At the same time, it was discovered that he had an extensive though patchy, retrograde amnesia, such that he did not remember the death of a favourite uncle three years before, nor anything of the period spent in the hospital three years before the operation, but did recall a few trivial incidents that had taken place just before his admission to the hospital. His early memories were seemingly vivid and intact, his speech was normal, and his social behaviour and emotional responses were entirely appropriate.[2]

Some 12 years later, the patient's condition was unchanged:

> . . . His mother states now, as she did in 1955, that he is unable to learn where objects constantly in use are kept; for example, although he mows the lawn regularly, and quite expertly, she still has to tell him where to find the lawnmower, even when he has been using it

---

[2]Milner, B.: Amnesia following operation on temporal lobes. *In* Wittey, C. M. W., and Zangwill, O. L. (Eds.): *Amnesia.* London, Butterworth & Co. (Publishers) Ltd., 1966, p. 113.

only the day before. His mother also observes that he will do the same jigsaw puzzles day after day without showing any practice effect, and read the same magazines over and over again without ever finding their contents familiar. The same forgetfulness applies to people he has met since the operation, even to those neighbours who have been visiting the house regularly for the past six years. He has not learned their names and he does not recognize any of them if he meets them in the street.[3]

From the series at the Montreal Neurological Institute, Milner describes other patients who showed similar but less marked defects after unilateral temporal lobe removals which included significant portions of the hippocampus. In each case there was evidence of damage to deep temporal structures, and presumably the hippocampus, on the side contralateral to the removal. These patients were thus left after surgery with only a diseased unilateral remnant of a bilateral system. The Wada technique (1949) provides further evidence of the memory loss (in this case of a temporary nature) following bilateral involvement of the temporal lobes. By this method, which is used extensively to determine the side on which speech is localized, Amytal Sodium (sodium amobarbital) is injected on separate occasions into the right and left common carotid arteries. In addition to the transient contralateral hemiplegia, hemianopia and hemianesthesia, a temporary dysphasia develops when the drug is administered to the hemisphere in which speech is localized. This is the primary clinical use of the Wada technique. However, it has also been shown that if the patient has one diseased temporal lobe, then administration of Amytal to the contralateral hemisphere is more likely to produce amnesia for stimuli presented during the period of hemianesthesia than if the drug is administered to the diseased hemisphere itself. Here again, there has presumably been bilateral disturbance of the hippocampal system; on one side it is due to temporal lobe disease, and on the other to the barbiturate. This demonstration is even more pronounced if the patient has already undergone a unilateral temporal lobe removal. On reviewing the several studies designed to specify the nature of the memory loss in these cases, Milner (1966) suggested that the defect lies in the process of consolidation—i.e., the transfer of information from the short-term memory "bank" within the brain, to longterm storage. The effect of lesions in the hippocampus may not be so much due to the failure of this structure itself to store information as it is to a failure of the hippocampus to integrate the mnemonic activity of cortical areas. According to this view, which is similar to one advanced earlier by Penfield and Jasper (1954), the hippocampus is analogous to the tape heads in a tape recorder; the stored data itself is kept on the "tape," to which the cerebral cortices correspond.

Studies involving the use of electroconvulsive shock, drugs and protein synthesis inhibitors in memory research have recently been reviewed by Jarvik (1968), McGaugh (1968), Barondes (1968) and Agranoff et al. (1968). Under some, but not all, conditions, the administration of a single electroconvulsive shock (ECS) can produce a retrograde amnesia for events in a conditioning trial that occurred prior to the ECS. Disagreement exists as to whether the amnesia extends backward in time for as little as 10 to 20 seconds (Chorover and Schiller, 1965) or for as long as several hours (Kopp et al., 1966); the core of the disagreement relates to the question of how much time the consolidation process requires. On

[3] Milner, B., 1966, pp. 113–114.

the other hand, McGaugh, reviewing studies in his and other laboratories, indicates that analeptic (convulsive) drugs such as strychnine and pentylenetetrazol may *facilitate* the learning of a maze or of various discrimination tasks; the enhancing effect is greater the closer in time (either pre- or posttrial) the drug administration is to the trial. There is evidence, as well, that ECS effects may be reduced by analeptic drugs under the proper conditions.

In contrast with these studies on the effects of agents on short-term memory or consolidation processes is the research represented by Barondes (1968) and by Agranoff et al. (1968). Working with mice and goldfish, respectively, these studies have shown that inhibitors of cerebral protein synthesis, such as actinomycin D, puromycin, cycloheximide and acetoxycycloheximide may impair memory. The impairment is not seen in short-term acquisition or retention of a task but is clearly manifest at three hours to four days afterwards. The studies using actinomycin D (and to some extent, puromycin) are somewhat difficult to interpret because the convulsive effects of these antibiotics may exert a longterm effect on the electrical activity of the brain. Some evidence suggests, in fact, that the hippocampus specifically may be directly involved in the effects of the antibiotics. The cyclohexamide drugs are not reported to have this effect, so the interpretation of their action is less clouded. That is to say, inhibition of protein synthesis in the hippocampus may be a significant factor in the mnemonic effects of these drugs, but convulsive activity in this or other related structures is apparently ruled out. Nevertheless the key role of the hippocampus is consistent with the studies by Milner described earlier.

Any conclusions to be drawn from this work are necessarily premature. Nevertheless, it may be said that the perturbation of the electrical activity of the brain (as afforded by ECS) during learning may disrupt consolidation of memory. Short-term memory, therefore, may depend upon electrical brain activity. This assumes, of course, that other effects of ECS, such as its aversive quality, can be ruled out. Long term storage may not involve EEG activity but depends instead upon structural (i.e., protein buildup) changes in the brain. However, this summary may be an oversimplification, on the basis of other available research related to the problem of memory. John (1966) has conducted a series of studies in which visual-evoked electrical potentials are monitored from various areas of the central nervous system during the acquisition, differentiation and generalization of various visually guided problem solving tasks in cats. Using slow, flickering lights as the conditioned stimuli in these experiments, John and Killam (1959) have shown that there is an accompanying frequency-specific pattern in the EEG of many brain areas (i.e., 10 cycles per second, if that is the signal for a response). The appropriate 10 c.p.s. rhythm in the EEG may even precede the appearance of the flickering light in later stages of training. Central to John's theory of memory is the notion that the brain, or certain key nuclei, may re-create the appropriate EEG activity associated with a response when it is necessary to recall it from storage. He notes "something about the system which is elaborated in memory gives it the property to re-create a temporal sequence of potentials in certain places when memory is active." This "constraint . . . must be met by any proposed biochemical theory of memory. . . . When the system of neurons is appropriately stimulated at another time, the pattern of activity elicited reflects the spatiotemporal characteristics of the excitation which produced the chemical changes in the first instance, rather than reflecting only the characteristics of the present situation" (John, 1966, p. 183). Ultimately, then, it would appear that any complete neuropsychological theory of memory must take into account simultaneously biochemical (e.g., protein synthetic) factors, the distribution and character of the EEG and the role and interrelation of certain key structures within the central nervous system.

DRIVE AND EMOTIONAL BEHAVIOR

The research which is included in this section falls within two broad subdivisions. One area has been concerned with the neuropsychological-neurophysiological mechanisms underlying the primary drive states of the organism, including hunger, thirst, fear, aggression, sex and beyond these to the fundamental processes involved in the reinforcement of behavior. This type of research falls within the domain of the physiologist as well as the psychologist and may be considered to be asking the question: What are the central mechanisms by which the basic needs for survival of the organism (and of the species) are met? The other area is more clinical-pathological in nature and is concerned with the problem of the disordered and deranged emotional behavior which seems to be a uniquely human affliction. The question here, which is broadly psychiatric in nature, is whether or not there are disturbances (anatomical, physiological, biochemical) within the brain which are necessary and sufficient to account for the disturbed behavior of psychosis and for the other major behavioral disorders. The first area falls with the realm of classic physiological psychology; the second one does not and is usually considered to be the domain of biological psychiatry. Thus, for example, a recent 932 page textbook of physiological psychology (Grossman, 1967) contains approximately two pages devoted specifically to the issue of psychobiological approaches to mental disease. Nevertheless, there are many points of contact between these two areas of study (if not between the investigators), and much of the research in both fields has been stimulated by the same influential papers, which include studies by Klüver and Bucy (1939), Papez (1937) and Hess (1957; this is an English translation of a work that appeared in German 20 or more years earlier). In the work by Klüver and Bucy mentioned earlier in the section on *temporal lobe function,* a complex syndrome of behavioral change was seen to follow bilateral removal of the temporal lobes of monkeys. In addition to the symptom of "psychic blindness" (difficulty in distinguishing between familiar objects on the basis of visual cues) the animals were described as follows: (1) They were changed from their normally aggressive state to one characterized by tameness and placidity, so that they could be approached and touched by the observer with impunity. (2) They exhibited markedly changed oral tendencies, so that they would indiscriminately and repeatedly mouth unpreferred foods, such as meat, and even nonfood objects, such as nails, feces, lighted matches and snakes. (3) They exhibited exaggerated sexual behavior, approaching male and female monkeys indiscriminately, and even attempted to copulate with other species (cats and dogs) as well as with inanimate objects such as brooms. (4) Their social behavior was radically altered; they treated other monkeys as inanimate objects (i.e., attempting to sit on them). Further, they acted as though they had forgotten their position in the pecking order or dominance hierarchy and were repeatedly punished by more dominant animals when they attempted to obtain food in a group-cage situation. Klüver (1951) considered this drastic alteration of behavior to be due to removal of the temporal lobe as a whole, and, as noted previously, he was skeptical of attempts to relate specific behavioral changes to specific loci of damage. Nevertheless, subsequent research, some of which is discussed later, suggests that the emotional-social-affective changes in the monkeys probably have little to do with the large temporal neocortical resection included within the lobectomy; these appear to be related more specifically to damage to deep subcortical structures within the temporal lobe. The classic paper of Papez (1937) provides a theoretical rationale as to why this should be the case.

Earlier anatomists used the term rhinencephalon (nosebrain) to describe the function of that system of structures within the forebrain which were apparently related to olfaction. These include the olfactory bulb itself, the olfactory tubercle and various other related cortical and subcortical tissue. Connections exist between these structures and other diencephalic areas; the presence of these connections plus the fact of contiguity suggested that the whole of the diencephalon was a nosebrain. On the basis of an extensive review of the literature, Papez proposed that there was a broader, more important role for this region of the brain: namely, the expression and experience of emotion. The Papez "circuit" included the hypothalamus, the anterior thalamic nuclei, the cingulate gyrus, the hippocampus and their interconnections. The inclusion of the cingulate gyrus was important, for this provided the cortical link necessary for emotion to be experienced. The link to the Klüver-Bucy phenomenon is readily seen, since the hippocampus is extensively damaged by a temporal lobectomy. Beginning in 1949, MacLean (1949, 1952, 1954, 1958) published a series of articles in which he called attention to the Papez theory and updated it considerably in terms of anatomical, physiological and behavioral evidence. The role of the amygdala in the system was emphasized, as was that of some other structures, but the major modifications of the Papez proposal concerned some of the implications of the theory. MacLean resurrected the term limbic system (originally proposed by Broca) to refer to the Papez circuit: the ring of structures around the midbrain and brain stem. He pointed out that the cortex of the limbic system was phylogenetically ancient, being either primitive paleocortex in the case of the hippocampus itself or mesocortex in the case of the cingulate and hippocampal gyri. The MacLean "limbic system" is presented in Figure 2–8. Furthermore, although the amount of neocortex had proliferated greatly in the higher as compared with lower mammals, paleo- and mesocortex had not. And yet these are the "higher" cerebral components of the emotion-handling machinery of the central nervous system! The fact that complex cognitive-affective decisions had to be made by a brain system that had changed little since the rabbit could account for the sorry state of human emotional affairs; in addition, the fact that the cortex most directly connected with the regulation of visceral and autonomic functions was meso- and not neocortex might have a bearing on human psychosomatic disease. MacLean later (1958) suggested a parcellation of function with the limbic system: the rostral frontotemporal-amygdaloid circuit was more concerned with feeding, fight and flight behavior (i.e., the preservation of the self); the more caudal circuit, comprising the septal

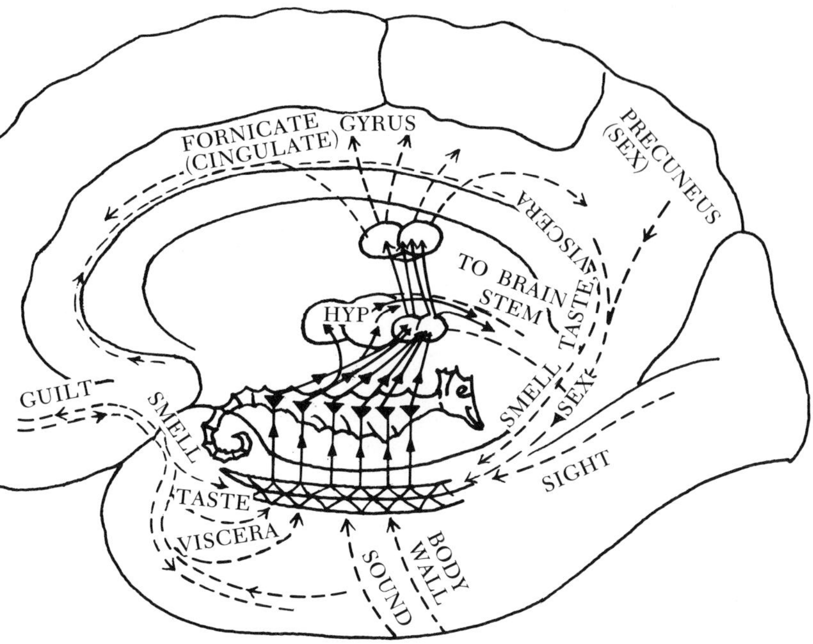

Figure 2–8 MacLean's limbic system (*ca.* 1949). Note the pre-eminent role and position afforded the hippocampus or "seahorse." (*From* MacLean, P. B.: *Psychosom. Med., 11*:345, 1949.)

region, hippocampus and cingulate gyrus, was more concerned with the expression, experience and effecting of states related to sexual behavior (i.e., the preservation of the species). Whether or not the MacLean theory is accepted, it is certainly compatible with, and provides a theoretical rationale for, the striking changes in affective behavior seen in the Klüver-Bucy preparations.

An alternative view of the limbic system complex has been provided by Pribram and Kruger (1954). According to this view, based again upon a review of anatomical, physiological and behavioral evidence, the Papez theory circuit is more appropriately subdivided into three major subsystems: (1) The first subsystem comprises those structures directly concerned with olfaction, such as the olfactory bulb and tubercle, the corticomedial area of the amygdala and related structures. (2) The second receives some afferents from the first and comprises the septal, subcallosal and frontotemporal areas, and the basolateral nuclei of the amygdala. (3) The third receives afferents from the second system only and consists of the major portion (in terms of mass) of the limbic system; it includes entorhinal cortex, the retrosplenial and cingulate gyri and the hippocampal formation. Pribram and Kruger concluded that the major role in the mediation of emotion was played by the second system, and that the first and third systems were more concerned with other matters. The three "systems" are illustrated in Figure 2–9. MacLean, and Pribram and Kruger are thus seen to differ with respect to the inclusion of the cingulate gyrus and hippocampus into the business of emotion.

The third work of germinal importance to be discussed is that of Hess. In the technique he developed and used extensively, cats were fitted with permanently implanted electrodes in various regions of the diencephalon. They were then stimu-

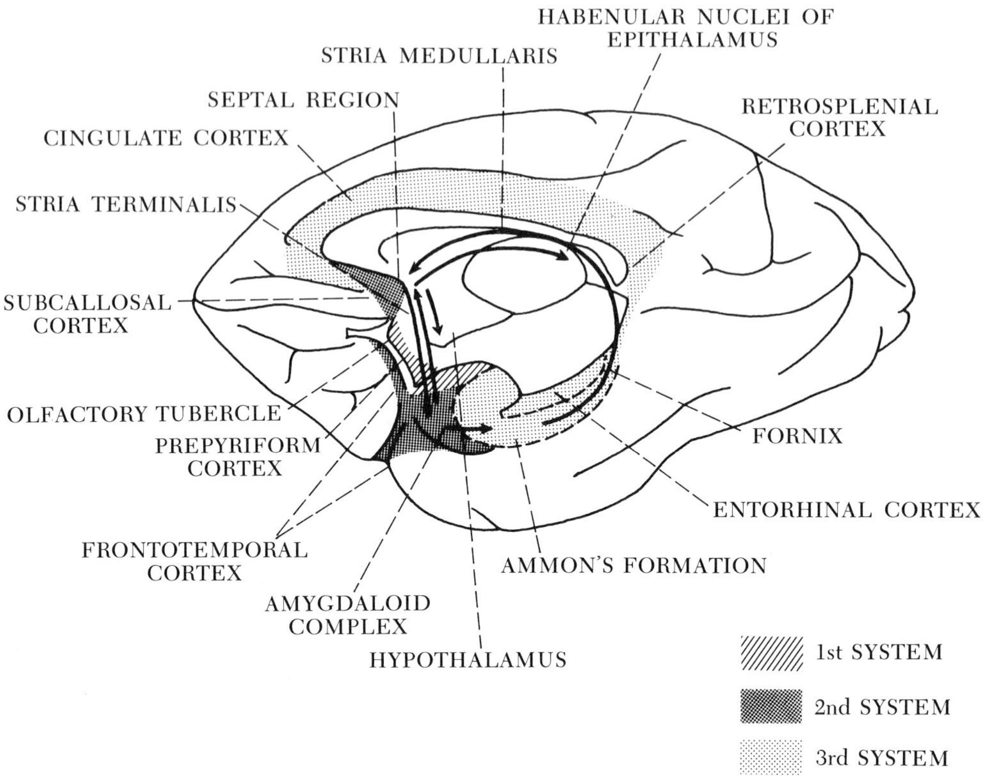

Figure 2–9 Pribram and Kruger's limbic system as seen on a mediobasal view of the right cerebral hemisphere of a monkey. The three rhinal systems are shown. The checkered area (second system) is afforded the pre-eminent role. Contrast this figure with Figure 2–8. (*From* Pribram, K., and Kruger, L., 1954, p. 116.)

lated systematically with low frequency pulses while in the conscious state, usually in a free-ranging situation. Hess made extensive and detailed observation of a wide variety of visceral, autonomic and affective behaviors that were elicited by stimulation, including feeding, drinking, micturition, defecation, vomiting, respiration, rage, arousal, flight and sleep. On the basis of a review of the neuroanatomical location of the various behaviors he had observed (which comprised hundreds of stimulation points), Hess concluded that they could best be summarized on the basis of a two-factor theory. There were, he said, two major systems localized within the diencephalon. One, which he labeled the *ergotropic*, was basically an adrenergic (epinephrine-dependent) system and had to do with the expenditure of energy—the mobilization of the organism for action (be it fight or flight). The second system, which he called the *trophotropic* was concerned with the preservation and conservation of energy. This cholinergic (acetylcholine-dependent) system acted antagonistically to the first and was brought into play when sleep occurred. This could be dramatically demonstrated by stimulation in the region of the medial thalamus: the cat assumed the natural posture associated with sleep and gradually went to sleep. Hess believed that the trophotropic "zone" was more rostrally localized; however, since there was a considerable degree of overlap between the points in the ergotropic and trophotropic systems, a case could not be made for the absolute spatial-anatomical localization or dominance of either one. What was involved instead was a complex, dynamic interplay between the two, resulting in the smooth ordering of adaptive behavior.

Neuropsychological Mechanisms Underlying Basic Drive States

Complete coverage of the area of research related to neural mechanisms underlying the basic drive states is clearly beyond the scope of this chapter. In his recent textbook of physiological psychology, for example, Grossman devotes 300 pages to the work in this area (Grossman, 1967, pp. 313–617). Consequently, what will be attempted here is a review of the broad outline of some of this research, and a few remarks concerning the goal and directions of the efforts.

A difficulty which must be borne in mind when considering research on drive and emotion that has been conducted with animals is that an important source of information about the effects of any neurological manipulation is absent: namely, the subjective report of the individual. While it is true that we can readily identify and classify various behaviors in animals into categories (e.g., feeding, drinking, aggressive, flight, copulatory), we can be relatively secure about the effects of an experimental treatment only when behavior is absent. Thus, it is clear that lesions in the lateral areas of the hypothalamus will reduce or abolish eating for greater or lesser periods of time. We are not quite sure that the animal is no longer *hungry*, for it may be that the treatment has simply caused him to forget how to eat. This dilemma about the overt, objective *versus* the covert, subjective efforts of a brain lesion (or other manipulation) is even more acute when the effect is to elicit some drive-related behavior. Without subjective reports, one is never certain that the treatment has not simply caused some part of the motor expression of a drive to be elicited in more or less automatic fashion, disconnected from the central experience of the emotion. Walter Cannon (1931) made essentially this criticism of the James-Lange theory of emotion, which held that the experience of the peripheral autonomic accompaniments of emotion were *themselves* the emotion. This criticism has a certain amount of force especially in relation to hypothalamic hyperphagia; Miller et al. (1950) showed that although a rat with destruction of the ventromedial hypothalamus would eat until it became obese, it would do so only if food were available *ad libitum*. On standard measures of hunger *drive*, such an animal would work less than normal rats to obtain food. Subsequent research confirmed this and led to the conception that hunger was not increased by the lesion; rather, it had impaired the mechanism which controls cessation of eating. Clearly, therefore, the possibility of some sort of disconnection of central from peripheral manifestations of drive-related behavior is no mere sophistical ploy but may aid in interpreting the results of experimental studies on drive states. But more than just a disconnection is implied; the issue is that behavior as complex as that usually considered as emotional is based on cognitive (memory, experience, interpretation) factors as well as the central and motor expression of some specific drive state, and it probably therefore includes a neuropsychological organization which involves many if not all levels of the neuraxis.

In general, the work that has been done seems to conform reasonably well with the theoretical assumption that manipulation of the structures within the limbic system (to use the least controversial term) will alter the maintenance and expression of drive-related behavior. A considerable amount of research has centered on the hypothalamus, which seems to play a key role in the regulation of eating (Teitelbaum, 1961), drinking (Andersson, 1953), sex behavior (Sawyer, 1960) and attack and flight behavior (Hunsperger, 1956). In addition to the methods of electrolytic lesions and electrical stimulation, some researchers (Grossman, 1964) have utilized the direct injection (via cannulae) of adrenergic (e.g., norepinephrine) and cholinergic (e.g., acetylcholine) substances into the hypothalamus, producing increased eating or drinking, respectively; or the local cooling of areas of the hypothalamus (Andersson and Larsson, 1961), which produces a reversible cessation of water intake. There are many reports, as well, of effects similar to these produced by lesions in other limbic system areas; thus, changes in feeding, drinking, aggressiveness and sexual behavior have been reported to follow destruction of the amygdala, hippocampus or areas of limbic cortex (Fonberg, 1963; Fuller, 1957; Grossman and Grossman, 1963; Rosvold et al., 1954; Schreiner and Kling, 1953). Altered aggressiveness also follows neocortical removals (Bard and Mountcastle, 1948). A considerable amount of evidence has been gathered, as well, on the role of what might be called peripheral factors in the genesis and display of these altered drive states; thus, the hyperphagic rat with lesions in the ventromedial hypothalamus is exquisitely sensitive to alterations in the taste of food (Teitelbaum, 1955) and may stop eating when substances such as quinine are added to its diet. These alterations may be without effect on the food intake of normal rats. Similarly, the "taming" seen in monkeys with amygdala lesions may be a function of the testing situation in which the animal is observed. Taming or loss of dominance in a group-cage situation may resemble increased aggressiveness and fearlessness in an individual-cage situation (Rosvold et al., 1954). Beach (1951) has described in detail and classified the stimuli which may affect the development and display of sexual behavior.

The facts that specific drive effects may be produced by lesions in widespread areas of the limbic system and that peripheral factors are also involved in the manifestation of lesion effects argue against any theoretical approach which assigns specific drive or motivational states to specific, narrow loci within the brain. The strategic role of the hypothalamus is probably to be understood in terms of its connections and pathways to and from almost all areas of the limbic system, as well as direct and indirect connections to the midbrain (Nauta, 1963). And the existence of peripheral factors may be a reflection of the complex neuropsychological system and social setting in which emotional behavior is embedded.

Earlier in this discussion it was noted that cognitive, experiential factors are involved in the total context in which emotion or drive-related behavior appears. It will be possible only to mention an extremely active area of research which bears on this statement, but it is clear that lesions or stimulation, or both, of many areas of the limbic system (i.e., the septal region, hippocampus, cingulate gyrus, amygdala) may affect the performance of tasks in which cognitive (as well as emotional) factors may be implicated. Some examples follow. Performance by monkeys on such procedures as avoidance learning, where the animal must learn to execute a response to avert punishment (usually an electric shock) is impaired by lesions in the amygdala (Weiskrantz, 1956). McCleary (1961) has shown that anterior and posterior cingulate gyrus lesions may have

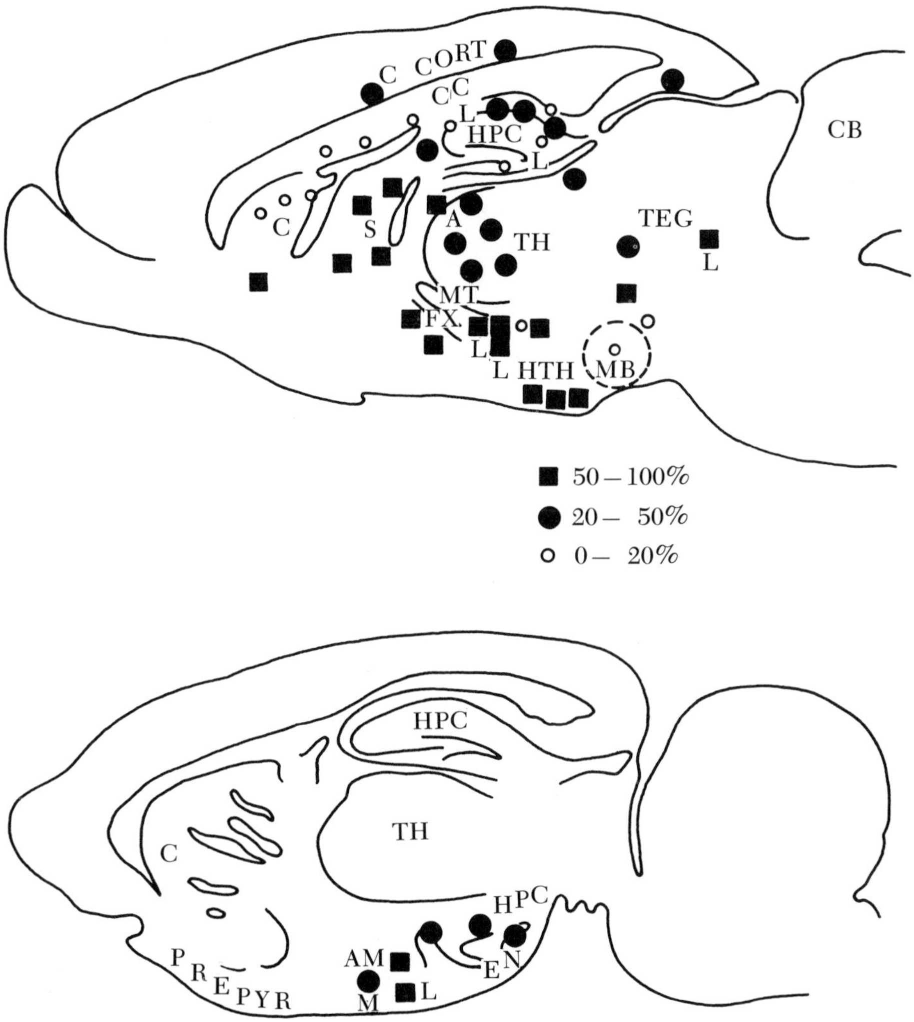

Figure 2–10 Medial and lateral sagittal sections of the rat brain showing loci of different rewarding effects with self-stimulation. The squares and circles indicate the percentage of bar-pressing produced during a 6-hour test period. Key: *A*, anterior thalamus; *AM*, amygdala; *C*, caudate nucleus; *CB*, cerebellum; *CC*, corpus callosum; *C CORT*, cingulate cortex; *EN*, entorhinal cortex; *FX*, fornix; *HPC*, hippocampus; *HTH*, hypothalamus; *MB*, mamillary body; *MT*, mamillothalamic tract; *PREPYR*, prepyriform cortex; *S*, septal region; *TEG*, tegmentum; *TH*, thalamus. The medial section (upper diagram) is near the midline; the lateral section (lower diagram) is 2 to 3 mm. more lateral. The letters *M* (medial) and *L* (lateral) near a given locus indicate that it is about 2 mm. medial or lateral to the plane shown. (*From* Olds, J., 1956, p. 283.)

differing but marked effects on the performance of avoidance responses in cats. King (1958) has shown that septal lesions may *enhance* the acquisition of avoidance responses in rats. Moreover, the clinical reports by Milner (1969) on the effects of hippocampal damage on memory in man are recalled. These examples emphasize that the assumption that only "emotional" effects may follow alterations in structures included in the limbic system is not supported. These observations must eventually be integrated into a complete description of the neuropsychological bases of emotional behavior.

The Self-Stimulation Phenomenon

No account of current studies of affective-emotional behavior would be complete without at least passing mention of the self-stimulation phenomenon. Olds and Milner (1954) reported that rats would learn various responses for the simple reward of delivering an electric shock to some part of the brain via an implanted electrode. Many studies followed this initial report, and subsequent research has established the following facts: (1) There are "punishing" as well as "rewarding" areas of the brain; rats will learn to perform responses to avoid stimulation in certain structures. These regions have been mapped in detail by Olds (1956), Lilly (1960) and others. One such map is illustrated in Figure 2–10. The structures which elicit the highest rates of self-stimulation are generally found within the limbic system. (2) There is considerable overlap between rewarding and punishing areas, and whether one or another phenomenon is displayed may depend on the spread of current, the parameters of stimulation employed and so forth. (3) The self-stimulation phenomenon is not unique to rats but is also seen in monkeys (Lilly, 1960) and in man (Sem-Jacobsen and Torkildsen, 1960). (4) As a reinforcer of behavior, self-stimulation of the brain is without peer: Lilly (1960) and Valenstein and Beer (1964) have shown that animals will perform a bar-press response for periods of days or weeks or until exhausted for the apparently rather meagre reward of a brain shock; animals can accumulate response totals in the tens or hundreds of thousands depending upon the manipulandum employed.

The relationship between the phenomenon of self-stimulation and other information on the central regulation of emotional behavior is problematical. Although the anatomical distribution of significant points is in conformity with the information from other (lesion) studies, and although self-stimulation seems in many ways to resemble other, more usual reinforcers, the considerable research effort expended on the phenomenon may not have taught us nearly as much about emotion as it has about self-stimulation.

Disordered Emotion in Man

Concerning the relation between disordered emotional behavior and brain function in man, there is no consistent, useful body of data that compares with the data available on disturbances in cognitive behavior. There are a few reports on the relation between schizophrenia and epilepsy, and a fairly voluminous literature on abnormal EEG phenomena in psychosis, but there are very few studies in which there is truly adequate specification or even more than a cursory description of the state of the brain associated with unusual or abnormal emotional manifestations. A few studies suggest that the bizarre behavioral effects of bilateral anterotemporal lobectomy as seen in monkeys (Klüver and Bucy,

1939) may be seen in man, as well. Terzian and Dalle Ore (1955) and Sawa et al., (1954) have described the effects of bilateral temporal lobectomy and bilateral amygdalectomy, respectively, in patients operated on for relief of epilepsy or for psychosurgical purposes. Postoperative symptoms of hypersexuality, increased oral tendencies and grossly inappropriate social behavior have been described in these cases; however, the significance of these symptoms is difficult to evaluate in view of the severely abnormal condition of the patients (i.e., uncontrolled epilepsy, schizophrenia) which led to the surgical therapy.

A systematic effort to relate the disordered emotional behavior of schizophrenia to cerebral pathology has been described by Heath and associates (Heath, 1954). Central to this approach has been the longterm implantation of electrodes in many areas of the brain of chronic schizophrenics. Heath has described abnormal EEG activity from the depth placements in these patients, particularly in the septal and deep frontotemporal regions. In some cases the presence of the abnormal activity has been described to be closely correlated with the appearance of bizarre delusional behavior. The most controversial part of Heath's work, perhaps, has been his report of a serum factor "taraxein" in the blood of schizophrenics. This serum factor is reportedly able to induce abnormal, schizophrenic-like behavior in control subjects. Other workers (Robins et al., 1957) have been unable to reproduce this phenomenon, although Heath has had continued success in his studies. In recent years he has indicated that this serum factor, when injected into monkeys, is capable of inducing abnormal EEG activity (spiking) in the septal area of the brain.

These few bits of evidence just described scarcely make a case for limbic system involvement in the regulation of emotional states in man; moreover, the evidence accumulates slowly, since most investigators do not have the temerity to perform bitemporal ablations in man or to implant depth electrodes merely for the purpose of identifying possible cerebral factors in mental disease. As a result, in most studies of schizophrenia the evaluation of brain function is based upon scalp EEG or upon neuropathological evaluation of a small number of cases. Some recent studies in this area have been reviewed by Mirsky (1969). The available data strongly suggest the presence of cerebral pathology in schizophrenia. Some of it is at least compatible with the animal research and theoretical views of Papez, MacLean, and Pribram and Kruger: the limbic system may subserve functions in man which are similar to those in other species that have been studied. However, other research also implicates a more fundamental cerebral defect in schizophrenia: a dysfunction in the midbrain and brain stem structures which subserve the processes of arousal and attentive behavior. Further discussion of this and of the possible anatomical pathways which could implicate and link both limbic and midbrain structures in the same pathophysiological states (Nauta, 1958) is found in the following section.

ATTENTION, ACTIVATION, AND SLEEP

Introduction and Definitions

Our current understanding of the cerebral mechanisms which underlie the processes of attention, consciousness and activation owes much to the contribution made by anatomists such as Horace Magoun, and to physiologists such as Frederic Bremer, Giuseppe Moruzzi and Herbert Jasper, as well as to psychologists such as Donald Lindsley. A related issue is the phenomenon of sleep. What process occurs in the brain that produces sleep? Is sleep a unitary phenomenon? Is sleep necessary? Is the process or processes that produce sleep the same as those involved in the variability in states of arousal that are encountered in waking behavior? What takes place centrally in the different clinical entities in which consciousness may be permanently lost (coma), in which consciousness is episodically and transiently impaired (petit mal epilepsy) or in which consciousness is chronically blunted (some forms of schizophrenia)? Are all these states related in some way? In part, a solution to these questions may be dependent upon a satisfactory definition of such terms as consciousness, wakefulness, activation, and attention, and on a clear statement of the relationship among them. A complete treatment of the problem would necessarily involve philosophical, and possibly even theological, considerations and will not be attempted here. Instead, the material of this section, as in the previous sections, will be concerned with biological (broadly speaking) efforts to come to grips with these terms, and with attempts to define consciousness and related concepts in terms of elemental physiological processes within the brain. From this point of view, a useful way of approaching consciousness is to consider it an abstraction based upon a series of neuropsychological events. In order for us to infer that consciousness exists, we are dependent upon the observation of some overt motor response to a specific environmental event. The chain of occurrences, therefore, involves the reception of a stimulus, some central processing of the stimulus (including a decision as to whether or not a motor response is appropriate) and the motor response itself. Often, the term consciousness is used to refer only to the central processing; however, this definition would limit the inquiry to the data of human introspection and eliminate the possibility of learning about the problem from animal studies. This definition could apply equally well to the term wakefulness. The difference between consciousness and wakefulness is illustrated by their opposites, which are not synonymous. The opposite of consciousness is unconsciousness, which usually implies some traumatic or pathological process such as coma. By contrast, the opposite of wakefulness is sleep, which is assumed to be a natural or normal phenomenon in which wakefulness (or consciousness) is reduced for some restorative, anabolic purpose. By this usage, it would be easier to reverse sleep to produce wakefulness than to reverse unconsciousness. It is not completely clear whether, and to what extent unconsciousness and sleep partake of the same physiological mechanisms, although they might be difficult to distinguish by neurophysiological means. In this context, activation refers to the ascension from a lower to a higher state of consciousness or wakefulness, such as from sleep to waking, or from consciousness to attentiveness (in terms of the distinction to be proposed later). Activation is beautifully demonstrated in the EEG—i.e., in the change from alpha to beta activity, or from the delta and theta of sleep to alpha). (See Fig. 2–11.)

It may be argued that the sequence of stimulus reception to central processing to motor response is a definition of attention rather than of consciousness. Although this may be true, we shall define attention for this discussion as the *focusing* of consciousness on some specific aspect of the environment, and add the stipulation that this function take place on the basis of training or learning. This distinction is not novel; it is similar to those proposed by Jung (1954) and by Hernández-Péon (1966). It should be added that the attention training for human subjects may involve only a simple verbal instruction such as "press the button when you see a red light." For animal subjects, the training may be a laborious process which involves learning to discriminate among stimuli that differ in terms of some dimension or quality. Clearly, we take advantage, in our human studies, of the extended prior educational experience of the subject. This must be built into animal subjects as part of the preparation for the experiment. However, the distinction between human and animal studies becomes less sharp as research is extended to include young subjects, or those with some obvious or inferred cerebral defect (epilepsy, brain damage, schizophrenia) which may produce severe deficiencies in attention capacity (Rosvold et al., 1956; Crosby, 1968; Fedio and Mirsky, 1969).

Two points from this discussion deserve emphasis: (1) The study of consciousness or attention must involve research on sensory input and motor output, as well as on central processing events. (2) The fact that learning is necessary for attention (by the present definition) means that

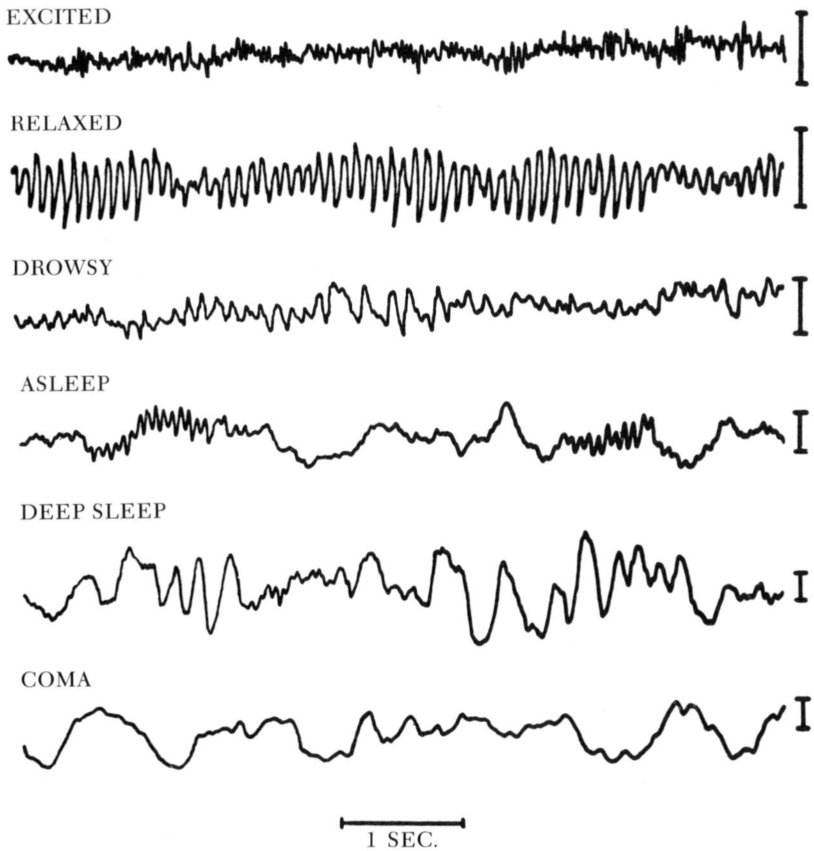

Figure 2–11 Sample EEG tracings from the human scalp. The calibration signal at the right of each tracing represents 50 microvolts. (*From* Penfield, W., and Jasper, H. H., 1954, p. 188.)

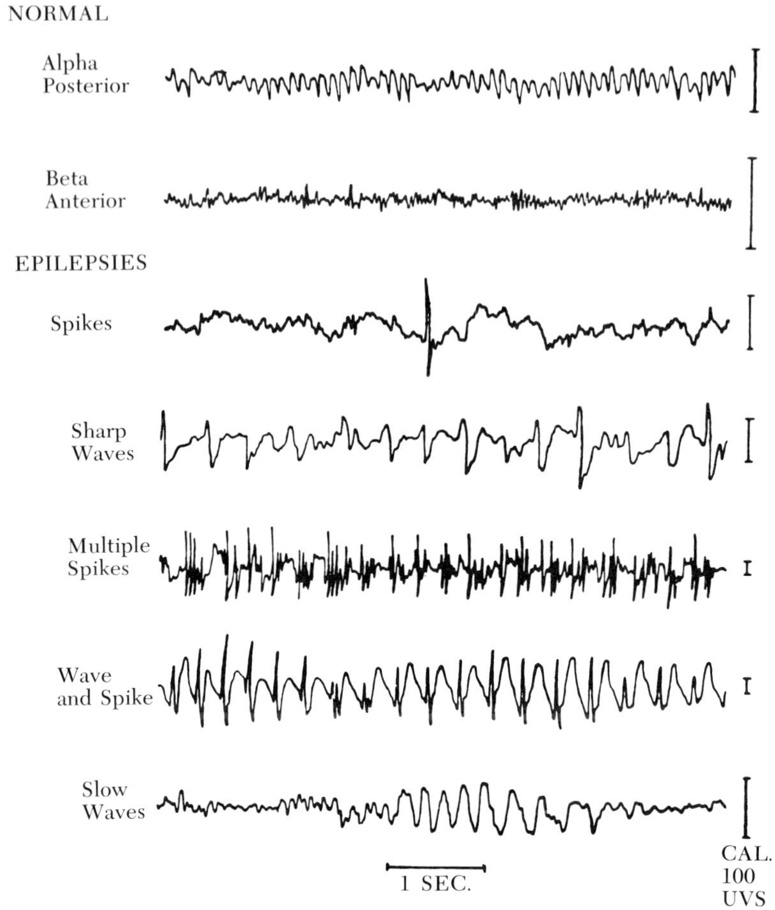

Figure 2–12 Examples of a few electroencephalographic patterns of epileptiform discharge in comparison with normal alpha and beta rhythms. Note particularly the high voltage of the epileptiform discharges. (*From* Penfield, W., and Jasper, H. H., 1954, p. 582.)

cortical function must be intimately involved in the process, even though most studies have focused on the subcortical contributions.

The Electroencephalogram

Before discussing the experimental work related to these questions it will be necessary to describe some of the phenomena of the electroencephalogram, since most of the research is predicated on the relationship between behavioral states and cerebral electrographic events. Often, in fact, it is the case that the *behavior* of the experimental preparation is impossible to observe, and the state of consciousness or wakefulness may only be inferred from the EEG; this is so because the conditions of the study are such as to effectively eliminate behavior.

For convenience and ease of communication, the EEG patterns are divided into frequency bands, designated by the letters alpha, beta, theta and delta. This follows the terminology of Hans Berger (1929), who first used the designation alpha to describe the frequency of the electrical activity seen in normal waking persons. Figure 2–11 illustrates some of the variations in frequency and amplitude seen in the normal (except for the "coma" segment) human adult electroencephalogram. The first sample, the so-called excited pattern, is representative of beta activity in which the frequency of the rhythmic oscillations varies between about 14 through 40 cycles per second (c.p.s.). As the person progresses through the several stages of sleep there is an increase in the amount of theta (4 through 7 c.p.s.) and delta (0.5 through 3 c.p.s.) activity. It is rare for any segment of EEG to contain activity in only one frequency band (i.e., only alpha activity), and most tracings, especially as analyzed by computer methods, reveal a wide dispersion of frequencies. There is a rough inverse correlation between frequency and amplitude in the normal EEG, so that the lower frequency delta and theta waves are invariably of higher amplitude than the alpha and beta waves. The higher amplitude waves are often described as synchronous or synchronized. This refers to the presumed increase in the simultaneity of firing of the individual neural elements whose summed activity comprises the EEG.

Missing from Figure 2–11 is the so-called paradoxical phase of sleep (Dement and Kleitman, 1957), which is usually accompanied by rapid eye movements and other bodily changes. However, the EEG recorded under such conditions is virtually identical to that seen in waking, active subjects and would closely resemble that seen in the "excited" segment.

Some examples of pathological EEG tracings seen in epilepsy are depicted in Figure 2–12. The chief differences between the pathological and the normal tracings lie in the presence of high voltage activity in the waking state, which may rise rapidly to a crescendo as seen in the so-called spike. Other examples of sharp waves are seen in Figure 2–12, as well as the particularly interesting form labeled wave and spike. This pattern, which when seen synchronously from many cerebral areas is characteristic of petit mal epilepsy, consists of the rapid oscillation between sharp (spike) and slow waves at a frequency of about 3 per second.

Cerebral Mechanisms in Consciousness

The pioneering work of Bremer (1935, 1937) made use of the several EEG patterns as indicative of sleep or wakefulness. In the animal preparations used in this research it was not possible to observe behavior directly because of a surgical section of the neuraxis, which interrupted the major motor pathways. Such sections are frequently used by neurophysiologists; the experiment is simplified by the reduction of motor artifacts. Moreover, the severing of the pain tracts reduces the requirement for anesthetic drugs which may have profound effects upon the electrical activity of the nervous system. The major thrust of the work of Bremer (and others) is summarized in Figure 2–13, which presents the several transections of the midbrain and brain stem upon which the earlier view of sleep was based. Depending upon whether the brain stem is intact, differences in the "behavior" of the preparation will be observed. If the section is made at the level of the first cervical vertebra (2, the encéphale isolé preparation), the brain stem is still connected to the forebrain. The sensory input to the brain is essentially normal, since the cranial nerves are intact. An animal prepared in this way will show the high voltage slow wave patterns of sleep alternating with the low voltage fast patterns of wakefulness; the animal thus displays at least in a rudimentary way the variability in consciousness (as indexed by the EEG) seen in normal animals. If the sec-

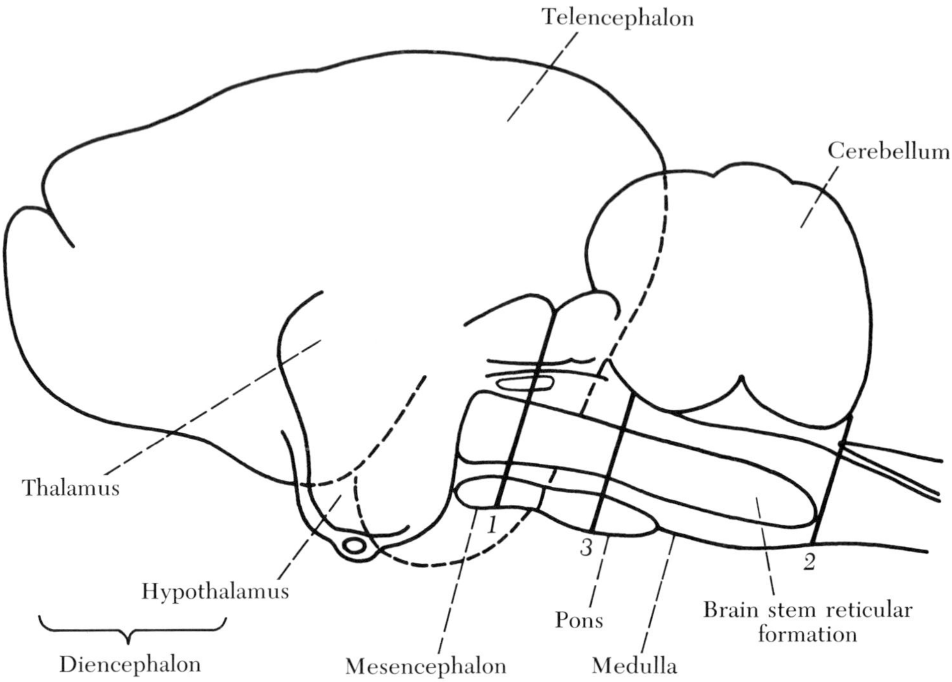

Figure 2–13 Diagrammatic representation of a cat brain, showing (*1*) the cerveau isolé, (*2*) the encéphale isolé and (*3*) the midpontine pretrigeminal preparation. (*From* Moruzzi, G.: The physiology of sleep. *Endeavour*, *22*:31, 1963.)

tion is made in the midbrain, at the midcollicular level (*1*, the cerveau isolé preparation) the brain stem is disconnected from the forebrain. The EEG manifests primarily sleep patterns with only relatively brief intervals of activity characteristic of wakefulness. In the cerveau isolé animal, the only cranial nerves intact are the optic (II), olfactory (I) and oculomotor (III). Bremer (1937) concluded that the near-continuous sleep of the cerveau isolé was the result of interruption of the total afferent inflow to the forebrain, which is necessary for it to maintain its vigilant state. The olfactory and visual inputs alone are clearly insufficient for this purpose. Bremer thus stressed the role of sensory input in wakefulness and the necessity of the integrity of the classic afferent (lemniscal) pathways. The results of later studies, however, have modified this view considerably. Moruzzi and Magoun (1949) showed that electrical stimulation of the reticular formation of the brain stem could reproduce the EEG patterns of wakefulness without involving the afferent pathways; the afferent pathways could be surgically destroyed without modifying the EEG arousal response to brain stem stimulation. In addition, more direct demonstrations (Lindsley et al., 1949) of the role of the medial (reticular) as opposed to the lateral (lemniscal) structures in wakefulness showed that the medial lesion could produce permanent comatose behavior; this was not observed following extensive destruction of lateral structures. This result is depicted in Figure 2–14. As a result of these and other studies, the concept of the *reticular activating system* was advanced; for wakefulness to be maintained it was necessary that this be intact, rather than the

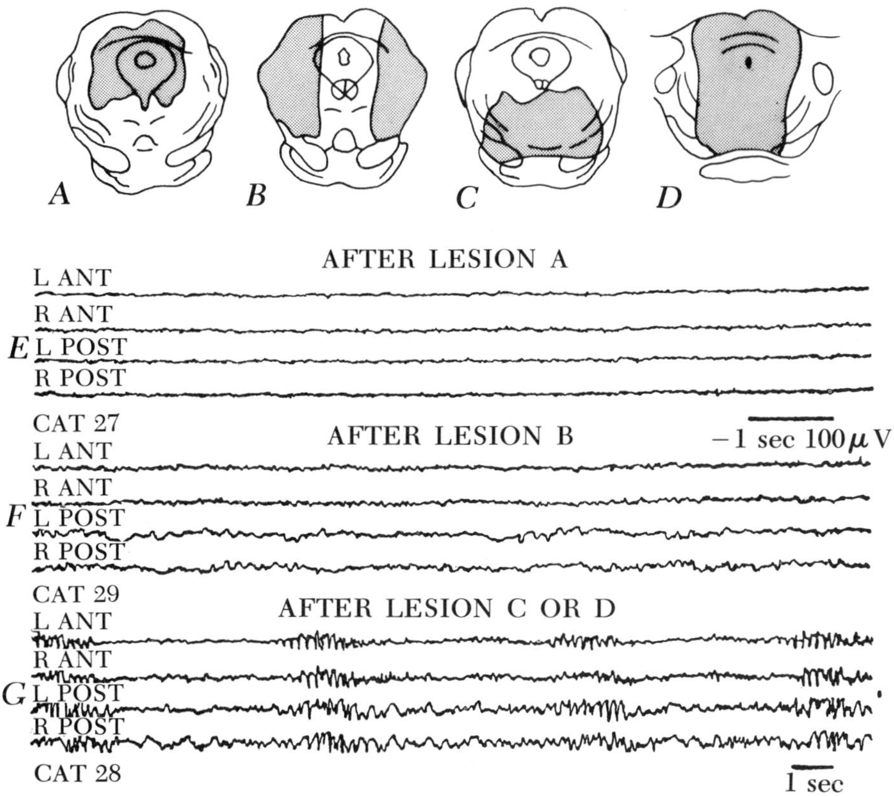

Figure 2–14 Four lesions in the midbrain of the cat are shown. In *A*, the lesion is in the central grey matter; in *B*, the lesion invades bilaterally the lemniscal, sensory pathways; in *C*, the lesion has destroyed the tegmentum (reticular substance); whereas in *D*, both the tegmentum and central grey are destroyed. The EEG pattern after lesion *A* is shown in tracing *E*; the EEG pattern after lesion *B* is seen in tracing *F*. Both tracings are normal. Only destruction of the tegmentum (*C* or *D*) produces the sleep pattern of the cerveau isolé. This is seen in tracing *B*. (*From* Moruzzi, G.: The physiology of sleep. *Endeavour*, *22*:33, 1963.)

sensory afferents.[4] This, then, was the key to the difference between the *cerveau isolé* and the *encéphale isolé* preparations. The remarkable function of the brain stem reticular formation is attributed to the fact that all ascending sensory pathways have collaterals which enter this system as they course rostrally to their eventual termination in the telencephalon.

Several other findings relevant to the cerebral regulation of wakefulness should be noted. First, there are several pathways by which the reticular formation of the brain stem influences the cortex. Although there are direct, long, monosynaptic connections from the brain stem to the cortex (Nauta and Kuypers, 1958), a main route is through polysynaptic connections to the diencephalic or thalamic portion of the activating sys-

---

[4]The research of Sprague et al. (1963) has raised some question about whether the localization studies concerned with the function of consciousness are in fact related to attention. Their results with chronic cat preparations suggested that lateral brain stem lesions may have more deleterious effects on attentive behavior than do medial brain stem lesions. Not all would concur, however, that their behavioral results (involving simple conditioning or discrimination tasks) were appropriately designed to study attention, or that permanent loss of some sensory capacity constitutes "inattention" to that sensory mode. More careful delineation of the behavior (and of the lesion) is necessary before complete clarity can be achieved in this area.

tem and thence to the cerebral hemispheres. The thalamic nuclei involved are referred to as the nonspecific or diffuse thalamic system because of their widespread manifold connections to the cortex. Included in this system are the intralaminar, midline and reticular nuclei (Ajmone Marsan, 1965). Ajmone Marsan, and Jasper and coworkers (Jasper, 1958) are largely responsible for demonstrating the role and importance of the thalamic contribution to the activating system. The studies of Hunter and Jasper (1949) and of Jasper and Droogleever-Fortuyn (1947) have suggested that the electrographic (spike and wave) and behavioral ("arrest" or "absence" reaction) signs of petit mal epilepsy can be simulated by direct stimulation of midline thalamic nuclei in animals. Hence, the specific role of thalamic structures in the phenomenon of altered consciousness (and in the maintenance of consciousness generally) in man may be indicated by this work.

The relationship between brain stem and diencephalic structures and the cerebral cortex is not only in the caudal-rostral direction, however. French et al. (1955) have provided evidence that there are corticofugal (i.e., downstream) connections as well, from the cortex *to* the subcortical way stations of the activating system. These reciprocal connections are illustrated in two classic schematic diagrams (Figs. 2–15 and 2–16), which depict the bidirectional nature of the relationship between cortext and subcortex. Clearly, the cortex itself participates in the regulation of its own activity and is not merely a passive recipient of information

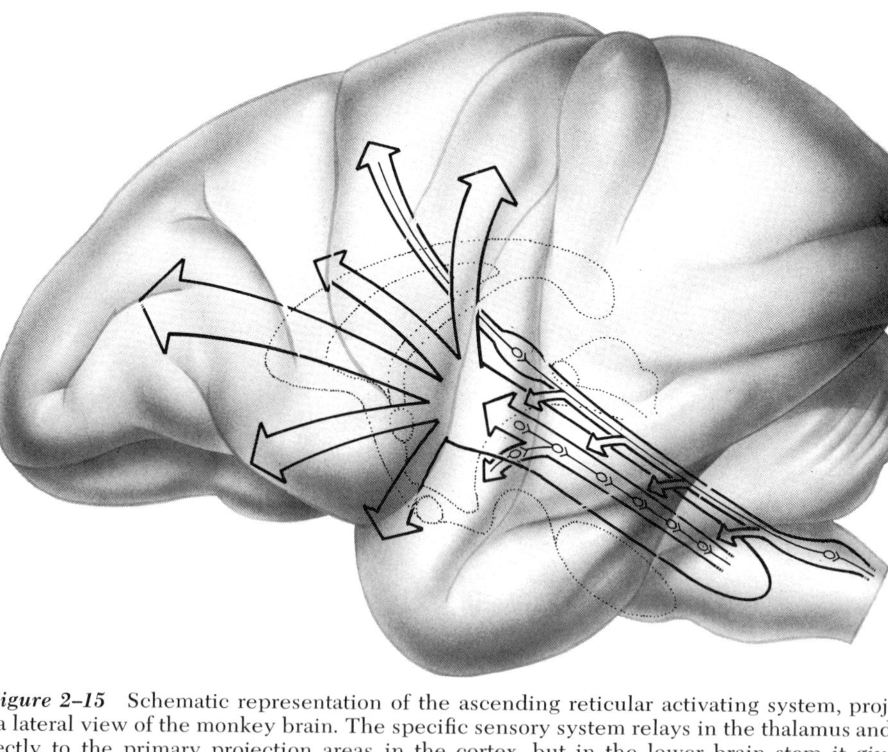

Figure 2–15 Schematic representation of the ascending reticular activating system, projected on a lateral view of the monkey brain. The specific sensory system relays in the thalamus and goes directly to the primary projection areas in the cortex, but in the lower brain stem it gives off collaterals to the unspecific sensory system, which projects diffusely upon the cortex. (*From* Magoun, H. W. *In* Adrian, E. D., Bremer, F., and Jasper, H. H. (Eds.): *Brain Mechanisms and Consciousness.* Oxford, England, Blackwell, 1954, p. 13.)

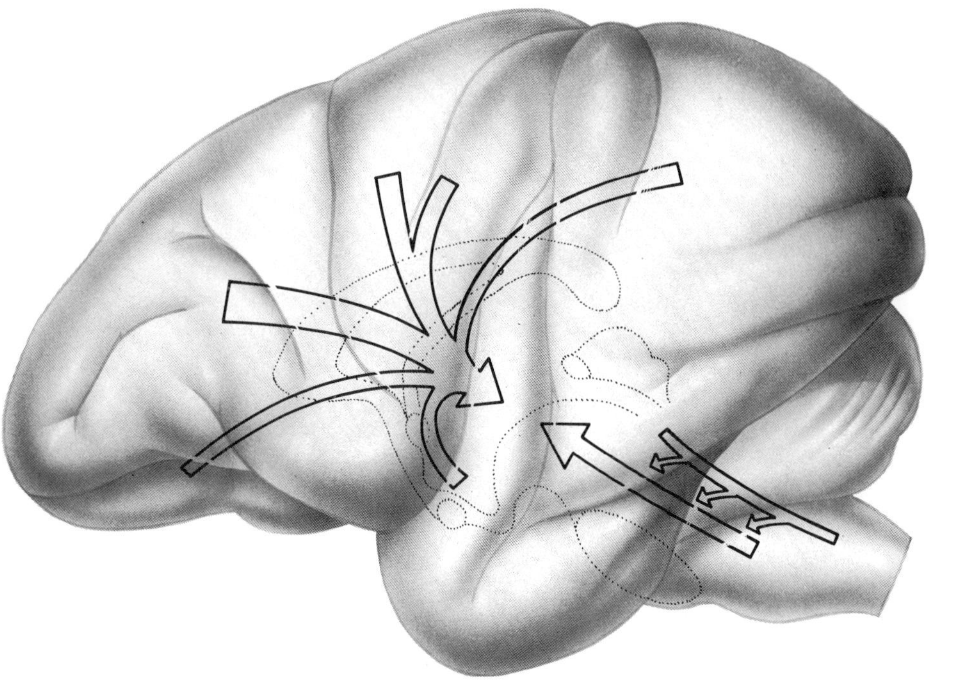

Figure 2–16 Schematic representation of corticofugal reticular connections, projected on a lateral view of the monkey brain. The reticular formation may be influenced either by peripheral or by corticofugal projections. (*From* French, J. D., Hernández-Peón, R., and Livingston, R. B., 1955, p. 92.)

from lower levels of the neuraxis. In functional terms, this means that the nature and quality of the stimulus (i.e., the meaning of the stimulus to the organism) can influence the way in which it is acted upon by the central nervous system. Hernández-Peón et al. (1956) have provided a dramatic instance of this in an oft-cited experiment with cats. The evoked sensory potential to an auditory stimulus, as recorded from the dorsal cochlear nucleus of a cat, has a characteristic form and amplitude. The amplitude of the stimulus is markedly reduced, however, when the cat is shown a pair of mice in a glass jar (Fig. 2–17). In interpreting this effect, Hernández-Peón believed that there is suppression of the auditory input in order to maximize the "attention" of the organism to this compelling, significant stimulus. The "significance" of the stimulus obviously lies in the learning experience of the cat, although unlearned "instinctual" factors may be involved as well. This extremely interesting experiment has generated considerable controversy. Some have maintained that the effect was due entirely to contraction of the middle ear muscles of the cat rather than to any central effect (Hugelin et al., 1960). However, later research by Moushegian et al. (1961) showed many of the same kinds of effects described by Hernández-Peón et al. in cats in whom middle ear muscles were destroyed. Marsh et al. (1962) have pointed out that evoked auditory potentials can vary greatly in amplitude and shape, depending upon the way the cat orients its head in relation to a sound source in an experimental chamber. None of this subsequent work has unequivocally shown that the Hernández-Péon effect was

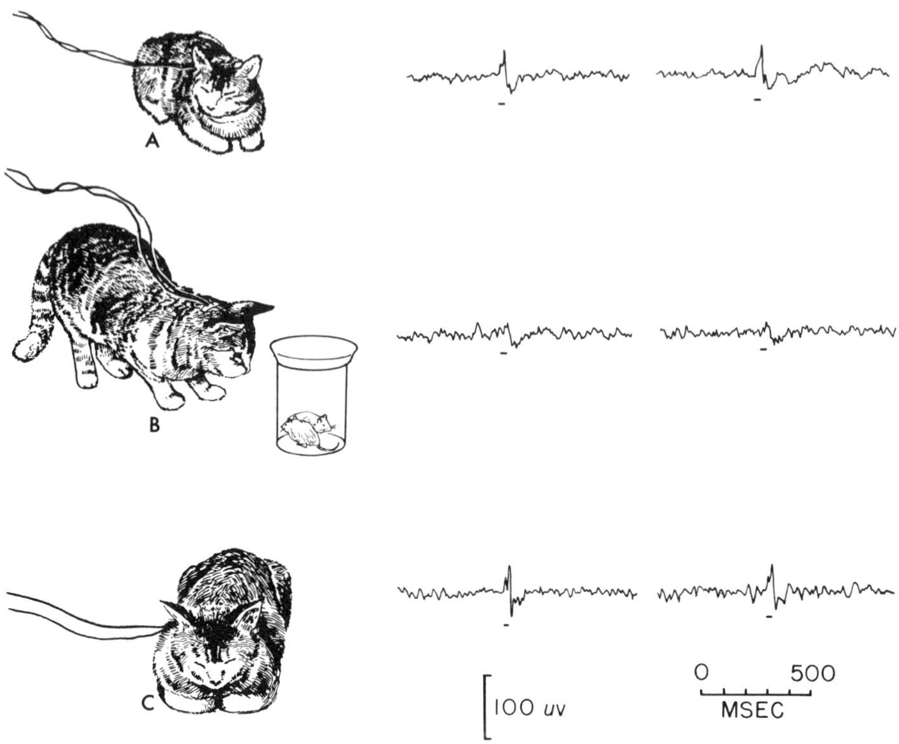

Figure 2–17 Blocking effects of distraction upon click-evoked potentials recorded from the dorsal cochlear nucleus. When the cat appeared to be attentively looking at a pair of mice placed inside a jar (B), the auditory potentials were significantly reduced as compared to those recorded during relaxed wakefulness (A and C). (*From* Hernández-Peón, R., Scherrer, H., and Jouvet, M., 1956, p. 331.)

in fact an artifact. Moreover, evoked potential changes in relation to attention (Tecce, 1970) have subsequently been described in many experiments. And the research of Hernández-Péon, incomplete as it was, was the pioneering effort in this area. It emphasized that "attention" may have overt physical meaning within the brain. The capacity of the cortex to gate or control selectively its own input may involve a direct effect on the receptor organ itself (Granit, 1959), as well as a relay through subcortical members of the activating system.

The role of brain stem and thalamic structures in activation has been described. And the characteristic way of demonstrating their functional role has been to show that high frequency stimulation in either locus can produce an excited or activated pattern in the EEG. There are other subcortical systems, however, which apparently act in opposition to the ascending activating system. The sleep-inducing effect of low frequency stimulation in the medial thalamus, described by Hess, has already been discussed. Akert et al. (1952) have shown that such stimulation is accompanied by the high voltage, low frequency synchronous activity characteristic of genuine sleep. In addition to this, however, Moruzzi and collaborators have described a brain stem system, with important centers in the pons and medulla, which, electrographically at least, acts in *opposition* to the ascending activating system (Battini et al., 1959; Battini et al., 1959). Thus, low frequency electrical stimulation in this region (Magnes et al., 1961) can induce synchronous high voltage slow activity in the cortex. Furthermore, if an animal is prepared with a section of the neuraxis at the midpontine level, and anterior to the region of the trigeminal nerve nucleus (although this is only a few millimeters posterior to the classic cerveau isolé cut) it will *not* show the near-continuous synchronous sleep activity of the cerveau isolé. The animal, in fact, appears to be in a chronic state of arousal. This result is interpreted as due to the destruction of the synchronizing center in the pons. The midpontine pretrigeminal preparation (or MPP) is illustrated in Figure 2–13 by the section marked *3*. The assumption is, therefore, that the regulation of consciousness (and its specific manifestation in attention) is under the multiple influence of opposing systems in the midline thalamus and the upper and lower brain stem, as well as subject to the control of cortical systems.

The inferences of consciousness mentioned in the foregoing discussion are clearly dependent upon the proposition that the EEG is an accurate index of the state of wakefulness; aside from a few manifestations of pupillary and oculomotor functioning, most of the animal preparations referred to are incapable of displaying behavior. The relation between the EEG and behavioral state is complex (see Mirsky and Bakay Pragay, 1967), and the precise behavioral equivalents of many of the physiological demonstrations by Moruzzi, Bremer and collaborators are yet to be provided. Nevertheless, it is reasonable to assume that the EEG provides a reasonably accurate index of behavior for a wide variety of conditions and to trust therefore to future study to provide the necessary behavioral concomitants of the subcortical synchronizing systems which have been described.

Sleep with Low Voltage Fast Activity

The optimism expressed in the conclusion of the previous section must be tempered somewhat by the evidence that the reduced consciousness or wakefulness of sleep is not inevitably accompanied by high voltage slow EEG activity. Dement and Kleitman (1957) described a stage of sleep in man which was accompanied by low voltage fast activity in the EEG, together with rapid eye movements as well as other autonomic changes. This stage of sleep was also described by Rimbaud et al. (1955), Dement (1958) and Jouvet (1961) in the cat and by Weitzman (1961) in the monkey. Jouvet labeled this the paradoxical phase, because of the simultaneous presence of rapid cortical activity (usually associated with alert wakefulness) and somnolence. The question as to whether or not this activity represents a deeper or higher level of consciousness than that represented by sleep with high voltage slow waves is still in question. Dement and Kleitman (1957) have argued that it represents a state of consciousness falling between deepest sleep and wakefulness; Jouvet (1961), on the other hand, maintains that it is the very deepest, most primitive state of sleep (*"l'archéosommeil"*), supporting his position with evidence based on increased arousal thresholds and the marked reduction in muscular activity which accompanies the paradoxical phase. Regardless of the precise level of consciousness that is represented, it is clear that increased fast activity may accompany widely differing states of consciousness. Therefore, any argument seeking to link a specific type of EEG activity with a specific behavioral state or effect must be qualified carefully.

Recent studies by Jouvet (1962) have sought to link the several stages of sleep to brain stem structures (*locus coeruleus, raphé nucleus*) which secrete specific types of catechol amines.

Study of Single Neural Units During Sleep and Arousal

The research on the mechanisms of consciousness based on macroelectrode recording (EEG from large aggregates of neurons) has been supplemented usefully in recent years by explorations employing microelectrode recordings. Several investigators have employed the technique of recording from single neural units in the brain in order to study the characteristics of the various stages of sleep and of wakefulness and arousal. In the study by Machne et al. (1955), the activity of brain stem units was studied during EEG synchrony (induced by drugs or lesions) and during arousal elicited by stimulation. Most often, it was observed that during EEG synchrony units fired in a patterned fashion, characterized by groups of spikes. This unit synchrony was disrupted by stimulation, which also had the effect of increasing the discharge rate of the units and of recruiting previously silent units. Although some of the units observed did not behave in this fashion, the results generally supported the notion that an aroused EEG is characterized by greater neural activity and that EEG synchrony is paralleled by unit synchrony and decreased neural activity. Generally similar results were reported by Jasper (1958) and by Hubel (1959).

Investigations of unit activity in unrestrained, unanesthetized animals, however, has not provided complete confirmation of the results of Machne and coworkers. Huttenlocher (1961) studied the behavior of single units in the brain stem during natural sleep and during waking under conditions of both evoked activity and spontaneous arousal. Although some units showed rapid continuous discharge during waking, and decreased spontaneous activity during sleep with EEG slow waves, the majority showed *more* spontaneous activity during slow wave sleep than during quiet waking. However, almost all units studied showed striking increases in firing rates during sleep with low voltage fast activity. The results obtained with respect to evoked activity were in the opposite direction but were in conformity with those obtained by Machne et al. and with those studies employing macroelectrode techniques. In most units, click stimuli produced the greatest unit firing during quiet waking. During slow wave sleep the firing rate was decreased, and during low voltage fast sleep it was decreased to zero.

The studies of Evarts (1957, 1960, 1961, 1962) have contributed extensive information about single unit activity. This work has shown that there are at least two populations of units: those with a relatively slow spontaneous firing rate, which tends to increase as the animal goes from wakefulness to sleep; and those with a relatively fast spontaneous rate, which shows the opposite effect. This finding has also been reported by Creutzfeldt and Jung (1961) in cat encéphale isolé preparations. Evarts has emphasized particularly, however, that most units show greater variance of spontaneous discharge rate during waking than during sleep. This increased variability rather than change in mean rate would appear to be the significant differentiation between sleep and wakefulness, since the altered variance was observed in the absence of changes in the mean firing rate. Evarts (1962) has also reported that no obvious differences exist in the effects between brain regions sampled in the visual cortex, in the suprasylvian association cortex and in the brain stem.

To the extent that one may generalize from samples of populations of single neurons to the activity of brain areas or systems it would appear that it is an oversimplification to describe sleep as a depression of the activity of the ascending reticular activating system, with a consequent reduction of cortical activity. Some of the units studied do conform to this description (i.e., show less activity during sleep with high voltage slow waves than during wakefulness); moreover, the response of most units to external stimulation seems to decrease as a function of decreasing level of wakefulness. However, many units increase in spontaneous firing frequency during slow wave sleep and almost all increase in activity markedly during the phase of sleep accompanied by low voltage fast waves.

The most nearly correct summary description of the present information is that some phases of sleep are characterized by a decrease in ongoing activity in some systems within the brain stem and cortex; concurrently, other systems within these brain areas become more active. During the paradoxical phase of sleep there is an almost uniform enhancement of spontaneous activity of all brain areas that have been sampled. Excluding this phase, however, sleep is characterized generally by greater rhythmicity and synchrony (which may be functionally tantamount to a reduction of activity) than is true of wakefulness.

This consideration of the findings of single unit studies leads to a conclusion which is not dissimilar to that reached previously, in the section *Cerebral Mechanisms in Consciousness*—namely, that consciousness (as well as synchrony in the EEG) is under the joint control of interrelated mechanisms in the cortex, thalamus, midbrain and brain stem. It is not clear to what extent these several mechanisms participate in the normal regulation of these processes, and to what extent they represent compensatory devices that come into play primarily after massive insult to the brain. However, the fact that at least some behavioral or electrographic indication reflecting conscious processes is possible after such insult (e.g., Adametz, 1959; Sprague et al., 1961, 1963; and Villablanca, 1962) indicates that compensation may occur and that it may involve the structures whose possible roles in the regulation of consciousness (and the EEG) have already been described.

Neuropsychological Studies of Impaired Attention in Man

Before discussing this research, it would be profitable at this juncture to describe the diagnostic terminology for epilepsy advanced by Penfield and Jasper (1954), since it is essential to an understanding of the results. On the basis of careful clinical and electroencephalographic studies and of neurosurgical treatment of hundreds of epileptic patients, Penfield and Jasper suggested that the older terminology of the epilepsies be replaced by one more diagnostic and descriptive of the locus of the disorder. According to the older usage, patients were divided essentially into three categories: grand mal, petit mal and psychomotor. Grand mal seizures were characterized by a tonic-clonic convulsion and accompanied by loss of consciousness and various autonomic phenomena (incontinence, salivation and so forth). They are also typically preceded by an aura (some perceptual or bodily sensation). Petit mal seizures are accompanied by little or no muscular involvement; the only convulsive manifestation is a brief staring spell during which consciousness is lost. Usually there is no aura or postseizure recall of the spell. In psychomotor seizures, the convulsive manifestation is a period of "automatic" behavior in which the patient might perform some meaningless act in repetitive fashion or engage in some skilled or coordinated activity (driving a car, fighting) for which he has no subsequent recall. There could be combinations of the several types of seizures in a single patient; other varieties of minor seizures exist as well. The view advanced by Penfield and Jasper is that to classify a patient in terms of his seizure type is not as useful for therapeutic purposes as a classification based on the locus (usually cortical) of the brain disorder. And this classification leans heavily upon the use of the EEG. Thus, the term psychomotor epilepsy is not as useful as the term temporal lobe epilepsy; grand mal epilepsy, similarly, should be replaced by frontal lobe epilepsy, parietal lobe epilepsy or some term based on the brain locus of the disorder, as well as this could be established by electrographic and other diagnostic means. Since Penfield and Jasper were convinced of the usefulness of neurosurgical therapy (in patients refractory to drug treatment) the location of the diseased or damaged area of the brain was a vital datum for them, and this helps to account for their emphasis. The problem arises as to how to fit petit mal seizures into this scheme. In petit mal and related disorders, in contrast to other types of convulsive illness, the evidence for a cortical focus is absent. Characteristically, the EEG shows a bilaterally synchronous and symmetrical discharge arising simultaneously from all regions of the brain (see Fig. 2–18). After reviewing relevant neurophysiological evidence, Penfield and Jasper concluded that the so-called nonfocal petit mal seizures were not cortical in origin, but arose instead from some subcortical focus lying deep within the "centrencephalon." This was defined broadly to include everything within the encephalon except the cerebral hemispheres and their dependencies. On the basis of the results of animal studies, they suggest that the focus of the disorder might actually lie in the midline thalamus (i.e., in the rostral diencephalic terminus of the diffuse ascending activating system). Electrical stimulation of the midline thalamic structures at low frequencies could reproduce in cats and monkeys the characteristic symmetrical and synchronous 3 per second spike and wave discharge that is the electrographic signature of petit mal epilepsy (Hunter and Jasper, 1949; Pollen et al., 1963). Penfield and Jasper reasoned that the mechanism by which the spike and wave discharge was manifested and propagated must be the same as the medial thalamic mechanism involved in the cortical recruiting response described earlier by Morison and Dempsey (1943). This line of reasoning was supported by the similarity in the several characteristics of the spike-wave and recruiting response phenomena. To promote the view that petit mal epilepsy was subcortical (if not thalamic) in nature, they coined the term centrencephalic epilepsy to replace petit mal epilepsy; this was consistent with their aim of substituting terminology that was descriptive of brain locus rather than of seizure pattern.

The approach of Penfield and Jasper has not been universally accepted (see, for example, Gibbs and Gibbs, 1952); nevertheless it has served to organize and prompt research efforts with epileptic patients and has provided a useful theoretical structure upon which to place various experimental findings. The studies by Brenda Milner, Kimura, Lansdell and others of patients with focal epileptic disorders (described in the section *Learning and Intellectual Behavior*) have in part stemmed from this theoretical position. But more pertinent to the material of the present section is the research on patients with centrencephalic epilepsy. In a series of studies with various populations of epileptic subjects, it has been established that those diagnosed as petit mal—i.e., centrencephalic or diffuse-unlocalized—are more likely to demonstrate impaired attentive behavior than those with a diagnosis of focal cortical epilepsy (Mirsky, et al., 1960; Lansdell and Mirsky, 1964). Focal temporal lobe or focal frontal lobe epileptic involvement was found generally to produce no impairment in attentive behavior; such patients were not different from controls. In fact, temporal lobe removals (Lansdell and Mirsky, 1964) produced no deficit on the measure of attentiveness, although the typical loss in verbal or performance I.Q. (depending on the side of the removal) was seen. In this research, the attentive behavior was studied by means of a special technique, the continuous performance test or CPT (Rosvold et al., 1956), in which letters of the alphabet were serially presented to the subject at the rate of about one per second for 5 to 10 minute periods. The subjects' task was to press a response key for a critical stimulus (i.e., the letter X) and to withhold pressing for other letters. Usually the stimulus was in view for 0.2 second or less, and the subject was allowed approximately 0.8 second in which to respond. An important characteristic of the task is that attentive effort must be sustained for long periods (i.e., 5 to 10 minutes). A recent study (Fedio and Mirsky, 1969) has extended the behavioral analysis of specific cognitive or attentive deficits in focal and centrencephalic epilepsy to a population of children. Three groups of patients matched in age and full scale I.Q. were studied; these were diagnosed as either left temporal, right temporal, or centrencephalic. A normal control group was also studied. The mean age of the subjects (between 10 and 11 years) was at least 10 years less than the adult populations studied previously by Mirsky et al. (1960) and by Lansdell and Mirsky (1964). The children, some of whom were as young as six years, showed the same specific patterns of impairment seen in adults (see section *Learning and Intellectual Behavior*): the left temporal focus is associated with loss in acquisition and retention of verbal tasks; the right temporal focus is accompanied by impaired acquisition and retention of visual-spatial tasks; and centrencephalic epilepsy is accompanied by significant impairment in attention as measured by the CPT. In addition to confirming the previous experimental work, this investigation shows that the specific behavioral defects associated with differing epileptogenic foci are present relatively early in life and are thus characteristic of epilepsy in childhood as well as in adulthood. The question of just how early in life the specific behavioral defects are seen must be the subject of additional research. Obviously such data are of great relevance to the issue of whether vicarious functioning or equipotentiality exist for these specific capacities in man. The question remains as to whether there is a point in development beyond which there can be no compensation for specific losses. Further, this may differ depending upon the function. The research involving monkeys on delayed-alternation function is particularly pertinent to this issue.

In an effort to provide greater neuropsychological specification of the impairment of the subjects with centrencephalic epilepsy, other research has involved the simultaneous recording of CPT and EEG in such patients (Mirsky and Van Buren, 1965). Generally, there is a close association between errors of omission on the task (failure to press for the letter X) and the appearance of the spike and wave EEG pattern

(Fig. 2–18), and many formal EEG characteristics of the spike-wave activity appear to be related to impaired performance. However, patients with centrencephalic epilepsy also perform more poorly on the CPT than focal epileptic controls, even in the absence of spike-wave bursts. The latter finding, that the scalp EEG was not perfectly correlated with omission error tendency, suggested a partial dissociation of the EEG and the behavior. This was borne out in the finding that this behavioral symptom tends to lead the convulsive EEG pattern in time (Fig. 2–19). The lack of a perfect correlation between scalp EEG and impaired attentiveness has prompted the study of animal models of centrencephalic epilepsy (Mirsky et al., 1966; Mirsky and Tecce, 1968) in which the seizure pattern is induced by the administration of a toxic drug, chlorambucil (Pradhan and Ajmone Marsan, 1963). The use of monkey subjects has made it possible to record simultaneously from cortical and subcortical placements in conjunction with attentive behavior. Such studies have suggested that for this model of the disease, the correspondence between direct intracerebral EEG recordings and attentive loss may be very close; it is not clear, however, that the model is in all re-

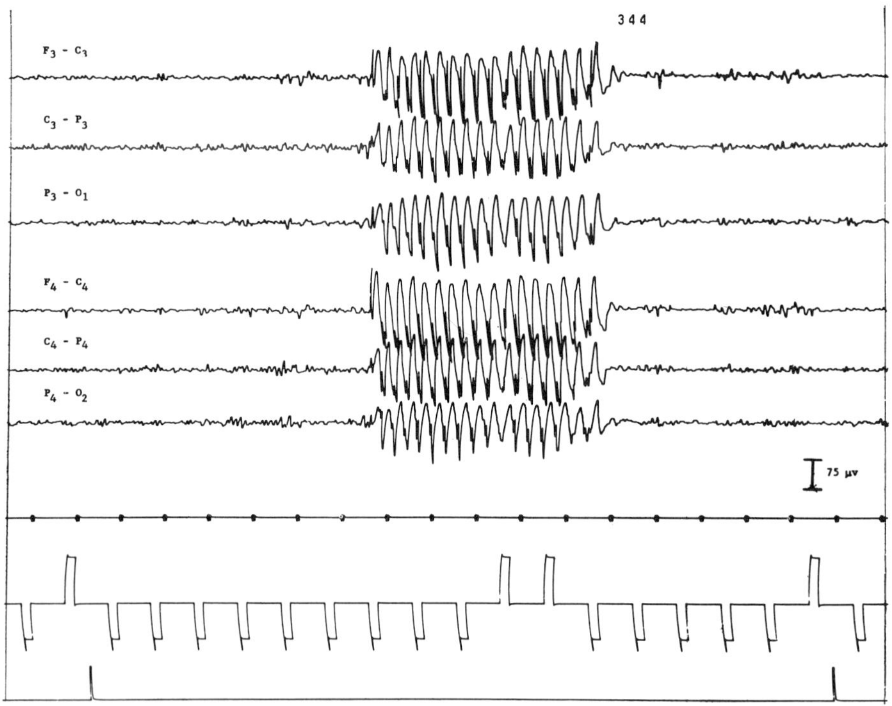

Figure 2–18 The relation between a burst of spike and wave activity and performance in a patient suffering from petit mal epilepsy. The top six channels in the tracing represent a standard anteroposterior EEG run, with electrode placements determined by the "10-20" system (Penfield and Jasper, 1954). The channel below this is a one second time mark. Below this are represented the stimuli (duration = 0.2 second) shown to the patient; those requiring a response (the letter X) are seen as deflections above the baseline; other letter stimuli appear as deflections below the baseline. The patient's response appears on the bottom-most channel as an upward deflection. In this sample, the patient responded correctly to X's presented before and after the spike and wave burst but failed to respond to the two occurring within the burst. (*From* Mirsky, A. F., and Tecce, J. J. *In* Brill, J. O. (Ed.): *Neuro-psychopharmacology.* The Hague, Netherlands, Excerpta Medica, 1968, p. 638.)

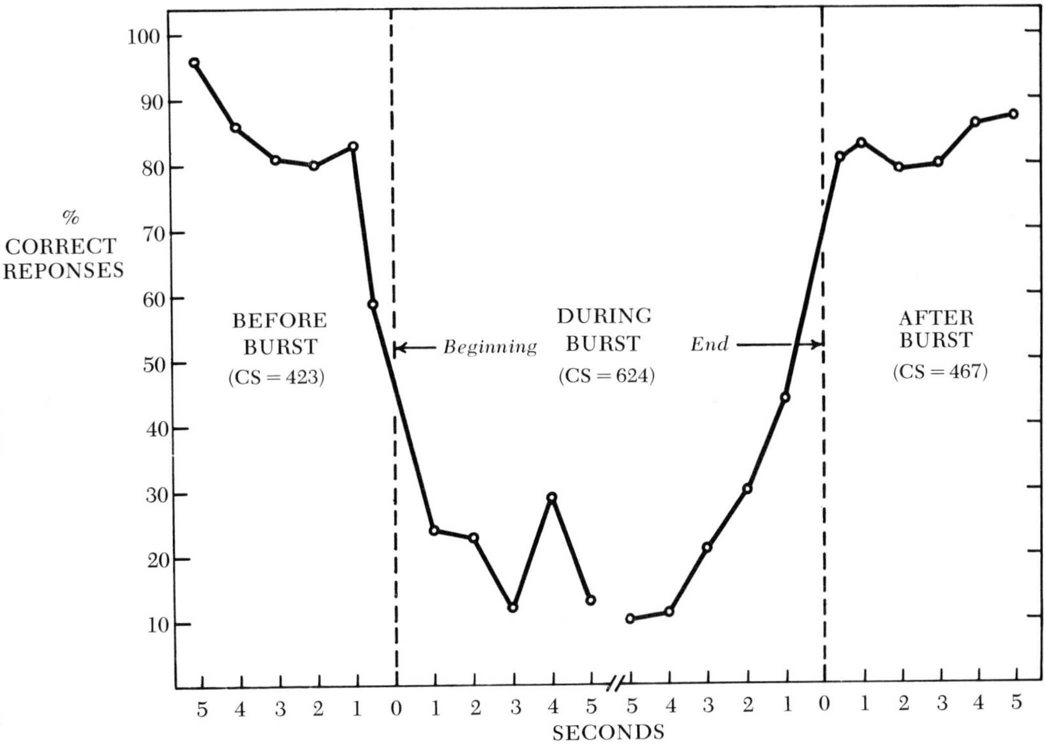

Figure 2–19 Relations between level of performance on the continuous performance test (CPT) and the onset, development and termination of the EEG burst. See text for description of CPT. The curve indicates a significant drop in performance before the burst is evident and a rise before it has ended. CS equals the number of X stimuli in the pooled data. Approximately 500 spike-wave bursts from 18 patients are represented. (Adapted from Mirsky and Van Buren, 1965. *From* Mirsky, A. F., and Tecce, J. J., 1968, p. 219.)

spects comparable to the human disease, and the question of the EEG-behavior dissocation in man remains open.

To turn from the question of centrencephalic epilepsy, it has been shown that various other clinical phenomena or experimental treatments may also be accompanied by impaired attentiveness (as measured by the CPT). Some of the experimental treatments include sleep deprivation and the administration of phenothiazine drugs, such as chlorpromazine. Mirsky and Kornetsky (1964) have argued that these experimental treatments share a common action on the midbrain and brain stem structures that are presumably pathologically involved in centrencephalic epilepsy, and that this accounts for the effect on attentive behavior that is seen. Some force is added to the argument by the fact that drugs such as LSD, meprobamate and low doses of barbiturates (which presumably act preferentially on the cortex) have a different behavioral effect from the centrencephalic epilepsy–sleep deprivation–chlorpromazine group. By contrast, the LSD–meprobamate–barbiturate group produces preferential impairment of tasks which may demand greater cognitive than attentive effort. This behavioral effect is compatible with their presumed action on the cerebral cortex (Mirsky and Kornetsky, 1964).

Other clinical conditions in which

impaired attentiveness (as indexed by the CPT) is seen include mental retardation, particularly that accompanied by overt evidence of brain damage (Rosvold et al., 1956; Crosby, 1969), phenylketonuria (Anderson and Seigel, 1967) and schizophrenia (Kornetsky, 1967). Although it is tempting to speculate that some disturbance or disruption of the brain stem–midbrain–diencephalic core of the nervous system is common to all of these, the evidence is lacking. The best argument, perhaps, can be made for interpreting the attentional defect in schizophrenia as the result of some subcortical dysfunction; some of the evidence for this is reviewed by Mirsky (1969). But the question which immediately arises concerns the other, more evident defects in emotional-affective behavior in schizophrenia. Such defects would seem more likely to be referable to dysfunction in the limbic system (see section *Drive and Emotional Behavior*) than in the midbrain or brain stem. The anatomical study by Nauta (1958), is an aid for a theoretical neuropsychological solution of this problem. Nauta described the extensive series of reciprocal connections between the limbic system and certain areas of the midbrain. He referred to these areas of the midbrain as the limbic-midbrain region. There is a possibility that some kind of disruption or disturbance at one terminus of this system (i.e., the midbrain) could rapidly be transmitted to the other (i.e., the limbic system) and thus provide the mechanism by which two neuropsychological substrata could be involved in the same clinical entity. The conditions under which this might occur are obscure, as is the possibility that it even takes place. However, a recent review by Towbin (1969) suggests that subtle defects of the brain can occur early in development and may provide the basis for later psychotic behavior. Towbin emphasizes that hypoxia during intrauterine life can produce a variety of infarctate lesions in deep cerebral loci, depending upon the gestational age of the fetus at the time of the hypoxic insult. Although he was largely concerned with the relation between prematurity and birth complications on the one hand, and their sequelae (palsy, epilepsy and mental retardation) on the other, he also states, "Manifestly, fetal and neonatal hypoxic cerebral damage results not only in the reduction but also in *distortion* [emphasis added] of the nervous system function. . . . Attention is being increasingly directed to . . . the high incidence of behavioral disorders in children with a history of complicated birth and prematurity." (Towbin, 1969, p. 160.) This line of reasoning does not establish the existence of either limbic or midbrain pathology in schizophrenia, but it does indicate a mechanism by which it might occur. The force of these findings, as well as the magnitude of the mental and public health problems resulting from schizophrenia, argues for a major research effort directed toward the neuropathogenesis of this disease. Such an effort must make fruitful use of the tools, methods and data of neuropsychology, much of which has been presented in review in this chapter.

SUMMARY

This chapter has presented a survey of some of the significant studies that have attempted to specify the role of central nervous system mechanisms in behavior. The categories of behavior selected—learning, emotion and attention—are traditional in psychology. All are of necessity involved in some degree in all behavior. This is reflected, perhaps, in the fact that many functions which have been investigated have been shown to be dependent upon brain "systems" with several vertical or horizontal, or both, components. The categories are not completely defensible from a logical or analytical point of view, but they do represent fairly accurately what the focus of interest in particular experiments or areas of investigation has been. The omission, in this presentation, of many significant and even elegant pieces of work is acknowledged. The excuse offered is that space did not permit a survey of all the research that has been done in the area of brain and behavior. Those portions which were selected can be said to have fulfilled one (or both) of two criteria:

1. The work relates to important areas of human behavioral function or dysfunction.
2. The work demonstrates or suggests useful correlations between human and infra-human studies.

The experience and biases of the author clearly relate to how the terms useful, significant and important are defined; their best definition, however, is provided by the examples of research which have been cited in the chapter.

The material on developmental issues or on experiments which have contrasted the effects of neural variables in young and mature subjects is sparsely represented in the chapter. Clearly, this area of research is in its infancy (from several points of view) and should increase in scope and importance in the future. This would appear to be a necessary direction for research related to human problems like schizophrenia, epilepsy and mental retardation, since many of the important neuropsychological events probably occur early in life and are obscured by later development. Remediation and the reversing of pathological directions may be possible, in some cases, only early in life and at no other time. If a prediction can be offered, it is that functional, "dynamic" research (as defined earlier), combined with the study of developmental processes, should be the most productive of information in years to come.

ACKNOWLEDGMENTS

Dr. Mirsky is a Research Scientist Awardee #KO5-MH 14,915 of the National Institute of Mental Health, Public Health Service. Part of the costs of preparing this paper, and of the research conducted by the author described in the section entitled *Attention, Activation and Sleep* was supported by grant #MH-12568 of the National Institute of Mental Health, Public Health Service. Part of the material included in this section appeared earlier in a publication by Mirsky and Kornetsky (1964). The author wishes also to acknowledge the competent editorial and secretarial assistance of Misses Margaret MacClymont, Kathleen Grimes and Judith Green.

REFERENCES

Abplanalp, J. M.: Electroencephalographic correlates of delayed-alteration and visual discrimination learning in monkeys. Unpublished Ph.D. Dissertation, Boston University, 1969.

Adametz, J. H.: Rate of recovery of functioning in cats with rostral reticular lesions. *J. Neurosurg., 16*:85–98, 1959.

Adey, W. R., Dunlop, C. W., and Hendrix, M. S.: Hippocampal slow waves: Distribution and phase relationships in the course of approach learning. *Arch. Neurol., 3*:74–90, 1960.

Agranoff, B. W., Davis, E. R., Lim, R., and Casola, L.: Biological effects in antimetabolities used in behavioral studies. *In* Efron, D. E. (Ed.): *Psychopharmacology. A Review of Progress 1957–1967.* Washington, D.C., U. S. Government Printing Office (Public Health Service Publication No. 1836), 1968, pp. 909–917.

Ajmone Marsan, C.: The thalamus. Data on its functional anatomy and on some aspects of thalamo-cortical integration. *Arch. Ital. Biol., 103*:847–882, 1965.

Akert, K., Koella, W. P., and Hess, R., Jr.: Sleep produced by electrical stimulation of the thalamus. *Amer. J. Physiol.*, *168*:260–267, 1952.

Anand, B. K., and Brobeck, J. R.: Hypothalamic control of food intake in rats and cats. *Yale J. Biol. Med.*, *24*:123–140, 1951.

Anand, B. K., Dua, S., and Schoenberg, K.: Hypothalamic control of food intake in cats and monkeys. *J. Physiol.*, *127*:143–152, 1955.

Anderson, V. E., and Siegel, F. S.: Behavior and unborn errors of metabolism. Presented at a symposium at the American Psychological Association in Washington, D.C., September 4, 1967.

Andersson, B.: The effect of injections of hypertonic NaCl-solutions into different parts of the hypothalamus of goats. *Acta Physiol. Scand.*, *28*:188–201, 1953.

Andersson, B., and Larsson, S.: The influence of local temperature changes in the preoptic area and rostral hypothalamus on regulation of food and water intake. *Acta Physiol. Scand.*, *52*:75–89, 1961.

Bakay Pragay, E., Mirsky, A. F., and Abplanalp, J. M.: The effects of chlorpromazine and secobarbital on matching from sample and discrimination tasks in monkeys. *Psychopharmacologia*, *16*:128–138, 1969.

Bard, P., and Mountcastle, V. P.: Some forebrain mechanisms involved in expression of rage with special reference to suppression of angry behavior. *Res. Publ. Ass. Res. Nerv. Ment. Dis.*, *27*:362–404, 1948.

Barondes, S. H.: Effects of inhibitors of cerebral protein synthesis on "long term" memory in mice. *In* Efron, D. E. (Ed.): *Psychopharmacology. A Review of Progress 1957–1967.* Washington, D.C., U. S. Government Printing Office (Public Health Service Publication No. 1836), 1968, pp. 905–908.

Battig, K., Rosvold, H. E., and Mishkin, M.: Comparison of the effects of frontal and caudate lesions on delayed response and alternation in monkeys. *J. Comp. Physiol. Psychol.*, *53*:400–404, 1960.

Battig, K., Rosvold, H. E., and Mishkin, M.: Comparison of the effects of frontal and caudate lesions on discrimination learning in monkeys. *J. Comp. Physiol. Psychol.*, *55*:458–463, 1962.

Battini, C., Palestini, M., Rossi, G. F., and Zanchetti, A.: EEG activation patterns in the midpontine pretrigeminal cat following sensory deafferentation. *Arch. Ital. Biol.*, *97*:26–32, 1959.

Battini, C., Moruzzi, G., Palestini, M., Rossi, G. F., and Zanchetti, A.: Effects of complete pontine transections on the sleep-wakefulness rhythm: The midpontine pretrigeminal preparation. *Arch. Ital. Biol.*, *97*:1–12, 1959.

Beach, F. A.: Instinctive behavior: Reproductive activities. *In* Stevens, S. S. (Ed.): *Handbook of Experimental Psychology.* New York, John Wiley & Sons, Inc., 1951, pp. 387–434.

Berger, H.: Über das elektrenkephalogramm des menschen. *Arch. Psychiat. Nervenkr.*, *87*:527–570, 1929.

Bremer, F.: Cerveau isolé et physiologie du sommeil. *C. R. Soc. Biol.*, *118*:1235–1242, 1935.

Bremer, F.: L'activité cérébrale au cours du sommeil et de la narcose. Contribution à l'étude de mécanisme du sommeil. *Bull. Acad. Belg.*, *2*:68–86, 1937.

Broadbent, D. E.: The role of auditory localization in attention and memory span. *J. Exp. Psychol.*, *47*:191–196, 1954.

Broca, P.: *Mémoires sur le Cerveau de l'Homme.* Paris, C. Reinwald, 1888.

Brush, E. S., Mishkin, M., and Rosvold, H. E.: Effects of object preferences and aversions on discrimination learning in monkeys with frontal lesions. *J. Comp. Physiol. Psychol.*, *54*:319–325, 1961.

Bures, J., and Buresova, O.: The use of Leão's spreading depression in the study of interhemispheric transfer of memory traces. *J. Comp. Physiol. Psychol.*, *53*:558–563, 1960.

Burns, J. T., House, R. F., French, F. C., and Miller, J. G.: Effects of magnesium pemoline and dextroamphetamine on human learning. *Science*, *155*:849–851, 1967.

Butter, C. M., Mishkin, M., and Rosvold, H. E.: Conditioning and extinction of a food-rewarded response after selective ablations of frontal cortex in monkeys. *Exp. Neurol.*, *7*:65–75, 1963.

Byck, R., and Dirlik, P.: Reversible section of the brain by a wall of cold. *Science*, *139*: 1216–1218, 1963.

Cannon, W. B.: Again the James-Lange and the thalamic theories of emotion. *Psychol. Rev.*, *38*:281–295, 1931.

Chorover, S. L., and Schiller, P. H.: Short-term retrograde amnesia (RA) in rats. *J. Comp. Physiol. Psychol.*, *59*:73–78, 1965.

Chow, K. L.: A retrograde cell degeneration study of the cortical projection field of the pulvinar in the monkey. *J. Comp. Neurol.*, *93*:313–340, 1950.

Chow, K. L.: Effects of combined destruction of frontal and posterior "associative areas" in monkeys. *J. Neurophysiol.*, *4*:59–71, 1951.

Chow, K. L., and Hutt, P. J.: The "association cortex" of macaca mulatta. A review of recent contributions of its anatomy and functions. *Brain*, *76*:625–677, 1953.

Creutzfeldt, O., and Jung, R.: Neuronal discharge in the cat's motor cortex during sleep and arousal. *In* Wolstenholme, G. E. W., and O'Connor, M. (Eds.): *Ciba Foundation Symposium: The Nature of Sleep.* Boston, Little, Brown and Company, 1961, pp. 131–170.

Crosby, K. G.: Attention and distractibility in

mentally retarded and average children. Unpublished Ed.D. Dissertation, Boston University, 1968.

Dement, W.: Occurrence of low voltage, fast electroencephalogram patterns during behavioral sleep in cat. *Electroenceph. Clin. Neurophysiol., 10*:291–296, 1958.

Dement, W., and Kleitman, N.: Cyclic variations in EEG during sleep and their relation to eye movements, body motility, and dreaming. *Electroenceph. Clin. Neurophysiol., 9*:673–690, 1957.

Doehring, D. G., Reitan, R. M., and Kløve, H.: Changes in patterns of intelligence test performance associated with hymonymous visual field defects. *J. Nerv. Ment. Dis., 132*:227–233, 1961.

Dorff, J. E., Mirsky, A. F., and Mishkin, M.: Effects of unilateral temporal lobe removals in man on tachistoscopic recognition in the left and right visual fields. *Neuropsychologia, 3*:39–51, 1965.

Evarts, E. V.: A review of the neurophysiological effects of lysergic acid diethylamide (LSD) and other psychotomimetic agents. *Ann. N. Y. Acad. Sci., 66*:479–495, 1957.

Evarts, E. V.: Effects of sleep and waking on spontaneous and evoked discharge of single units in visual cortex. *Fed. Proc., 19*:828–837, 1960.

Evarts, E. V.: Effects of sleep and waking on activity of single units in the unrestrained cat. *In* Wolstenholme, G. E. W., and O'Connor, M. (Eds.): *Ciba Foundation Symposium: The Nature of Sleep.* Boston, Little, Brown and Company, 1961.

Evarts, E. V.: Activity of neurons in visual cortex of the cat during sleep with low voltage fast activity. *J. Neurophysiol., 25*:812–816, 1962.

Farley, B. G., and Clarke, W. A.: Simulation of self-organizing systems by digital computer. *Trans. IRE, Vol. PGIT-4,* 76–84, 1954.

Fedio, P., and Mirsky, A. F.: Selective intellectual deficits in children with temporal lobe or centrencephalic epilepsy. *Neuropsychologia, 7*:287–300, 1969.

Flourens, P.: *Recherches Expérimentale sur les Propriétés et les Fonctions du Système Nerveux dans les Animaux Vertèbres.* Paris, Crevot, 1824.

Fonberg, E.: The inhibitory role of amygdala stimulation. *Acta Biol. Exp. (Warsz), 23*:171–180, 1963.

Freeman, H., and Watts, J. W.: *Psychosurgery.* Springfield, Illinois, Charles C Thomas Publisher, 1942.

French, J. D., Hernández-Péon, R., and Livingston, R. B.: Projections from cortex to cephalic brain stem (reticular formation) in monkey. *J. Neurophysiol., 18*:44–55 and 74–95, 1955.

Fuller, J. L., Rosvold, H. E., and Pribram, K. H.: The effects on affective and cognitive behavior in the dog of lesions of the pyriform amygdala-hippocampal complex. *J. Comp. Physiol. Psychol., 50*:89–96, 1957.

Fulton, J. F., and Jacobsen, C. F.: The functions of the frontal lobes. A comparative study in monkeys, chimpanzees and man. *Advanc. Mod. Biol. (Moscow), 4*:113–123, 1935. (Abtracts from the Second Intertional Congress, London, pp. 70–71, 1935.)

Gall, F. J., and Spurzheim, G.: *Anatomie et Physiologie du Système Nerveux en Général et du Cerveau en Particulier.* Paris, Schoell, 1810–1819.

Geschwind, N., and Levitsky, W.: Human brain: Left right asymmetries in temporal speech region. *Science, 161*:186–187, 1968.

Gibbs, F. A., and Gibbs, E. L.: *Atlas of Electroencephalography.* 2 Vols. Reading, Massachusetts, Addison-Wesley Publishing Co., Inc., 1952.

Goldman, P. Rosvold, H. E., and Mishkin, M.: Personal communication, 1969.

Goldstein, K. (Ed.): *Human Nature in the Light of Psychopathology.* Cambridge, Massachusetts, Harvard University Press, 1951.

Goldstein, K., and Scheerer, M.: Abstraction and concrete behavior. An experimental study with special tests. *Psychol. Monogr., 53*:1–151, 1941.

Granit, R.: Neural activity in the retina. *In* Field, J. (Ed.): *Handbook of Physiology.* Vol. I: *Neurophysiology.* Washington, D.C., American Physiological Society, pp. 693–712, 1959.

Grant, D. A., and Berg, E. A.: A behavioral analysis of degree of reinforcement and ease of shifting to new responses in a Weigl-type card sorting problem. *J. Exp. Psychol., 38*:404–411, 1948.

Grossman, S. P.: Eating or drinking elicited by direct adrenergic or cholinergic stimulation of hypothalamus. *Science, 132*:301–302, 1960.

Grossman, S. P.: Behavioral effects of direct chemical stimulation of central nervous system structures. *Int. J. Neuropharmacol, 3*:45–58, 1964.

Grossman, S. P.: *A Textbook of Physiological Psychology.* New York, John Wiley & Sons, Inc., 1967.

Grossman, S. P., and Grossman, L.: Food and water intake following lesions on electrical stimulation of the amygdala. *Amer. J. Physiol., 205*:761–765, 1963.

Halstead, W. C.: *Brain and Intelligence.* Chicago, University of Chicago Press, 1947.

Harlow, H. F.: Effects of induction age and size of frontal lobe lesions on learning in rhesus monkeys. *In* Isaacson, R. L. (Ed.): *The Neuropsychology of Development.* New York, John Wiley & Sons, 1968, pp. 79–120.

Harlow, H. F., Akert, K., and Schiltz, K. A.: The effects of bilateral prefrontal lesions on learned behavior of neonatal, infant and preadolescent monkeys. *In* Warren, J. M., and

Akert, K. (Eds.): *The Frontal Granular Cortex and Behavior.* New York, McGraw-Hill Book Company, 1964, pp. 126–148.

Heath, R. G. (Ed.): *Studies in Schizophrenia.* Cambridge, Massachusetts, Harvard University Press, 1954.

Hebb, D. O.: *The Organization of Behavior. A Neuropsychological Theory.* New York, John Wiley & Sons, Inc., 1949.

Hebb, D. O., and Williams, K.: A method of rating animal intelligence. *J. Genet. Psychol., 34*:59–65, 1946.

Held, R., and Hein, A. V.: Adaptation of disarranged hand-eye coordination contingent upon reafferent stimulation. *Percept. Motor Skills, 8*:87–90, 1958.

Hernández-Péon, R.: Physiological mechanisms in attention. *In* Russell, R. W., (Ed): *Frontiers in Physiological Psychology.* New York, Academic Press, Inc., 1966, pp. 121–144.

Hernández-Péon, R., Scherrer, H., and Jouvet, M.: Modification of electrical activity in cochlear nucleus during "attention" in unanesthetized cats. *Science, 123*:331–332, 1956.

Heron, W.: Perception as a function of retinal locus and attention. *Amer. J. Psychol., 70*: 38–48, 1957.

Heron, W., Doane, K. K., and Scott, J. H.: Visual disturbances after prolonged perceptual isolation. *Canad. J. Psychol., 10*:13–18, 1956.

Hess, W. R.: *Functional Organization of the Diencephalon.* New York, Grune & Stratton, Inc., 1957.

Horsley, V., and Clarke, R. H.: The structure and function of the cerebellum examined by a new method. *Brain, 31*:45–124, 1908.

Hubel, D. H.: Single unit activity in striate cortex of unrestrained cats. *J. Physiol., 147*: 226–238, 1959.

Hugelin, A., Dumont, S., and Paillas, N.: Tympanic muscles and control of auditory input during arousal. *Science, 131*:1371–1372, 1960.

Hunsperger, R. W.: Affektreaktionen auf elektrische reizung im hirnstamm der katze. *Helvet. Physiol. et Pharmacol. Acta, 14*:70–92, 1956.

Hunter, J., and Jasper, H. H.: Effects of thalamic stimulation in unanesthetized animals. The arrest reaction and petit-mal like seizure activation patterns and generalized convulsions. *Electroenceph. Clin. Neurophysiol., 1*:305–324, 1949.

Huttenlocher, P. R.: Evoked and spontaneous activity in single units of medial brain stem during natural sleep and waking. *J. Neurophysiol., 24*:451–468, 1961.

Jackson, H.: *In* Taylor, J. (Ed.): *Selected Writings of John Hughlings Jackson.* London, Hodder and Stoughton Ltd., 1931.

Jacobsen, C. F., and Nissen, H. W.: Studies of cerebral functions in primates. IV. The effects of frontal lobe lesions on the delayed alternation habit in monkeys. *J. Comp. Physiol., 23*:101–112, 1937.

Jarvik, M. E.: Consolidation of memory. *In* Efron, D. E., (Ed.): *Psychopharmacology, A Review of Progress 1957–1967.* Washington, D. C., U. S. Government Printing Office (Public Health Service Publication No. 1836), 1968, pp. 885–890.

Jasper, H. H.: Recent advances in our understanding of ascending activites of the reticular system. *In* Jasper, H. H. (Ed.): *Reticular Formation of the Brain.* Boston, Little, Brown and Company, 1958, pp. 319–331.

Jasper, H. H., and Droogleever-Fortuyn, J.: Experimental studies of the functional anatomy of petit-mal epilepsy. *Res. Publ. Ass. Res. Nerv. Ment. Dis., 26*:272–298, 1947.

John, E. R.: Neural processes during learning. *In* Russell, R. W., (Ed.): *Frontiers in Physiological Psychology.* New York, Academic Press, Inc., 1966, pp. 149–184.

John, E. R., and Killam, K. F.: Electrophysiological correlates of avoidance conditioning in the cat. *J. Pharmacol. Exp. Ther., 125*:252–274, 1959.

Jouvet, M.: Telencephalic and rhombencephalic sleep in the cat. *In* Wolstenholme, G., and O'Connor, M., (Eds.): *Ciba Foundation Symposium. The Nature of Sleep.* Boston, Little, Brown and Company, 1961, pp. 188–208.

Jouvet, M.: Recherches sur les structures nerveuses et les mécanismes responsable des différentes phases du sommeil physiologique. *Arch. Ital. Biol., 100*:125–206, 1962.

Jung, R.: Correlation of bioelectrical and autonomic phenomena with alterations of consciousness and arousal in man. *In* Adrian, E. D., Bremer, F., Jasper, H. H., and Delafresnaye, J. F. (Eds.): *Brain Mechanisms and Consciousness.* Springfield, Illinois, Charles C Thomas, 1954, pp. 31–344.

Kennard, M. A.: Age and other factors in motor recovery from precentral lesions in monkeys. *Amer. J. Physiol., 115*:138–146, 1936.

Kennard, M. A.: Reorganization of motor function in cerebral cortex of monkeys deprived of motor and premotor areas in infancy. *J. Neurophysiol., 1*:477–496, 1938.

Kennard, M. A.: Cortical reorganization of motor function: Studies on a series of monkeys of various ages from infancy to maturity. *Arch. Neurol. & Psychiat., 48*:227–240, 1942.

Kimura, D.: Cerebral dominance and the perception of verbal stimuli. *Canad. J. Psychol., 15*:156–165, 1961.

Kimura, D.: Right temporal lobe damage. *Arch. Neurol., 8*:264–271, 1963.

King, F. A.: Effects of septal and amygdaloid lesions on emotional behavior and conditioned avoidance responses in the rat. *J. Nerv. Ment. Dis., 126*:57–63, 1958.

Kling, A., and Tucker, T. J.: Effects of combined lesions of frontal granular cortex and caudate nucleus in the neonatal monkey. *Brain Res.*, *6*:428–439, 1967.

Klüver, H.: Functional differences between the occipital and temporal lobes with special reference to the interrelations of behavior and extracerebral mechanisms. *In* Jeffress, L. A. (Ed.): *Cerebral Mechanisms in Behavior. The Hixon Symposium.* New York, John Wiley & Sons, Inc., 1951, pp. 147–199.

Klüver, H.: Neurobiology of normal and abnormal perception. *In* Hoch, P., and Zubin, J. (Eds.): *Psychopathology of Perception.* New York, Grune & Stratton, Inc., 1965, pp. 1–40.

Klüver, H., and Bucy, C. P.: Preliminary analysis of functions of the temporal lobe. *Arch. Neurol. & Psychiat.*, *42*:979–1000, 1939.

Köhler, W.: *Gestalt Psychology. An Introduction to New Concepts in Modern Psychology.* New York, Liveright, 1947.

Kopeloff, N., Whittier, J. R., Pacella, B. L., and Kopeloff, L. M.: The epileptogenic effect of subcortical alumina cream in the rhesus monkey. *Electroenceph. Clin. Neurophysiol.*, *2*:163–168, 1950.

Kopp, R., Bohdanecky, Z., and Jarvik, M. E.: A long temporal gradient of retrograde amnesia for a well discriminated stimulus. *Science*, *153*:1547–1549, 1966.

Kornetsky, C.: Attention dysfunction and drugs in schizophrenia. *In* Brill, J. O. (Ed.): *Neuro-Psycho-Pharmacology.* The Hague, Netherlands, Morton and Co., 1967, pp. 948–954.

Krech, D., Rosenzweig, M. R., and Bennett, E. L.: Environmental impoverishment, social isolation and changes in brain chemistry and anatomy. *Physiol. Behav.*, *1*:99–104, 1966.

Krech, D., Rosenzweig, M. R., and Bennett, E. L.: Relations between brain chemistry and problem solving among rats raised in enriched and impoverished environments. *J. Comp. Physiol. Psychol.*, *55*:801–807, 1962.

Lansdell, H.: Effects of brain damage on intelligence in rats. *J. Comp. Physiol. Psychol.*, *46*:461–464, 1953.

Lansdell, H.: Effect of extent of temporal lobe ablations on two lateralized deficits. *Physiol. Behav.*, *3*:271–273, 1968.

Lansdell, H., and Mirsky, A. F.: The effects of focal and non-focal epilepsy on the continuous performance test. *Exp. Neurol.*, *2*:463–469, 1964.

Larsson, S.: On the hypothalamic organization of the nervous mechanism regulating food intake. *Acta Physiol. Scand.*, *32*(*Suppl. 115*): 1–63, 1954.

Lashley, K. S.: *Brain Mechanisms and Intelligence. A Study of Injuries to the Brain.* Chicago, University of Chicago Press, 1929.

Lashley, K. S.: The problem of serial order in behavior. *In* Jeffress, L. A. (Ed.): *Cerebral Mechanisms in Behavior. The Hixon Symposium.* New York, John Wiley and Sons, Inc., pp. 112–146.

Lashley, K. S., Chow, K. L., and Semmes, J.: An examination of the electrical field of cerebral integration. *Psychol. Rev.*, *58*:123–136, 1951.

Leão, A. A. P.: Spreading depression of activity in the cerebral cortex. *J. Neurophysiol.*, *7*:359–390, 1944.

Lele, P. P.: A simple method for production of trackless focal lesions with focused ultrasound: Physical factors. *J. Physiol. (Lond.)*, *160*:494–512, 1962.

Lilly, J. C.: Learning motivated by subcortical stimulation: The "start" and the "stop" patterns of behavior. *In* Ramey, E. R., and O'Doherty, D. S. (Eds.): *Electrical Studies on the Unanesthetized Brain.* New York, Hoeber Medical Division, Harper & Row, Publishers, 1960, pp. 78–105.

Lilly, J. C.: The balanced pulse-pair waveform. *In* Sheer, D. E. (Ed.): *Electrical Stimulation of the Brain.* Austin, University of Texas Press, 1961, pp. 60–64.

Lindsley, D. B., Bowden, J. W., and Magoun, H. W.: Effect upon EEG of acute injury to the brain stem activating system. *Electroenceph. Clin. Neurophysiol.*, *1*:475–486, 1949.

Machne, X., Calma, I., and Magoun, H. W.: Unit activity of central cephalic brain stem in EEG arousal. *J. Neurophysiol.*, *18*:547–558, 1955.

MacLean, P. D.: Psychosomatic disease and the "visceral brain." *Psychosom. Med.*, *11*: 338–353, 1949.

MacLean, P. D.: Some psychiatric implications of physiological studies on frontotemporal portion of limbic system (visceral brain). *Electroenceph. Clin. Neurophysiol.*, *4*:407–418, 1952.

MacLean, P. D.: The limbic system and its hippocampal formation: Studies in animals and their possible implications to man. *J. Neurosurg.*, *2*:29–44, 1954.

MacLean, P. D.: The limbic system with respect to self-preservation and the preservation of the species. *J. Nerv. Ment. Dis.*, *127*: 1–11, 1958.

McCleary, R. A.: Response specificity in the behavioral effects of limbic system lesions in the cat. *J. Comp. Physiol. Psychol.*, *54*: 605–613, 1961.

McCulloch, W. S., and Pitts, W. A.: A logical calculus of the ideas immanent in nervous activity. *Bull. Math. Biophys.*, *5*:115–133, 1943.

McGaugh, J. L.: Drug facilitation of learning and memory. *In* Efron, D. E. (ed.): *Psychopharmacology, A Review of Progress 1957–1967.* Washington, D. C., U. S. Government Printing Office (Public Health Service Publication No. 1836), 1968, pp. 891–904.

McGaugh, J. L., and Petrinovich, L.: Effects of drugs on learning and memory. *Int. Rev. Neurobiol.*, *8*:139–196, 1965.

Magnes, J., Moruzzi, G., and Pompeiano, O.: Synchronization of the EEG produced by low-frequency electrical stimulation of the solitary tract. *Arch. Ital. Biol.*, *99*:33–67, 1961.

Marsh, J. T., Worden, F. G., and Hicks, L.: Some effects of room acoustics on evoked auditory potentials. *Science*, *137*:280–282, 1962.

Melzack, R.: Effects of early perceptual restriction of simple visual discrimination. *Science*, *137*:978–979, 1962.

Mettler, F. A. (Ed.): *Selective Partial Ablation of the Frontal Cortex. A Correlative Study of the Effects on Human Psychotic Subjects.* New York, Hoeber Medical Division, Harper & Row, Publishers, 1949.

Mettler, F. A. (Ed.): *Psychosurgical Problems.* New York, The Blakiston Company, 1952.

Michael, R. P.: Oestrogens in the central nervous system. *Brit. Med. Bull.*, *21*:87–90, 1965.

Miller, G. A., Galanter, E., and Pribram, K. H.: *Plans and the Structure of Behavior.* New York, Holt, Rinehart & Winston, Inc., 1960.

Miller, N. E., Bailey, C. J., and Stevenson, J. A. F.: "Decreased hunger" but increased food intake resulting from hypothalamic lesions. *Science*, *112*:256–259, 1950.

Milner, B.: Psychological defects produced by temporal lobe excision. *Pub. Ass. Res. Nerv. Ment. Dis.*, *36*:244–257, 1958.

Milner, B.: Laterality effects in audition. *In* Mountcastle, V. P. (Ed.): *Interhemispheric Relations and Cerebral Dominance.* Baltimore, The Johns Hopkins Press, 1962, pp. 177–195.

Milner, B.: Effects of different brain lesions on card sorting. *Arch. Neurol.*, *9*:90–100, 1963.

Milner, B.: Amnesia following operation on the temporal lobes. *In* Whittey, C. W. M., and Zangwill, O. L. (Eds.): *Amnesia.* London, Butterworth & Co. (Publishers) Ltd., 1966, pp. 109–133.

Milner, B.: The memory defect in bilateral hippocampal lesions. *Psychiatric Research Reports 11*, American Psychiatric Association, December, 1969, pp. 43–52.

Milner, P.: The cell assembly: Mark II. *Psychol. Rev.*, *64*:242–252, 1957.

Mirsky, A. F.: Neuropsychological bases of schizophrenia. *In* Rosenzweig, M. (Ed.): *Annual Review of Psychology.* Palo Alto, Annual Reviews Inc., 1969, Vol. XX, pp. 321–348.

Mirsky, A. F., and Bakay Pragay, E.: The relation of EEG and performance in altered states of consciousness. *In* Kety, S. S., Evarts, E. V., and Williams, H. L. (Eds.): *Sleep and Altered States of Consciousness.* Baltimore, The Williams and Wilkins Co., 1967, pp. 514–534.

Mirsky, A. F., Bloch-Rojas, S., and McNary, W. F.: Experimental "petit mal" epilepsy produced with chlorambucil. *Acta Biol. Exp.* (Warsz.), *25*:55–61, 1966.

Mirsky, A. F., and Kornetsky, C.: On the dissimilar effects of drugs on the digit symbol substitution and continuous performance tests. *Psychopharmacologia*, 5:161–177, 1964.

Mirsky, A. F., and Kornetsky, C.: The effect of centrally acting drugs on attention. *In* Efron, D. E. (Ed.): *Psychopharmacology, A Review of Progress 1957–1967.* Washington, D. C., U. S. Government Printing Office (Public Health Service Publication No. 1836), 1968, pp. 91–104.

Mirsky, A. F., Primac, D. W., Ajmone Marsan, C., Rosvold, H. E., and Stevens, J. R.: A comparison of the psychological test performance of patients with focal and nonfocal epilepsy. *Exp. Neurol.*, *2*:75–89, 1960.

Mirsky, A. F., and Tecce, J. J.: The analysis of visual evoked potentials during spike and wave EEG activity. *Epilepsia*, *9*:211–220, 1968.

Mirsky, A. F., and Van Buren, J. M.: On the nature of the "absence" in centrencephalic epilsepsy: A study of some behavioral, electroencephalographic and autonomic factors. *Electroenceph. Clin. Neurophysiol.*, *18*:334–348, 1965.

Mishkin, M.: Effects of small frontal lesions on delayed alternation in monkeys. *J. Neurophysiol.*, *60*:615–622, 1957.

Mishkin, M.: Visual discrimination following partial ablations of the temporal lobe. II. Ventral surface vs. hippocampus. *J. Comp. Physiol. Psychol.*, *47*:187–193, 1954.

Mishkin, M.: Perseveration of central sets after frontal lesions in monkeys. *In* Warren, J. M., and Akert, K. (Eds.): *The Frontal Granular Cortex and Behavior.* New York, McGraw-Hill Book Company, 1964, pp. 219–241.

Mishkin, M.: Visual mechanisms beyond the striate cortex. *In* Russell, R. W. (Ed.): *Frontiers in Physiological Psychology.* New York, Academic Press, Inc., 1966, pp. 93–119.

Mishkin, M., and Forgays, D. G.: Word recognition as a function of retinal location. *J. Exp. Psychol.*, *43*:43–48, 1952.

Mishkin, M., and Pribram, K. H.: Visual discrimination performance following partial ablations of the temporal lobe. I. Ventral vs. lateral. *J. Comp. Physiol. Psychol.*, *47*:14–20, 1954.

Mishkin, M., Prockop, E. S., and Rosvold, H. E.: One-trial object-discrimination learning in monkeys with frontal lesions. *J. Comp. Physiol. Psychol.*, *55*:178–181, 1962.

Moniz, E.: *Tentative Operatoires dan le Traitement de Certaines Psychoses.* Paris, Masson, 1936.

Morison, R. S., and Dempsey, E. W.: Mechanism of thalamo-cortical augmentation and repetition. *Amer. J. Physiol.*, *138*:297–308, 1943.

Moruzzi, G., and Magoun, H. W.: Brain stem reticular formation and activation of the EEG. *Electroenceph. Clin. Neurophysiol.*, *1*:455–473, 1949.

Moushegian, G., Rupert, A., Marsh, J. T., and

Galambos, R.: Evoked cortical potentials in absence of middle ear muscles. *Science, 133*:582–583, 1961.
Nauta, W. J. H.: Hippocampal projections and related neural pathways to the midbrain in the cat. *Brain, 81*:319–340, 1958.
Nauta, W. J. H.: Central nervous organization and the endocrine motor system. *In* Nalbanov, A. V. (Ed.): *Advances in Neuroendocrinology.* Urbana, Illinois, University of Illinois Press, 1963, pp. 5–28.
Nauta, W. J. H., and Kuypers, G. J. M.: Some ascending pathways in the brain stem reticular formation. *In* Jasper, H. H., Proctor, L. D., Knighton, R. S., Noshay, W. C., and Costello, R. T. (Eds.): *Reticular Formation of the Brain.* Boston, Little, Brown and Company, 1958, pp. 3–30.
Neff, W. D.: Neural mechanisms of auditory discrimination. *In* Rosenblith, W. A., (Ed.): *Sensory Communication.* New York, John Wiley and Sons, Inc., 1961, pp. 259–278.
Lorente de Nó, R.: Cerebral cortex: Architecture. *In* Fulton, J. F. (Ed.): *Physiology of the Nervous System.* New York, Oxford University Press, Inc., 1943, pp. 274–301.
Olds, J.: A preliminary mapping of electrical reinforcing effects in the rat brain. *J. Comp. Physiol. Psychol., 49*:281–285, 1956.
Olds, J., and Milner, P.: Positive reinforcement produced by electrical stimulation of the septal area and other regions of the rat brain. *J. Comp. Physiol. Psychol., 47*:419–427, 1954.
Olds, J., Mink, W. D., and Best, P. J.: Conditioned responses of hippocampal and other neurons. *Electroenceph. Clin. Neurophysiol., 26*:159–166, 1969.
Papez, J. W.: A proposed mechanism of emotion. *Arch. Neurol. Psychiat. (Chicago), 38*:725–743, 1937.
Pavlov, I. P.: *Conditioned reflexes. An investigation of the physiological activity of the cerebral cortex.* (Trans. and edited by G. V. Anrep.) New York, Dover Publications, Inc., 1960.
Penfield, W., and Jasper, H. H.: *Epilepsy and the Functional Anatomy of the Human Brain.* Boston, Little, Brown and Company, 1954.
Pollen, D. A., Perot, P., and Reid, K.: Experimental bilateral wave and spike from thalamic stimulation in relation to level of arousal. *Electroenceph. Clin. Neurophysiol., 15*: 1017–1028, 1963.
Porteus, S. D., and Peters, H.: Maze test validation and psychosurgery. *Genet. Psychol. Monogr., 36*:3–86, 1947.
Pradhan, S. N., and Ajmone Marsan, C.: Chlorambucil toxicity and EEG "centrencephalic" patterns. *Epilepsia, 4*:1–14, 1963.
Pribram, H., and Barry, J.: Further behavioral analysis of the parieto-temporo-preoccipital cortex. *J. Neurophysiol., 19*:99–106, 1956.
Pribram, K. H.: Neocortical function in behavior. *In* Harlow, H. (Ed.): *Biological and Biochemical Bases of Behavior.* Madison, University of Wisconsin Press, 1958, pp. 151–172.
Pribram, K. H., and Kruger, L.: Functions of the "olfactory brain." *Ann. N. Y. Acad. Sci., 58*:109–138, 1954.
Pribram, K. H., Mishkin, M., Rosvold, H. E., and Kaplan, S. J.: Effects on delayed response performance of lesions of dorsolateral and ventromedial frontal cortex of baboons. *J. Comp. Physiol. Psychol., 45*:565–575, 1952.
Reitan, R. M.: Psychological deficits resulting from cerebral lesions in man. *In* Warren, J. M., and Akert, K. (Eds.): *The Frontal Granular Cortex and Behavior.* New York, McGraw-Hill Book Company, 1964, pp. 295–312.
Riesen, A. H.: Stimulation as a requirement for growth and function in behavioral development. *In* Fishe, D. W., and Maddi, S. R. (Eds.): *Functions of Varied Experience.* Homewood, Illinois, Dorsey Press, 1961, pp. 57–80.
Rimbaud, L., Passouant, P., and Cadilhac, J.: Participation de l'hippocampi à la régulation des états de veille et de sommeil. *Rev. Neurol., 93*:303–308, 1955.
Robins, E., Smith, K., and Lowe, I. P.: Discussion of clinical studies with taraxein. *In* Abramson, H. A. (Ed.): *Neuropharmacology, Transactions of the Fourth Conference.* New York, Josia Macy, Jr. Foundation, 1957, pp. 123–135.
Ross, A. O.: Brain injury and intellectual performance. *J. Consult. Psychol., 22*:151–152, 1958.
Rosvold, H. E.: The effects of electroconvulsive shock on gestation and maternal behavior. I and II. *J. Comp. Physiol. Psychol., 42*:118–136 and 207–219, 1949.
Rosvold, H. E., and Delgado, J. M. R.: The effect on delayed-alternation test performance of stimulating or destroying electrically structures within the frontal lobes of the monkey brain. *J. Comp. Physiol. Psychol., 49*:365–372, 1956.
Rosvold, H. E., Mirsky, A. F., and Pribram, K. H.: Influence of amygdalectomy on social behavior in monkeys. *J. Comp. Physiol. Psychol., 47*:173–178, 1954.
Rosvold, H. E., Mirsky, A. F., Sarason, I., Bransome, E. D., and Beck, L. H.: A continuous performance test of brain damage. *J. Consult. Psychol., 20*:343–350, 1956.
Rosvold, H. E., Szwarcbart, M. K., Mirsky, A. F., and Mishkin, M.: The effect of frontal-lobe damage on delayed-response performance in chimpanzees. *J. Comp. Physiol. Psychol., 54*:368–374, 1961.
Rothballer, A. B., Jarvik, M. E., and Jacobs, G. B.: Effects of intracarotid and intravertebral amobarbital and physostigmine in conscious, intact cats. *In* Kety, S. S., and Elkes,

J. (Eds.): *Regional Neurochemistry.* New York, Pergamon Press, Inc., 1961, pp. 442–454.

Rowe, S. N.: Mental changes following removal of the right cerebral hemisphere for brain tumor. *Amer. J. Psychiat., 94*:605–614, 1937.

Sawa, M., Yukiharu, U., Masaya, A., and Toshio, H.: Preliminary report on the amygdaloidectomy on the psychotic patients, with interpretation of oral-emotional manifestations in schizophrenics. *Folia Psychiat. Neurol. Jap., 7*:309–316, 1954.

Sawyer, C. H.: Reproductive behavior. *In* Fridd, J. (Ed.): *Handbook of Physiology.* Section 1: Neurophysiology. Baltimore, Waverly Press, Inc., 1960, Vol. II, pp. 1225–1240.

Schreiner, L. H., and Kling, A.: Behavioral changes following rhinencephalic injury in cat. *J. Neurophysiol., 16*:643–659, 1953.

Scoville, W. B., and Milner, B.: Loss of recent memory after bilateral hippocampal lesions. *J. Neurol. Neurosurg. Psychiat., 20*:11–21, 1957.

Sem-Jacobsen, C. W., and Torkildsen, A.: Depth recording and electrical stimulation in the human brain. *In* Ramey, E. R., and O'Doherty, D. S. (Eds.): *Electrical Studies on the Unanesthetized Brain.* New York, Hoeber Medical Division, Harper & Row, Publishers, pp. 275–287.

Semmes, J., Weinstein, S., Ghent, L., and Teuber, H. L.: *Somatosensory Changes after Penetrating Brain Wounds in Man.* Cambridge, Massachusetts, Harvard University Press, 1960.

Sherrington, C. S.: *The Integrative Action of the Nervous System.* New Haven, Yale University Press, 1947.

Skinner, B. F.: *Behavior of Organisms: An Experimental Approach.* New York, Appleton-Century-Crofts, 1938.

Sperry, R. W., Miner, N., and Myers, R. E.: Visual pattern perception following subpial slicing and tantalum wire implantations in the visual cortex. *J. Comp. Physiol. Psychol., 48*:50–58, 1955.

Sprague, J. M., Chambers, W. W., and Stellar, E.: Attention, affective and adaptive behavior in the cat. *Science, 133*:165–173, 1961.

Sprague, J. M., Levitt, M., Robson, K., Liu, C. N., Stellar, E., and Chambers, W. W.: A neuroanatomical and behavioral analysis of the syndromes resulting from midbrain lemniscal and reticular lesions in the cat. *Arch. Ital. Biol., 101*:225–295, 1963.

Stamm, J. S.: Retardation and facilitation of learning by stimulation of frontal cortex in monkeys. *In* Warren, J. M., and Akert, K. (Eds.): *The Frontal Granular Cortex and Behavior.* New York, McGraw-Hill Book Company, 1964, pp. 102–125.

Stone, C. P.: Effects of electroconvulsive shock on daily activity of albino rats in revolving drums. *Proc. Soc. Exp. Biol. Med., 61*:150–151, 1946.

Tecce, J. J.: Attention and evoked potentials in man. *In* Mostofsky, D. I. (Ed.): *Attention: Contemporary Theory and Analysis.* New York, Appleton-Century-Crofts, 1970, pp. 331–365.

Teitelbaum, P.: Sensory control of hypothalamus hyperphagia. *J. Comp. Physiol. Psychol., 48*:158–163, 1955.

Teitelbaum, P.: Disturbances in feeding and drinking behavior after hypothalamic lesions. *In* Jones, M. R. (Ed.): *Nebraska Symposium on Motivation.* Lincoln, Nebraska, University of Nebraska Press, 1961, pp. 39–65.

Terzian, H., and Dalle Ore, G.: Syndrome of Klüver and Bucy reproduced in man by bilateral removal of the temporal lobes. *Neurology, 5*:373–380, 1955.

Teuber, H. L., Battersby, W. S., and Bender, M. B.: Performance of complex visual tasks after cerebral lesions. *J. Nerv. Ment. Dis., 114*:413–429, 1951.

Teuber, H. L., and Mishkin, M.: Judgment of visual and postural vertical after brain injury. *J. Psychol., 38*:161–175, 1954.

Teuber, H. L., and Weinstein, S.: Performance on a formboard-task after penetrating brain injury. *J. Psychol., 38*:177–190, 1954.

Toman, J. P.: Some aspects of central nervous pharmacology. *In* Cutting, W. C. (Ed.): *Annual Review of Pharmacology.* Palo Alto, Annual Reviews, Inc., 1963, Vol. III, pp. 153–184.

Towbin, A.: Mental retardation due to germinal matrix infarction. *Science, 164*:156–161, 1969.

U. S. War Department, Adjutant General's Office, Classification and Replacement Brain, Pers. Res. Sec. The Army general classification test. *Psychol. Bull., 42*:760–768, 1945.

Valenstein, E. S., and Beer, B.: Continuous opportunity for reinforcing brain stimulation. *J. Exp. Anal. Behav., 7*:183–184, 1964.

Villablanca, J.: Electroencephalogram in the permanently isolated forebrain of the cat. *Science, 138*:44–46, 1962.

Wada, J.: (A new method for the determination of the side of cerebral speech dominance. A preliminary report on the intracarotid injection of sodium amytal in man.) *Med. Biol.* (Tokyo), *14*:221–222, 1949.

Weinstein, S.: Deficits concomitant with aphasia or lesions of either cerebral hemisphere. *Cortex, 1*:154–169, 1964.

Weinstein, S., and Teuber, H. L.: Effects of penetrating brain injury on intelligence test scores. *Science, 125*:1036–1037, 1957.

Weiskrantz, L.: Behavioral changes associated with ablations of the amygdaloid complex in monkey. *J. Comp. Physiol. Psychol., 49*:381–391, 1956.

Weiskrantz, L., Mihailovic, L., and Gross, C. G.: Effects of stimulation of frontal cortex and hippocampus on behavior in monkey. *Brain, 85*:487–504, 1962.

Weitzman, E.: Note on EEG and eye movements during behavioral sleep in monkeys. *Electroenceph. Clin. Neurophysiol., 13*:790–794, 1961.

Wilson, W. A., Jr., and Mishkin, M.: Comparison of the effects of inferotemporal and lateral occipital lesions on visually guided behavior in monkeys. *J. Comp. Physiol. Psychol., 52*:10–17, 1959.

Windle, W. F.: Respiratory distress: Relation to prematurity and other factors in newborn monkeys. *Science, 143*:1345–1346, 1964.

3 PERCEPTION

Ronald H. Forgus

Since physicians have the responsibility of keeping people healthy, they are constantly faced with the task of diagnosing and remediating a physical or psychological dysfunction. It is within this context of adaptive behavior that this chapter is cast —that is, perception as related to the processes involved in man's adaptation to his environment.

PERCEPTION AND ADAPTIVE BEHAVIOR

It almost goes without saying that the individual must receive reliable information from the environment in order to cope and to adapt effectively. The process of perception mediated through the senses and the brain is involved with how this information is obtained, maintained and utilized.

Definition of Perception

For our purposes, perception is defined as the process of information extraction. Late in this chapter we will present a model to elaborate the functions involved in this process. At this point it is necessary to emphasize that from the vast array of physical energy which impinges upon the individual's senses, only the energy from which the nervous system can code significant *information* will initiate an effective perceptual process.

Phylogenetic Perspective for Adaptive Behavior

It is quite logical to conceive of the perceptual process in stimulus-response terms. Thus we could simply write behavioral laws which relate the information contained in the stimulus complex to the nature of the organism's responses. This is in fact what has been done with great accuracy and predictability in lower animals by ethologists and animal psychologists. For example, Tinbergen and Perdeck (1950) have shown that the mechanism through which the fledgling herring gull pecks food from its mother's beak is effected by a very simple *built-in* reflex system. The releaser stimulus (which invariably gives rise to the built-in pecking response) is a segregated red against a yellow background—for example, a red tongue against a yellow beak or any synthetic simulation thereof.

Just as nature has provided for the regulation of eating in the herring gull, adaptive behavioral patterns have ensured for other survival needs through evolutionary development in lower animals. Thus, ethologists such as Lorenz (1958) have shown how such adaptive behavior as spawning, imprinting and aggression (as well as its inhibition) is controlled by instinctive patterns which are chains of reflexive-tropistic reactions.

Needless to say, this kind of universal predictability for all members of a species is by no means true for the human organism; on the contrary, we are characterized by wide individual differences in the ways we go about coping with and adapting to environmental demands. Our adaptive behavioral patterns are far less fixed by genetic determination and are far more subject to postnatal modification. As a result of this greater modifiability, man has developed the capacity to perceive—that is, to extract information from—a very wide range of stimuli or stimulus patterns. Just think, for example, of the ability of humans to recognize literally thousands of different faces, to read, to solve mathematical problems, to appreciate beauty and so on. Yet, evidence which we will analyze later in the chapter indicates that the perceptual abilities of human infants are somewhat limited, and that the wider range of discrimination develops with age, primarily as a result of learning or practice. We therefore say that while some *built-in* or *wired-in programs* are necessary for the adaptive process to commence, these programs become modified as a result of learning.

For example, the newborn human is capable of making a preferential response to a differentiated rather than a homogeneous stimulus; this built-in program becomes modified by subsequent sensory stimulation and experience into more sophisticated perceptions such as the recognition of specific human faces. It is within the context of these *modified programs* that we can better understand both the extensive range of human perceptions and the wide individual differences within this range. To this task we now proceed.

THE HIERARCHICAL ORGANIZATION OF PERCEPTION

The concept of modified programs implies that we cannot make a clear-cut distinction between perception and so-called pure sensation, since, following experience, no pure sensation can exist. Rather, the total act of perception is a multistage process, beginning with simple stages which become increasingly more complex.

One reason that classic philosophical theory failed to realize the integration of sensation into perception was the absence of the analytical tools of modern experimental psychology. One of these tools is the *tachistoscope,* which presents the stimulus for varying durations and thereby makes it possible to study stages within the total perceptual process.

When the total process of perception is broken down in this manner, it can be ordered into a hierarchy, beginning at the primitive stage of perception and extending through the most sophisticated stage, with each successive progression in the hierarchy involving the *extraction and segregation of more information* from the stimulus energy. This order, listed from the simplest to the most complex task, conforms to the following sequence:

1. The *detection* of the stimulus energy and a discrimination of change in stimulus energy; i.e., simply being aware of whether a stimulus is present and whether there is a single change in the stimulus.
2. The discrimination of a unified brightness or *figural unity* as separate from the background; e.g., seeing a homogeneous white patch emerge from a black background without further elaboration of the white patch.
3. The *resolution* of *finer details,* which gives rise to a more *differentiated* perception; e.g., the figure is more than a homogeneous brightness and has some additional features.
4. The *identification* or recognition of a *form* or *pattern;* e.g., the additional features are integrated into a recognizable identity.

5. The *manipulation* of the identified form; i.e., what you do with the total information you have processed. This happens, for example, in *problem solving, conceptual thought* and *social perception.*

There are experimental studies which support this notion that perception is not a unitary task but rather is an integration over a set of hierarchically ordered substages. We have classified these studies into the following categories, along with a very brief description within each category.

Studies of the Threshold Determination for Light and Form

A number of studies have found that progressively more energy is required for each successive task of the hierarchy to take place (Davies, 1905; Dickinson, 1926; Wever, 1927; Freeman, 1929; Helson and Fehrer, 1932; Bridgen, 1933; Douglas, 1947). Representative of these studies is the finding of Helson and Fehrer that the recognition of form (Task 4) requires 25 times as much light energy as the just-discriminable detection of light (Task 1), and that the perception of vague form (Task 2) requires a value of 15 times as much light energy.

Studies of the Role of Learning

A number of studies indicate that learning is necessary for the higher stages, especially Tasks 4 and 5, but plays essentially no role in Task 1. This applies throughout the phylogenetic scale. Most of the evidence was brought together by Hebb (1937a, 1937b). He initiated this kind of research by comparing the discrimination ability of rats who were reared in the dark with that of rats who were reared under normal conditions. He found that while the two groups were equivalent in brightness discrimination (Task 1), the dark-reared rats were inferior in pattern perception (Task 4).

In his work with primates, Riesen (1947) found that there was little difference between dark-reared and normally reared chimpanzees in brightness and color discrimination (Task 1), whereas the animals deprived of light experience were grossly inferior in form discrimination (Task 4). The fact that similar results (Riesen, 1958) were found when the deprived group was raised in diffuse light rather than in darkness rules out an explanation based solely on organic atrophy, and points to the importance of experience. In fact, in some cases the deprived chimpanzees required three to four weeks of learning before they could discriminate between two identities even though this discrimination was instrumental in preventing an electric shock.

Senden (1932, 1960) collected similar reports from clinical observations of human adults who underwent surgical removal of congenital cataracts and were consequently first capable of vision after reaching adulthood. Again it was found that while brightness perception appeared to be normal, discrimination and recognition of form identity required much learning, sometimes two months or longer.

This research with three different species indicates that learning is important for the development of higher order perception across a wide range of mammals. However, we would expect that man is capable of more sophisticated perceptions because of his wider range of experience and his more complex cortex. These differences in cognitive abilities between lower and higher animals, and also between young children and older ones, probably involve progressing from the generalization of concrete parts to the generalization of relationships. Nevertheless, it is testimony to the extreme modifiability of the mammalian nervous system that Forgus (1954, 1956) was able to demonstrate, even in rats, how these pattern generalizations and abstractions can be improved by more differentiated visual exposure during early experience.

Studies of the Development of Perception

The findings from the aforementioned studies on deprivation and enrichment have been corroborated by research dealing with the growth of perception as the young child develops.

Fantz (1965) used a technique whereby he could directly observe and photograph the attentional process of young infants while they were presented with pairs of stimuli. Three kinds of results were obtained:

1. In general, the infants preferred heterogeneous to homogeneous patterns. For example, when given a choice between three stimulus patterns, 8-week-old infants would fixate, during a one-minute test, a bull's-eye for 20 seconds, a horizontally striped pattern for 10 seconds and a homogeneously colored rectangle for only a brief glance; whereas infants under 2 weeks of age preferred the intermediate complexity of the striped pattern.

2. The infants preferred looking at a pattern of a human face rather than at printed matter, and looking at a bull's-eye rather than homogeneously colored disks, in that order. The pattern, not color or brightness, was important.

3. The adaptive significance of attending to certain forms was indicated by the fact that order of preference was (1) a human face, (2) a scrambled-face pattern and (3) an oval which was black at the top and reddish at the bottom. It is important to note that a human infant's preference for the human face is age-dependent and does not emerge until 8 to 10 weeks of age.

While the work of Fantz suggests that the progressive growth of the ability to recognize form or pattern requires experience, it also points out that this capacity has an innate foundation, since very young infants still prefer some degree of complexity. It is reasonable to assert—in fact it seems that it is logically necessary—that *there can be no adaptive behavior without some built-in coding ability* to program or to discriminate some degree of heterogeneity (pattern) from homogeneity. If such innate, wired-in programs were not present at birth, no reactions would be possible, and without reactivity there could be no learning.

Evidence that the cerebral cortex contains cells which have the capacity to code specific attributes and dimensions of the form of the stimulus in the informational complex has been obtained in painstaking research conducted by Hubel and Wiesel (1959, 1962, 1968). Very fine, small electrodes were implanted in single cells of the visual cortex of both cats and monkeys, so that recordings could be taken from these electrodes while various kinds of stimuli were presented to the eye (retina) of the intact animal. The differential pattern of responsiveness indicated that the visual cortex consists of different categories of neural cells, each category being maximally sensitive to a particular kind of stimulus dimension. Some cells respond to both location and orientation, some to only one of these, others to edge, still others to movement and so on. Furthermore, within the class of orientation, the cells are specific with respect to one dimension of orientation. For example, a "vertical" cell will respond maximally if a line or bar is presented in the vertical orientation but will respond very weakly if a line is presented in the horizontal position.

It seems reasonable to infer from the work on single-cell recording that there is an innate foundation for coding the specific elements of form because of the way specific cells respond. What experience probably creates is the patterning of these cells into the necessary cortical organization required for form, identity and relational perception. (See Hebb's theoretical discussion on the growth of the cell assembly, 1949.)

The interaction between these innate-maturational and learning determiners of form perception is nicely seen in additional data from Fantz (1961). After establishing that the perception of form (sphere *versus* pyramid) was largely innate in chicks, Fantz raised monkeys in darkness for periods ranging from one to eleven weeks. When the monkeys reared under these reduced conditions for the shorter periods were brought into a normal environment, they generally exhibited good spatial orientation after a few hours or days, and they also showed the usual interest in patterned objects. But those left in the dark for the longer periods were completely disoriented in space when brought into the light for the first time. "These older infant monkeys bumped into things, fell off tables, could not locate objects visually—for all practical purposes they were blind" (Fantz, 1961, p. 5). Contrasted with the younger monkeys, who preferred patterned objects, the older monkeys appeared to be more interested in color, brightness and size, and it took some of them weeks to "learn to see."

What conclusions can be drawn? Obviously, innate ability cannot be the whole answer. Otherwise the dark-reared animals would not have been so highly disoriented. Maturation is not enough either, since otherwise the younger animals would not have been superior to the older ones. Nor can learning stand alone, since the older animals required a longer time to learn to perceive form and space than did the younger monkeys. Evidently, there is an interesting interaction between learning and the preceding developmental history of the organism, such that the *amount of training interacts with the time at which the training originates to determine maximal effectiveness in facilitating the growth of form perception.*

A COGNITIVE DEFINITION OF PERCEPTION

The previous section reviewed data which make clear that neither a purely nativistic nor a purely empirical theory of perception is tenable. However, the debate in psychology concerning the relative importance of these two determiners of cognition has a long history, which goes back to Plato and Aristotle and can be traced through Descartes, Locke, Hume and Kant.

The logical core of this debate was brought into sharp focus by the Gestalt psychologists (see Wertheimer, 1923; Koffka, 1935), who asserted that if experience influenced perceptual organization, there already existed certain intrinsic laws which governed the way stimuli are organized, and that these Gestalt laws of perceptual organization are prior to experience and thus direct the influence of experience.

These laws were first described by Max Wertheimer (1923). One could go into a set of elaborated illustrations of these laws, but they are all based on what Wertheimer called the *Law of Prägnanz,* which states that stimulus elements will be grouped into organizations which are as regular, symmetric, simple, inclusive, continuous and unified as possible. The other laws of perceptual organization should be considered as subsidiary to the leading principle of Prägnanz; they merely describe how the latter is attained. They include the laws of closure, inclusiveness,

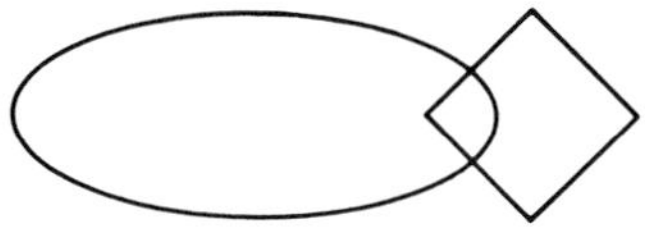

An example of closure:

Seen as an oblong and a square.

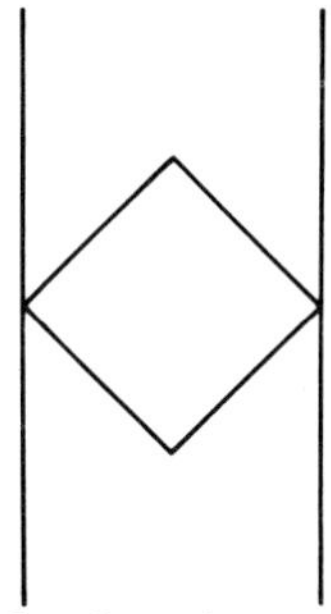

Example of good continuation:

Seen as a diamond in the middle of two lines—not a W on top of an M.

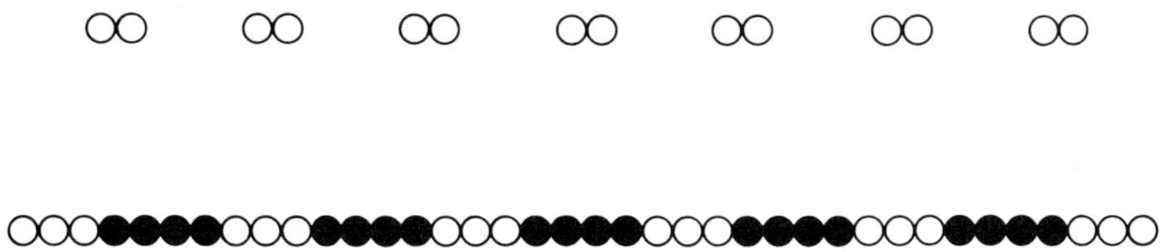

In the top row, segregation is achieved by the law of proximity, whereas in the bottom row the spaces between dots are uniform and segregation is achieved by similarity.

Figure 3–1 Examples of Gestalt laws of perceptual organization.

good continuation and direction, proximity and similarity, examples of which are shown in Figure 3–1.

Since we cannot illustrate these laws more fully here, the interested reader can consult Koffka (1935) or Forgus (1966, pp. 112–131). It should be added, however, that while the early Gestalt theorists left open the possibility that past experience leaves effects or a *trace* which could alter subsequent perception, their major emphasis was on the immediate *isomorphic* relationship between external stimulus patterns and brain field organizations. However, the evidence reviewed in the last section indicates that any comprehensive theory of perception must assign a more central role to learning.

It was not until Hebb (1949) published his most influential neuropsychological theory, and until the implications of information theory (Shannon and Weaver, 1949) and information processing (Broadbent, 1958) for psychology were realized, that psychologists conceptualized more adequate ways to explain how innate coding of certain gross stimulus dimensions can be modified into a variety of complex perception systems. Thus, perception has innate components which become elaborated with learning and experience.

Definition of Perception as a Superset

At the beginning of this chapter we defined perception simply as the process of information extraction. We would now like to elaborate this definition, taking into account what we have so far developed about how learning is related to perception.

One can apply the mathematical construct of *SET* to conceptualize the organization of the perceptual process. A set is defined as a collection of items which have some relational or directional property. There can be 1, 2, 3 . . . or N items in the set. A further elaboration of this definition in Webster's dictionary states that *to set* is to "fix something mentally or to direct with a purpose."

It is in the context of the mathematical definition of set, buttressed by the evidence that the process of information extraction is universally involved in man's adaptive behavior, that this author was led to the conviction that perception must be related to the general problem of cognitive development. Looked at in this way, perception becomes the *basic* process in the acquisition of cognition and should throw light on the development of, for example, reading, language and learning disorders as well as on perceptual handicaps. In fact, we can conceive of a *family of sets* and relate perception to motivation, emotion and personality.

But, to get back to cognition as such, *we will thus define perception as a superset, with learning and thinking as subsets under the perceptual process.* This relationship between learning and thinking in the complex process of perception is shown in Figure 3–2.

The direction of the arrows in Figure 3–2 can be used to understand why the author holds the rather strong and unconventional view that learning and thinking are subordinate to the superset of perception. The process begins with the stimulus being coded by the organism. This first stage, which is traditionally called perception, also leads to learning and, subsequently, to thinking. Clearly, therefore, we can have no learning or thinking without perception. One could therefore parsimoniously view learning and thinking as extensions of the perceptual process, with the traditional separations of these three divisions of the cognitive process being arbitrary cut-off points.

To elaborate further on Figure 3–2, the work on the perception of brightness and figure/ground separation indicates that the organism's ability to react to these stimuli is innate. The nervous system reactivity *modifies cortical cell organization,* so that learning and, later, thinking can develop. We can thus understand how developmental experience in the perceptual realm produces the family of sets which provides the structural foundation for the hierarchical organization of perception, from the primitive level of sensory discrimination, on through learning and finally to thought.

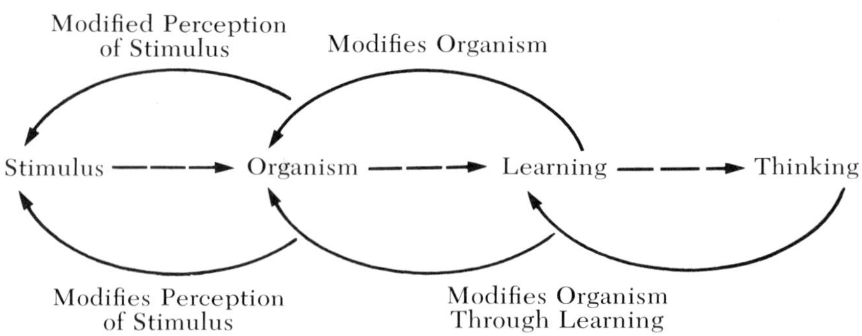

Figure 3–2 The relationship of learning and thinking in the complex process of perception. After stimulus information is extracted and stored as learning, it influences thinking. Thought modifies the organism, because new learning occurs. Thus, the perception of stimuli is modified. The process involves two-way relationships.

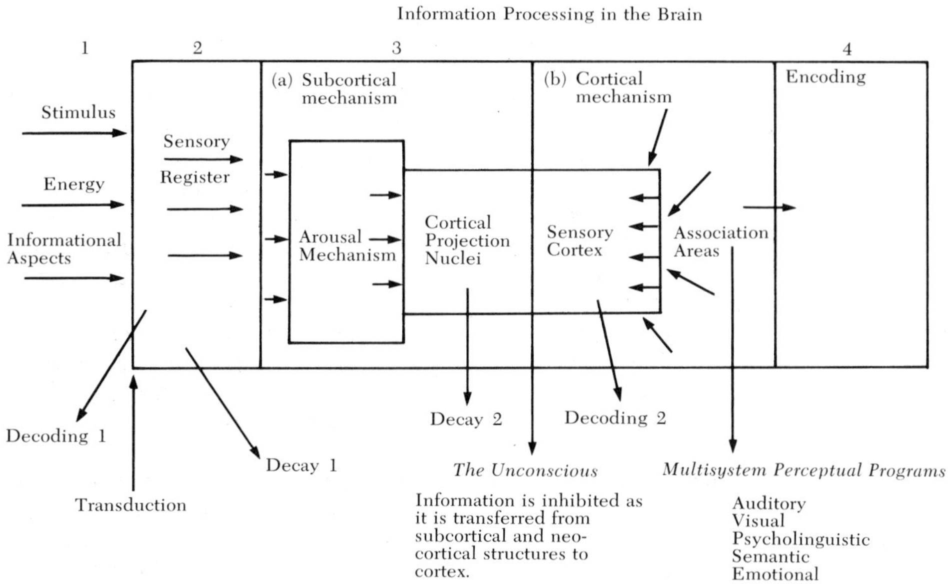

Figure 3–3 A model of the information extraction process. See text for explanation.

The relationship between the subsystems in the cognitive process is, however, by no means unidirectional. A good example of how the process works in the other direction is the way stereotyped thinking inhibits future learning and constricts the information coming from a message. An example of experimental verification of the fact that learning can be either facilitated or inhibited by thinking sets is given in a study by Forgus and Schwartz (1957).

A Model to Explain How the Perceptual Process Works

Having defined perception as a family of sets, we now present a model to explain how the subsets or subsystems within this superset are organized. This model is schematized in Figure 3–3.

The stages in this process of perception are as follows:

1. *First,* there must of course be the potential *informational aspects of stimulus energy* (for example, the dimensions of intensity and hue contain relatively simple information in comparison with the shape of contours).

2. These informational aspects must be transduced into units which the nervous system can meaningfully use (Lowenstein, 1966). This *second* stage of transduction and analysis takes place within the *sensory register* and seems to be primarily in units of the physical attributes of intensity, frequency, location, orientation, extension and so on (*Decoding 1*). We note in passing that some decay (*Decay 1*) can take place in Stage 2. Later in this chapter when we discuss research on the sensory register and sensory masking, we will see that if the transduced information is not passed on within one-fourth to three-fourths of a second following registration, it will be lost. That is, the registration is quite transient.

3. Two things can happen to transduced stimulation as it is passed on to the *third* stage of information processing:

(a) *Gross stimulation* from all the senses congregates at the midregion (called the Ascending Reticular Activating System or ARAS) of the brain stem, where the coming together acts as some kind of amplification. From here, impulses diffusely bombard the cerebral cortex in general in order to arouse it. If the *arousal* level does not reach a sufficient (but still indeterminate) intensity, integrated perception and thought is not possible, as we know from the work on relative deprivation of sensory stimulation (Heron et al., 1956; Heron, 1957) and also from our own experience of the time required to "get going" after we wake from sleep.

(b) More *specific information* is directed to the *projection nuclei* of the diencephalon (thalamic region), and from here it is projected to primary sensory areas of the cortex (e.g., occipital lobe for vision, part of the temporal lobe for audition, part of the parietal lobe for somesthetic perception and so on). We note again in passing that some decay (*Decay 2*) can take place at Stage 3a either because of channel overloading (i.e., more signals congregating at the projection nuclei than can be passed on to the primary sensory areas of the cortex) or because of a state of overarousal (i.e., too much diffuse bombardment of the cortex, so that organized perceptual processing is disrupted).

For certain kinds of information (e.g., brightness perception), the perceptual processing is complete when the information reaches the sensory cortex (*Decoding 2*).

For other kinds of information, the association areas of the cortex provide *contextual models* or *sets* as a reference against which the incoming information is judged or tested before the information processing is complete. These models consist of modified programs which have been stored in the association cortex and encompass a variety of *interacting systems*, such as auditory, visual, psycholinguistic, semantic and emotional. In connection with the latter, for example, we note that these associational programs can even block the information, and thereby prevent its being fully processed as it enters the cortex from the subcortex and neocortex. We thus have a clarifying explanation of "unconscious motivation" and "repression" as the results of limitations that are imposed by these associational programs on perceptual processing.

4. While it is not necessary for perception to show up in overt behavior, if it does, motor encoding of the processed information must have taken place.

Since most perceptions in experienced human beings involve such high level organizations as form, symbols, reading and social perception, which are filled with complex meaning, it is most plausible to believe that the significant perceptions necessary for us to cope wih our complex world are organized at the highest level—i.e., elaborations of stage 3b. Since these elaborations within stage 3b involve the directional intervention of experiential sets which are stored in the association areas of the cerebral cortex, it would be heuristic to describe a brain model that accounts for their operation. This model is based on the work of such people as Sokolov (1960), Pribram (1963) and Hebb (1949).

Sokolov and Pribram have theorized that in the *experienced* organism, cortical sets do focus attention toward certain kinds of information, and Hebb (1949) has hypothesized how past experience builds up the cell assemblies which constitute these sets.

This view of brain functioning has been brought together and extended in a book, by Miller, Galanter and Pribram (1960), and is called the TOTE model. What it states, in brief, is that before information can be let into the rest of the system from the sensory register, a *T*est stimulus is sent down to select or to gate information which is relevant to this test, much the same way that a thermostat turns the furnace on only if it is below a certain temperature. The gated information is *O*perated upon by the longterm storage sets and *T*ested again to see if it is a better match and if the perception is complete and might *E*xit in behavior. The significance of this model is that it asserts that the flow of information in perception is not simply in the afferent direction. Instead, ongoing cortical events often precede and therefore selectively filter incoming information.

We move now to a more detailed description of events within each stage of the informational process.

The Sensory Register

The reader can probably remember times when more information seemed to have reached the perceptual system than he was able to report—e.g., when viewing a complex picture, or speed reading.

An ingenious experiment by Sperling (1960) offers strong empirical support for this belief. He tachistoscopically presented a display of three rows of letters under two conditions of reporting. In one condition the subject was required to specify the units in a particular row in turn, while in other trials the subject was asked for the entire display. He found that when the subjects were asked to read out the item in a single row, their percentage of accuracy was higher than when they were required to read out the entire display. Sperling noted that this result indicated that more information gets into the system, at least in the sensory register—that is, the number of items which can be reported is grossly below the receptive capacity of the system (see Miller, 1956a).

An implication of Sperling's experiment is that if information is not used very quickly, it is lost. This inference is given powerful support by Turvey's investigation (1967), in which eight subjects were asked to participate for four days in an experiment that used the Sperling (1960) procedure of partial report. The stimulus array consisted of three rows of five digits each. Stimuli were presented for 50 milliseconds. After a delay of 0, 300 or 700 milliseconds, an auditory poststimulus cue was sounded. Subjects then reported as much as they could remember of *one* of the three rows.

One slide was repeated 54 times, with 54 other slides of a series interspersed between repetitions. The result was that there was no cumulative effect of the 54 repetitions. Accuracy for both the repeated and the nonrepeated slides, averaged over cue delays, remained at roughly 50 per cent.

It can be concluded that there appears to be no residual of an uncoded stimulus trace. That is, if sufficient time is not allowed for registered information to pass on to higher storage systems, there can be no effect of practice or of repeated presentations.

Data consistent with this interpretation of the discrepancy between received information and reported information come from the studies of a kind of stimulus interference called *visual masking*. To demonstrate this phenomenon, we first present a stimulus, S_1 (e.g., a letter) for a short duration, and remove it. Then, following a short interstimulus interval, (less than 300 milliseconds) we present a second but *different* stimulus, S_2 (e.g., a number) on the same retinal locus as the first stimulus. What happens is that the second stimulus masks the first one: in other words, the subject has difficulty in reporting the identity of S_1.

While some people have tried to account for masking on the basis of temporal neural (cell) summation, it is clear from the work of Averbach and Coriell (1961) that spatial summation (or integration) occurs as well.

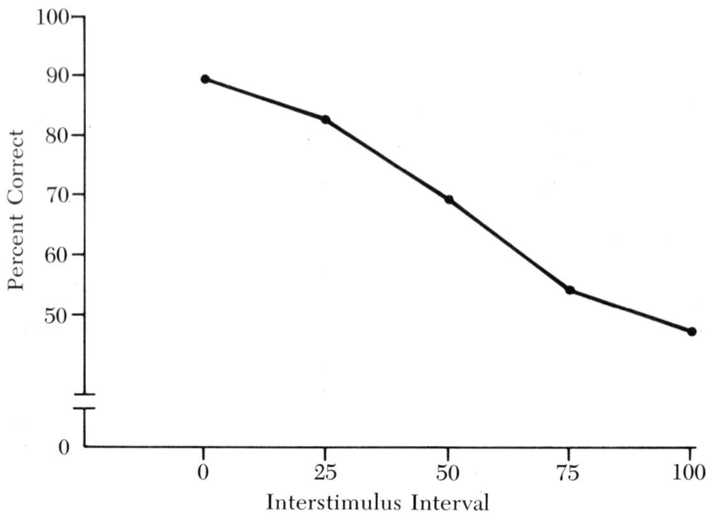

Figure 3–4 Results of the experiment of Eriksen and Collins (1967).

They presented two rows of letters for a brief duration. After removing this stimulus field they presented a large ring around the position where one of the letters had been located. However, the ring was much larger than the letter, so it could not involve the same cells. Yet the letter was masked.

An experiment by Eriksen and Collins (1967) clarifies the process underlying both spatial and temporal summation. In this study, five subjects were asked to participate for five days in a "masking" experiment. Stimuli consisted of dot patterns which, when *superimposed,* formed a three-letter nonsense syllable. Stimulus 1 was presented for six milliseconds. After a delay of 0, 25, 50, 75 or 100 milliseconds, stimulus 2 (spatially "superimposed") was presented for a duration of six milliseconds. The subject's task on each trial was to recognize the nonsense syllable formed by the superimposition of stimuli 1 and 2. The results are presented in Figure 3–4.

Eriksen and Collins interpreted their data to mean that masking effects must be, at least in part, a function of spatial and temporal summation. This explanation of summation in terms of an "additive" process is more warranted if one looks at the slope of the graph, than the "subtraction" assumption of Averbach and Coriell, who concluded that the second stimulus "erased" the effect of the first. The fact of temporal and spatial summation shows that two stimuli, presented in temporal and spatial disparity, can coexist. This phenomenon has functional utility, such as in motion picture viewing, but can also have inhibiting effects when the second stimulus makes resolution of the first stimulus more difficult.

The fact that there is a discrepancy between the amount of information received and reported, the fact that more time is required for memory storage than for reception and the fact that the additive effects of spatial and temporal summation in masking is time-dependent all suggest that events in the sensory register are organized, in part at least, at a level higher than the sense receptor.

Multisystem Integration and the Role of Memory

From what has been said so far in this section, we can infer that difficulties in perceiving could be related to a variety of reasons—namely, interference in connection with the reception of the stimulus and interference in connection with the simultaneous processing by the cortex of multidimensional stimulus information. All this suggests that effective perception requires *focused attention,* a long enough period for *sensory registration* and active *rehearsal* of decoded material before new information is let in. Effective organization of cognitive and general personality functioning requires the integration of these multisystem perceptual programs. Examples of research illustrating that such integration does take place was reported by Conrad (1964), who investigated the relationship between auditory and visual systems.

In the first experiment of Conrad's project, 300 subjects were asked to listen to letters of the entire alphabet spoken in a background of white noise (white noise is homogeneous sound energy which has no informative aspect), and to write down which letter they thought was being spoken at a particular time. Stimulus material was taped, and subjects were run in groups of 30. Letters were presented every five seconds. Subjects were required to write a letter for every stimulus presentation; no blanks were allowed.

In this first experiment the overall accuracy was 39 per cent. A confusion matrix was constructed in which the letters the subjects guessed and their associated frequency were tallied as a function of the particular letter presented. Errors were systematic—that is, they bore a "sound-alike" relationship to the presented stimulus.

In a second experiment, 387 additional subjects were asked to view sequences of six letters presented by a movie camera at a rate of one letter every three-fourths second. Each letter was exposed for a duration of five milliseconds. As in Experiment 1, subjects were asked to write down which letters they thought had appeared, and were instructed to leave no blanks.

In the second experiment the following letters were employed as presenting stimuli:

B C P T V F M N S X

The overall accuracy was 60 per cent. A confusion matrix was constructed as in Experiment 1. The correlation between the cell frequencies in this confusion matrix and the corresponding cells in the matrix in Experiment 1 was 0.64. Errors again bore a systematic—a "sound-alike"—relationship to the presented stimulus.

The implications of these two experiments are clear: *The decoding system employed need not correspond to the sense modality of the stimulus input.*

Another example of multisystem interaction can be inferred from an experiment conducted by Forgus and DeWolfe (1969). In this study the authors interviewed 49 actively hallucinating male and female schizophrenic patients. All of the interviews were tape-recorded, so that the themes of the hallucinations could be analyzed. A reliable manual for categorizing the hallucinatory themes was constructed using the hallucinations of a representative 10 males and 7 females. The two researchers agreed on the major theme for 30 of the 32 remaining subjects, indicating significant interjudge reliability (the correlation coefficient was 0.93).

Twenty-seven (of the 30) patients who were still in the hospital at this stage of the study heard a taped story which contained a composite of the themes present in the hallucinations.

In 18 of 23 subjects on whose dominant recall themes the two researchers agreed, the major hallucinatory theme category predicted the patient's dominant recall theme.

A plausible conclusion of this study is that hallucinatory themes are a reliable index of the relatively constricted nature of the decoding systems of schizophrenics. This cognitive constriction in turn is related to their relatively poor ability to cope with anxiety-provoking stimuli. It is not too large a step to generalize from this study, dealing with extreme thought disorder, to the delusional systems of neurotics and the delusions and paralogical systems of everyday life, which inhibit interpersonal communication and personality functioning. A note of caution is in order here. The author realizes that there have been other speculative interpretations of hallucinations, and that some investigations have concerned themselves with the relationship between hallucinations and brain chemistry. There has, however, been little scientific research on this problem, and most theories about hallucinations have been developed from *post hoc* interpretations of psychoanalysis. The Forgus and DeWolfe study was an attempt to bring the scientific investigation of hallucinations within methodological reach, and it suggests ways that the subsystems (in this case auditory and emotional) are related in the perceptual process.

A third example of subsystem research deals with the experimental demonstration that memory, part of the subset learning, plays a crucial role in the completion of many perceptual tasks. For example, whenever we read, recognize a person or identify an object, it is clear that at some point a representation of a stimulus is brought into contact with information that is stored in memory.

Memory involves practice. An experimental demonstration that practice facilitates processing of information can be seen in the data from Hebb (1961). In this study a set of 24 series of nine-digit numbers was presented to 40 subjects. Each series was *read aloud* at a rate of about one digit per second, and the subject's task was to repeat the series in exactly the same order. Every third trial (apparently from the beginning of the experiment) contained the same series of digits. The results of Hebb's experiment are presented in

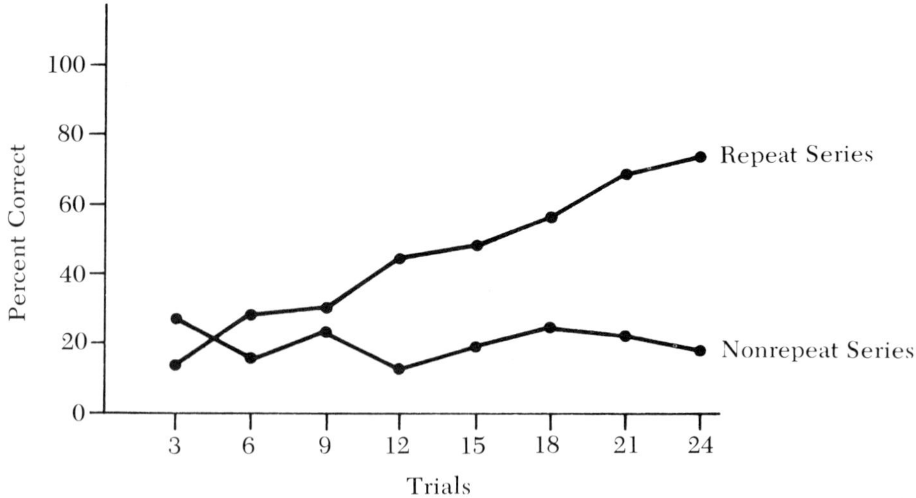

Figure 3–5 Results of Hebb's experiment (1961).

Figure 3–5. Hebb's data were replicated by Melton (1963) in a more extensive and well-controlled study.

It is important to highlight the fact that Hebb's study showed that practice was effective, whereas in the study of Turvey, previously described (p. 171), this was not the case. The shorter time exposures in the Turvey experiment were not sufficient for the completion of perceptual operations.

The fact that Hebb obtained an effect from repetition implies that the results of perceptual activity do leave a trace. How are these traces utilized?

Sternberg (1966, 1967) employed a memory search task to investigate this question. In a memory search task, the memory set is defined prior to the presentation of a test stimulus. The subject's task is to decide whether the test stimulus is a member of the memory set, and make an appropriate response. For example, a subject might be instructed to respond "yes" if the stimulus that appears is a 4 or a 7, and "no" if it is any other number. In a series of experiments of this type, where the number of items in the memory set (M) was the major independent variable and the reaction time (RT) was the major dependent variable, Sternberg found that for each unit increase in the size of M, the subject's RT for both "yes" and "no" responses increased 35 milliseconds. He hypothesized that the functional units of information processing in this task were unitary replicas of the memory set (rather than subfeatures of it). The 35 milliseconds became his estimate of the time required to process each memory set item. Further, Sternberg compared this figure with that obtained by Landauer (1962) for subvocal speech (at most, one item per 100 milliseconds), and rejected the explanation of subvocal speech as a sufficient mechanism for the task.

The fact that the unit of information processing in Sternberg's data seemed to be the whole identity, and the fact that 35 milliseconds were required for additional processing of each new unit suggest that the processing must take place centrally rather than peripherally.

Selected Comparisons of Lower and Higher Perceptual Tasks

Space precludes a full treatment of the extended range of perceptual phenomena. The following representative comparisons will hopefully give the reader more insight into the kinds of principles which must be considered in order to arrive at a more adequate understanding of a particular perceptual phenomenon, or to make a more accurate diagnosis of a specific perceptual problem or perceptually related behavioral disorder.

Brightness *versus* Size Constancy. The perceptual world seems to remain fairly constant in spite of large-scale variations in the energy patterns which reach the retina. Some relationships we see in the environment, therefore, remain *invariant* with respect to changes in physical energy. We refer to these perceived invariant properties as perceptual constancies.

The first constant property of perception is organized at the level of Task 2 of the hierarchy and, therefore, primarily at the level of the sensory register. This property, brightness constancy, is determined by the relative *reflectances* or *albedos* of objects. Since the ratio between relative albedo is constant, objects retain their relative whiteness, greyness or blackness despite changes in incident illumination from intense to twilight or shadow conditions.

The other constancies, such as size and shape, as suggested by the two experimental paradigms which follow, are organized at the level of Tasks 3 and 4 of the hierarchy. Apparently the subjects require experience to realize that retinal size and shape can be "corrected back" to objective size and shape by taking distance or spatial orientation into account.

In the first experiment on size constancy, Gilinsky (1955) determined the effects of attitudes on the reported sizes of objects. Four standard isosceles triangles were exposed, one at a time, at various distances directly in front of the subject; and a variable triangle—a triangle whose altitude could be altered—was located at a distance of 1200 feet from the subject.

Judgments of the heights of each standard triangle, at various predetermined distances up to 4000 feet, were made under two sets of conditions: (1) under the *objective* instructions, the subject was asked to alter the variable triangle until it equaled the objective size of the standard, despite appearances to the contrary. (2) Under *retinal* instructions, the subject was told to alter the size of the variable until it equaled the size of the standard as it appeared at the moment, even though he knew it was bigger.

It is quite clear from an inspection of the average results, which are presented in Figure 3–6, that the two sets of instructions gave rise to two diametrically different-sized matches. It can be seen that the objective instructions followed the prediction of the size-constancy law, while the retinal instructions followed the law of visual angle, slight overestimations being obtained in both cases. It is indeed remarkable that the human organism is capable of giving two widely differing reports of size under the same physical conditions of retinal stimulation. We can only conclude that cognitive intervention can affect size-constancy judgments.

By contrast, a brightness-constancy experiment by Gelb (1929) indicated the futility of trying to affect brightness perception through knowledge or cognitive intervention. In a room where several objects were faintly lit by a ceiling light, a rotating *black* disk, illuminated by an intense but concealed lantern, was placed in the foreground. The beam of the light fell exactly on the area of the disk, no additional light being projected onto the background. Under these conditions, subjects reported seeing a

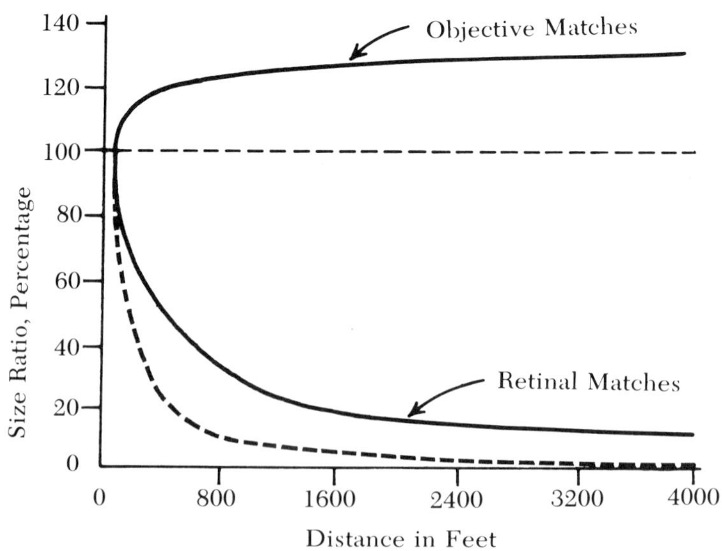

Figure 3–6 Objective and retinal matches as ratios of the variable to the size of the standard. (After Gilinsky, A. S., 1955, p. 183.)

white disk standing in dim light, and this impression was very compelling. When a small piece of white paper was now brought into the beam, next to the rotating disk, the disk was instantly reported as "turning into" its objective color, black, with the beam correspondingly becoming very intense. When the comparison white paper was withdrawn the black disk turned "white" again. This cycle can be repeated many times with the same predictable results; *knowledge makes no difference.*

Let us compare these two dramatic demonstrations, which we believe typify the differences between perceptions which are sense-dominated and those which are influenced by intervention from cognitive sets.

In the size-constancy effect it is important to note that the observer can give *either* constancy or retinal matches under conditions of adequate cues to distance perception. Should cues to distance be removed, he will obviously be able to give only one perception—that based on retinal size (not corrected by perceived distance). In brightness constancy, however, the subject can give only *one* discrimination in each of the conditions: a sensing of the illumination when he is not able to compare the reflectance or albedo, or a perception of objective whiteness when he can compare the brightness of an object with at least one other object—or a common background. A judgmental process is evidently involved in the size-constancy process but not in brightness constancy.

Attaining Figural Stability. A favorite demonstration to which the Gestalt followers refer is the work of Rubin (1921) on figure/ground fluctuation. He asserted that either the figure or the ground can be made more permanent by certain physical manipulations, such as differentiating the colors of the different parts or by asking the subject to look at one part consistently.

Subsequent and more precisely controlled work of Rock and Kremen (1957) and Hochberg (1964), however, place the attention variable in a broader context. This capturing of attention can be effected through stimulus factors such as increasing the differentiation between figure and ground; by changing from a two-dimensional border between figure/ground to a three-dimensional border or edge, so that eye movement fluctuation can be controlled; or, centrally, by providing a contextual set for directing the aspect which is given pre-eminence. The fact that we can obtain figural stability through central (cortical) direction implies that we are moving out of Task 2 toward Task 3 and above.

Form and Space Perception. The growth of form perception has already been described. Two notes should be added here. First, a variety of perceptual organizations require learning (or at least experience) for their appearance. Thus, Gregory and Wallace (1963) have shown that experience is even necessary for the perception of the visual illusions. For example, the congenitally blind person when first given vision *failed* to show the following illusory effects: (a) the normal reporting of curved lines in the Hering illusion, (b) nonparallel lines in the Zöllner illusion and displacement of slanted line in the Poggendorf illusion and (c) the perception of depth and reversal in the Necker cue and staircase illusion. Examples of these illusions are shown in Figure 3–7.

Depth Perception. Since the perception of depth (three-dimensional space and distance) requires the discrimination of pattern, it involves a kind of form perception. However, because it falls short of recognizing an identity, its complexity falls between Tasks 3 and 4 in the perceptual hierarchy.

In order for this ability to develop, there must be a rudimentary founda-

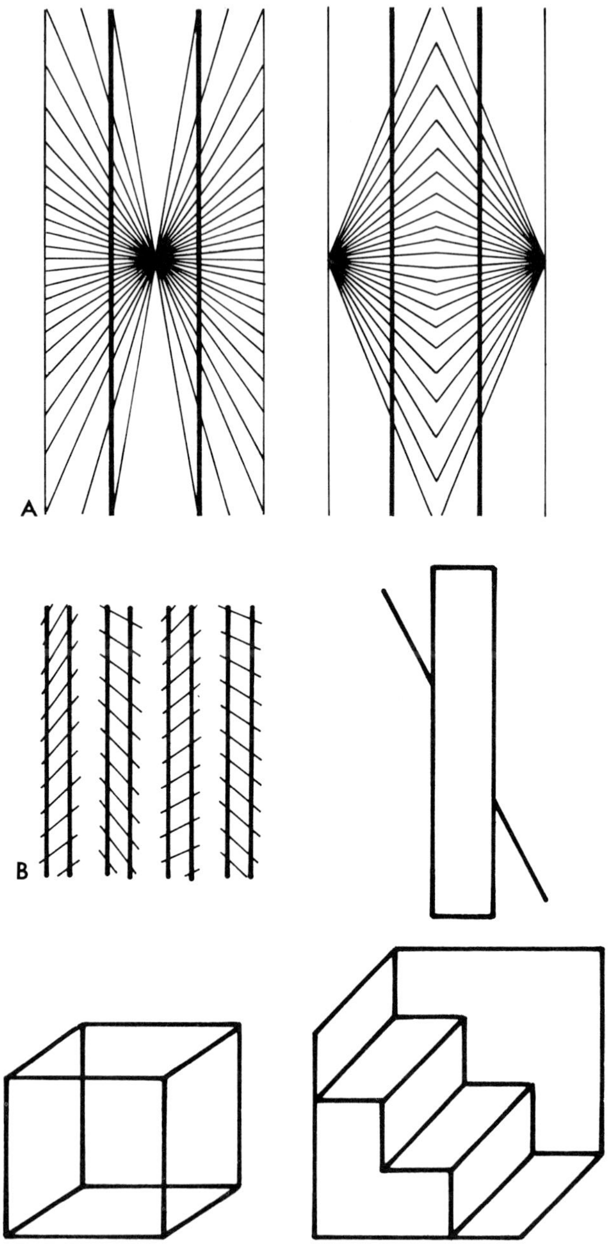

Figure 3–7 Varieties of illusory effects. In a study by Gregory and Wallace (1963) on the perception of a congenitally blind person who was given sight via surgery, interesting data were reported. The normal reporting of curved lines in the Hering illusion (A), of nonparallel lines in the Zöllner illusion and displacement of the slanted line in the Poggendorf illusion (B) and the perception of depth and reversal in the Necker cube and staircase illusion (C) were all absent. Instead, the subject reported these lines as straight and saw no depth or reversal.

tion before experience can take effect. That this is so was supported in an experiment by Gibson and Walk (1960). These investigators found that a variety of mammalian infants—for example, kittens, goats and 6- to 14-month-old human babies—could discriminate depth because they would not crawl over a glass top which was over a steep descent (the "visual cliff"), whereas they would crawl on a glass top which was over a shallow space.

However, when they compared young animals who were raised in the dark with young animals raised under normal (having exposure to patterned light) conditions, they noticed an interesting and informative difference. The dark-reared animals could only make the depth discrimination when the cue of motion parallax was allowed to operate. The reader can see the operation of this cue for himself by fixating a distant point when he is in a moving vehicle. He will notice that near objects move faster across his visual field than more distant objects. Similarly, when these young infants, without experience, crawl or move their heads, nearer areas move faster than more distance ones.

The experimenter can synthetically destroy the effectiveness of this cue by making the distant patterns correspondingly bigger than the nearer ones, so that differential displacement is destroyed. When this was done in these experiments, the inexperienced animals "froze"—that is, they could not make a depth discrimination. But the experienced animals could still make the discrimination. Evidently, they were responding to the fact that certain patterns (e.g., pattern density) vary with distance.

One can draw the conclusion that motion parallax is an innate cue which enables the newborn infant to explore space with his eyes and head and, when he begins to crawl, with his body. *Motion parallax* is one of the class called *primary cues* to distance and depth, the others consisting of the nervous system reaction to differences in *accommodation* of the lens, *convergence* of the eyes and *binocular disparity* in retinal images. These other primary cues are probably also functional shortly after birth, although they might require some time for full maturation. Ling (1942), for example, in a longitudinal study of the human infant from birth to six months, found that convergence was not completely functional until about eight weeks of age.

The experience connected with spatial exploration, made possible by the functional operation of the primary cues, gives rise to the *secondary cues*, which result from *learned* discrimination of *pattern gradients*. These pattern dimensions are based on the two laws of optical geometry: the visual angle, which refers to the relative vertical size of the retinal image, and the linear perspective, which refers to the relative horizontal size (this is demonstrated in the visual impression of railroad tracks seeming to converge with increased distance from the eye). These pattern cues consist of changes or gradients in relative size, texture, density and interposition. Artists use these cues effectively when creating the impression of three dimensions on a two-dimensional surface. These cues are also operating when we see depth in a two-dimensional photograph.

We end this brief discussion of depth perception by noting that the primary cues are effective at relatively short distances. Binocular disparity or stereoscopic vision, the favored cue of the ophthalmologist and the primary cue which is effective for the greatest distance, begins to lose its discriminable power between 300 and 600 yards. Conversely, the secondary cues, so typical of the amazing flexibility and adaptability enabled by learned programs, are effective well beyond a mile. This takes on added significance in the age of space and high speed.

SOCIAL AND PERSONALITY EFFECTS ON PERCEPTION

In spite of Freud's assertion that motives influence perception, and although a few psychologists had tried to study the influence of personal values on the perception of size and number (Ansbacher 1937; Stephens 1931, 1936), the Gestalt theory, which emphasized objective stimulus determiners, dominated perceptual research until the provocative experiment of Bruner and Goodman (1947) and the theoretical article of Bruner and Postman (1948) started a new trend.

The essential thesis of Bruner and Postman was that the perceiver will tend to accentuate positively valued objects and de-accentuate negatively valued objects in perceptual judgments. The work of Bruner and Goodman, and the controversy to which it gave rise, ended in equivocal theoretical interpretations.

Equivocation also exists when one attempts to interpret the "dirty word" experiments of McGinnies (1949), who found that subjects had *higher* recognition thresholds for dirty words as opposed to neutral words. Yet we know from personal experience that when threatened, some individuals attack rather than withdraw. So one might intuit that certain individuals should be more vigilant and thus have lower recognition thresholds for emotionally toned stimuli.

The fact that there is, indeed, an interaction between personality motives and response to emotionally laden stimulation was neatly demonstrated in classic experiments performed by Lazarus et al. (1951) and evaluated by Eriksen (1963). These experiments and the theoretical logic on which they are based can be supported by clinical observations. First, we know that there are wide individual differences in the kinds of stimuli which are anxiety-provoking. Secondly, while some individuals repress or withdraw in the face of threat (defensive individuals), others project, intellectualize or counterattack (vigilant individuals).

In one study, Eriksen (1951a) first measured the associative responses of psychiatric patients to words that had meanings related to dependence, aggression and homosexuality. Then he measured the recognition thresholds of these patients when pictures similar to these themes, in addition to other pictures, were exposed for varying durations. He found that those patients who showed a high degree of disturbance and avoidance to words in the three emotional categories also exhibited higher recognition thresholds to related pictures. Furthermore, in other studies, Eriksen (1951b) and Lazarus et al. (1951) found that subjects who freely gave aggressive and sexual content in Thematic Apperception Test (TAT) stories or in sentence completion tests also exhibited vigilance or heightened sensitivity to visual or auditory stimuli in these semantic categories.

So the objective meaning of the stimulus is not the sole determinant of its perceptual report, but rather it is the subjective significance, as it interacts with the subject's characteristic mode of dealing with anxiety, that determines whether reactions to particular information will be *sensitized* or *repressed*. This fact, too, throws light on the baffling problem of why some individuals have selective but, in this light, predictable difficulties in spelling or perceiving certain kinds of words.

In the work of Eriksen and in its clinical counterpart, the social and personality factors are part of the *independent variable*—that is, these factors are considered as part of the complex system of interacting variables which determine the course of the perceptual process and therefore the direction of the final perceptual act, the latter representing the *dependent variable,* or that which is to be explained.

We also have the case, however, where the social or personal event is the dependent variable. An example would be interpersonal perception, the perception of other people's behavior and the clues the clinician picks up when he conducts a diagnostic interview. While all of us engaged in practice do this every day (for that matter, so do most people in everyday interpersonal interaction), very little experimental data exists to throw light, without equivocation, on how this can be done with reliability. Attempts in this direction were made by Michotte (1946, 1950), Heider and Simmel (1944), and Heider (1958), and there is a good review of the work on the perception of persons by Bruner and Tagiuri (1954).

THE PERCEPTUAL ASPECTS OF BEHAVIORAL DYSFUNCTION

The conceptual theory described in this chapter, and the analysis of the experimental research which supports it, suggest specific ways that a knowledge of perception, defined in a cognitive context and related to adaptive behavior, can be of use to physicians in the diagnosis, treatment and prevention of *learning disorders* and *personality abnormalities.*

Specific Learning Disabilities

There are certain severe syndromes of gross perceptual handicaps caused by organic dysfunction of the senses, the peripheral nervous system, parts of the subcortex or the cerebral cortex. For most of these—such as aphasia, blindness or deafness—the prognosis is variable, and the afflicted require specific kinds of remediation, the details of which are beyond the scope of this chapter.

There exists, however, an assorted and baffling array of highly specific and peculiar disabilities which has given rise to controversial "theories," most of which seem still to be stabs in the dark. Many of these defects are found in children who, in spite of normal or superior IQ's, display peculiar anomalies such as alexia (difficulties with reading), mirror-reading, mirror-writing, inconsistent spelling and selective retention.

While adequate basic knowledge or sound theory is lacking, it would appear that we will make more headway in diagnosis, treatment and significant research if we use, as a *guide,* what we already know; namely, that the process of perception or information extraction does consist of a sequence of *stages,* as we outlined in the first part of this chapter (p. 169). Thus, if we are going to trouble-shoot effectively and efficiently, we should be guided by the following systems, which we here summarize. If a child is substandard for his age in reading, for example, the problem could be related to one or more of the following stages in perception:

1. *The sensory register:* Examination of the organic and physical function should be conducted. This consists of tests of acuity, depth perception and eye dominance. If the physical performance is satisfactory, then we look for other causes. For the average individual, stimulus material is preserved in the sensory register for a duration ranging from one-fourth to three-fourths second. Consequently, should we find an individual in whom decay takes place more rapidly, *receptive* disorders should be investigated.

2. *The multisystem perceptual systems and the role of memory:* This final stage is of unusual importance for at least two reasons. First, *attention* is influenced not only by certain stimulus factors, such as contrast,

but also by central sets which focus attention in such a way as to test incoming stimulus information against certain standards or schemata. In fact, it seems that in the experienced individual these standards sensitize or inhibit the information entering the higher perceptual system from the sensory register.

The second important aspect involves the more complex pattern of the individual's attitudes, values, biases and personality dispositions. These affect the rehearsal or memory *storage* and search function.

Both the attentional and personality aspects can be studied independent of the usual perceptual tasks, by means of personality evaluations such as the clinical interview and the TAT.

3. *Motor encoding:* While perception does not have to be expressed in overt behavior, the individual is frequently called upon to do so when, for example, he writes or speaks. It is thus important to determine whether problems of expression are caused by blocking and interference in the perceptual system, or by difficulties in transferring (encoding) the final outcome or "decision" of the perceptual process into expressed action.

It is hoped that current research into the nature of human perceptual systems will result in improved techniques for diagnosing perceptual and cognitive disabilities. To illustrate one way in which this might be accomplished, consider the research previously reported by Sternberg (p. 175). In these experiments, Sternberg recorded the amount of time it took a subject to decide whether a test stimulus was a member of a predetermined memory set. By varying the number of items in the memory set (M), Sternberg was able to isolate two components of this reaction-time function: (1) a component that varied with M, which Sternberg interpreted as a measure of the time required to process items in memory, and (2) a component that was independent of M, which Sternberg interpreted as time required for operations occurring both prior to memory processing (stimulus input) and subsequent to memory processing (response selection and execution). What has this to do with diagnosis? It is a well-established fact that people who are labeled "schizophrenic" have slower overall reaction times than people not so labeled (Shakow, 1963). With a technique such as Sternberg's, it should be possible to establish more precisely, both for an individual and in general, the locus of the deficits giving rise to the overall slower reaction time. In so doing, a better understanding of the nature of the disability would be obtained.

Specific Tests

With the exception of the personality measurement, which usually requires the expert evaluation of clinical psychologists, standard tests of perceptual abilities together with standard age norms are available. The following are three of the best:

1. *The Frostig Developmental Test of Visual Perception,* ordered from Consulting Psychologists' Press, 577 College Avenue, Palo Alto, California.
2. *The Illinois Test of Psycholinguistic Abilities,* ordered from Follett Publishing Company, 1010 West Washington Boulevard, Chicago, Illinois.
3. *The Denver Developmental Screening Test,* ordered from University of Colorado Medical Center, Denver, Colorado.

The Frostig Test provides developmental norms in perceptual development for preschool and school ages. The Illinois Test of Psycholinguistic Abilities has extensive norms from pre-school to adolescent years for separate abilities, including receptive (visual and auditory), associational (higher processing systems) and motor encoding (e.g., speech). The

Denver Developmental Screening Test has norms from infancy to age 6 for motor, language and social-personal development.

PERCEPTUAL DIRECTION OF PERSONALITY STYLE AND MOTIVES

In describing one of the ways in which memory influences perception, we alluded to the fact that personal attitudes and personality dispositions can influence the way we respond to input communication or the way we go about processing information. Some psychologists (e.g., Witkin, 1950) have, in fact, argued strongly that we can use differences or selectivity in perception as a reliable index of personality functioning. Witkin's distinction between field-independent and field-dependent perceivers, Kagan's (1966) distinction between reflective and impulsive personality styles and Gardner and Long's (1966) distinction between extensive and narrow scanners are important examples of this kind of theorizing. While this work is new, the potential power it has for improving diagnostic treatment and preventative procedures is vast and exciting. The data suggest that personality styles are related, through perception, to cognitive styles. These styles develop as a result of learning during socialization.

The centrality of cognitive functioning was originally emphasized by Alfred Adler when he defined *life style* as a cognitive blueprint—an internal standard which is used as a reference for processing information related to interactions with the external world, especially its interpersonal aspect. I will end this chapter by giving a few examples of how behavioral disorders which are typical in children can be better understood by relating them to the core of the individual's life style or cognitive blueprint.

It is a truism that human beings are amazingly variable individuals. For this reason, attempts to look for single or unitary causes of particular behavioral syndromes are doomed to failure. This, perhaps, is the greatest reason for the failure of the promise of libidinal theory, despite the great insight, genius and perceptiveness of Freud. One fact does seem common for all human children, however; if they have learned to depend on and to trust their parents, this provides a new motive to obtain their favor. The interaction between the model provided by the parents, the comparison with siblings, and the contingencies of reinforcement produce the foundation for the development of the child's *perception* of how to go about getting that favor, which is eventually integrated into his perception of self and identity.

If he is fortunate in the way these three variables interacted, he will perceive self goals and self-other relationships in terms of self-regard (esteem), success and the anticipation of positive relatedness and fulfillment. If socialization practices are misguided, he will unfortunately learn to perceive self goals distortedly, in terms of warding off the *anxiety* connected with loss of favor. The *center* or *focal* point of this distortion is revealed through the content of *distorted* perception. Let me illustrate briefly with an example which, though by no means the full story of the personality involved, nevertheless demonstrates how the distorted centeredness of self is caused by the anxiety connected with loss of favor or status.

A young girl, aged 9, is referred by a pediatrician because the teachers consider her a learning problem. Her spelling is substandard, and they report that she "for no reason and without warning or cause tunes out." In addition, her parents find her to be a recluse. In spite of an above average IQ, her grades are borderline-fail.

The Illinois Test of Psycholinguistic Abilities reveals adequate sensory reception and decoding, and motor encoding. However, substandard performance in perceptual associations suggests problems with the memory component of perception. Closer inspection of her incorrect spelling reveals that it is highly and predictably selective, semantically related to succorant motives such as love, care, food and so forth. Thus, she could spell longer and more difficult words which were unrelated to succorance and yet miss on simple words which denoted succorance. Further personality analysis, including use of the projective themes of the TAT, revealed, among other things, repetitive concern that her parents are so wrapped up in their own problems and needs that they could not notice her desires and wants. Hence, she resorts to incompetency and "having difficulties," so that they will notice her, care for her and, in this way, give her some recognition. Interestingly enough, verifying evidence came from watching her performance on the block design part of the Weschler Intelligence Scale for Children and while she was solving arithmetical problems. On the block designs she would get half the pattern right and then "err" on one block of the mirror half. Similarly, in arithmetic she would get the problem almost correct and then "err" on the last step.

The importance of the above description is *not* that the girl has succorant needs or needs for recognition. All human beings do. The important point is that she has developed *misguided standards* by which she judges whether she is being recognized. This distorted way in which she goes about processing information about her relationships with older people, especially with respect to satisfying the goal of recognition, is what has to be changed.

As complex, varied and diverse as the systems are in this case, they can be economically understood in the context of the *cognitive* standards which direct the *information-seeking* components of motives. Such economy is needed for the very reason that our channel processing capacity is limited. If we cannot process that many isolated items, then, as Miller (1965a) recommends, we have to "chunk" the items into larger multicomponent units; that, precisely, is what life styles and cognitive sets are.

SUMMARY

In this chapter we analyzed perception from the vantage point of its central role in guiding man's adaptive behavior to his environment.

In so doing, we presented an information-extraction model, which proposes, with compelling experimental evidence, that the perceptual process is a stage-like, ordinal, hierarchical system.

After comparing the organization of lower and higher stages in the hierarchy, we concluded with an application of this model, in developmental stage perspective, to the diagnosis of perceptual, learning and personality disorders, pointing out the central importance of learned experience.

ACKNOWLEDGMENTS

I would like to acknowledge my warm thanks to my Lake Forest College friend and colleague, Stephen Checkosky, for reviewing and discussing the section on the information processing model, and for his valuable contributions.

REFERENCES

Ansbacher, H.: Perception of number as affected by the monetary value of the objects. *Arch. Psychol.*, New York, No. 215, 1937.

Aronfreed, J. M., Messick, S. A., and Diggory, J. C.: Reexamining emotionality and perceptual defense. *J. Personality, 21*:517–528, 1953.

Attneave, F.: Some informational aspects of visual perception. *Psychol. Rev., 61*:183–193, 1954.

Averbach, E., and Coriell, A. S.: Short-term memory in vision. *Bell System Technical Journal, 40*:309–328, 1961.

Beach, F. A., and Jaynes, J.: Effects of early experience upon the behavior of animals. *Psychol. Bull., 51*:239–263, 1954.

Biederman, I., and Checkosky, S.: Processing and redundant information. *J. Exp. Psychol.,* In Press.

Bridgen, R. F.: A tachistoscopic study of the differentiation of perception. *Psychol. Monogr., 44*:153–166, 1933.

Broadbent, D.: *Perception and Communication.* London, Pergamon Press Ltd., 1958.

Brown, J. L., et al.: Relation of threshold criterion to the functional receptors of the eye. *J. Opt. Soc. Amer., 47*:198–204, 1957.

Brown, J. L., et al.: Spectral energy for the resolution of acuity. *J. Opt. Soc. Amer., 50*: 950–960, 1960.

Bruner, J. S.: *The Process of Education.* Cambridge, Massachusetts, Harvard University Press, 1961.

Bruner, J. S., and Goodman, C. C.: Value and need as organizing factors in perception. *J. Abnorm. Soc. Psychol., 42*:33–44, 1947.

Bruner, J. S., and Postman, L.: An approach to social perception. *In* Dennis, W. (Ed.): *Current Trends in Social Psychology.* Pittsburgh, University of Pittsburgh Press, 1948.

Bruner, J. S., and Tagiuri, R.: The perception of people. *In* Lindzey, G. (Ed.): *Handbook of Social Psychology.* Reading, Massachusetts, Addison-Wesley Publishing Co., Inc., 1954.

Carter, L. F., and Schooler, K.: Value, need and other factors in perception. *Psychol. Rev., 56*:200–207, 1949.

Conrad, R.: Acoustic confusion in immediate memory. *Brit. J. Psychol., 55*:75–84, 1964.

Davies, A. E.: An analysis of elementary psychic process. *Psychol. Rev., 12*:166–206, 1905.

Dickinson, C. A.: Experience and visual perception. *Amer. J. Psychol., 37*:330–344, 1926.

Douglas, A. G.: A tachistoscopic study of the order of emergence in the process of perception. *Psychol. Monogr., 61,* No. 6, 1947.

Eriksen, C. W.: Perceptual defense as a function of unacceptable needs. *J. Abnorm. Soc. Psychol., 46*:557–564, 1951a.

Eriksen, C. W.: Some implications for TAT interpretations arising from need and perception experiments. *J. Personality, 19*:283–288, 1951b.

Eriksen, C. W.: Perception and personality. *In* Wepman, J. M., and Heine, R. W. (Eds.): *Concepts of Personality.* Chicago, Aldine Publishing Company, 1963.

Eriksen, C. W., and Brown, C. T.: An experimental and theoretical analysis of perceptual defense. *J. Abnorm. Soc. Psychol., 52*: 224–230, 1956.

Eriksen, C. W., and Collins, J. F.: Some temporal characteristics of visual pattern perception. *J. Exp. Psychol., 74*:476–484, 1967.

Fantz, R. L.: The origin of form perception. *Sci. Amer., 204*:66–72, 1961.

Fantz, R. L.: Visual perception from birth as shown by pattern selectivity. *Ann. N.Y. Acad. Sci., 118*:793–814, 1965.

Forgus, R. H.: The effect of early perceptual learning on the behavioural organization of adult rats. *J. Comp. Physiol. Psychol., 47*: 331–336, 1954.

Forgus, R. H.: Influence of early experience on maze-learning with and without visual cues. *Canad. J. Psychol.,* 9:231–238, 1955.

Forgus, R. H.: Advantages of early over later perceptual experience in improving form discrimination. *Canad. J. Psychol., 10*:147–155, 1956.

Forgus, R. H.: The effect of different kinds of form pre-exposure on form discrimination learning. *J. Comp. Physiol. Psychol., 51*:75–78, 1958a.

Forgus, R. H.: The interaction between form pre-exposure and test requirements in determining discrimination learning. *J. Comp. Physiol. Psychol., 51*:588–591, 1958b.

Forgus, R. H.: *Perception: The Basic Process in Cognitive Development.* New York, McGraw-Hill Book Company, 1966.

Forgus, R. H.: The hierarchical organization of perception. *Int. J. Neurol., 6*:138–146, 1967.

Forgus, R. H., and DeWolfe, A. S.: Perceptual selectivity in hallucinatory schizophrenics. *J. Abnorm. Psychol., 74*:288–292, 1969.

Forgus, R. H., and Schwartz, R. J.: Efficient retention and transfer as affected by learning method. *J. Psychol., 43*:135–139, 1957.

Freeman, G. L.: An experimental study of the perception of objects. *J. Exp. Psychol., 12*: 241–258, 1929.

Gardner, R. W., and Long, R. I.: Cognitive controls and inhibition: A study of individual consistencies. *Brit. J. Psychol., 53*:381–388, 1962. Reprinted in Vernon, M. D. (Ed.): *Experiments in Visual Perception.* Baltimore, Penguin Books, Inc., 1966.

Gelb, A.: Die "Farbenkonstanz" der Sendinge. *Hand. Norm. Path. Physiol., 12(1)*:594–678, 1929.

Gellerman, L. W.: Chance order of alternating stimuli in visual discrimination experiments. *J. Genet. Psychol., 42*:207–208, 1933.

Gibson, E. J., and Walk, R. O.: The "visual cliff." *Sci. Amer., 202*:64–71, 1960.

Gibson, J. J., and Gibson, E. J.: Perceptual learning: Differentiation or enrichment. *Psychol. Rev., 62*:32–41, 1955.

Gilinsky, A. S.: The effect of attitude on the perception of size. *Amer. J. Psychol., 68*:173–192, 1955.

Gollin, E.: Developmental studies of visual recognition of incomplete objects. *Percept. Motor Skills, 11*:289–298, 1960.
Green, R. T., and Courtis, M. C.: Information theory and figure perception: The metaphor that failed. *Acta Psychol. (Amst.), 25*:12–36, 1966.
Gregory, R. L., and Wallace, J. G.: Recovery from early blindness. *Expt. Psychol. Sci. Monogr.*, No. 2, 1963.
Gurewitz, E. M.: *The Molecular Basis of Memory.* Englewood Cliffs, New Jersey, Prentice-Hall, Inc., 1969.
Haaf, R. A., and Bell, R. Q.: A facial dimension in visual discrimination by human infants. *Child Develop., 38*:893–899, 1967.
Hake, H. W.: *Contributions of psychology to the study of pattern vision.* U.S.A.F. WADC-TR-57-621, October, 1957.
Haynes, H., White, B. L., and Held, R.: Visual accommodation in human infants. *Science, 148*:528–530, 1965.
Hebb, D. O.: The innate organization of visual activity. I. Perception of figures by rats reared in total darkness. *J. Genet. Psychol., 47*:181–188, 1937a.
Hebb, D. O.: The innate organization of visual activity. II. Transfer of response in the discrimination of brightness and size by rats reared in total darkness. *J. Comp. Psychol., 24*:277–299, 1937b.
Hebb, D. O.: *The Organization of Behavior.* New York, John Wiley & Sons, Inc., 1949.
Hebb, D. O.: *In* Delafresnaye, J. F. (Ed.): *Brain Mechanisms and Learning.* New York, Oxford University Press, Inc., 1961.
Heider, F.: *The Psychology of Interpersonal Relations.* New York, John Wiley & Sons, Inc., 1958.
Heider, F., and Simmel, M. L.: An experimental study of apparent behavior. *Amer. J. Psychol., 57*:243–249, 1944.
Heinemann, E. S.: Simultaneous brightness induction as a function of inducing-and-test-field brightness. *J. Exp. Psychol., 50*:89–96, 1955.
Helson, H., and Fehrer, E. V.: The role of form in perception. *Amer. J. Psychol., 44*:79–102, 1932.
Heron, W.: The pathology of boredom. *Sci. Amer., 196*:52–56, 1957.
Heron, W., et al.: Visual disturbances after prolonged perceptual isolation. *Canad. J. Psychol., 10*:13–18, 1956.
Hochberg, J. E.: *Perception.* Englewood Cliffs, New Jersey, Prentice-Hall, Inc., 1964.
Hochberg, J. E., and Silverstein, A. A.: A quantitative index of stimulus similarity: Proximity vs. differences in brightness. *Amer. J. Psychol., 69*:456–458, 1956.
Hubel, D. H., and Wiesel, T. N.: Receptive fields of single neurones in the cat's striate cortex. *J. Physiol., 148*:574–591, 1959.
Hubel, D. H., and Wiesel, T. N.: Receptive fields, binocular interaction and functional architecture in the cat's visual cortex. *J. Physiol., 160*:106–154, 1962.
Hubel, D. H., and Wiesel, T. N.: Receptive fields of cells in striate cortex of very young, visually inexperienced kittens. *J. Physiol., 26*:994–1002, 1963.
Hubel, D. H., and Wiesel, T. N.: Receptive fields and functional architecture of monkey striate cortex. *J. Physiol., 195*:215–243, 1968.
Hyman, R., and Hake, H. W.: *Form recognition as a function of the number of forms which can be presented for recognition.* U.S.A.F. WADC-TR-54-164, May, 1954.
Ives, W. C., and Schilling, C. W.: *Object identification with Hect-Schlaer Adaptometer.* Night Vision Board, U.S. Submarine Base. New London, Connecticut, 524-1 (102) WC1 Fgl/aam. December 26, 1941.
Kagan, J.: Developmental studies in reflection and analysis. *In* Kidd, O. H., and Rivoire, J. L. (Eds.): *Perceptual Development in Children.* New York, International Universities Press, 1966.
Koffka, K.: *The Principles of Gestalt Psychology.* New York, Harcourt Brace Jovanovich, Inc., 1935.
Kohler, W., and Wallach, H.: Figural aftereffects: An investigation of visual processes. *Proc. Amer. Philos. Soc., 88*:269–357, 1944.
Landauer, T. K.: Rate of implicit speech. *Percept. Motor Skills, 15*:646–647, 1962.
Lashley, K. S.: The mechanism of vision; XV Preliminary studies on the rat's capacity for detail vision. *J. Genet. Psychol., 18*:123–193, 1938.
Lazarus, R. S., Eriksen, C. W., and Fonda, C. P.: Personality dynamics in auditory perceptual recognition. *J. Personality, 19*:471–482, 1951.
Lorenz, K. Z.: *The evolution of behaviour. Sci. Amer., 199*:67–83, 1958.
Ling, B. C. I.: A genetic study of sustained visual fixation and associated behaviour in the human infant from birth to 6 months. *J. Genet. Psychol., 61*:227–277, 1942.
Lowenstein, O.: *The Human Senses.* Baltimore, Penguin Books, Inc., 1966.
McCall, R. B., and Kagan, J.: Attention in the infant: Effects of complexity, contour, perimeter and familiarity. *Child Develop., 38*:939–952, 1967.
McGinnies, E.: Emotionality and perceptual defense. *Psychol. Rev., 56*:244–251, 1949.
Melton, A. W.: Implications of short-term memory for a general theory of memory. *J. Ver. Learn. Verb. Behav., 2*:1–21, 1963.
Michotte, A.: *La perception de la causalité.* Louvain (Belgium) Institu Supérieur de Philosophie, 1946.
Michotte, A.: The emotions regarded as functional connections. *In* Reymert, M. L. (Ed.): *The International Symposium on Feelings and Emotions.* New York, McGraw-Hill Book Company, 1950.
Miles, W. R.: Light sensitivity and form per-

ception in dark adaptation. *J. Opt. Soc. Amer., 43*:560–566, 1953.
Miller, G. A.: The magical number, seven, plus or minus two: Some limits on our capacity for processing information. *Psychol. Rev., 63*:81–97, 1956a.
Miller, G. A.: Information and memory. *Sci. Amer., 195*:42–46, 1956b.
Miller, G. A., Galanter, E., and Pribram, K.: *Plans and the Structure of Behavior.* New York, Holt, Rinehart & Winston, Inc., 1960.
Milner, B.: Neuropsychological evidence for differing memory processes. *XVIII International Congress of Psychology,* Moscow, 1966.
Penfield, W.: The permanent record of the stream of consciousness. *Acta Psychol. (Amst.), 11*:47–69, 1956.
Piaget, J.: *The Origins of Intelligence in Children.* New York, International Universities Press, 1952.
Piaget, J.: *The Construction of Reality in the Child.* New York, Basic Books, Inc., Publishers, 1954.
Piaget, J., and Inhelder, B.: *La représentation de l'espace chez l'enfant.* Paris, Presses Universitaires de France, 1948.
Pribram, K.: Reinforcement revisited: A structural view. *Nebraska Symposium on Motivation,* 1963.
Pritchard, R. M., et al.: Visual perception approached by the method of stabilized images. *Canad. J. Psychol., 14*:67–77, 1960.
Riesen, A. H.: The development of visual perception in man and chimpanzee. *Science, 106*:107–108, 1947.
Riesen, A. H.: Arrested vision. *Science, 183*: 16–19, 1950.
Riesen, A. H.: Plasticity of behavior: Psychological aspects. *In* Harlow, H. F., and Woolsey, E. N. (Eds.): *Biological and Biochemical Bases of Behaviour.* Madison, Wisconsin, University of Wisconsin Press, 1958.
Rock, I., and Kremen, I.: A reexamination of Rubin's figural after-effect. *J. Exp. Psychol., 53*:23–30, 1957.
Rubin, E.: *Visuelle wahrgenommene Figuren.* Copenhagen, Gyldendalske Boghandel, Nordisk Forlag A/S, 1921.
Salapatek, P.: Visual scanning of geometric figures by the human newborn. *J. Comp. Physiol. Psychol., 66*:247–258, 1968.
Salapatek, P., and Kessen, W.: Visual scanning of triangles by the human newborn. *J. Exp. Child Psychol., 3*:113–122, 1966.
Senden, M. Von: *Raum und Gestalt auffassung bei operierten blindgeborenen vor und nach der Operation.* Leipzig, Otto Wilhelm Barth-Verlag GMBH, 1932. (Translated by P. Heath: *Space and Sight,* London, Methuen & Co., Ltd., 1960.)
Shakow, D.: Psychological deficit in schizophrenia. *Behav. Sci., 8*:275–305, 1963.
Shannon, C. E., and Weaver, W.: *The Mathematical Theory of Communication.* Urbana, Illinois, University of Illinois Press, 1949.
Sokolov, E.: *In* Brazier, M. A. B. (Ed.): *The Central Nervous System and Behavior: Transactions of the Third Conference.* New York, Josiah Macy Jr. Foundation, 1960.
Sokolov, E.: The modeling properties of the nervous system. *In* Cole, M., and Maltzman, I. (Eds.): *A Handbook of Contemporary Soviet Psychology.* New York, Basic Books, Inc., Publishers, 1969.
Sperling, G.: The information available in brief visual presentations. *Psychol. Monogr., 74,* No. 498, 1960.
Stephens, J. M.: The influence of different stimuli upon preceding bonds: An examination of the law of effect. *Teachers Coll. Contr. Educ.,* 1931, p. 493.
Stephens, J. M.: The perception of small differences as affected by self-interest. *Amer. J. Psychol., 58*:480–484, 1936.
Sternberg, S.: High-speed scanning in human memory. *Science, 153*:652–654, 1966.
Sternberg, S.: Two operations in character-recognition: Some evidence from reaction time measurements. *Perception and Psychophysics, 2*:45–53, 1967.
Tinbergen, W.: *The Study of Instinct.* Oxford, Fairhaven, New Jersey, 1952.
Tinbergen, N., and Perdeck, A. C.: On the stimulus situation releasing the begging response in the newly hatched herring-gull chick. *Behaviour, 3*:1–38, 1950.
Turvey, M. T.: Repetition and the preperceptual information store. *J. Exp. Psychol., 74*:289–293, 1967.
Wertheimer, M.: Untersuchen zu Lehre von Gestalt. *I. Psychol. Forsch., 1*:47–58, 1923; *4*:301–350, 1923.
Wever, E. G.: Figure and ground in the visual perception of form. *Amer. J. Psychol., 38*: 194–226, 1927.
White, B. L., and Held, R.: Plasticity of sensory motor development. *In* Rosenblith, J. F., and Allinsmith, W. (Eds.): *Readings in Child Development and Educational Psychology,* 2nd Ed. Boston, Allyn & Bacon, Inc., 1966.
Wiesel, T. N., and Hubel, D. H.: Single-cell responses in striate cortex of kittens deprived of vision in one eye. *J. Neurophysiol., 26*:1013–1017, 1963.
Wiesel, T. N., and Hubel, D. H.: Extent of recovery from the effects of visual deprivation in kittens. *J. Neurophysiol., 28*:1060–1072, 1965.
Witkin, H. A.: Individual differences in the ease of perception of embedded figures. *J. Personality, 19*:1–16, 1950.
Zigler, M. J., Cook, B., Miller, D., and Wemple, L.: The perception of form in peripheral vision. *Amer. J. Psychol., 42*:246–259, 1930.

4 CHILDREN'S LEARNING

Sheldon H. White, and
Harold D. Fishbein

The psychological analysis of learning and thinking is in a period of great change. Early in this century, two significant bodies of activity were developed and became popular among psychologists—the stimulus-response analysis of learning and the psychometrics of intelligence. The elaborate development of these approaches tended to be pre-emptive. Until recently, for a majority of psychologists, learning was what the learning psychologists studied and intelligence was what the intelligence tests tested. Today, however, the basic assumptions under which these approaches were developed are widely rejected. There are newer concepts of human learning and adaptive processes, and a reconsideration of children's learning is in order.

This chapter takes the following course: First we will give a brief description of the research usually designated as basic experimental research on children's learning, outlining the historic rationale for that approach but suggesting that the resultant body of research is limited in scope and view. We will then attempt to sketch the beginnings of a broader, more adequate picture of the processes of human learning, where man is seen as adapting to the environment through a set of psychobiological and psychosocial subsystems. These subsystems regulate the growth of his cognitive structure, his social interactions and his mood and tension. Each of the subsystems may "remember" aspects of the environment in the course of its regulatory function, or it may incorporate aspects of experience in its development. The term learning is consequently seen as encompassing a series of remembering functions or organizational functions arising in the coordination of the human's behavior to the environment.

Our discussion will then briefly turn back to traditional learning analysis and take up an interesting practical elaboration of the stimulus-response conception of learning: the field of behavior modification. Behavior modification has been used with some positive results in the management of a variety of childhood behavior problems. The work is of direct interest in its own right, but it offers a paradox. Behavior, modification techniques achieve their success with a surprisingly simple conception of human behavioral problems.

Our consideration of behavior

modification will serve as a bridge between "basic" *versus* "natural" analyses of learning. Questions about basic processes in learning generally move toward a more refined examination of events—toward moment-to-moment analysis of the interchanges between behavior and environment, and toward a coordination of behavior with neuropsychological events taking place on a time scale of milliseconds. But our ordinary concerns about how children learn are generally on a time scale of months or years. In the next major section of the chapter, we will be concerned with psychological attempts to define broad trends and broad influences on human learning. Historically, the psychometric work on the measurement of intelligence and, more recently, certain broad theories about cognitive development have tried to describe these larger movements.

The last section will summarize the relationship between our present knowledge of children's learning and current intervention in child development. At present, the demands for help in the development of various governmental programs directed at optimal child development have placed an enormous overload on our knowledge base and on that small cadre of individuals committed to the development of that knowledge base. In this final section we will try to indicate the kinds of research that are most needed in the future.

RESEARCH ON CHILDREN'S LEARNING

Children's learning has for some time been directly studied with a group of special procedures designed for the experimental study of lower animals or adult humans. The extensive use of these procedures has been associated with an American tradition of stimulus-response analysis and learning theory building. The most widely used procedures are described in the following paragraphs. (For a more complete description of such procedures, see Spiker, 1960.)

Experimental Procedures for the Study of Children's Learning

Classical (Pavlovian) Conditioning

Classical conditioning is demonstrated by the elicitation of a new response (the conditioned response) to a stimulus (the conditioned stimulus) which prior to conditioning did not elicit that response. The emergence of the conditioned response depends upon a contingent relation, in time, between the conditioned stimulus and an unconditioned stimulus (a stimulus which reflexively produces an unconditioned response). The conditioned response usually resembles part of the unconditioned response.

For example, in an experiment on learning in infants by Lipsitt and Kaye (1964), the conditioned stimulus was a tone, the unconditioned stimulus was a pacifier, and the unconditioned response was sucking. After 10 presentations of the tone with the pacifier, presentation of the tone came to elicit a sucking reaction. (For a fuller account of classical conditioning work with children, see Reese and Lipsitt, 1970, and Stevenson, 1970. For a description of classical conditioning in general, see Kimble, 1961.)

Instrumental Conditioning: Operant Conditioning

While classical conditioning depends upon contingent time arrangements between two external stimuli, instrumental or operant conditioning depends upon contingent time relations between responses and subsequent stimuli. Classical conditioning is usually linked with the modification of emotional or vegetative functions; instrumental or operant conditioning is generally believed to determine more goal-oriented, executive functioning.

Operant and instrumental conditioning are slightly different, but they are often considered together. In both, positive or negative reinforcement is administered contingent upon, and immediately after, a response selected by the experimenter. Depending upon the response consequence, the subsequent frequency of the response is either increased or decreased. For example, Weisberg (1963) increased the vocalization rate of 3-month-old institutionalized infants by contingently reacting to vocalization—by briefly touching the infant's chin, smiling and talking to him following vocalization. (For a fuller account of instrumental and operant conditioning with children, see Reese and Lipsitt, 1970. The literature on animal research is vast and not completely summarized anywhere, but a general idea is given by Kimble, 1961, and Reynolds, 1968.)

Discrimination Learning

This procedure is a variant of instrumental conditioning. Typically, the child is shown two stimuli, and he may choose one or the other. The choice of one stimulus is rewarded; choice of the other is not. The child is repeatedly shown the pair of stimuli, choosing each time, until a criterial string of correct choices suggests that he has learned the discrimination. For example, Hill (1965) gave one-year-olds two objects: a small green triangle and a tall red cylinder, one of which consistently concealed candy. He found that about half the children learned to choose consistently the object having the reward within 100 trials. (See Fellows, 1968, and Reese and Lipsitt, 1970, for accounts of discrimination learning in children. See Riley, 1968, for a more general treatment.)

Probability Learning

In most learning procedures, the desired response is invariably rewarded and other responses are not rewarded. However, in the paradigm for probability learning—generally, a variant of the discrimination procedure—one response choice is only probabilistically more correct than another. (See Stevenson, 1970.)

Concept Attainment

Concept attainment is a variant of discrimination learning. In the usual discrimination learning procedure, a single stimulus—an object, a visual pattern, a tone—defines the correct and incorrect choice. In concept-attainment experiments, the presenting stimuli are "noisy," that is, they contain relevant and irrelevant features. Some aspect of the stimulus defines its correctness. The child must selectively ignore part of the presenting material. The correct "concept" may be a visual part-element, such as the color, form, numerosity of the stimulus display, or perhaps some category-name that applies to the stimulus. (See, for example, Osler and Kofsky, 1966.)

Certain variants of concept attainment are sometimes used. In *Oddity Learning,* the child must learn to select from a set of stimuli the one stimulus that differs from the set. (See, for example, Gollin and Shirk, 1966.) In *Matching-from-Sample,* the child must learn to select from a set of stimuli the one stimulus that matches a sample placed at a specific locus. (See, for example, Fellows, 1968.)

Verbal Learning

There are a family of procedures here, but the two most common are

Paired-Associates Learning and *Rote Serial Learning.* These are the classic memory drum-techniques. In paired-associates learning, the subject is presented with a list of words; for each word he must learn another word as an associate. He sees the stimulus word, has a few seconds to deliver the associated response word and then is shown the correct response word. In rote serial learning, the subject is trying to learn an *n*-item word list in order. He sees the first word on the list, has a few seconds to deliver the second word, is then shown the second word, tries to guess the third word, and so forth. This procedure is generally used with older, literate children, although picture variants have occasionally been used for preschool children. (See Goulet, 1968.)

USE OF THE EXPERIMENTAL PROCEDURES

The procedures just described are the windows through which the child psychologist has taken a controlled view of children's learning. The number of formats is small, but this is deceptive because each generic format may be expressed in a great variety of specific procedures. There is not just one, or even a circumscribed number, of exact physical arrangements for classical conditioning. A great number of conditioned and unconditioned stimuli may be arranged into a classical conditioning configuration; furthermore, there are myriad possibilities for variation of the physical or procedural details of the routine. This brings great richness and versatility to the procedures. Each may be used with a great variety of stimuli, response arrangements, types of subject, motivational conditions and systematic procedural variation. There are hybrid procedures. There are sequential "transfer" series, in which seriated tasks are presented to the subject; the child's response to the second task indicates the nature of what he has learned in the first task. Undoubtedly, the ability to exploit these formats so flexibly has led to their popularity and continued usage. They are good experimental tools. Some have exploited the laboratory formats sensitively and ingeniously to develop significant analyses of motivation, sensory processes, attention, individual differences and so forth.

But if we are concerned with a complete picture of children's learning, we must consider the specialization of this body of techniques as a whole. All are fairly quick, involving a child for one or two 20-minute sessions. All are presented to children working alone, usually in an environment shielded from distractions. The stimuli and loci of responses are well demarcated from their background. The learning proceeds on a trial-by-trial basis and is registered by changes on one or a few response indices. All of these conditions restrict the experimental study of learning to a certain range and form of phenomena. Micro-events, events occurring in that interval of time between the appearance of the stimulus and the delivery of the response, are not recorded. Similarly, learning on the macro-scale, the evolution of human learning over periods of weeks and months, is not studied. Within the time frame of the experiment, the experimenter notes only those behavior changes that the system is designed to register.

These restrictions have been so severe that to date no full-scale account of children's learning has been developed from the research literature. Periodic reviews of the accumulated research literature (Munn, 1957; White, 1963, 1970b) have instead found somewhat segregated clusters of research work. Three topics of presently ongoing activity are the following:

1. As part of a general resurgence of research on infancy, there has been a new interest in the learning capacities of the infant. We have not looked very hard at learning in infancy, although various arguments about optimal infant care make assumptions about the infant's capacity for learning. To date, the new wave of work has largely been devoted to meeting the special technical problems of research with infants, and to providing a series of exploratory studies of infant learning using the kinds of experimental procedures described in the preceding test (Papousek, 1967; Reese and Lipsitt, 1970).

2. There has been an extended examination of preschool children's handling of the simple two-choice discrimination problem. The way children handle this simple problem is not so simple. One can identify a number of interacting factors involved in the child's attempts at solution—factors like right and wrong placements of the child's attention, strategies, stereotypes and the influence of discrimination learning sets, which act as a kind of cumulative wisdom about problems-of-this-type. In the complex nature of the child's attempts to solve this problem, we may see something of the essential nature of higher order human problem solving. The analytical literature has been concerned with trying to construct rough formal models of the processes involved in the child's approach to these problems (Fellows, 1968).

3. There is now a literature on social factors in learning, generally concerned with identifying the effect of a specified social stimulus or influence in the context of one of the standard learning procedures. This literature is of several kinds. It has been shown that short-term social deprivation or satiation immediately influences the sensitivity of the child to "social reinforcement." A number of explanations for this are being tested (Gewirtz, 1967). Laboratory learning procedures have now been used as a baseline for assessment of the relative efficacy of various sources of social reinforcement—male or female, adult or peer, friend or stranger (Stevenson, 1965). And finally, there has been a growing amount of work on imitational and observational induction of learning in children (Bandura, 1965; Aronfreed, 1969).

These three clusters of activity typify the present drift of research on children's learning. The experimental literature dealing with this area is not unified. We have a literature of selected topics, a literature that has moved away from its ancestral premise of a complete and close-knit stimulus-response analysis of learning to become a literature of segregated clusters of work. The great range and flexibility of the laboratory learning procedures allows them to be used to explore newer, often antibehavioristic issues of psychological analysis, like attention, planning, inference, language, curiosity, anxiety, imitation and social influence. But the question of how one can understand human learning still remains. What seems more and more likely is that this now must be approached by a speculative synthesis, deriving evidence from a variety of experimental and observational procedures now extant.

THE MECHANISMS OF HUMAN LEARNING: THE LEARNING THEORY PERSPECTIVE AND THE ADAPTATIONAL PERSPECTIVE

The learning theory movement that extended from the 1920's to the mid 1950's was an historically important organizer of American psychological activities. Some, only dimly aware of the special meaning of the term "learning theory" as used by psychologists, have imagined learning theory to be a comprehensive attack on the psychological nature of learning. Others, better acquainted with the restrictions inherent in the tradition, have denounced it as an impossibly mechanistic misconception of the nature of animal learning. Both judgments miss the point. Learning theory in its historical inception was an experiment in the scientific development of psychology, involving self-conscious restrictions of scope and plausibility (White, 1970a).

A full account of the genesis and elaboration of the learning theory movement in psychology cannot be given here, but enough must be said to account for certain influences on current work and thinking about children's learning. In back of the development of learning theory there rested a Pandora's box of fundamental issues: philosophical issues about the nature of human knowledge, biological issues about the role of consciousness in human adaptation and programmatic issues about the possibility of systematic development of Psychology by organized scientific procedure. The learning theory movement was, historically, a pre-emptive resolution of these issues.

During the late 19th century, the classic philosophical issue of empiricism *versus* rationalism was still being debated. There was a British group of philosopher-psychologists who were essentially concerned with elaborating on empiricistic associationism—the notion that human knowledge is developed entirely through experience (without any innate ideas) by associationistic processes that progressively bind sensation to sensation and idea to idea to attain the complexities of adult thought. With the advent of Darwin and Spencer and evolutionary thinking in the middle of the 19th century, this traditional associationism was blended with biological ideas. It became, eventually, an associationism of reflexes, or an associationism of stimulus-response links. I. M. Sechenov, a teacher of Pavlov, transformed associationism into reflexology. He envisioned the brain as a nested system of reflex units, with reflexes of the higher centers exerting inhibitory regulation over the lower reflexes (Sechenov, 1863). Pavlov, at the turn of this century, began his studies of the influence of "psychic stimuli" on the gastric and salivary reflexes of dogs, and this, in the light of Sechenov's projection, was seen as an event of fundamental importance. The simple reflex, the elementary stimulus-response connection, could be modified in Pavlov's laboratory under controlled conditions, and thus the dynamics of the fundamental building block of behavior could be studied in a controlled way. This generated a great interest in the scientific study of stimulus-response connection as a basic analysis of psychological function.

The American adoption of Pavlov's program was fostered by a concern to make Psychology less speculative, more solidly grounded on behavior facts alone (White, 1970a). The subsequent phase of the learning theory movement—the learning theories of E. C. Tolman, C. L. Hull and B. F. Skinner (Hilgard and Bower, 1966)—gradually discarded Pavlov's "neurologizing" of what was manifestly observable; namely, behavior stimulus-response connections. A stimulus-response psychology developed, which, like reflexology, projected a total analysis of behavior in terms of nested stimulus-response linkages, but which, unlike reflexology, treated the organism itself as a black box and tried to develop the stimulus-response network from a formal analysis of behavior. This explanation oversimplifies the history, but it does suggest the special interests that laid down a special distribution of laboratory effort and a special concentration on particular kinds of studies.

It was assumed that certain laboratory procedures—notably, classical and instrumental conditioning—would get at basic processes of stimulus-response condition. These processes were to be studied in detail in the laboratory. Controlling variables were to be precisely (some hoped, quantitatively) defined. At the same time, progressively more complex and more natural domains of human behavior were to be interpreted as stimulus-response systems. It was hoped that the laboratory and life would ultimately meet in bridging synthetic theories. (For an account of the learning theories, see Hilgard and Bower, 1966. For an account of some of the elaborate parametric analyses of classical and instrumental conditioning, conceived as the basic learning mechanisms, see Kimble, 1961.) There were as a result many and diverse prospectuses of stimulus-response analyses of natural human phenomena. (See Miller and Dollard, 1941, for accounts of social learning and imitation through stimulus-response processes.)

The body of direct experimental research on children's learning today represents a fragmented residue of this program, a body of procedures floating free of their original theoretical core and placed in the service of emergent, newer conceptions of human learning.

Human Learning as Adaptation

Psychologists are now moving toward another outlook on human learning. It is new in that it departs from the outlook of the last several decades, but not so new in that it picks up an evolutionary, psychobiological perspective which is ancestral to the learning theories but which was lost as they became specialized. The most direct impetus toward our new perspective has been the repeated successes of various experimental, naturalistic and clinical studies in demonstrating forms of human learning and adaptation not found in the laboratory. A secondary impetus has been the gradual growth of our information about brain and behavior relationships to a point where it is logically inconceivable to sustain a model of learning in terms of hookups among stimuli, responses and reinforcers.

We have much new work on sensory information-processing to discount what was once called the "doctrine of immaculate perception" and to suggest that a "stimulus" is an endpoint of human thinking and learning as well as a beginning (Neisser, 1967; Vernon, 1970). We have Piaget's studies of the child's development of conceptual operations to show that a child's learning is by no means simply reactive to his experience. Rather, it involves an intricate interaction between experience and pre-existing cognitive structures that fit or do not fit with it (Piaget and Inhelder, 1969; Piaget, 1970). The ethologists and anthropologists have been doing naturalistic observations of animal social organization, and their work has led us to think about children's socialization in new ways (Scott, 1968; Hess, 1970). What is most interesting about the current ethological work is its apparent ability to capture the essence of some basic Freudian insights about child development and to re-express them in less metaphoric and more researchable terms (Bowlby, 1969). At a more basic level, there has been a great growth of information about brain and behavior (Harlow and Woolsey, 1958; Eccles, 1966; Grossman, 1967; Quarton et al., 1967), and we are now more sensitive to the complex engineering of thought.

All of this information attacks an old root metaphor. Once, we imagined a parsimoniously simple biological creature with a minimum set of "primary drives"—hunger, thirst, sex and so forth—the drive systems representing the survival goals for the creature in a threatening, objective world. That creature's job was to learn to find its way about in that objective world, to locate and remember the stimulus signals for all those things in the world that reduced the primary drives. The creature was alone, joining with other creatures only because they came to be "secondary reinforcers" for the reduction of its primary drives. The creature was passive, reacting to stimuli as they came. In this simple creature, primary drive reduction served as a kind of natural selection principle, causing adaptive behavior to survive.

This, the old root metaphor, is being supplanted by a vision of an innately more complex creature engaged in a much more delicate and richer process of adaptation to its environment.

Learning in the Context of Adaptational Systems

The most significant new analyses of children's learning are not intended as explanations of learning *per se*. Piaget's writings in a broad way, and Bowlby's (1969) recent treatment of children's attachment in a specific way, set forth an account of the pattern of children's adaptation to their environment which seems most faithful to the flow of psychological events in real time. We will speak about the writings of these two authors in more detail later; the present discussion follows them in spirit rather than in specific details or terminology.

Human psychology no less than human physiology is organized in the context of adaptation; that is to say, human behavior is determined according to mechanisms which, on the average and in the long run, maintain certain kinds of states of the organism and reject others. Generally, we have tended to think of the motives or the needs of the human as tensions, or disturbing factors, that seek relief. The importance of envisioning human behavior in an adaptational context is the understanding that behavior systems, as systems, work toward future states, goals or criteria. This is teleology, the explanation of the present in terms of the future, but it is fundamental to the understanding of human behavior systems to see that they are designed to express an implicit, probabilistic purposiveness.

Although the first of the major learning theories, set forth in Tolman's *Purposive Behavior in Animals and Men* (1932), was an attempt to deal with purposes in behavioristic terms, subsequent learning theories tended to minimize purpose, plan and goal as unscientific in psychological discourse. A large part of the present reorientation comes because of the reassertion that behavior must be understood as goal-oriented.

Bowlby has admirably expressed this notion:

> A teleological theory is one that not only recognizes that an active biological system, whether physiological or behavioral, tends in a species' environment of adaptedness to result in a predictable outcome that is usually of value to the species, but accounts for its reaching that outcome by supposing that in some way the outcome is itself an immediate cause of the physiological reaction, or of the behavior, that leads to it. . . . The immediate causes of a system's activation are one thing; the function of that system is quite another. Functions are the special consequences that arise from the way a system is constructed; causes are the factors that lead the system to become active or inactive on any one occasion.

When this distinction is applied to the problem of instinctive behavior, it is seen that the causes of any behavior are those factors that activate that particular behavioral system; whereas the function of that behavior derives from the structure of the system, which is such that, when it is in action in its environment of evolutionary adaptedness, a consequence that promotes survival commonly follows.[1]

For the purposes of discussion, we should distinguish between a "regulational subsystem" and an "adaptational subsystem." Human learning can be discussed in terms of three major adaptational subsystems: a cognitive system, a social system and a mood-tension system.

A regulational system "hunts" certain values or states or criteria, which in effect are its "motives" for activity. The simple analogy in human physiology is the regulational system which hunts, for instance, a fixed body temperature, a pH level of the blood or an oxygen tension of the blood. The existence of any regulational system implies the presence of (1) some target state or criterion that serves as the "goal" of the system, (2) momentary-state detectors that establish the present value and (3) regulational activities so designed that momentary states differing critically from the target state will trigger mechanisms that are designed to be corrective. We describe nothing other than the well-known negative feedback control system of cybernetics, quite familiar as a regulational model in contemporary discussions. Somewhat new is the effort by present-day psychologists to reconstrue human psychological affairs in these regulational terms. (See Fig. 4–1.)

The special, tricky point about human psychological regulatory systems is that they are not completely fixed in form or function. Rather, they are open, and they are elaborated during the course of growth and development. Herein lies what is a bit new: our distinction between a regulational system and an adaptational system. An adaptational system may be reprogrammed during the course of its activities. Imagine a second-order set of activities whose function it is to alter the definition of a target state,

[1]Bowlby, J.: *Attachment and Loss.* Vol. I: *Attachment.* New York, Basic Books, Inc., 1969, Vol. I, pp. 124–126.

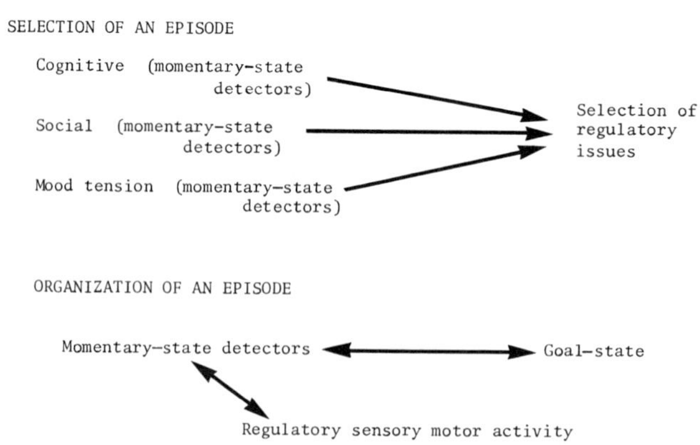

Figure 4–1 A sketch of the multiple regulatory scheme discussed in the text. We assume (1) that the child's multiple regulation agenda includes cognitive, social and mood-tension issues; (2) that the purposive behavior of the child is, effectively, a "one-channel" vehicle directed by one goal at a time; (3) that the selection of which goal is to direct behavior is a continuous issue. We do *not* assume any physiological or psychological separation of the three domains beyond the taxonomy of purposes. If one looks at children who are engaged in learning over real time, one sees that the apparent direction of their activities toward the task is intermittent and episodic, interrupted by segments of activity that seem to represent episodes of social or mood-tension management. The figure does not reflect the alterations in the system with growth and experience that lead to adaptation.

the nature or precision of the momentary-state detectors or the number or efficiency of the regulational activities. This system would, in effect, progressively reorganize regulational systems; this system would be an "adaptive" system and, insofar as we can approximate that traditional term in this new terminology, this adaptive system would be that capacity we have called "learning."

We usually think of an equilibratory or homeostatic system as tending toward a steady state, a return from change to an enduring norm. What we have here called a regulational subsystem has this maintenance property. It is the special, intriguing property of children's psychology that while a regulatory agenda is maintained, the components of the regulatory system—the definition of target state, the momentary state detectors and the regulational activities—are changed by that great complex of factors called growth and learning. The elegance of Piaget's intricate theory of cognitive development is, precisely, the working out of this shifting regulatory pattern for one of our three major subsystems. Piaget's analysis shows an equilibrium-seeking cognitive structure, impelled by the very dynamics that cause it to seek equilibrium, growing larger, more complex and more sophisticated. In effect, each time the child solves one problem, by the very same act he recognizes new problems. We speak, then, of an adaptational subsystem of regulatory activities and momentary-state detectors progressively reprogrammed during the course of development, so that enduring values or target states are hunted in progressively more sophisticated ways.

Somewhere in the midst of this scheme are what have been called mechanisms of learning: classical conditioning, imitation, habituation, instrumental conditioning and so forth. What are they? What part do they play? They are, in the context of our discussion, those design features of the organism that modify a regulational subsystem into that higher-order, more labile entity that we here call an adaptational subsystem. They are reprogramming mechanisms that if stimulated in a certain way will produce a certain change in the program of the organism's behavior. We do not know how many mechanisms there are, and though there are frequent pleas for a good taxonomy of types of learning, the indications are that we are a long way from a defined set of pure and distinct types. Indeed, the custom of speaking as though there were discoverable distinct types of learning may be simply an engrained bad habit of psychological discourse. What may be nearer the truth is that certain kinds of environmental influences produce discriminable adaptation syndromes to which we have assigned special names and special measurement procedures that exaggerate their distinctness.

Cognitive Regulation

Generally speaking, our understanding of human knowledge has been greatly dominated by the style of discourse that treats knowledge as conterminous with immediate behavior change. Consequently, there only begins to be a direct discussion of how knowledge, in the larger sense, is adapted or learned. Certain arguments, strongly developed in the recent literature, have begun to address the development of knowledge in children and should have important implications for our approach to training or educating children. The major new themes are (1) an emphasis of the spontaneity of children's approach to learning, (2) the argument that humans possess not one, but several, knowledge systems and (3) the notion that one fundamental way in which learning can be construed is as a differentiative process. No acceptable blend of these new themes exists as yet. The closest approximation to it is Piaget's quasi-embryological account of the successive stages of the child's logical and objective thought, but Piaget is least clear about exactly why the age changes that are found in children's thought occur. He insists that his observed progressions are not to be simply assigned to either learning or maturation, but he leaves open what he calls "the American question"—the persistent American interest in establishing where and how much difference training makes in his scheme (Athey and Rubadeau, 1970; Flavell, 1970). Piaget, and a good many other writers nowadays, offer some implicit assumptions about children's learning that are distinctly different from the conventional assumptions of much recent writing.

Spontaneous Motivation. As suggested earlier, one very interesting feature of Piaget's theory of cognitive development is the thesis that cognitive structure, in seeking to come to terms with the environment, grows and elaborates itself. The cognitive structure is in effect "disturbed" by new information that is slightly discrepant from that-which-can-be-dealt-with, and it changes to encompass the new information. With that change, the system is prepared to recognize a new order of discrepancy and to be stimulated to grow still further. In a rather elegant and abstract way, Piaget proposes an equilibrium-seeking system of cognitive regulation that by the simple rules of its operation is steadily led to adapt itself to new information, to enlarge and complicate itself and thus to learn. It is this special analysis, more than any other, that leads us to speak about the growth of knowledge as related to cognitive regulatory mechanisms (see, particularly, Piaget, 1970).

The thesis that learning does not have to be dependent on motives or rewards immediately in the situation has been developed in a number of ways recently. There has been an abundance of research on animals showing that learning is guided by simple curiosity or an "exploratory drive." Robert White (1959), in a well-known paper, has developed the argument that children are strongly stimulated to learn and develop by a simple need to be competent and to master. This is very new in the literature on learning, although it is a commonplace and irresistible impression when one watches children. Probably, our heavy emphasis on data from animals and children in artificial experimental situations has been misleading in that it has led us to see all learning as critically dependent upon items such as drive reductions or reinforcers.

There is now a parallel argument about children in school. It claims that the traditional schools, like the traditional experiments, create an environment where the motivation for learning artificially becomes a serious, chronic issue. A diversified contemporary movement toward educational reform advocates the release of the child to pursue learning through discovery (Bruner, 1961, 1966), the institution of open classrooms, or the design of technology to permit "autotelic" (self-purposing) teaching of the child. There is much force to these arguments. It is impossible to fully resist a line of argument that contains some of the most sensitive, convincing writing about children's learning to be found (see Holt, 1967). But there is an opposite trend in educational reform that insists on a high degree of preorganization for the child, and an environment that is replete with reinforcements. This kind of thinking, too, has its evidence and its justifications.

No one has ever demonstrated that *all* human learning proceeds spontaneously or nonspontaneously, and one can be suspicious of any argument that makes prescriptive claims for learning or training in general. There is good reason to believe that what we generally and loosely speak of as "knowing" refers not to a singular but to a plural cognitive structure.

Knowledge Systems. Ordinary discourse treats "knowing" in intellectual terms and often in specifically verbal terms. We know when we have "the concept" of something. Set against this, there has been already mentioned technical psychological discourse that insists that knowledge resides in behaviors. These apparent oppositions can probably be reconciled if we accept the proposition that human knowledge is an expression of several psychobiological systems that are integrated but not perfectly correlated in function.

Bruner (1964) has discussed a distinction among *enactive, ikonic* and *symbolic* human representational systems. He points out that the child may represent meaning to the world in terms of what he does to it, in images, or encoded in symbols. There is an ordering of the prominance of these representational systems in the developing child. Very early in life the child's intelligence seems to be predominantly a motor affair; Piaget speaks of the first 18 or 24 months of life as the period of sensory-motor intelligence. In the preschool years, literal visual imagery seems to play an unusually strong part in the child's thinking. Then, in the school years there is a move toward symbolized interpretations of the world. There is some argument about whether the essence of these higher thought processes is only word symbols, but there is general agreement that some sort of abstractive system comes into play for interpreting and reasoning about experience. All of the major developmental theorists—Piaget, Werner, Freud, Vygotsky—appear to concur about this order of prominence of the representational systems.

What seems true from infancy onward is that some number of essential systems coexist in the human, and that these systems are not alike in their susceptibility to experience or training, so that they are not always "in phase" with one another in what they know of the world. Children at age 4 are as acute as adults in their ability to discriminate a diagonal from a nondiagonal, but they are unable to draw a diagonal. There are a number of cases where knowing-in-perception precedes knowing-in-performance in children (Maccoby and Bee, 1965). During the course of language development, there seems to be a sequence from imitation to comprehension to production (Fraser et al., 1963). These special experimental demonstrations find their counterpart in ordinary experience. From time to time we are all aware that we know something intuitively that we cannot express in words, or vice versa.

We do not know how many semiautonomous representational systems there are, but a respectable variety of psychological literatures has suggested diversity of knowledge. The factor analytic approach to mental testing has regularly differentiated mental abilities given names like spatial ability, verbal ability, numerical ability and so forth. The patterns of such mental abilities differ among children of differing ethnic groups (Stodolsky and Lesser, 1967). Are we talking about different abilities or different knowledge systems? There is a century-old supposition of a distinction between visual-minded *versus* auditory-minded kinds of thinkers (Bissell et al., 1971). Studies of the consequences of brain damage regularly produce evidence for some fragmentation in the neurological organization of knowledge. The brain-damaged patient may write a word that he cannot read, or he may be able to utter a word in one context of conversation but not in another.

Because of such evidence, one must regard broadside arguments or claims about human learning with reservation. We do not, in truth, know that there is a conflict between optimal learning through reinforcement and optimal learning through discovery. The different techniques may optimize different aspects of learning. More generally, all questions about optimization of the child's training or environment depend upon some kind of understanding of the articulation of knowledge and knowledge systems in the child and their sensitivities to experience.

Learning as Differentiation. Quite often we discuss learning in terms of an empty-full metaphor. Learning adds on something—an idea, a behavior, a fact, a skill. The opposite of learned is ignorant, and a synonym for learning is acquisition. There is another way to address the process of learning that rests on a confused-unconfused metaphor. Learning organizes what is initially incoherent.

This perspective is quite useful in a basic sense, and it is of special importance in discussions of children's learning. In the basic sense, it is more realistic to think of the environment as a diffuse flux of physical energy impinging upon the receptors, than it is to suppose an environment somehow packeted as stimuli. "Stimulus" has always been a somewhat mysterious term in psychological theory, precisely because it entails a separation of some part of the sensory flux from a remainder, and this separation does not occur "out there" but by means of the work of the organism. The organism organizes its sensory environment into stimuli and nonstimuli by its patterns of selective orientation, attention and action, and learning that changes those patterns changes the stimuli received by the environment. It must also be true that as the child extends his cognitive structure by learning, he progressively makes coherent more and more of the flux of his experience.

Piaget's interpretation of the child's cognitive development rests on the premise that children find their objective world through experience.

> From the most elementary sensorimotor actions (such as pushing and pulling) to the most sophisticated intellectual operations, which are interiorized actions, carried out mentally (e.g., joining together, putting in order, putting into one-to-one correspondence), knowledge is constantly linked with actions or operations, that is, with *transformations.*
>
> Hence the limit between subject and object is in no way determined beforehand, and, what is more important, is not stable. Indeed, in every action the subject and the objects are fused. The subject needs objective information to become aware of his own actions, of course, but he also needs many subjective components. Without long practice or the construction of refined instruments of analysis and coordination, it will be impossible for him to know what belongs to the object, what belongs to himself as an active subject, and what belongs to the action itself taken as the transformation of an initial state into a final one. Knowledge, then, at its origin, neither arises from objects nor from the subject, but from interactions—at first inextricable—between the subject and those objects.[2]

The notion that learning organizes experience into coherence is by no means unique to Piaget. It has been developed by such other theorists as James Mark Baldwin, George Herbert Mead, Freud and Werner. To get a feeling for the idea, one can imagine what one's sense of the world would be if one could not make fundamental distinctions like the following:

There is a "me" and a "not me," and some sensations have to do with what is inside "me" and others pertain to what is outside "me."

---

[2]Piaget, J.: Piaget's theory. *In* Mussen, P. H. (Ed.): *Carmichael's Manual of Child Psychology,* 3rd ed. New York, John Wiley & Sons, Inc., 1970, p. 704.

There is a clear difference between the chair I am seeing and the chair I am conjuring up in my imagination.

There are separate and enduring objects in this world.

Any perceived change has a cause. Some other change occurred to precipitate it.

There is a distinction between what I feel or know about a thing and what others feel or know about it.

To imagine these distinctions not made is, for adults, to imagine confusion in thought. Piaget's analysis presumes that the child does not make them, and that cognitive adaptation brings about a progressive construction of reality. The organization is by no means solely intellectual; the world is organized by action as well as by thought.

We presume, then, that the child's confusion is extreme because he is unable to recognize the "obvious." Following the analysis into the movement of the older child's thought, we recognize that progressively more subtle kinds of confusions exist and are resolved by the development of cognitive organization. There is a resolution of egocentrism, confusion of the objective and the subjective, implicit in every stage of cognitive growth. Indeed, that problem is in us and is implicit in our own cognitive growth. Piaget's genetic epistemology envisions the historical movement of scientific thought as embodying principles of progression like those of childhood thought development and, again, he is not the first genetic psychologist to have made this proposal. When a scientist employs some technique of observation (his sensory motor scheme) he is always concerned with separating artifacts of method. He, like the child, is trying to separate himself (the observing) from the observed. When the cell biologist tries to discriminate which parts of his observations are due to staining or preparation artifacts and which are in the preparation, he is working with a sophisticated expression of the egocentrism issue. He resolves his problem with transformational techniques, mixed pairings of procedures and preparations, which are formally quite analogous to the transformational procedures by which the infant arrives at a stable, objective world.

Social Regulation

In this section we will consider the development of a second adaptational system that moderates the child's social interaction. Why speak of this as a second system? It seems likely that the child's basic social and emotional needs are at the heart of an organized system—an equilibrium-seeking system that adapts through growth and experience, and whose processes may be distinct from (at times, competitive with) the processes of cognitive adaptation. Certain issues of children's social adaptation have been singled out in the psychological literature: (1) infant-mother interaction, (2) the processes of imitation and identification, (3) moral development and (4) social influences on aggression. These are only samplings of the broad issues of children's socialization.

The child at birth is acultural, amoral, unattached and gifted with only a few simple reflexes such as crying, smiling, eye contact and vocalization, through which he makes contact with others. Within a very few months after birth, he forms a primary social bond with his family. From this slim, strong bond a vast elaboration ensues, during which the child becomes "socialized." He learns to play and to work with others. He will imitatively absorb. There come to be people he accepts as like himself, and others whom he begins to regard as strangers. He develops moral and ethical codes, and he develops certain deep schemes for normative and idealized behavior that are special to his cultural background. He may have intuitive notions of the social "rightness" of Democracy, Achievement, *Machismo*, Soul, Socialist Brotherhood, Godliness or Courtesy. Our discussion here attempts to highlight the special issues of learning involved in the articulation of that socialization.

Infant-Mother Interaction. During infancy, when the infant's behavior is not sufficient to sustain life, survival is a matter of cooperation of the infant with the caretaker. We have begun to look at the infant's capacity to modify its behavior in accord with stimuli in the objective environment, as noted above, but the central story of infancy is a social story involving the mother and the child. Consequently, research on infancy has been extensively concerned with developing information about the adaptations in the child relative to what the mother does, and to an attachment process that seems to bind the mother and the infant together emotionally and as an inter-regulating system.

There have been several decades of largely fruitless attempts to establish stable consequences to the child of parental methods of feeding, weaning, toilet training or punishment. Similarly, attempts to categorize the attitudes or the behavior of parents have not been convincing. Maccoby (1968) lists some of the proposed names for discrete parental attitudes that have emerged from factor analytic studies: Warmth, Permissiveness, Child-rearing anxiety, Sex anxiety, Inhibitory demands and discipline, Responsible child-rearing orientation, Physical punishment, Dependence encouragement, Democratic attitudes, Authoritarian control, Punishment, General family conflict, Firm discipline, Independence-achievement orientation and Seclusiveness. Although claims are regularly made in popular child rearing literature about the consequences of parental attitudes such as these, and though such claims may well be valid, we do not have hard-edged evidence to support or elaborate them. A common weakness of discussions of parental practices is that they regularly treat parental behavior as though it were all cause and no effect. A more adequate discourse developed in recent literature treats the processes of child rearing as a dyadic adaptational system.

It has been shown that from birth children differ with respect to sensory thresholds, general activity or muscular tension, disposition toward crying and various other psychophysiological characteristics (Lipsitt, 1970). In one well-known study, infant characteristics, such as activity level, tendency to approach or withdraw, general adaptability, attention span, distractibility and persistence, were shown to be reliably different from one child to the next over the first two years of life (Thomas et al., 1963). Babies differ, just as mothers do, and it is likely that during early infancy there is an intercalibration of the idiosyncratic mother and the idiosyncratic child. In this intercalibration, in this organization of the two into a caretaking rhythm and style, we have a first elaboration of the influence of learning on the child's life, but it is a mutual organization of the mother's and the child's behavior, so that it is impossible to say who is cause and who is effect (Escalona, 1968).

There is some reason to believe that the infant and the mother may be designed for this collaboration, designed to come to love one another and to send and receive signals that maintain the caretaking. At the heart of the arguments is the ethological analysis of social behavior in animals, most specifically an extension of the ideas developed from the study of *imprinting* in animals to the study of *attachment* in human infancy.

Imprinting was first described by Konrad Lorenz in 1935, and is now widely known, as a hard-edged developmental phenomenon. During early life, the young gosling or duckling passes through a critical period, a brief span of a few hours during which certain sign stimuli conforming to innate specifications will release following behavior. The following behavior, in turn, brings about an imprinting of the nestling upon the followed object, a social bond that becomes experientially irreversible at the close of the critical period. The nestling then follows the object and, in the general pattern of its behavior, treats the object as it would its natural mother. It emits distress calls if separated from the object and later, upon reaching maturity, will show courtship and sexual display to it. In birds it is evident that imprinting must provide the mechanism by which the newborn locates its mother and its species. Some very special kind of learning is involved that is unlike any other in the extreme innate limitation of time and circumstance, and in its irreversibility.

Lorenz's original description of a critical period phenomenon has been somewhat moderated by subsequent work with animals. Many now prefer to speak of a "sensitive period" with somewhat softer boundaries. Bowlby's recent volume provides a summary of current thinking about imprinting in animals (Bowlby, 1969, pp. 169–170) and a parallel summary of our present evidence of a similar attachment mechanism in human development:

i. In human infants social responses of every kind are first elicited by a wide variety of stimuli and are later elicited by a much narrower array, confined after some months to stimuli arising from one or a few particular individuals.

ii. There is evidence of a marked bias to respond socially to certain kinds of stimuli more than others.

iii. The more experience of social interaction an infant has with a person the stronger his attachment to that person becomes.

iv. The fact that learning to discriminate different faces commonly follows periods of attentive staring and listening suggests that exposure learning may be playing a part.

v. In most infants attachment behavior to a preferred figure develops during the first year of life. It seems probable that there is a sensitive period in that year during which attachment behavior develops most readily.

vi. It is unlikely that any sensitive phase begins before about six weeks and it may be some weeks later.

vii. After about six months, and markedly so after eight or nine months, babies are more likely to respond to strange figures with fear responses, and more likely also to respond to them with strong fear responses, than they are when they are younger. Because of the growing frequency and strength of such fear responses, the development of attachment to a new figure becomes increasingly difficult towards the end of the first year and subsequently.

viii. Once a child has become strongly attached to a particular figure, he tends to prefer that figure to all others, and such preference tends to persist despite separation.[3]

Bowlby's monographic treatment of attachment is of significance in several ways. The work organizes a considerable body of recent work on infant-attachment and mother-infant relations. It views those processes in the large in an evolutionary framework, and in the fine grain as an ever-adjusting regulative, equilibrium-seeking system. Bowlby sees this kind of analysis as the beginning of a recodification of psychoanalytic theory in terms ostensibly quite foreign to that system, but maintaining and containing the dynamic argu-

---

[3]Bowlby, J.: *Attachment and Loss, Vol. I: Attachment.* New York, Basic Books, Inc., 1969, pp. 222–223.

ments metaphorically set forth by Freud and at the same time allowing for their development through programmatic research. This newer kind of analysis may subsume, as well, an extensive psychological literature on dependency in the recent past.

There is a kind of prospectus for the research work on attachment in the much better developed work on *imprinting* in animals, and if the homologies continue to develop as they have been developing, we may well complete the subsumption of the Freudian dynamics by establishing connections between attachment formation in early childhood and later social and sexual adjustment. We now know that rhesus monkeys who are socially isolated in infancy show serious adulthood disturbances in social, sexual and maternal behavior, and we have long known that various kinds of abnormal childhood environments produce disturbances in adult humans. It is possible that the research on attachment will allow us to get closer to the sources of these problems.

Imitation, Shaping and Identification. If the story of infant social regulation is that of a behavior duet between caretaker and child, organized around an attachment bond between them, the story of preschool social regulation seems to be based upon *shaping* and *imitation,* both tending to produce in the child an *identification* with selected individuals and groups in his social environment. The term "Shaping" means yes-no signals from the parent that guide the child's behavior. These are the "social reinforcements" whose effects are now being studied in the learning laboratory. There have been many arguments about how the child's behavior is, or might be, trained by shaping, and later, in the section entitled *Behavior Modification,* we will consider intervention efforts guided by such arguments.

Until about 10 years ago, our accounts of children's learning tended to underplay imitation as a factor, not because imitation was unknown but because so much research was concentrated in studies of the solitary child. When imitation was discussed, it was not considered as a force in the child's development but rather as a special phenomenon to be accounted for by stimulus-response principles (Miller and Dollard, 1941). Recently there has been an upsurge in experimental studies of children's imitation (Bandura, 1965; Aronfreed, 1969). There are still attempts to show that the imitative phenomenon may somehow be subsumed as a special case of reinforcement principles (Baer and Sherman, 1964), but in his excellent survey of the literature on children's imitation, Aronfreed expresses some reasonable skepticism: "The extensions of contemporary concepts of learning to the phenomena of imitation are not persuasive contradictions or even amplifications of the flat assumption that children imitate because they are constructed to do so" (1969, p. 212).

What role does imitation play in the child's life? We usually think of imitation as a "monkey see, monkey do" phenomenon, in which the child's behavior mirrors that of the model. But imitation is more complex and more subtle in its effects than this. In the first place, faithful transmission of a complex pattern of observed behaviors into practice is a rarity, not often seen until the child comes near the end of the preschool years. The child seems to absorb into his own behavior certain aspects of a model's behavior that are understandable to him—that is, within range of his own constructive repertory for behavior. Piaget speaks of imitation as a device for bringing about *accommodation,* an extension of the pre-existing action schemes.

What does the model do for the child?

1. The model's behavior may pro-

vide patterns of movement, gesture, rhythm, posture and language which the child can absorb into his own behavior.

2. The model may test the permissiveness of the environment for the child. Punishment of a model for a particular behavior inhibits similar behavior in the child. Demonstrated permission or reward encourages it (Bandura et al., 1961, Walters and Parke, 1964).

3. Under certain circumstances the model may teach the child how he (the child) feels about something, a curious and interesting phenomenon. There have been experiments in which an adult subject injected with epinephrine, an arousing drug that is sometimes said to bring about "white emotion," has apparently been induced to regard his own stirred-up feelings as rage or elation depending upon the arbitrarily chosen behavior of another individual, a stooge, in the same room with him (Schacter and Singer, 1962). We really do not know how much naturally occurring human emotional states are innately labeled for the emoter as they occur. There is reason to believe they are not always so labeled and, therefore, that these experiments in social emotional contagion may be prototypic for natural human affairs.

How does a person become a model for the child? The child will, in some sense and to some extent, imitate anyone; experiments on imitation are typically conducted with models who have no particular emotional meaning for the child. But there have been some experiments showing that individuals who are associated with gratifications for the child will be selected as models. Furthermore, since the phenomenon of "identification with the aggressor" has been identified as a sort of paradoxical effect (prisoners in Nazi concentration camps imitating their jailers, in a classic autobiographical account by Bettelheim) one might conclude that any individual with whom the child associates some strong emotion will gain status as a model.

We speak now about identification. Freud first used the term identification to refer to the male child's tendency to model himself on the like-sexed parent as part of the resolution of the Oedipus conflict. This notion has since been applied generically, and the term identification is now used to encompass the child's affiliation with a broad group of social models. The person or persons identified with, chosen by the child as like himself or like what he wants to be, are imitated. However, there is a chicken-egg problem. Does the child imitate because he identifies or identify because he imitates (Kohlberg, 1966)? The issue is fundamentally the question of the relationship between the imitative behaviors and the child's "self-concept"—his awareness of his own pattern of social similarities and uniquenesses, and his feelings about them.

The natural workings of imitation and shaping in the preschool years bring about an implicit social identification whether or not the child is aware of it. The child learns to speak, not English generally, but some dialect of English, and he picks up group-specific gestures, habits, attitudes and etiquette. This brings about a behavioral and emotional determination of a distinctive self-concept before the usual age at which an aware self-concept is said to be formed. In this sense, identification is not a new or a special issue when it arises; it is, in part, the recognition of a *fait accompli*. What may then happen is that the imitative process gets caught up in the next wave of development, when the child's perception of self and society becomes expressed in terms of dimensions ("People differ in height—I am short"), theorized and mythicized.

Moral Development. During the late preschool years, parents begin to introduce the child into that great basis of all human morality, the game of "taking turns." Then, in the school years, there is evidence that the child begins to be intellectually aware of an issue of reciprocity or social balance between himself and others. Kohlberg's (1964) theory of moral development, elaborating earlier findings of Piaget (1962), traces the child's comprehension of social reciprocity through six major stages of development, each stage representing an elaboration and a subtilization of the preceding stage. These are conceived of as universal stages, and there is evidence for a similar set of age progressions throughout a good sample of cultures.

A child's stage is assessed through a set of questions that pose ethical quandaries. "Should a man steal a drug to help his dying wife?" The child answers yes or no, but that is not important. What is important is his explanation of his answer. As children grow older, they move from explanations based upon fear of consequences toward, first, explanations based upon what the rules and laws say and then, finally, a principled level that regards rules and laws themselves as derived from basic principles of justice. These stages seem to represent a cognitive rather than a moral development in that they imply a deeper and deeper understanding of the premise that humans have reciprocal rights and claims upon one another. But Kohlberg has argued that they represent much more than intellectualization because, in fact, they predict the moral behavior of children.

One might say, quite generally, that at about 6 or 7 years of age the child's thinking begins to be expressed in terms of dimensions and continua. He becomes aware of rules and rule systems He shows a first apprehension of formal systems of relationships among variables (White, 1968, 1970b). This has far-reaching ramifications in his ability to think about abstract space, time, cause-effect relationships, number and so forth, and it has a profound influence on his approach to social interaction as well. The child becomes sensitive to his "social contract," the set of rules that define normative and ideal human interaction for this culture. One reflection of this is written into the English Common law: the doctrine that children first know right from wrong—may first be considered guilty of a crime—at age 7. In a variety of cultures there are indications that children are first held to social rules at this time.

At such higher age levels, when the child's thought begins to become "theorized," a new and important social factor in learning emerges. The child's thought is stimulated by a dialectical process, involving a reconciliation of his own expressed thoughts with those of others. We know very little about this dialectical process, and yet a variety of developmental theorists have suggested its importance. Interestingly, Turiel (1966) has offered evidence suggesting that the child may be induced to advance in moral stage if he is placed in discussion with another child whose thinking is at a level that is one (but not two) stage above his own.

The child's assimilation of a social contract at this time may involve more than his understanding of reciprocity. Humans who share a culture are apt to share normative myths defining a wide range of culturally preferred behaviors, outlooks and styles. The cowboy story and the detective story may express such normative myths for our culture, endlessly reiterating the style of the good man and the bad man and perhaps outlining the right way and the wrong way to deal with aggression. The "message" of such modern myths is not very different from the stories of knightly deeds quite popular in Europe a few centuries ago. McClelland (1951) has identified a characteristic called need achievement, not found in all cultures but found in ours and emergent in children at about 6 or 7 years of age. According to McClelland, a cultural belief in need achievement can be traced in the themes of its children's books. Need achievement may be a residue of a second kind of normative myth in our culture, the myth typified by the Horatio Alger stories.

Social Influences on Aggression. In our discussion of social regulation in the developing child, we have emphasized in infancy an attachment mechanism mediating the caretaking dyad. Then, in the preschool period, we have seen social regulation developed by shaping and by imitative behaviors, with identification serving as a half-cognitive, half-emotional substrate. Finally, in the school years, there is the emergence of symbolized understanding of social regulation, embodied in a system of moral judgments and in the understanding of norm-defining cultural myths.

Two of the perennial issues of human interaction are sex and aggression. The development of the sexual impulse from childhood to adulthood has been treated by Freud, and his analysis of the transformations of the sexual impulse from infant cathexis to adult sublimations is not dissimilar from what might be projected in terms of the regulational systems offered in this chapter.

A full treatment of the elaboration of the aggressive impulse and its controls in childhood has not yet been offered. Lorenz (1967) has offered an analysis of the problem of aggression in human society that has one important similarity to Freud's analysis of the problem of sex. Both men see society plagued by instinctive urges that are controlled by the structures of civilization but, being too much held back, occasionally burst forth with pathological force. This similarity is quite important, particularly since the two men differ so radically in the scientific frame of reference that led them to advance their arguments.

We do not have a counterpart to Freud for tracing human aggression, its regulation and adaptation during human growth. However, there is one line of work on the social learning of aggression that is of great interest. Some of the research on imitation has been the basis for much discussion of the effect of televised aggression and violence on the behavior of children. It has been repeatedly shown that children exposed to models who take aggressive and destructive action against toys will themselves be stimulated toward the same actions. Some have offered these experiments as the basis for an argument that television transmits violence into the behavior of children in our society. Others argue that the experiments do not support the larger conclusion, because they only demonstrate an imitation of limited, socially acceptable forms of aggression. And there is even a counterargument to the effect that televised violence, through catharsis, may *reduce* overt social violence. (For a summary of the arguments, see Maccoby, 1964.)

Regulation of Mood and Tension

There is a third great regulational issue in human learning, an issue having to do with the child's sense of ease and sense of moment-to-moment control over himself and the situation. From many and diverse sources we have evidence that tension states in the human, variously called activation, arousal, drive or anxiety, strongly influence his ability to learn and to adapt. These tension states have sometimes been conceived of as deriving from subject needs or hungers, or from psychodynamic mechanisms. Ordinarily, we speak of these tensions as the "motivators" of learning, but it may be rather important to see human tension states as independent regulational issues, presenting their own agenda that, in an important sense, competes with cognitive and social regulation for the child's behavior.

We will not discuss at length the nature of this system or its adaptation during development. Much has been written about children's adjustment and maladjustment, their psychodynamics, their patterns of fear and avoidance or their more and less favorable personality traits. Generally, this literature has taken the position that stable and enduring habits, traits or symptoms residing in the child interfere with his adjustment to the environment. One might see the problem of stress in another light.

The child, whom we now presume to be striving toward competence and mastery, may also be thought to have a very good sense of the edges of his competence and the domain of his incompetence. He does this not by any rational calculation of his own resources and of the demands of the situation, but simply by taking prudent steps when he feels growing tension, aggravation or confusion. He effects a kind of behavior homeostasis designed to keep the situation within bounds. This is true for all children. All children will try to circumvent, deny or avoid situations that arouse more stress than they can handle. We know, from all kinds of formal and information observations, that stress and stress management offer a running counterpoint to the cognitive and social issues in diverse learning situations. In experimental situations we have identified something called "failure set," where the child simply gives up on his experimental learning problem. In the schools we have something called "learning blocks," where the child simply gives up in the classroom. Currently, a growing program of behavior modification is an attempt to deal with problems like this by giving simplified, structured, organized training to the child.

BEHAVIOR MODIFICATION

If the theory of learning derived from traditional stimulus-response analysis has more and more been ruled out of the theoretical arena, the opposite has been true in the practical sense. Within the last decade there has been a progressively enlarging extension of stimulus-response analysis to behavior engineering, behavior modification and behavior therapy. The rationale for this work is quite simply stated in traditional stimulus-response terms, but the apparent simplicity may be deceptive.

Skinner's book *Science and Human Behavior* (1953) is a kind of prolegomenon to the approach. Two small volumes by Bijou and Baer (1961, 1965) present its relationship to child development. The latter works make an enormous endeavor to treat child development in objective, behavioristic and scientific terms. A great deal of effort is made to separate those problems that are psychological—i.e., purely behavioral—from those that are not. A lexicon of purely objective and behavioral terms is offered, and then a good number of the issues of child development care are translated into this vocabulary. Most of the current work on behavior modification (almost all of which is with children) comes from this kind of viewpoint (see, for example, the collections of reports offered in Krasner and Ullmann, 1965; Ullmann and Krasner, 1965; Bijou and Baer, 1967). There are also some other species of behavior therapy (Wolpe et al., 1964).

The viewpoint asserts that undesirable behavior is just that—undesirable behavior. All of the various flora and fauna of psychopathology may be viewed as sets of undesirable response patterns in the repertoire of the subject, sensitive to the reinforcement principles by which responses are increased or decreased in the laboratory. They may be extinguished by the removal of some maintaining reinforcement in the environment. Alternative and more desirable responses may be developed by appropriate reinforcement. Behavior modification is a generalized system of psychotherapy by shaping through reinforcement.

The following brief descriptions of two studies will be useful in characterizing this approach.

Poor Reading

Staats and Butterfield (1965) have reported on reading training that was given to a delinquent Mexican-American boy. When training was initiated, the boy was 14 years old and read at the second grade level. He was failing in every grade and was generally disliked as a troublemaker in school; the promotions he had had were "just to get rid of him." Like his four older brothers, he was regularly in trouble for juvenile misdemeanors. His Wechsler-Bellevue verbal score was 77, and his principal regarded him as mentally retarded.

The behavior modification procedure developed for the boy used tokens as rewards, the tokens being convertible for cash. There was a blue token worth 1/10 cent, a white token worth 1/5 cent and a red token worth 1/2 cent. These tokens were used to provide systematic rewards for performance on Science Research Associates reading kits. There were vocabulary cards. The boy had to pronounce the word on each card, receiving a white token if he was correct, and a blue token if he was incorrect. There was oral reading of paragraphs with, again, a white token if correct and blue token if there was an error. Then there was silent story reading. During this, the boy was rewarded on a V. I. 15 (Variable Interval 15 reward) schedule for attentive behavior; that is, he received a token over intervals varying from 1 second to 30 seconds and averaging 15 seconds if he steadily maintained concentration on the reading. There was an extra token if he read without moving his lips. Then he was asked comprehension questions on the story with, again, tokens for being correct and for avoiding spelling errors.

This kind of training was given for a total of 40 hours extending through four and one-half months. The boy, who had begun at the second grade level, reached the 4.3 grade level on the California Reading Test. There were some side effects: The training extended over a school term and, during that term, the boy got a C in physical education, a D in shop, a D in English and a D in mathematics—an unprepossessing grade picture, but these were the first courses the boy had ever passed in school. Official demerits for misbehaviors—he received 10 per month before the training began—went down to zero the last two months of the training. Unfortunately, after this promising start, the study was terminated because the boy shot out lights and windows of the school with a BB gun and was brought to court for malicious mischief. He was sent to a school for juvenile delinquents and then, because he was creating disturbances, he was sent to an industrial school for juvenile delinquents.

Stuttering

Goldiamond (1965) has reported on his development of a laboratory treatment for stuttering. In a sequence of case studies, the first few essentially showed that the rate of nonfluencies delivered by stutterers reading from text in the laboratory could be manipulated, moved up or down, by contingent reinforcements. Another study showed that repeated exposure to the laboratory did not produce a reduction in stuttering. This was a critical adaptation control for the therapy studies that followed. Finally, a treatment that had three stages was evolved. In the first stage, the stutterers read aloud, experiencing delayed auditory feedback whenever they delivered a nonfluency. This produced a gradual elimination of stuttering accompanied by a drastic reduction in reading rate. In the second stage, this low rate of clear reading was maintained while the delayed auditory feedback was gradually faded out, until the subject could read clearly without it. In the third stage, the rate of reading was gradually speeded up by manipulation of the speed with which the pages were presented and by the use of monetary rewards. Using this kind of procedure, Goldiamond was able to eliminate stuttering in the laboratory for each of the eight cases. There was some, but not universal, extension of the stuttering pattern to situations outside the laboratory. Interestingly, the elimination of stuttering in this procedure was mediated by a new "voice" (a new intonation and rhythm) developed during the course of the training. This is consistent with a general phenomenon in stuttering. There are bilinguals who stutter in only one of their languages. Even severe stutterers may be quite fluent if they speak in dialect or if they sing. Essentially, the behavior modification procedure of Goldiamond seems to have developed for the stutterer another voice in which he could be fluent.

The reports by Staats and Butterfield and by Goldiamond are representative of the general approach of most behavior modification studies. The presenting problem is analyzed as one, or usually a set, of undesirable behaviors. Ideally, there will be objective, countable behaviors. An estimate of their presenting rate will be obtained. Behavior modifiers are quite conscientious about this and at times will follow a child about for days, noting the rate of the undesirable behavior and, if possible, noting the presence of environmental events that seem to initiate or reward the behavior.

At the same time there will be an establishment of a reinforcer. The behavior modifier will attempt to show that something he can control in the child's environment—e.g., candy, money, toys, praise, isolation, television—will be worked for by the child. The behavior modifier will then attempt a strategic use of his information to reduce the rate of the undesirable behavior in the child. He obtains this objectively determined rate reduction quite often.

In work with diagnostically normal children, there have been reports of obtained improvement in cases of regressed crawling (Harris, et al., 1964), vomiting (Wolf et al., 1965), mutism (Kerr et al., 1965), prolonged crying (Hart et al., 1964), isolation or timidity in play (Allen et al., 1964; Johnston et al., 1966), tantrums (Williams, 1959; Wolf et al., 1964) and stuttering (Goldiamond, 1965). Behavior modification has been applied to various diagnostic groups, and there has been some demonstrated improvement of behavior problems of handicapped children (Meyerson et al., 1967), brain-injured patients (Hall and Broden, 1967), retarded patients (Bensberg, 1965; Birnbrauer et al., 1965; Minge and Ball, 1967, Wiesen et al., 1967), autistic patients (Wolf et al., 1964) and schizophrenic patients (Hingtgen et al., 1965; Lovaas et al., 1967). Behavior modification techniques have been brought into education and have been used for remediation of reading problems (Staats et al., 1964; Staats and Butterfield, 1965) and for the betterment of the classroom group's functioning (Zimmerman and Zimmerman, 1962; Brown and Elliott, 1965; Mithaug and Burgess, 1967; Quay et al., 1967). Gelfand and Hartmann (1968) offer a recent critical review of behavior modification using children.

Almost all of the work done to date has been addressed to individual problems, but some has been addressed toward the collective behavior of a group. For example, Brown and Elliott (1965) were interested in the possibility that nursery school teachers, sensitive to acts of aggression in their classroom, may inadvertently encourage it. For two weeks they counted observable acts of aggression in a nursery school. For the next two weeks they asked the teachers to cooperate in a program of systematic inattention to all acts that did not threaten injury. For another two weeks they released the teachers from constraint, and then for the following two weeks they reinstated it. This special ABAB treatment design strongly suggested that the teachers were encouraging aggression by reinforcing it with attention. The rate of aggression was relatively high during both periods when the teachers were behaving naturally, and lower during both periods when the teachers were systematically ignoring it.

There are now a number of programs that attempt a modification of group functioning on an even larger scale. Tharp and Wetzel (1969) describe a consultative program in which children from ages 6 to 16 were referred to their Behavior Project for Misbehaviors at school or home, or for poor academic achievement. The general target of the program was predelinquency. A good assortment of problems was encountered among the 77 children, and 168 "behaviors" were treated by *ad hoc* behavior modification routines. Several different kinds of estimates of the program's efficacy were obtained. These generally showed a positive pattern, but one important criterion, school grades, was unchanged. The authors attribute this to the imperfections of school grading procedures. It is unfortunate that they did not include school achievement test scores as criteria.

An even more complex social intervention has been reported by Ayllon and Azrin (1968). A wide variety of the activities and routines of an institution for chronic mental patients was shown to be susceptible to reinforcement procedures. The authors note that parallel efforts directed at handicapped populations are now under way.

THE EFFECTIVENESS OF BEHAVIOR MODIFICATION

Although one can find antecedent efforts stretching back for several decades, extensive work on behavior modification has only been conducted during the last decade. Strong claims are made for its power and versatility, but the time is not yet here for a definitive judgment about it. It is difficult to ignore the positive results reported by behavior modifiers. Nevertheless, it is still possible to reserve judgment about whether these positive results signify that we have arrived at a substantial system of practical therapy. There are some technical problems in the data (Gelfand and Hartmann, 1968). Furthermore, it seems likely that there is something more complicated going on in behavior modification than the reinforcement of desirable behaviors.

On the subject of efficacy, the teachings of psychoanalysis are very much in the general culture, and so the first criticism behavior modifiers usually confront is the argument that their behavior treatments are too superficial. Because their methods remove symptoms, there will necessarily be symptom substitution with new undesirable behaviors erupting as the old ones are suppressed, a kind of conservation of psychopathology. The behavior modifiers have some answers to this. First, a good number of them have reported unsuccessful attempts to find symptom substitution in the subsequent life histories of their treated patients. Second, they argue that the general belief that there is such a thing as symptom-substitution has not been solidly supported by objective evidence. Third, they argue that there is no real evidence to support either the hypotheses or the techniques of the traditional kinds of psychotherapies. All of the intellectual paraphernalia of traditional psychotherapy—the diagnostic nomenclatures, the various psychodynamic explanations of disorder—they dismiss as empty and obfuscatory, simply an assertion in a roundabout way that the patient is classified as disordered because he manifests undesirable behaviors. They argue that the effectiveness of traditional psychotherapy has not been clearly demonstrated.

The debate thus goes back and forth. Let us quickly note that the behavior modifiers have engaged in some tortuous reasoning themselves; for instance, the argument that all behavior patterns that are influenceable by reinforcement (e.g., rocking or head banging in children) are *ipso facto* learned behaviors, the elaborate speculative arguments of a "reinforcement history" underlying such disorders as childhood autism (Ferster, 1961), the claim that mental retardation is simply a set of undesirable behaviors. All in all, it is highly unlikely that we will presently be able to discount the efficacy of either behavior modification or psychoanalysis in terms of first principles. Let us return to the primary criteria of efficacy most accepted by the behavior modifiers themselves, the data of behavior change itself.

Considering only the studies just cited, there have already been enough reports of efficacy to indicate that behavior modification might prove to be practical and should be taken seriously. Some of the reports can be discounted. Behavior modification has "cured" various nursery school problems like crying, shyness and regressed crawling, but one suspects that a technology of behavior modification isn't needed to do this. Children spontaneously grow out of these problems, or else sensitive parents or teachers help the children to get over them (generally using approximations of the techniques adopted by the behavior modifiers). The best that one can say for this level of problem is that behavior modification may offer a cookbook kind of approach that can help the less sensitive parent or teacher to work with the child's problems. At the other end of the spectrum of disorder, there are the reports of success with some deficits of retarded, psychotic or autistic children. The work with autistic children has been most dramatic. Extremely arduous programs of behavior modification have produced some amelioration of autistic symptoms, improvements not usually obtainable in other ways. But one must seriously question whether these reports of improvement are much more than a *tour de force* of the method, whether there is any real promise of a wholesale remediation of autism through behavior modification. However, if we lower our therapeutic signs a little, we might improve the management or the comfort, or both, of a severely disturbed child through behavior modification.

There is a middle sort of problem, severe enough that it may offer a substantial and lasting problem to the child, that can be reached by behavior modification. The two kinds of work outlined above, Staats and Butterfield's work with a nonreading Mexican-American boy and Goldiamond's work with stutterers, were selected to illustrate both the promise and the problems now found at this middle level of work. Both programs produced improvements substantial enough to be practical, but both programs were somewhat flawed. Goldiamond's complete suppression of stuttering in the laboratory did not always lead to nonstuttering outside the laboratory, and there is some reason to believe that there were some undesirable personality changes in the subjects with their new voices. Referring to the other report, we note that the remarkable upsurge in reading seen in the program was cut off because of the boy's other behavior problems. Generally, work at this middle level of behavior problems, so far, gives a kind of qualified impression of efficacy. The obstacles to complete success may be minor and merely a matter of further elaboration of the technique, or they may not be minor. But there is now no question that behavior modification works part of the way at least, and this presents an interesting problem. Why?

We have previously argued that the stimulus-response-reinforcement analysis of learning has been recognized as inadequate, and has been supplanted by a much more elaborate kind of analysis of learning. Yet the behavior modifiers have been ostensibly successful without any of this auxiliary theoretical apparatus. It is interesting that so simple a recipe can offer a practical guide. Of course, the exact pattern of the results of behavior modification does not fully follow the recipe. In the Staats and Butterfield work, the improvement of the boy's reading was quite in line with what was expected, but other beneficial efforts of the training were not—the general improvement of the boy's course work and the marked reduction of the boy's school demerits for misconduct, for example. In the Goldiamond work there were a number of features of the course of the behavior modification—the gradual slowing of the speech to achieve nonstuttering, the transition to a new voice—indicating that something more complicated was happening then the extinction of stuttering.

One might venture the suspicion that something much more is going on in behavior modification than reinforcement. Behavior modification is an importation into natural situations of some thinking about learning derived from experimental studies of learning. To apply that thinking, behavior modifiers must construe or, at times, arrange natural situations. They must identify stimuli, responses and reinforcers. These are the basic terms of the experimental analysis of behavior. To apply the techniques of behavior modification in the solution of some behavior problem, one very often has to exercise considerable thought and ingenuity. One might guess that this effort accomplishes for the child what he himself is not able to do: (1) structures the learning problem, breaking it down into a series of step-by-step subproblems and (2) reduces the noise and uncertainty of the environment. This is done as a means to an end, to arrange things so that appropriate stimuli and responses can be identified and responses can be delivered, but it may be true that the arrangement is the heart of the method.

Why does such structure and noise-reduction help? It may help precisely because it reduces tension in the child, the kind of tension that may be a normal "cost factor" in human encounters with the issues of learning and growth. In most natural environments, one must find the stimuli, find and decide among the possibilities of response, endure the irregularity or at times the misleadingness of the reinforcers. To do this may require, quite literally, the mobilization and management of tension. For some children, behavior modification procedures may reduce this cost in tension; for others, it may circumvent a catastrophic reaction that causes them to try to deny or to circumvent the adaptational issue. This is not to say that the reinforcement training in behavior modification is not genuine training. But what may be most significant about such procedures is not the principle of the stick and the carrot, hardly a twentieth century discovery, but the medium within which that principle has been embedded.

LONGTERM TRENDS IN HUMAN ADAPTATION

We have thus far been concerned with the effort to obtain some kind of basic understanding of the processes involved in children's learning, and with a contemporary effort to use one picture of these processes as a basis for programs of training and therapy. All of this has to do with the basic nature of learning or adaptation. There are questions of larger scope, having to do with the natural course of the child's adaptation through the course of development, his capacity to adapt and the establishment of the best environment for development. Let us transpose our questions about human learning to a more natural scale. Instead of asking about stimuli and responses, let's ask about antecedents and consequents. What are the consequences of various kinds of child stimulation or child care for the intellectual development of the child? Are there critical periods—stages, points of readiness—for particular kinds of learning? Is there one main sequence of intellectual development for all children? If there is or if there is not, how can one best adapt school (Head Start and day care centers) to it? All of these questions depend for their answer on some degree of structured understanding of the relatively finer processes, and we have already seen how one kind of understanding at the lower level has percolated some proposals about intervention in child development. But our ability to make nontrivial, nonrhetorical contact between the finer level and the natural level is still generally spotty. We have only recently begun to develop some broad estimates of the course of development through childhood and adolescence.

The Question of Sensitive Periods

Thompson (1966), and Thompson and Grusec (1970) have offered an interesting hypothesis about shifting zones of learning during development. They note that it is generally true that neonates begin life with sensory and response systems rather undifferentiated, and that sensory systems usually differentiate before response systems. This being so, they propose that one should therefore find three sequenced zones of adaptation during ontogenesis: (1) a temperament adaptation zone (undifferentiated input, undifferentiated output), (2) an affective-meaning zone (differentiated input, undifferentiated output), and (3) an instrumental-meaning zone (differentiated input, differentiated output). This is a speculative hypothesis but nevertheless worth mentioning because it puts together some assumptions that again and again crop up in the psychological literature; namely, that temperament, if it is formed by experience at all, is formed very early; that human emotional learning and cathexes are most powerfully established in the preschool years; and that it is the middle and later years of childhood that see the strongest manifestation of rational and instrumental kinds of learning. Freud, for one, believed in such a sequence.

What little evidence there is about the availability of various learning mechanisms with age does not contradict such a hypothesis. Habituation, which Thompson believes to be a mechanism of temperament adaptation, is found in infants in the first few days of life (Bartoshuk, 1962a and b). Habituation is a process by which general behavioral and psychophysiological reactivity to a novel stimulus is damped out with repeated presentations of the stimulus. The infant becomes "bored" by the stimulus. Classic conditioning, which Thompson believes to be a second zone mechanism for affective meaning, now seems to be fully organized in the infant at about three months of age (Sameroff, 1969). On the basis of an absolute minimum of evidence, we are now led to believe that classical conditioning may rise to a maximum at 7 years of age (Mateer, 1918), and that later in life there begins a decline such that there may be no clinical conditioning at all in human old age (Braun and Geiselhart, 1959). Another mechanism that seems likely to be a second zone mechanism, the attachment process which binds the child to his caretaker, is held by some to be maximally operative between 6 weeks and 6 months of age. We do not have any clear-cut developmental studies for Thompson's third zone learning mechanisms, but here, even without the evidence, the hypothesis seems most plausible. There are many complex kinds of knowledge and action patterns that one cannot even begin to try to teach to children until they enter the grade school years.

A good deal of popular or professional psychological argument has held that there are maturational readinesses or optimal periods for learning, and that attempts to train or retrain children must respect these landmarks. A long time ago William James, in his *Talks to Teachers on Psychology,* held that there were fixed age-zones for the development of children's talents, and that teachers should capitalize on them in their approach to children (1900, p. 61):

> In children we observe a ripening of impulse and interests in a certain determinate order. Creeping, walking, climbing, imitating vocal sounds, constructing, drawing, calculating, possess the child in succession; and in some children the possession, while it lasts, may be of a semi-frantic and exclusive sort. Later, the interest in any one of these things may wholly fade away. Of course the proper pedagogic moment to work skill in, and to clench the useful habit, is when the native impulse is most acutely present. Crowd on the athletic opportunities, the mental arithmetic, the verse-learning, the drawing, the botany, or what not, the moment you have reason to think the hour is ripe. In this way you economize time and deepen skill; for many an infant prodigy, artistic or mathematical, has a flowering epoch of but a few months.

Freud, in his theory of psychosexual development, held that there was a series of stages during early childhood—the oral, anal and genital periods—during which certain kinds of instinctual needs had to be gratified in the child's encounters with his environment or else "fixations" would occur and later present problems in adulthood.

We have, so far, no conclusive evidence for the existence of Jamesian or Freudian special periods for human learning. Nevertheless, as with so many other psychological issues, the absence of significant confirmatory data does not necessarily mean that the arguments for such critical periods are groundless or invalid. For one thing, a good many psychologists have been disinclined to consider instinctivist arguments about human development. For another, it is difficult, even given the willingness, to mount a decisive test of a critical period hypothesis in human development. The ethologists have now given us definite evidence for critical periods in birds (Hess, 1959, 1964), and subsequently a good number of critical period phenomena have been identified in the ontogenesis of laboratory animals (Denenberg, 1964).

At the moment there are two elaborated arguments for the existence of critical periods in humans. One is an argument for a critical period of social attachment in infancy extending from 6 weeks to 6 months of age (Gray, 1958; Scott, 1963). The other is an argument that a critical period for the organization of human language exists between 2 and 12 years of age (Lenneberg, 1967). Neither offers a case for a dramatic, hard-edged, now-or-never kind of critical period, the kind that sometimes crops up in public discussions of critical periods. Rather, in both cases there seem to be "optimal periods" with somewhat blurred edges.

Related to this are suppositions about "readiness" for certain kinds of formal educational training. Originally, the notion of readiness was based on the assumption that there was a fairly fixed maturational schedule determining the growth of the child's learning capacities, and that training applied too early for this schedule would either fail or be unduly difficult. The model experiment, almost always in discussions of readiness, is McGraw's (1935) stair climbing experiment. Two twins, Johnny and Jimmy, were seen before the age at which they would normally climb stairs. Johnny was given extensive training in stair climbing and Jimmy was not. Johnny showed steady improvement, but Jimmy, at some point, launched into stair climbing spontaneously and rather rapidly improved to a level about equal to that of his trained twin. The idea, then, was that the early training in stair climbing, applied before "readiness," was inappropriate and misguided.

Obviously, there are "readinesses" in early human ontogenesis. The child has some kind of maturational schedule dictating when he will walk, toilet train, begin speaking and develop various kinds of sensory motor competences, and reasonable parents or caretakers will constrain themselves in training the child according to an intuitive understanding of this. McGraw's experiment applies to this level of child development. But what has been controversial has been an extension of the readiness idea to formal education, usually the notion of reading readiness in the first grade. Generally, many public schools have been persuaded that some kind of developmental readiness is an issue for the teaching of reading. They have used one of several commercial tests for diagnosis of reading readiness and, presumably, have moderated their approach to the child according to the results of such tests. But we do not understand exactly what maturational factors lie behind reading readiness. The issues presented by reading failure in the first grade, "dyslexia" or "reading disability," are quite complicated. Children may do poorly in first grade reading because of inadequate instruction, because their sociological background has not prepared them to be at all involved in reading, because they are bilingual, because they are slow or retarded, because of emotional problems or because they have the Gerstmann syndrome indicative of a constitutional dyslexia—or, perhaps, they are developmentally immature. The reading readiness tests do not discriminate among most of these problems. What complicates any discussion of reading readiness today are the wide-branching possible causes of first grade reading problems. Somewhere in the midst of this complex of factors, not as easy to sort out in practice as they are to categorize here, there may or may not be a genuine developmental issue for school reading.

THE QUESTION OF STAGES

We have little direct and conclusive information that will allow us to mark off age zones for human learning that arise directly out of maturational factors. That is not to say that such zones do not exist, but only that our present evidence does not permit us to be conclusive in our judgment about them. Nevertheless, there is good reason to believe that more adequate information about the neuropsychology of development would have much relevance for our understanding of children's learning (McGraw, 1945; Milner, 1967; Lenneberg, 1967; White, 1970b).

It is becoming more and more common for developmental psychologists to speak about stages in children's growth. On what basis can stages be distinguished? Generally, we have marked off age zones according to *social stages, actuarial stages* or *quasi-embryological stages.* These three ways of deriving stages of development are not perfectly distinct from one another. All represent devices for depicting successive states of the child arrived at by combinations of growth and experience. They are useful in describing longterm trends in the child's development, and in developing some kind of organized picture of the successive attainments of the child and the successive issues that arise for him. They offer useful, rough, heuristic landmarks of development.

Social Stages

Society expects certain accomplishments, certain competences and certain behaviors from humans at certain ages. There is a time to be toilet trained, a time to go to school, a time for this or that kind of self-discipline, a time for legal responsibility and so forth. The social expectations are formal, embedded in codes of the law and the church and the school, and they are informal, embedded in the myriad ways in which people affirm their expectations about other people. These social institutions and mores are by no means passive factors in human development. On the whole, they are designed to bring the expectations of society into phase with the development of the child, but they exert their special kind of demand upon him.

There is an old custom of marking off "ages of man." It seems to be associated with the definition or rationalization of cultural expectations about children. Phillippe Aries' book, *Centuries of Childhood* (1962), discusses medieval ideas and practices concerning children. His description is interesting because it reveals a social conception of childhood in some ways quite variant from our own and in other ways quite similar. Other and diverse contrasts in the social handling and staging of childhood are to be found in various studies of the development of children in non-Western cultures (Cohen, 1964; Whiting, 1962).

The point of such social stagings for any discussion of human learning is that the formal and informal curricula of society are keyed to such social expectations. The first grade is, in some sense, a "critical period" for that-which-is-taught-in-the-first-grade. Schools, and other human institutions, allow for a good deal of variance in human growth, but they are not sufficiently pliant to avoid losing some children in the steady sequence of the school's curriculum. Consequently, there are circumstances in which the child's inability to keep pace with the school will cause him to be set aside formally (by assignment to a special class) or informally. The curriculum of American education does, of course, represent a well-articulated and well-known set of expectations. It is possible to disagree with the human validity or meaning of such expectations, and precisely such disagreement is to be found in the many-faceted contemporary movement toward educational reform. (See, for example, the excellent series of policy papers compiled by the Committee on Education and Labor, *Needs of Elementary and Secondary Education for the Seventies*, 1970).

One may see educational or other social expectations about children in terms of the kinds or amounts of work demanded of them. One may see readiness for schooling as largely a matter of prerequisite intellectual skills. That has been the norm in educational discussions. Readiness tests, intelligence tests and the policy of Head Start, if not its practice, are keyed to this notion that children succeed or fail in society largely through their ability or inability to cumulate knowledge and skills. But one can be suspicious of this kind of interpretation for a variety of reasons. For one thing, in the preceding discussion of the fine grain of human learning, we have been at pains to emphasize that the child's encounter with a learning situation is an exercise not only in cognitive adaptation, but in social and emotional adaptation as well. We have seen that in one provocative behavioral modification study, Staats and coworkers produced, at least for a short time, a sudden, marked acceleration in the intellectual skills of a Mexican-American boy, and that they did this by a change in the environmental setting in which the boy was asked to engage in learning. We have just begun to recognize the force and the relevance of the social settings in which various expectations of children are enforced. Jackson, in his book *Life in Classrooms* (1968), has written an account of the child in the measured, routinized, bureaucratic environment, emphasizing the importance of the routines and the controls involved in schooling.

It is quite probable that the major force of social stages for the child arises from expectations about his maturity in a personal and social sense, in his ability to show self-discipline, understanding, initiative, resourcefulness, responsibility and so forth. We have only begun to explore how children enter into social situations. There is presently a movement toward the study of *behavioral ecology*. Roger Barker and coworkers at the University of Kansas have been concerned with an intensive analysis of the child's minute-by-minute encounters with the people and institutions of his social environment. The intent is to fully explore the child's commerce with his psychosocial environment, to record completely the behavior settings in which he engages with others, the agents who act upon him by providing "environmental force units" that direct him toward certain goals or end-states. It is quite probable that some kind of detailed analysis like this will be necessary to fully understand the various implications of the social stages of childhood (see Barker and Wright, 1955; Barker, 1963).

At the heart of the sequence of social stages, one must probably find a sequential set of issues presented to the child, a set of tasks that he must solve in order to progressively enter into commerce with other humans. Erik Erikson has presented a scheme for stages of development of interpersonal relationships. These represent, from the perspective of the individual, the tasks of socialization and the inner dynamics activating the broad human response to social stagings. (Erikson, 1950; see also an outline of Erikson's analysis in Maier, 1965.)

Actuarial Stages

Another device for marking off segments of growth, not usually conceived of as a stage analysis but nevertheless having the properties and force of one, arises from various kinds of normative testing of children. Since the turn of the century, with the beginning of the child study movement, there have been an enormous volume and variety of normative sampling of index characteristics of children's physical growth, their language, reasoning, intelligence and so forth. This huge volume of studies has been largely devoted to developing statistical expectations about development—what might be expected of the average child, what might be expected to be a common or rare deviation from this average growth pattern.

By far the most important of the normative efforts, and the one most directly relevant to our present attitudes and beliefs about the longterm course of children's learning, is the work that led into what we now speak of as intelligence testing. Intelligence testing has been and is a bootstraps operation; that is, we have no solid basis for affirming that our tests measure that human quality called intelligence. Intelligence tests are essentially numerical expressions of an individual's relative ranking in a peer group with respect to a set of problems that, in the judgment of the test designer, represents intelligence. Such testing rests on an actuarial scheme of mental development. One samples the problem-solving capacity of many children and establishes expectancies about successive ages. At age 5, a certain set of performance is expected; at age 6, another set and so on. In this way, "mental ages" are defined.

Almost all of our research-derived expectations about the child's behavior and development are actuarial in nature. We define the child's development as proper or improper by finding some way to make a numerical comparison of his progress with that of a large sample of his peers. Actuarial stages are not bad as an approximation. They are derived from resultants, indices, odd measurements or performances, but they are expressions of realities in child development. Implicitly, they acknowledge the general cumulation of children's maturation and experience. But there are fundamental problems with actuarial stages, and such problems are well illustrated by the variety of current controversies about intelligence testing. First, actuarial stages rest on plausibility plus coincidence. We proceed forward without much understanding. There is no really persuasive reason why the set of intelligence measures at ages 5 and 12 should both be considered measures of intelligence or, for that matter, measures of the same thing at all. We say they are alike because they look alike (plausibility) and because they tend to show correlations (coincidence). When a child shows "drift" in his IQ score as he grows up, and many children do, is this some kind of unevenness in the growth of the child or is this an expression of the haphazardness of our estimation of him? A second, serious, problem with actuarial stages is one of establishing the proper statistical reference group for any given child. Most of the major normative studies of child development were done in the 1930's, a time when one could comfortably assume that what was true for the white, middle-class child was adequate as a reference standard for all children. One could believe then that America was, or was about to become, a melting pot. We believe now in the existence and relative durability of subcultures in our society, and thus for a variety of developmental issues, notoriously the issue of intelligence estimation, we have serious questions about existing actuarial stagings of mental development.

The problem is posed most sharply and critically in the case of intelligence testing, of course, because those tests are used to make decisions about a child that have serious implications for his life chances. But all actuarial stages are built by techniques that are susceptible to the same flaws as intelligence tests, and the use of such stages to establish expectancies or diagnoses for children exposes one to corresponding problems.

Quasi-embryological Stages

We have said that over the short run, psychologists have more and more been inclined to construe the pattern of human learning as part of an adaptational flow. We will now argue that over the long run, over segments of weeks and months and years of the life span, psychologists have tended more and more to discuss the progression of events in a quasi-embryological framework. A dominant and sophisticated contemporary force in bringing about this kind of perspective on development is, again, Piaget (1970), who is responsible for our best present estimate of stages of cognitive development. (For a treatment of the issues of stages in socialization, see Kohlberg, 1969.)

The great importance of this approach to the development of the child is that it views the child's progress not just as a saltatory progression through heterogeneous times of maturational readiness, not in terms of promotions on the social ladder, not in terms of norms or average expectancies; rather, it tries to see the child's progress, his learning, his social adjustment and his competence as growth. Life is continuous. Life is organized. Everything the child does is in some sense an expression of an existing organization of thought and actions. It feeds back to that organization and is expressed in reorganization. It is not very difficult to express this in the abstract, but it is terribly difficult to work it out in actual, concrete cases of development.

This view of development was strongly advocated by Arnold Gesell, the psychologist-pediatrician. His book, *The Embryology of Behavior* (1945), was largely ignored at a time when the fashion in psychological theorizing went in other directions. It has now become relevant. Exactly the same might be said about another great landmark of the past decades, Werner's *Comparative Psychology of Mental Development* (1948), now only slowly taking its proper place in psychological discussions. In an autobiographical memoir, Gesell sees human learning as growth (1952, p. 153):

> Huxley was right when he insisted that the study of embryology subtends the entire life cycle. The higher as well as lower orders of behavior were built by evolutionary processes, and they survive only through embryological (ontogenetic) processes however much they bear the final impress of acculturation. Learning is essentially growth; and even creative behavior is dependent upon the same kind of neuronic growth which fashions the capacities of the archaic motor system, *in utero* and *ex utero*. The performance of genius belongs to a hierarchical continuum because there is only one physiology of development. There is but one embryology of behavior.

There are antecedents to Gesell and Werner and Piaget. The great thesis of mental development's being akin to embryology is to be found in Herbert Spencer's writings. Spencer, a philosopher, sociologist and psychologist, was a contemporary of Charles Darwin and an important source of many of our evolutionary conceptions of human development. Our broad schemes of thought in psychology, neurology and psychiatry owe much to his influence, which was large and pervasive near the turn of this century. The conception of human mental development as a progressive differentiation and hierarchical integration of thought structure was broadly set forth by Spencer. Then, in cycle after cycle, the conception has been worked out and detailed by developmental theorists. Gesell and Werner and Piaget represent a kind of middle level of development of this kind of view, each keyed to facts and observations, empiricism of the twentieth century, but each still at a middle level of abstractness. Now, stimulated by them, there is a new flurry of quasi-embryological analysis. Various contemporary writings are concerned with working out developmental sequences in smaller or more specialized aspects of human ontogenesis: Kohlberg's (1964) analysis of stages in moral ideology in childhood, Brown and Bellugi's (1964) treatment of early syntactical development, Perry's (1970) system of stages in the college student's adaptation to college and Werner and Kaplan's (1963) analysis of the ontogenesis of human symbolization.

A recent analysis by Fischer (1970) is of considerable importance and contemporary relevance. Fischer, studying animals in rather typical psychological learning situations, has proposed a structured, staged sequence of development in the course of their learning. His analysis is new, and its viability will be determined after a period of consideration and probing by others. If it holds, as well it may, it may represent a kind of historic turnabout. Where it has been almost axiomatic among many psychologists that one must eventually expect to use learning theory—the fine-grained analysis—to account for developmental theory, the broad-grained analysis—Fischer's analysis—poses as a kind of paradox the notion that developmental process provides the fine structure of laboratory learning. This is much like Gesell's point expressed in the quotation just given.

SUMMARY

In the preceding pages we have offerred a sketch of the contemporary psychological analysis of children's learning. We have spent much time discussing the form of our analysis of children's learning, and relatively little time in exposition of substantive facts and conclusions about children's learning. That is not to say that facts about children's learning do not exist in abundance. They exist in the context of the laboratory paradigms outlined early in this chapter, and as a group they have the strengths and the weaknesses characteristic of the data yielded by this approach. They are small, precise, discrete facts, very provocative and suggestive but not, in their totality, forming a broad picture or a deep understanding of what one would naturally or practically or basically want to know about the nature of children's learning. What seems most important right now is that our approach to children's learning is in the throes of what the analysts of scientific history would call a "paradigm shift." We are looking at children's learning in a new way, and as a result old facts are becoming less relevant and less interesting—in a way, less factual—and a new realm of phenomena is coming actively under consideration.

We have spoken of the dynamics of children's learning in terms of adaptations. We have spoken of the cumulation or progressive reorganization produced by experience in the terms of a quasi-embryological view of development. We have discussed concurrent human regulational systems—one concerned with cognition, another concerned with social interaction and still another concerned with the child's mood and tension. Are there three systems? Surely not. There is some number larger than one, and the point being emphasized is that there is pluralism. Any child faced with something to be learned has multiple agenda to deal with. This is true of the child in an isolated room confronted with a laboratory gadget and an experimenter. It is true of a school classroom. It is true of a child in a play group in the park. In practical terms, we are most often concerned about a child's learning when there is some shortcoming or failure in the learning. The pluralism is of central importance here. In a way, the child who has successfully solved a learning task that we have set before him is a much simpler case than the child who has not. We know one thing for sure about the successful child, and we are not terribly concerned about the rest. But when the child fails, it may take the most sophisticated and enlightened analysis of learning possible to state the precise terms of the failure. One need not look far to assert this. Any experimenter who has observed children in a laboratory learning situation, and who has recorded the objective evidences of failures homogeneously and monotonously—"100 trials, no criterion, 100 trials no criterion. . . ." —knows that every child has failed differently, has struggled with the problem differently. If this is true of the highly controlled and simplified setting of the laboratory problem, one can only try to imagine what failure to meet the criteria of the first grade or high school might imply.

What about practical problems, real problems of children failing to learn? Over the past decade there has been an explosive confrontation with the problems of children in our society. One after another, the government programs have come forth—Head Start, Follow Through, Title I, and now, coming forward, the various proposals for national day care centers. All these confront the problem of the education of the disadvantaged children of our society. In and around the special programs and the special allocations for the disadvantaged child, there are pervasive and pressing issues of educational reform. We are no longer comfortable with the educational procedures of the recent past. There are mounting problems of costs, of disorders, of student disaffection, of more and more apparent unfairness to diverse groups of children in our society. When we look into our educational procedures to try to understand what might or might not be wrong, we find that we do not fully understand them and that perhaps no one has ever fully understood them. There seems to have been a time when one did not have to understand them, when one could tolerate a certain amount of genial or not-so-genial inefficiency to produce the limited number of highly educated people our society called for. Now we live in a time when one has to have a relatively large amount of education, a high school diploma, just to get by in our society, and we live in a time when every single segment of our educational system from the preschool to the medical school is subject to soul-searching and criticism.

Developmental psychologists have participated in the policy and planning having to do with children's learning, working from the kind of knowledge base outlined in this chapter. The knowledge base is inadequate, woefully inadequate. Still, practical problems demand attempts at solution, ready or not. If one must make educated guesses in devising programs of children's learning, then developmental psychologists are the most educated kinds of guessers our society has available. The interaction of professors and policy has been awkward at times. It is no easy matter to move from an arena where relevance does not much count and where the rules are the rules of evidence, into a new arena where relevance is the central issue and the rules are the rules of advocacy. The professors have had to learn to deal with the politicians and the politicians have had to learn to deal with the professors. Amidst all this, the developmental psychologist has been forced to assemble his information in new ways, to estimate and to argue on new grounds (White, 1967, 1969, 1970c, 1970d). The backwash of all this, its effect on our knowledge base, has been to the good. The great demands placed upon our knowledge of children's learning have stimulated a maturation of our approach, a reappraisal, the very kind of paradigm shifts we have been discussing. There is interdisciplinary communication and a communication between the theoretical and the practical that have been much missed in the past few decades.

What do we now need for our consideration of children's learning? What will best develop our knowledge and our understanding?

At the more basic or micro-level of analysis, we need more information about the neural substrate of thought and we need more understanding of the processes governing attention, mood and emotion. We need more understanding of the temporal integration of human behavior, and we need to know much more about the role of plans in directed human activity. We need to look more closely at moment-to-moment processes at work during the construction of those behavior changes that we call learning, and we need to look at them in such a way to understand the multiple regulatory agenda that govern the encounters with problems.

At the longterm level of analysis, we need to extend and more rigorously probe the various stage conceptions of segments or aspects of human development. We need to test our various estimations of the course of human development against cross-cultural analysis, and against the special configurations of thought pathology one finds in such disorders as dyslexia, aphasia, autism and the various sensory deficit conditions. Beyond pathology, we need a clinical psychology of learning, perhaps of the sort that may develop from the present work on behavior modification. We need, from time to time, to look at learning through wider windows. Generally, we need to do much looking at the processes and the problems of humans learning over longer segments of time and in more natural behavioral settings.

Finally, because of our new interface with social action problems, an interface that should and will last, we need to find ways to look at those problems directly and to estimate the consequences of various attempts to ameliorate them. All too often we have had to respond to the initial stimulus of a social problem by some trumped-up interpretation derived from the literature. "Cultural deprivation," itself a rather interpretive name for a problem, has been variously estimated as an issue of sensory deprivation, sensory overstimulation, breakdown of the family and critical periods. Now there is time and much need to look directly and long at the problems, and at the programs we have developed to deal with them. New institutional arrangements may be necessary for this, large interdisciplinary arrangements. But in real life—as, for that matter, in basic analysis—the topics and the issues of human learning are abstractions from the topics and the issues of human development, abstractions at some cost. We cannot really look at a whole child, but perhaps we can find ways to maintain our study of the abstracted issues while remaining conscious of the whole and responsible to it.

REFERENCES

Allen, K. E., Hart, B. M., Buell, J. S., Harris, F. R., and Wolf, M. M.: Effects of social reinforcement on isolate behavior of a nursery school child. *Child Develop.,* *35*:511–518, 1964.

Aries, P.: *Centuries of Childhood: A Social History of Family Life.* New York, Alfred A. Knopf, Inc., 1962.

Aronfreed, J.: The problem of imitation. *In* Lipsitt, L. P., and Reese, H. W. (Eds.): *Advances in Child Development and Behavior,* Vol. IV. New York, Academic Press, Inc., 1969.

Athey, I. J., and Rubadeau, D. O.: *Educational Implications of Piaget's Theory.* Waltham, Massachusetts, Ginn/Blaisdell, 1970.

Ayllon, T., and Azrin, N.: *The Token Economy: A Motivational System for Therapy and Rehabilitation.* New York, Appleton-Century-Crofts, 1968.

Baer, P. M., and Sherman, J. A.: Reinforcement control of generalized imitation in young children. *J. Exp. Child Psychol., 1*: 37–49, 1964.

Bandura, A.: Vicarious processes: A case of no-trial learning. *In* Berkowitz, L. (Ed.): *Advances in Experimental Social Psychology,* Vol. II, New York, Academic Press, Inc., 1965.

Bandura, A., Ross, D., and Ross, S. A.: Transmission of aggression through imitation of aggressive models. *J. Abnorm. Soc. Psychol., 63*:575–582, 1961.

Barker, R. G.: *The Stream of Behavior: Explorations of Its Structure and Content.* New York, Appleton-Century-Crofts, 1963.

Barker, R. G., and Wright, H. F.: *Midwest and Its Children.* New York, Harper & Row, Publishers, 1955.

Bartoshuk, A. K.: Human neonatal cardiac acceleration to sound: Habituation and dishabituation. *Percept. Motor Skills, 15*:15–27, 1962A.

Bartoshuk, A. K.: Response decrement with repeated elicitation of human neonatal cardiac acceleration to sound. *J. Comp. Physiol. Psychol., 55*:9–13, 1962b.

Bensberg, G. J., Colwell, C. N., and Cassel, R. H.: Teaching the profoundly retarded self-help activities by behavior shaping techniques. *Amer. J. Ment. Defic., 69*:674–679, 1965.

Bijou, S. W., and Baer, D. M.: *Child Development,* Vol. I: *A Systematic and Empirical Theory.* New York, Appleton-Century-Crofts, 1961.

Bijou, S. W., and Baer, D. M.: *Child Development,* Vol. II: *Universal Stage of Infancy.* New York, Appleton-Century-Crofts, 1965.

Bijou, S. W., and Baer, D. M.: *Child Development: Readings in Experimental Analysis.* New York, Appleton-Century-Crofts, 1967.

Birnbrauer, J. S., Wolf, M. M., Kidder, J. D., and Taque, C. E.: Classroom behavior of retarded pupils with token reinforcement. *J. Exp. Child Psychol., 2*:219–235, 1965.

Bissell, J., Zivin, G., and White, S. H.: Sensory modalities in learning. *In* Lesser, G. S. (Ed.): *Psychology and Educational Practice.* Chicago, Scott, Foresman and Company, 1971.

Bowlby, J.: *Attachment and Loss,* Vol. I: *Attachment.* New York, Basic Books, Inc., Publishers, 1969.

Braun, H. W., and Geiselhart, R.: Age differences in the acquisition and extinction of the conditioned eyelid response. *J. Exp. Psychol., 57*:386–388, 1959.

Brown, R., and Bellugi, U.: Three processes in the child's acquisition of syntax. *Harvard Educational Review, 34*:133–151, 1964.

Brown, R., and Elliott, R.: Control of aggression in a nursery school class. *J. Exp. Child Psychol., 2*:103–107, 1965.

Bruner, J. S.: *The Process of Education.* Cambridge, Massachusetts, Harvard University Press, 1961.

Bruner, J. S.: The course of cognitive growth. *Amer. Psychol., 19*:1–15, 1964.

Bruner, J. S.: *Toward a Theory of Instruction.* Cambridge, Massachusetts, Harvard University Press, 1966.

Cohen, Y. A.: *The Transition from Childhood to Adolescence: Cross-cultural Studies of Initiation Ceremonies, Legal Systems and Incest Taboos.* Chicago, Aldine Publishing Company, 1964.

Committee on Education and Labor: *Needs of Elementary Education for the Seventies: A Compendium of Policy Papers.* Washington, D.C. U. S. Government Printing Office, 1970.

Denenberg, V. H.: A theory of infantile stimulation. *Psychol. Rev., 71*:335–351, 1964.

Eccles, J. C.: *Brain and Conscious Experience.* New York, Springer-Verlag New York Inc., 1966.

Erikson, E. H.: *Childhood and Society.* New York, W. W. Norton & Company, Inc., 1950.

Escalona, S. D.: *The Roots of Individuality: Normal Patterns of Development in Infancy.* Chicago, Aldine Publishing Company, 1968.

Fellows, B. J.: *The Discrimination Process and Development.* London, Pergamon Press, Inc., 1968.

Ferster, C. B.: Positive reinforcement and behavioral deficits of autistic children. *Child Devel., 32*:437–456, 1961.

Fischer, K. W.: The structure and development of sensory-motor actions. Unpublished Ph.D. Dissertation, Harvard University, 1970.

Flavell, J. H.: Concept development. *In* Mussen, P. H. (Ed.): *Carmichael's Manual of Child Psychology,* 3rd ed. New York, John Wiley & Sons, Inc., 1970.

Fraser, C., Bellugi, U., and Brown, R.: Control of grammar in imitation, comprehension and production. *Journal of Verbal Learning and Verbal Behavior, 2*:121–135, 1963.

Gelfand, D. M., and Hartmann, D. P.: Behavior therapy with children: A review and evaluation of research methodology. *Psychol. Bull.*, *69*:204–215, 1968.

Gesell, A.: *The Embryology of Behavior.* New York, Harper & Row, Publishers, 1945.

Gesell, A.: *In* Murchison, C. (Ed.): *A History of Psychology in Autobiography.* Worcester, Massachusetts, Clark University Press, 1952.

Gewirtz, J. L.: Deprivation and satiation of social stimuli as determinants of their reinforcing efficacy. *In* Hill, J. P. (Ed.): *Minnesota Symposium on Child Psychology,* Vol. I. Minneapolis, University of Minnesota Press, 1967.

Goldiamond, I.: Stuttering and fluency as manipulatable operant response classes. *In* Krasner, L., and Ullman, L. P. (Eds.): *Research in Behavior Modification.* New York, Holt, Rinehart & Winston, Inc., 1965.

Gollin, E. S., and Shirk, E. J.: A developmental study of oddity-problem learning in young children. *Child Devel.*, *37*:213–217, 1966.

Goulet, L. R.: Verbal learning in children: Implications for developmental research. *Psychol. Bull.*, *69*:359–376, 1968.

Gray, P. H.: Theory and evidence of imprinting in human infants. *J. Psychol.*, *46*:155–166, 1958.

Grossman, S. P.: *A Textbook of Physiological Psychology.* New York, John Wiley & Sons, Inc., 1967.

Hall, R. V., and Broden, M.: Behavior changes in brain-injured children through social reinforcement. *J. Exp. Child Psychol.*, *5*:463–479, 1967.

Harlow, H. F., and Woolsey, C. N.: *Biological and Biochemical Bases of Behavior.* Madison, Wisconsin, University of Wisconsin Press, 1958.

Harris, F. R., Johnston, M. K., Kelley, C. S., and Wolf, M. M.: Effects of positive social reinforcement on regressed crawling of a nursery school child. *J. Educ. Psych.*, *55*:35–41, 1964.

Hart, B. M., Allen, K. E., Buell, J. S., Harris, F. R., and Wolf, M. M.: Effects of social reinforcement on operant crying. *J. Exp. Child Psych.*, *1*:145–153, 1964.

Hess, E. H.: Imprinting. *Science, 130*:133–141, 1959.

Hess, E. H.: Imprinting in birds. *Science, 146*:1128–1139, 1964.

Hess, E. H.: Ethology and developmental psychology. *In* Mussen, P. H. (Ed.): *Carmichael's Manual of Child Psychology,* 3rd ed. New York, John Wiley & Sons, Inc., 1970.

Hilgard, E. R., and Bower, G. H.: *Theories of Learning,* 3rd ed. New York, Appleton-Century-Crofts, 1966.

Hill, S. D.: The performance of young children on three discrimination-learning tasks. *Child Devel.*, *36*:425–435, 1965.

Hingtgen, J. N., Sanders, B. J., and DeMyer, M. K.: Shaping cooperative responses in early childhood schizophrenics. *In* Ullman, L. P., and Krasner, L. (Eds.): *Case Studies in Behavior Modification.* New York, Holt, Rinehart & Winston, Inc., 1965.

Holt, J.: *How Children Learn.* New York, Pitman Publishing Corp., 1967.

Jackson, P. W.: *Life in Classrooms.* New York, Holt, Rinehart & Winston, Inc., 1968.

James, W.: Talks to Teachers on Psychology. London, Longmans Green & Co. Ltd., 1939 (orig. 1900).

Johnston, M. K., Kelley, S. C., Harris, F. R., and Wolf, M. M.: An application of reinforcement principles to development of motor skills in a young child. *Child Devel., 37*: 379–387, 1966.

Kerr, N., Meyerson, L., and Michael, J. A.: A procedure for shaping vocalizations in a mute child. *In* Ullman, L. P., and Krasner, L. (Eds.): *Case Studies in Behavior Modification.* New York, Holt, Rinehart & Winston, Inc., 1965.

Kimble, G. A.: *Hilgard and Marquis' Conditioning and Learning,* 2nd ed. New York, Appleton-Century-Crofts, 1961.

Kohlberg, L.: Development of moral character and moral ideology. *In* Hoffman, M. L., and Hoffman, L. W. (Eds.): *Review of Child Development Research,* Vol. I. New York, Russell Sage Foundation, 1964.

Kohlberg, L.: A cognitive-developmental analysis of children's sex-role concepts and attitudes. *In* Maccoby, E. E. (Ed.): *The Development of Sex Differences.* Stanford, Stanford University Press, 1966.

Kohlberg, L.: Stage and sequence: The cognitive-developmental approach to socialization. *In* Goslin, D. A. (Ed.): *Handbook of Socialization Theory and Research.* New York, Rand McNally & Co., 1969.

Krasner, L., and Ullmann, L. P.: *Research in Behavior Modification.* New York, Holt, Rinehart & Winston, Inc., 1965.

Lenneberg, E. H.: *Biological Foundations of Language.* New York, John Wiley & Sons, Inc., 1967.

Lipsitt, L. P.: The experiential origins of human behavior. *In* Goulet, L. R., and Baltes, P. R. (Eds.): *Life-span Developmental Psychology.* New York, Academic Press, Inc., 1970.

Lipsitt, L. P., and Kaye, H.: Conditioned sucking in the human newborn. *Psychonomic Science, 1*:29–30, 1964.

Lorenz, L.: *On Aggression.* New York, Bantam Books, Inc., 1967.

Lovaas, O. I.: A behavior therapy approach to the treatment of childhood schizophrenia. *In* Hill, J. P. (Ed.): *Minnesota Symposia on Child Psychology,* Vol. I. Minneapolis, University of Minnesota Press, 1967.

Maccoby, E. E.: Effects of the mass media. *In* Hoffman, M. L., and Hoffman, L. W. (Eds.): *Review of Child Development Research,* Vol. I. New York, Russell Sage Foundation, 1964.

Maccoby, E. E.: The development of moral values and behavior in childhood. *In* Clausen, J. A. (Ed.): *Socialization and Society.* Boston, Little, Brown and Company, 1968.

Maccoby, E. E., and Bee, H. L.: Some speculations concerning the lag between perceiving and performing. *Child Devel., 36*:367–378, 1965.

Maier, H. W.: *Three Theories of Child Development.* New York, Harper & Row, Publishers, 1965.

Mateer, F.: *Child behavior: A Critical and Experimental Study of Young Children by the Method of Conditioned Reflexes.* Boston, (Badger), Humphries, Bruce, Inc., 1918.

McClelland, D. C.: *The Achieving Society,* New York, The Free Press, 1967 (orig. 1951).

McGraw, M. B.: *Growth: A Study of Johnny and Jimmy.* New York, Appleton-Century-Crofts, 1935.

McGraw, M. B.: *The Neuromuscular Maturation of the Human Infant.* New York, Hafner Publishing Co., Inc., 1966 (orig. 1945).

Meyerson, L., Kerr, N., and Michael, J. L.: Behavior modification in rehabilitation. *In* Bijou, S. W., and Baer, P. M. (Eds.): *Child Development: Readings in Experimental Analysis.* New York, Appleton-Century-Crofts, 1967.

Miller, N. E., and Dollard, J.: *Social Learning and Imitation.* New Haven, Yale University Press, 1941.

Milner, E.: *Human Neural and Behavioral Development: A Relational Inquiry, with Implications for Personality.* Springfield, Illinois, Charles C Thomas, Publisher, 1967.

Minge, M. R., and Ball, T. S.: Teaching of self-help skills to profoundly retarded patients. *Amer. J. Ment. Defic., 71*:864–868, 1967.

Mithaug, D. E., and Burgess, R. L.: Effects of different reinforcement procedures in the establishment of a group response. *J. Exper. Child Psychol., 5*:441–454, 1967.

Munn, N. L.: Learning in Children. *In* Carmichael, L. (Ed.): *Manual of Child Psychology,* 2nd ed. New York, John Wiley & Sons, Inc., 1957.

Neisser, U.: *Cognitive Psychology.* New York, Appleton-Century-Crofts, 1967.

Osler, S. F., and Kofsky, E.: Structure and strategy in concept attainment. *J. Exp. Child Psychol., 4*:198–209, 1966.

Papousek, H.: Experimental studies of appetitional behavior in human newborns and infants. *In* Stevenson, H. W., Hess, E. H., and Rheingold, H. L. (Eds.): *Early Behavior: Comparative and Developmental Approaches.* New York, John Wiley & Sons, Inc., 1967.

Perry, W. G.: *Forms of Intellectual and Ethical Development in the College Years: A Scheme.* New York, Holt, Rinehart & Winston, Inc., 1970.

Piaget, J.: *The Moral Judgment of the Child.* New York, P. F. Collier, Inc., 1962.

Piaget, J.: Piaget's theory. *In* Mussen, P. H. (Ed.): *Carmichael's Manual of Child Psychology,* 3rd ed. New York, John Wiley & Sons, 1970.

Piaget, J., and Inhelder, B.: *The Psychology of the Child.* New York, Basic Books, Inc., Publishers, 1969.

Quarton, G. C., Melnechuk, T., and Schmitt, F. O.: *The Neurosciences: A Study Program.* New York, The Rockefeller University Press, 1967.

Quay, H. C., Sprague, R. L., Werry, J. S., and McQueen, M. M.: Conditioning visual orientation of conduct problem children in the classroom. *J. Exp. Child Psych., 5*:512–517, 1967.

Reese, H. W., and Lipsitt, L. P.: *Experimental Child Psychology.* New York, Academic Press, Inc., 1970.

Reynolds, G. S.: *A Primer of Operant Conditioning.* Glenview, Illinois, Scott, Foresman and Company, 1968.

Riley, D. A.: *Discrimination Learning.* Boston, Allyn & Bacon, Inc., 1968.

Sameroff, A.: Can conditioned responses be established in the newborn infant? Unpublished manuscript, 1969.

Schachter, S., and Singer, J. E.: Cognitive, social, and physiological determinants of emotional state. *Psychol. Rev., 69*:379–399, 1962.

Scott, J. P.: The process of primary socialization in canine and human infants. *Monogr. Soc. Res. Child Develop., 28*:1–47, 1963.

Scott, J. P.: *Early Experience and the Organization of Behavior.* Belmont, California, Brooks/Cole Publishing Co., 1968.

Sechenov, I. M.: Reflexes of the brain. *In* Sechenov, I. M.: *Selected Works.* Moscow and Leningrad, State Publishing House for Biological and Medical Literature, 1935 (orig. 1863).

Skinner, B. F.: *Science and Human Behavior.* New York, The Macmillan Company, 1953.

Spiker, C. C.: Research methods in children's learning. *In* Mussen, P. H. (Ed.): *Handbook of Research Methods in Child Development.* New York, John Wiley & Sons, Inc., 1960.

Staats, A. W., and Butterfield, W. H.: Treatment of nonreading in a culturally deprived juvenile delinquent: An application of reinforcement principles. *Child Develop., 36*: 925–942, 1965.

Staats, A. W., Finley, J. R., Minke, K. A., and Wolf, M. M.: Reinforcement variables in the control of unit reading responses. *J. Exp. Anal. Behav., 7*:139–149, 1964.

Stevenson, H. W.: Social reinforcement of children's behavior. *In* Lipsitt, L. P., and

Spiker, C. C. (Eds.): *Advances in Child Development and Behavior,* Vol. II. New York, Academic Press, Inc., 1965.

Stevenson, H. W.: Learning in children. *In* Mussen, P. H. (Ed.): *Carmichael's Manual of Child Psychology,* 3rd ed. New York, John Wiley & Sons, Inc., 1970.

Stodolsky, S. S., and Lesser, G.: Learning patterns in the disadvantaged. *Harvard Educational Review, 37*:546–593, 1967.

Tharp, R. G., and Wetzel, R. J.: *Behavior Modification in the Natural Environment.* New York, Academic Press, Inc., 1969.

Thomas, A., Chess, S., Birch, H. G., Hertzig, M., and Korn, S.: *Behavioral Individuality in Early Childhood.* New York, New York University Press, 1963.

Thompson, W. R.: Early experiential and genetic influences on flexibility. *In* Harvey, O. J. (Ed.): *Experience, Structure, and Adaptability.* New York, Springer Publishing Co., Inc., 1966.

Thompson, W. R., and Grusec, J. E.: Studies of early experience. *In* Mussen, P. H. (Ed.): *Carmichael's Manual of Child Psychology,* 3rd ed. New York, John Wiley & Sons, Inc., 1970.

Tolman, E. C.: *Purposive Behavior in Animals and Men.* New York, Century House, Inc., 1932.

Ullmann, L. P., and Krasner, L.: *Case Studies in Behavior Modification.* New York, Holt, Rinehart & Winston, Inc., 1965.

Vernon, M. D.: *Perception Through Experience.* New York, Barnes & Noble, Inc., 1970.

Walters, R. H., and Parke, R. D.: Influence of response consequences to a social model on resistance to deviation. *J. Exp. Child Psychol., 1*:269–280, 1964.

Weisberg, P.: Social and nonsocial conditioning of infant vocalizations. *Child Develop., 34*:377–388, 1963.

Werner, H.: *Comparative Psychology of Mental Development.* New York, Science Editions, 1961 (orig. 1948).

Werner, H., and Kaplan, B.: *Symbol Formation: An Organismic-Developmental Approach to Language and the Expression of Thought.* New York, John Wiley & Sons, Inc., 1963.

White, R. W.: Motivation reconsidered: The concept of competence. *Psychol. Rev., 66*: 297–333, 1959.

White, S. H.: Learning. *In* Stevenson, H. W. (Ed.): *Child Psychology: Sixty-second Yearbook of the National Society for the Study of Education.* Chicago, University of Chicago Press, 1963.

White, S. H.: Some educated guesses about cognitive development in the preschool years. *In* Hess, R., and Bear, R. (Eds.): *Early Education: Current Theory, Research, and Practice.* Chicago, Aldine Publishing Company, 1967.

White, S. H.: Changes in learning processes in the late preschool years. Paper presented at symposium, "Early Learning." American Educational Research Association Convention, Chicago, January, 1968.

White, S. H.: Plausibilities and possibilities in early education. *Pediatrics, 44*:901–904, 1969.

White, S. H.: The learning theory tradition and child psychology. *In* Mussen, P. H. (Ed.): *Carmichael's Manual of Child Psychology,* 3rd ed. New York, John Wiley & Sons, Inc., 1970a.

White, S. H.: Some general outlines of the matrix of developmental changes between five and seven years. *Bulletin of the Orton Society, 20*:41–57, 1970b.

White, S. H.: The national impact study of Head Start. *In* Hellmuth, J. (Ed.): *The Disadvantaged Child.* Vol. III. New York, Brunner/Mazel, Inc., 1970c.

White, S. H.: Human research and human affairs. Paper presented at symposium, "The developmental sciences: State and fate of research funding." AAAS Convention, Chicago, December, 1970d.

Whiting, B.: *Patterns of Child Rearing.* New York, John Wiley & Sons, Inc., 1962.

Wiesen, A. E., Hartley, G., Richardson, C., and Roske, A.: The retarded child as a reinforcing agent. *J. Exp. Child Psych., 5*:109–113, 1967.

Williams, C. D.: The elimination of tantrum behavior by extinction procedures. *J. Abnorm. Soc. Psychol., 59*:269, 1959.

Wolf, M. M., Risley, T. R., and Mees, H. I.: Application of operant conditioning procedures to the behavior problems of an autistic child. *Behav. Res. Ther., 1*:305–312, 1964.

Wolf, M. M., Birnbrauer, J. S., Williams, T., and Lawler, J.: A note on apparent extinction of the vomiting behavior of a retarded child. *In* Ullmann, L. P., and Krasner, L. (Eds.): *Case Studies in Behavior Modification.* New York, Holt, Rinehart & Winston, Inc., 1965.

Wolpe, J., Salter, A., and Reyna, L. J. (Eds.): *The Conditioning Therapists.* New York, Holt, Rinehart & Winston, Inc., 1964.

Zimmerman, E. H., and Zimmerman, J.: The alteration of behavior in a special classroom situation. *J. Exper. Anal. Behav., 5*:59–60, 1962.

5 DEVELOPMENTAL BEHAVIORAL GENETICS

Benson E. Ginsburg

There has been a certain reluctance on the part of many scientists, ranging from the biochemist, the geneticist and the neurophysiologist, to the developmental psychologist, sociologist and educator, to accept behavioral genetics as a legitimate discipline having important interrelations with their own fields. In the limiting instances—those in which gross genetic anomalies such as trisomy 21 or phenylketonuria impose limitations on mental and behavioral development—the role of a chromosomal aberration or of a gene mutation as a causal factor is acknowledged.

At the population level, behavioral differences between species and subspecies, based on multiple genetic differences, are likewise recognized. No one is surprised to find heritable differences in behavioral patterns between distinct but related groups of birds (Hinde, 1959; Dilger, 1962) or fruit flies (Bastock, 1956; Hirsch, 1959; Manning, 1959; Benzer, 1967; Dobzhansky, 1967; Ikeda and Kaplan, 1970) or even strains of mice (Scott, 1942; Lindzey, 1951; Ginsburg, 1958; McClearn, 1961; Thiessen and Nealey, 1962; Fuller, 1964; Bruell, 1965; Sidman et al., 1965), though the latter represent replicated individual differences of the kind that separate you from me.

The presumptions, though seldom overtly stated, are that taxonomic groups may differ genetically in their behavioral capacities, and that infrahuman individuals within the same species or subspecies may, similarly, exhibit such genetically based differences, but that we humans are somehow less at the mercy of our genes, except, as mentioned, in extreme cases. Happily, even these are correctable with appropriate treatment—now or in the future. Such extreme cases can occur at either end of the spectrum and include the genius as well as the idiot, since we seem to be unable to create geniuses out of common genetic fabric exposed to uncommon advantages, or to overcome mental deficiency without resorting to biological interventions, as in the case of the cretin or the phenylketonuric.

Importance of Primary Causal Factors in Genetic Abnormalities

The criterion implied in the above instances is that what is genetic should not be labile to environmental manipulation. Yet, not all environmental manipulations are given equal weight in this context. To supply thyroid hormone to a cretin in order to compensate for a biological deficiency, or to withhold phenylalanine from an individual who metabolizes it in a peculiar fashion detrimental to his own development, can be easily conceptualized as compensating for a chemical imbalance at a critical time during development. This is much like providing insulin to a diabetic. The fact that a genetic predisposition is involved in all of these instances becomes almost an ancillary point. The chemical imbalance might as well have resulted from infection or from other environmental stresses in individuals of normal genetic makeup. From a palliative point of view that seeks to identify and treat a syndrome, the primary causal factor is of less practical importance than the intervening mechanisms by means of which the effects are produced. It is these mechanisms which must be identified and manipulated by the proper means at the proper time in order to achieve normality. If an endocrine gland is not secreting its proper level of hormone beginning at the time of development when it should normally do so, the hormone may be supplied by the physician or investigator, and the deficient individual will respond whether his deficiency is genetic or the result of infection, radiation damage or (in the case of the thyroid) an inadequate iodine supply.

The causes underlying the manipulable mechanisms are, however, important in two respects: One is prevention of the abnormality, and the second is correction of the primary defect, thereby restoring the affected individual to a normal state rather than having to rely on continuing compensatory measures.

In the first instance, when a known mode of inheritance exists, genetic counseling can prevent the abnormality. Where an infectious organism is the primary cause, inoculation, hygienic safeguards or prompt treatment may prevent or minimize the damage. Where other environmental agencies are the prime causes (e.g., radiation, toxic substances, vitamin and mineral deficiencies) control may involve considerable logistic problems, but these are, in principle, solvable.

The re-engineering of an affected individual is another matter. Many changes are irreversible, or become so after a certain time. Even if the thyroid gland of a cretin could be restored to normal function after a certain time, irreversible damage would already have occurred in terms of growth, body proportions and mental function. Eventually, organ transplants may become feasible and, if done in time, could bring dramatic results. The brain would continue to present a peculiar problem even if its transplantation were possible, since what is desired is not the identity and capacities of some other individual, but the derivation of the maximal potential—at least that usually considered normal—of a particular, individual brain. The underlying assumption is that there is no stage at which the brain is a *tabula rasa* that will be inscribed in accordance with its life experience, but that each brain brings its own, unique, interacting potential into play such that my brain in your body, even if transplanted as an early anlage and subjected to your set of life experiences, would result in a consciousness of self and set of behaviors and capacities different from what you have now.

ALTERATION OF BIOLOGICAL CAPACITIES FOR BEHAVIOR

We come, therefore, to the realization that if we wish to understand and to be able to alter biological capacities for behavior, the understanding that we seek must relate the genetic potential, through developmental processes, to ultimate behavior. From the biological and genetic point of view, four approaches suggest themselves:

1. Selective breeding.
2. Providing an optimal environment.
3. Altering the genes themselves.
4. Changing the activation pattern of the genetic potential.

Selective Breeding

Ample evidence exists to indicate that behavioral capacities, no less than morphological ones, are subject to genetic variation and selection (Scott, 1942; Bastock, 1956; Hirsch, 1959; McClearn, 1961; Thiessen and Nealey, 1962; Fuller, 1964; Vandenberg, 1965; Benzer, 1967; Dobzhansky, 1967; Ginsburg, 1967; Manning, 1967; Collins, 1968, 1969; Wimer et al., 1969). These range from aggressiveness to emotionality to learning ability. The genetic bases for various behavioral potentials include single genes (Grüneberg, 1947; Stern, 1960; Sidman et al., 1965; McKusick, 1966; Ginsburg, 1967), multiple genic differences (Fuller et al., 1950; Hirsch, 1967) and chromosomal differences (Lejeune et al., 1959; Hirsch, 1967; Ginsburg, 1971; Razavi, 1971). In sum, there is nothing that is in principle different between the genetic basis for behavioral phenotypes and that for any other phenotypes, and it is therefore to be expected that the principles and findings of population genetics apply as much to behavior as to any other highly adaptive aspect of phenotype (Dobzhansky, 1967). What may be different is the relationship between the encoded genotype and the expressed phenotype if, as is often assumed, more degrees of freedom exist between the genome and behavior—especially the behavior of a human being—than between genes and physiology or morphology. This notion will be examined in the ensuing section (*Providing an Optimal Environment*).

Selection experiments based on behavioral criteria have been performed using dogs, rabbits, mice, chickens, guinea pigs, fruit flies and many other organisms (see Tryon, 1929; Roderick, 1960; Ginsburg, 1966, 1967; Benzer, 1967; Dobzhansky, 1967; Hirsch, 1967). The behavioral criteria have included simple responses to light and gravity, aggressiveness and learning ability. With varying degree of selection, results begin to be achieved within three to four generations. After six to seven generations, these are generally quite marked. In the fruit fly, *Drosophila*, Dobzhansky and Spassky (Dobzhansky, 1967) selected for positive and negative geotaxis. They continued the selection for 18 generations, by which time the populations differed significantly and dramatically in this behavior. Using these populations as a base, they then tried breeding them with no further selection. Another sample was subjected to reverse selection. After only six generations of reverse selection, the differences achieved in 18 generations of selection were virtually wiped out. Merely relaxing selection, without instituting any reverse selection, resulted in a loss of about half the gains that were made during the selection experiments.

These results are instructive in a number of respects: They demonstrate that far from taking eons of time, selection acts relatively quickly. At the same time, a population of sufficient size to retain appreciable genetic variability retains its plasticity. Reverse selection can restore it to its previous phenotypic profile, or a change in the criteria for selection can move it to quite another profile. The interpretation of the recidivistic effects of merely relaxing selection that Dobzhansky has offered is that the longterm effects of natural selection have again taken over after the comparatively short period of imposed artificial selection, and that the population is returning to its natural range of phenotypes. Lerner (1954), who has analyzed this phenomenon *in extenso,* has termed it "genetic homeostasis." It has also been argued that in naturally evolved wild populations, by contrast with domesticated and cultivated forms, selection has favored the normative phenotype by buffering it, so that a relatively wide array of genetic variability is assimilated to a much narrower range of phenotypic expression than occurs with domesticated varieties (Ginsburg, 1968). This creates a potential for evolving along new lines under continual selection pressure on an evolutionary time scale by conserving genetic variability and masking it by means of phenotypic buffering. Genetic variability is thereby protected from the effects of short-term selection, which would otherwise restrict the genetic plasticity of the population, since selection can only act by favoring some genetic combinations over others. In the meantime, it keeps the population within its range of evolved adaptive phenotypes.

Insofar as a relaxation of selection may return the population to a situation of random mating (which would not usually be found in nature) (Ginsburg, 1968), this, too, would change the array of genotypes and phenotypes relatively quickly and would tend to keep these constant after a new equilibrium had been reached (Wright, 1939).

Selection, therefore, can alter the array of behavioral phenotypes in a relatively short time without closing the door to further genetic change. This, of course, is a general statement drawn primarily from examples that are polygenic and complex. Even rigorous selection would not be able to eliminate a gene with a high mutation rate—especially if it did not always come to phenotypic expression. Those who are interested in exploring these models in detail are referred to a number of recent books on quantitative and population genetics by Li (1955), Kempthorne (1957), Lerner (1958), Falconer (1960), Wright (1968) and Crow and Kimura (1970).

The Nature of the Human Gene Pool. That the principles just discussed apply to man is evidenced by familial data on psychoses (Kallman, 1938, 1946; Rosenthal, 1966; Gottesman and Shields, 1967; Elston and Campbell, 1970), intelligence (Burt, 1958), musical and mathematical ability, personality types (Gottesman, 1963; Brazelton, et al., 1969) and the association of chromosomal anomalies with mental deficiency (Lejeune et al., 1959) and with deviant behavior (Razavi, 1971), to cite a representative series of examples. Man is not and never has been a panmictic species. The author has argued elsewhere (Ginsburg, 1968) that social behavior in vertebrates as well as in other groups has as its major adaptive value the avoidance of random breeding, and the concomitant partitioning of the gene pool of a population into a network of partial isolates, within each of which genetic exchange is much freer than it is between them. This is a situation which, as Wright (1939) has reasoned, provides conditions conducive to rapid evolution. Different genes would be expected to exist in differing proportions in various segments of such a subdivided gene pool. Those genes that are rare in one gene pool might be common in another. The genes with which they are most likely to combine will also be different. Since the genetic contribution to phenotype is not determined by an individual gene but by the interactions of any given gene with the total genome, genes that do not usually find themselves in favorable phenotypic combinations in one segment of the gene pool may achieve more favorable expression in another. These favorable gene complexes, which will differ across the geographic range of a species, will eventually be "tried out" against each other. During this process, new genetic combinations may be created, some of which may have a greater adaptive advantage than any of the previous ones. The new genetic combinations would be expected to spread through the species via the combined processes of the replacement of more poorly adapted individuals by those who are better adapted, and the spread of favorable gene combinations through genetic exchange among various segments of the gene pool.

The human species provides an excellent example of a subdivided but interbreeding gene pool. It is geographically ubiquitous and has had to adapt to a wide variety of climatic conditions. While there is no biological barrier to interbreeding, geographic and cultural barriers have effectively partitioned the species so that it has evolved as a reticulum of partially isolated groups. Moreover, the size and composition of these groups has been changing. From the theoretical point of view, such a history would be conducive to rapid evolution and could result in at least temporary differentiation of different groups within the species reticulum. Such differentiation has, of course, occurred with respect to pigmentation, body type, sickling anemia, blood type distribution and a variety of other characteristics, but all in all, genetic differences in adaptation to diverse ecological niches are relatively few (Goldschmidt, 1963; Baker and Weiner, 1966).

In the behavioral realm, such differences, if they exist, are even more difficult to assess. Freedman and Freedman (1969) have shown that Oriental and Caucasian babies differ in measurable responses. Brazelton's studies with Yucatan Indian infants suggest that from a very early age they do not respond like Caucasian babies to different levels of stimulation and that the infant may, therefore, program the mother to adjust her activities to its response levels.

Recently, Jensen (1969) has suggested that there are important ethnic differences in intelligence and that these occur on a genetic basis. This is a hypothesis that has been put forward many times since the dawn of the Darwinian era, as Hirsch (1971) has indicated. In its most recent incarnation, it is based on differences in IQ test performance between Negroes and whites without regard to the fact that neither group consists of an unpartitioned gene pool, or to the further circumstance that American Negroes have received 20 to 30 per cent of their genes from the white population (Stern, 1960) and that we are, therefore, closer to being brothers under the skin than phenotypic appearance would suggest.

It might be argued, all the same, that the appropriate conceptual model to which to refer the data supporting admixture between Negroes and Caucasians is that of the natural, rather than the domesticated species, where it seems most probable that the normative phenotype will be maintained despite the introduction of new genes from a related but phenotypically different population. The hypothesis that there are systematic racial differences in intelligence that are genetic in origin cannot be critically tested by comparing the performance of the groups in question on actual tests, regardless of how we try to equate our comparisons. As Hirsch (1971), Li (1971) and Vandenberg (1971) have all pointed out, heritability statistics cannot be interpreted to mean that some fixed proportion of the characteristic to which the statistic is applied is immutable from the moment of conception—except for environmental accidents which can diminish but not improve it. Suppose that you or I could live our lives over again under the altered circumstance of being differently reared in a similar cultural context, but by different parents. Animal research using genetic replicates indicates that this would make a substantial difference even on traits having high heritabilities (Ginsburg, 1966). Work with monozygotic twins raised in similar environments indicates that as far as IQ is concerned such circumstances can account for up to 20 points on the standard scales, a difference which exceeds that separating the means of the populations reported on by Jensen (see Shields, 1962; Bloom, 1964; Smilansky, *in* Bloom, 1969; Ginsburg, 1971). There is, therefore, a certain amount of slippage between genotype and phenotype, and its magnitude for IQ measures is sufficient to cast serious doubt on the presumption that a genetic explanation must be involved to account for the mean differences in performance reported by Jensen.

A second argument that has as long a history as that of genetic racial differences in intelligence is that of the purported dysgenic effect of the disadvantaged, and especially those with lower IQ's, leaving more progeny than the rest of the population. Given the imperfect relationship between genetic potential and the IQ achieved, the relationship between phenotypic selection and its effect on the gene pool is possibly not what is feared. Even assuming that there is a sufficient connection to produce an effect, Li (1971) has reasoned (as has the author: see Ginsburg, 1971) that given the polygenic additive model that we have for intelligence, the population of most effective breeders would represent all of the multiple heterozygotes containing the genetic potential to reconstitute the entire array of genetic potential for intelligence contained in the population at large. If this is analogous to what happened to the Negro population during the period of slavery, it is not a history that suggests a deterioration in the genetic potential of that gene pool.

The gene pool, however, represents only a potential for a population. The way in which the gene pool actually assorts will determine one dimension in the effectiveness with which that potential is utilized. The other dimension is that of maximizing the potential inherent in each genotype by providing an optimal environment.

In dealing the genetic cards, positive phenotypic assortative mating (in which individuals of similar ability, stature, coloring and so forth would choose each other as mates more often than they would choose individuals of substantially differing phenotypes) would be expected to increase the expressed phenotypic variance of a population and, if sustained, to expose the genetic diversity contained in its gene pool to the effects of additional selective factors. The frequency of what would otherwise be chance combinations of genes under random mating would be much enhanced. Affording equal and optimal opportunities to all subdivisions of the human population would not only permit each individual to attain the best potential inherent in his genotype, but could also produce a shift in the proportion of those genotypes that are affected by the mating preferences of the interbreeding group. It is thus not necessary for any fairly large and genetically diverse population to go outside of its own gene pool in order to change its normative array of phenotypes relatively quickly (Ginsburg and Laughlin, 1966, 1968).

Unfortunately, we lack sufficient hard data to demonstrate the precise nature and magnitude of the differences in the makeup of the human gene pool as we encounter it across the geographic range of our species. Physical anthropologists have catalogued the accessible variations and their distribution. There are some characteristics that are encountered much more frequently in certain populations than in others, and many fewer than are unique to a particular group. Those that are clearly adaptive to a given ecological niche are relatively rare, and as a consequence the species has remained flexible. In the behavioral realm one would also expect to find statistical differences in the array of measurable capacities from one group to another, and one would not expect to find that the same characteristic had the same genetic basis every time it was encountered. It is perfectly conceivable that there could be more than one genetic predisposition for schizophrenia, for example, and that populations in which this condition was manifest might differ in which "schizophrenia genes" they contained. There is, however, nothing to suggest that—with the exception of marker genes that have been so important in mating selection as to have become virtually fixed, and some peculiarly adaptive traits that have become indigenous to a particular population—the human species is not genetically equipotential from a behavioral point of view in all of its larger subdivisions. It should be borne in mind that equipotential does not mean identical.

Providing an Optimal Environment

In the limiting case, providing an optimal environment would require that a different set of conditions be available for each uniquely different genotype. Fortunately, from the point of view of setting practical goals for understanding and for practice, each species and variety of organism does not represent an unordered array of variability along each dimension in which variation can occur, but rather a clustered organization of its potential to vary, around evolved phenotypic norms. Although it remains true that as long as individual differences exist, the fine grain solution to the equation of the optimal environment could be unique for each genotype, solutions of greater generality are applicable, with some loss of accuracy, to clusters of genotypes and phenotypes and, therefore, to groups. Where these clusters are with respect to behavioral dimensions is not always obvious.

Phenotype as a Product of Environmental Circumstances. Our group has been involved in studies of aggressive behavior in mice, rabbits and various canids. Within each of these forms, using standardized conditions of rearing, there are demonstrable genetic differences in aggressiveness as measured by a variety of criteria. It has now been shown that preweaning experiences can play a large role in altering the later personality profile of an individual with respect to aggressive behavior (Fisher, 1955; Denenberg, 1962; Ginsburg, 1966, 1967). However, even within the same species, manipulations that will drastically alter the behavior of some genotypes may either not affect others at all, or affect them quite differently (Ginsburg, 1958, 1966, 1967; Jumonville, 1968). Further analyses have demonstrated that one genetic basis for the behavior in question is the makeup of the Y chromosome, while another appears to be an autosomal gene (Ginsburg, 1971). Other studies suggest that the Y-chromosome effect is mediated by means of testosterone levels (Walter and Hamilton, 1970). Work with humans indicates that there are close analogies between the biological correlates of aggressive behavior in mice and men (Ginsburg, 1970, 1971).

In addition to the Y-chromosome effect, various chromosomal anomalies in man that constitute sex mosaics produce a highly disproportionate incidence of sexual offenders involving aggressive acts among persons imprisoned for such actions (Razavi, 1971). Since there are usually physical developmental anomalies associated with these chromosomal conditions, it may be argued that the affected individual's anomalous gender role and the feelings associated with these circumstances account for the later behavioral phenomena, and that these are, therefore, socially induced responses that are not otherwise biologically driven. Even where an altered hormonal balance or other biological mechanism is involved, the relationship between the biological condition and the behavior may well be more flexible in the human subject, where ideational dimensions can intervene, than in the closest corresponding animal analogues. Despite the availability of the ideational dimension to the affected human, the prison statistics do not indicate that he is that much better off, with respect to being able to alter his behavior, than his animal homologue, even though the potential is there. The combination of delayed detection and an uncontrollable social milieu seems usually to provide the circumstances most inimical to the development of normal behavior. If, therefore, it is the affected individual whose actions and development must be reprogrammed under social circumstances that are unfavorable, the method that would hold the most promise would be correction of the underlying biological anomaly, which would at one and the same time alter the social responses that are, behaviorally speaking, teratogenic, and ameliorate the biological tendencies for anomalous behavior by intervention at the nonideational level of mechanism.

However, even at this level, the phenotype does not stand in any unitary relationship to the key biological processes affected. In our work with genetic susceptibility to convulsive seizures, we have shown that an agent that is palliative for one genotype may not be so for another, even though the same behavior is involved (Ginsburg, 1963, 1966, 1967). Moreover, the identical brain lesion will have different effects, depending on the genotype (Maxson, 1966). So will differences in behavioral history and variations in diet (Maxson, 1966). The overall phenotype embraces this spectrum of biological variation. The most effective simple method of controlling the phenotypic reaction in a given population will depend upon the proportion in which each separate genotype comprising the phenotype which embraces them all appears.

When it comes to similar studies in the human realm, we may expect to find homologies in underlying mechanisms identified through animal studies. In population isolates, especially those that are relatively small and to some extent consanguineous, one would expect to find a more common genetic basis for any aspect of phenotype than would obtain when diverse gene pools are compared. Studies of population isolates, should, therefore, be undertaken on a comparative basis in order to provide data comparable to those obtained from animal studies.

The paucity of data suggesting that man has evolved important biological adaptations to a diversity of ecological niches suggests that much of the variations we observe in our own species may have been random and not of particular adaptive value. If we evolved our distinctive behavioral adaptations in common before spreading all over the globe, and if, as seems necessary, the adaptive value of "intelligence" was high and genetic exchange occurred between groups, then it appears unlikely that basic qualitative differences could exist and be maintained to the present time between subdivisions of our species. The argument that differences in selection and mating patterns could have produced such differences secondarily has already been referred to and deemed unlikely for any sizeable gene pool under conditions of selection and mating that we know to have occurred. On this basis, though one might expect differences in frequency distribution of IQ among different population groups, one would not expect large differences in the means of such groups to be due to biological factors unless the possibility of environmental interventions had first been ruled out. Given, that the Jensen data, which have been used to make the contrary argument, were not based on interbreeding gene pools but on an ethnic taxonomy that has no identifiable relationship to the breeding structure, and that differences in the way whites and Negroes are reared, fed, motivated and educated could not be adequately assessed, the hypothesis that the reported differences are most probably genetic is not demonstrated. The results of the Smilansky studies (see Bloom, 1969) comparing European and Oriental populations in Israel under a set of circumstances in which environmental differences have been controlled, suggest that the mean differences separating these index populations under circumstances where the motivational, nutritional, cultural and economic environments differ, must be largely referred to these factors rather than to biological ones (see also Ginsburg, 1971).

The same array of genotypes may express themselves quite differently in one set of environmental circumstances than in another. Providing an optimal environment, therefore, may result in rapid and significant change in the distribution of many phenotypes within a population. The change in average stature with better nutritional conditions, especially during the last 25 years, is an example of this. It is at least as tenable a hypothesis as Jensen's that the change in IQ of those populations in the United States that have been the product of a deprivation experiment would be as markedly affected as stature has been, were the relevant environmental circumstances to be altered.

Altering the Genes Themselves

It is now over 15 years since the scientific community was made aware of the structure of the gene and the relationship of this structure to its properties as a self-replicating entity as well as to its properties as a directive agent in development. We now know how genes code for sequences of amino acids, at least in simple organisms, and there have been successes in achieving an alteration in this coding by incorporating new elements into the genic structure itself by means of viral action. Such activities, plus advances on the synthetic side, suggest that it may one day be possible to climb the ladder of the DNA double helix to new heights represented by the possibility of correcting deficiencies in genetic coding, so that a normal individual would result in place of a defective one. We are not here considering the improvement of the species by second guessing how to restructure the genotype. This would be fraught with most of the same pitfalls that would attend a eugenic selection program. There are important political, personal and social considerations involved, and even more fundamental, we do not yet possess the omniscience to know what to program for. Where, however, there is a known genetic defect as in the case of phenylketonuria, or an adverse chromosomal anomaly, the problem becomes a therapeutic one, and only deficient knowledge and inadequate technology stand in the way of improving the human condition for those unfortunate enough to possess a genetic defect.

Although the gleam of hope is on the horizon, the level of technology and knowledge needed to achieve the directed alteration of the genes has not yet been realized. Like the solution of the cancer problem (in which it might well be involved) the giant breakthrough could come next week—or not until the next century. In the meantime we must look to other means while encouraging research to make this one possible in the future.

Changing the Activation Pattern of the Existing Genetic Potential

In conceptualizing the manner in which genes control and interact with developmental processes, based on studies with mammalian materials, two categories of genetic predisposition may be identified: One is that in which the genetic potential is restricted, such that the normal degrees of freedom inherent in the genetic mechanism do not exist. The other is that in which a broad potential inherent in the genotype receives its individuation as development proceeds through the selective activation and/or suppression of genic activity.

In the first instance, biological engineering, given the present state of the art, might seek to create or modify an enzymatic capacity or product at appropriate times during development to correct, perhaps continuingly, an accessible genetic defect in some compensatory way. In the second instance, the attempt would be to selectively activate those aspects of the genetic potential leading to the desired phenotype. The intervention would have to occur at the appropriate point in development, would probably only be necessary once and would lead to as lasting a change (from the point of view of the individual affected) as a gene mutation. From the point of view of the next generation, however, no change in the genome will have been produced, as would have occurred with a mutation. Since genes affect each other's activity, one class of mutations would consist of genes that preprogram the selective activation patterns of other genes during development, thus insuring a particular phenotypic outcome over a relatively broad range of circumstances. By studying the processes controlled by such genes, and the times and sites at which the changes occur that differentiate the mutants from the normal, it should, in theory, be possible to intervene in order to produce a phenocopy in either direction.

Selective Activation of Genic Activity in Mice. In our own work with the mouse, we believe that we have an illustration of such a system and of its manipulation to create phenocopies either of the mutant from the normal, or of the reverse (Ginsburg et al., 1967; Sze, 1970). Since the processes involved in mammalian systems may not be the same as those in microbial preparations, terminology having conceptual connotations based on microbiological findings have been avoided.

During the course of the work with sound-induced convulsive seizures, a number of mutations affecting this response have been identified (Cowen, 1966; Maxson, 1966; Ginsburg, 1967; Sze, 1969, 1970). Two of these, both predisposing to seizures, have arisen from the same inbred strain (C57BL/6) which is itself seizure-resistant under normal circumstances. Each of these mutations represents a one gene difference from the parent stock correlated with an associated behavioral phenomenon. This is as simple and controlled a difference as one is likely to find in a mammal. It has the additional advantage that each of the genotypes under investigation can be replicated at will.

Although it is possible to manipulate the seizures in these and other genotypes in a variety of ways, most (e.g., the manipulation of biogenic amine levels) are not genotype-specific. Pretreatment with monosodium glutamate does, however, distinguish the genotypes in question from other seizure-prone stocks and allies them with the DBA strain. We therefore investigated the glutamic acid metabolism of these and other selected genotypes.

The salient finding for these purposes was that glutamic acid decarboxylase (GAD) in brain has a higher activity in DBA mice than it does in C57BL/6 animals. When the activity is plotted against age during the postpartum preweaning period, the curves are parallel. Moreover, the difference in activity is a reflection of a difference in the amount of the protein moiety of the enzyme (Sze, 1969). The process controlled by the enzyme—the decarboxylation of glutamic acid—results in the formation of gamma aminobutyric acid (GABA), a substance associated with neural inhibition. The two mutants that predispose to seizures on the C57BL/6 background each show a departure from the GAD curve of the parent strain. Each of these occurs at a circumscribed time during development, and the change is completed within about a day. In each case, the change effected is that of departing from the curve it has been following up to that point, and abruptly adjusting to the level of another curve which it then continues to follow. In one instance the initial path was indistinguishable from the normal DBA curve and the change was to the level characteristic of C57BL/6. In the other instance, the reverse occurred (Sze, 1969, 1970). It appears that it is not the absolute activity of the system but rather the fact that it has abruptly changed which is the predisposing phenomenon.

Henry (1967, 1970) and Jumonville (1968) have shown that exposing the seizure-resistant C57BL/6 animals to sound on day 18 or 19 renders them seizure-susceptible when they are tested at 28 days of age. This is a time (19 days) when the GAD curve is rising rapidly, and Sze (1969, 1970) has demonstrated that the sound priming produces a change in the GABA level and that the manipulation of the GABA level by means of a single administration of amino oxyacetic acid (AOAA) at the same vulnerable period of development will also alter the behavior. Using these methods, a phenocopy of either the seizure-prone or the normal condition can be created in the genetic stock of opposite predisposition by a single treatment.

These findings suggest that priming by audible sound at an appropriate time during development can produce a phenocopy of a particular mode of seizure susceptibility on the C57BL/6 genetic background that can also be preprogrammed by genetic mutation. On this hypothesis, both the mutation and the sound stimulation have the effect of activating a potential in the genotype at an appropriate time during development in such a way that the behavior is thereafter changed. Since the GAD-GABA system occurs in other forms, including man, and appears to have similar functions across taxonomic categories, the major findings resulting from the work with mice should be applicable to other species (see Roberts, 1967). Analogously, other neural transmitters might be expected to yield to comparable genetic and environmental programming and to be involved in the determination of behavioral capacities. In the case in question—and in others, if the analogy holds—it is important to note that the neurochemical changes have occurred some time before the shift in behavior, by which time the neurochemical changes are no longer evident.

The study of developmental effects of gene mutations on neural processes may, on this basis, be expected to provide an understanding of how, where and when such processes can vary to bring about later changes in behavior. This understanding, in turn, can lead to the production of phenocopies by means of appropriate manipulations at given times during development that will result in permanent effects for the individual. In the genetic realm, it is the closest that we can now come to biological engineering. Assortative mating patterns, enhanced opportunities, including access to better health and nutritional facilities as well as to better motivational and educational opportunities, and genetic counseling can be expected to improve the human condition at other levels. The most imminent and promising breakthrough, however, appears to be at the level of developmental behavioral genetics.

SUMMARY

At first blush it would appear that acceptance of the thesis of genetic determination of behavioral capacities implies that the best that environment can do is permit an individual to reach his genetic limits. Given the fact that populations differ in their gene pools, just as individuals differ in their genomes, a corollary of this implication is that even under optimal conditions, races or varieties within a species may be expected to differ normatively in their behavioral potentials.

This chapter stresses the fact that at the individual level the genome is not merely a blueprint that will be translated into an organism that may be larger or smaller, depending on nutrition, or smarter or duller, depending on experience. Instead, the genome contains alternative sets of instructions that can be activated or suppressed at crucial stages such that the final product may be quite different in a qualitative sense even where the encoded genotype is the same. Widely different genotypes may thus be brought to equipotentiality and identical genotypes may be made to diverge.

At the population level, the degree of freedom between an encoded genotype and the varieties of phenotypic expression it may attain necessitates a dynamic interpretation of what alternative phenotypic norms a population might achieve without further genetic differentiation. Moreover, the population may have genetic ways of attaining a given phenotypic norm that are different from those open to other populations of the same species with which it overlaps phenotypically. Thus it is possible for a fruit fly to have white eyes because of the presence of a sex-linked recessive gene. The combination of two separate autosomal genes will also produce white eyes. The two populations of white-eyed flies would be phenotypically identical but genetically quite different. The probability of exploiting several genetic routes to the same phenotype is enhanced in proportion to the adaptability of that phenotype.

On the other hand, mice of identical genotype may either be seizure-prone or not, depending on the sound levels to which they are exposed on the 18th day postpartum. Another genotype may not show this lability. We do not need to be genetically identical to become phenotypically identical, nor will genetic similarity insure phenotypic homogeneity. We are only beginning to understand the critical factors and processes involved, and they offer hope for a very positive type of bioengineering that depends not on altering the structure of the gene but rather depends on the differential activation of genetic alternatives represented in the encoded genomes of most individuals.

Finally, adaptive traits within a species will tend to converge and overlap phenotypically even though the subpopulations exhibiting such convergence differ genetically with respect to the characteristics in question.

ACKNOWLEDGMENTS

The researches of the author reported herein were supported by research grants Nos. MH-03361 and MH-17088 from the National Institutes of Mental Health, and by grant 17-302 from the Psychiatric Training and Research Fund, State of Illinois Department of Mental Health.

REFERENCES

Baker, P. T., and Weiner, J. S. (Eds.): *The Biology of Human Adaptability.* New York, Oxford University Press, Inc., 1966.

Bastock, M.: A gene mutation which changes a behavior pattern. *Evolution, 10*:421–439, 1956.

Benzer, S.: Behavioral mutants of *Drosophila* isolated by countercurrent distribution. *Proc. Nat. Acad. Sci. U.S.A.*, 58:1112–1119, 1967.

Blooms, B. S.: *Stability and Change in Human Characteristics.* New York, John Wiley & Sons, Inc., 1964.

Bloom, B. S.: The Jensen article. *Harvard Educational Review*, 39:419–421, 1969.

Brazelton, T. B., Robey, J. S., and Collier, G. A.: Infant development in the Zinacanteco Indians of Southern Mexico. *Pediatrics, 44*:274–290, 1969.

Bruell, J. H.: Mode of inheritance of response timing in mice. *J. Comp. Physiol. Psychol., 60*:147–148, 1965.

Burt, C.: The inheritance of mental ability. *Amer. Psychol., 13*:1–15, 1958.

Collins, R. C.: On the inheritance of handedness: I. Laterality in inbred mice. *J. Hered.*, 59:9–12, 1968.

Collins, R. C.: On the inheritance of handedness: II. Selection for sinistrality in mice. *J. Hered., 60*:117–119, 1969.

Cowen, J. S.: A hippocampal anomaly associated with hereditary susceptibility to sound induced seizures. M.S. Dissertation, University of Chicago, 1966.

Crow, J. F., and Kimura, M.: *An Introduction to Population Genetics.* New York, Harper & Row Publishers, 1970.

Denenberg, V. H.: The effects of early experience. *In* Hafez, E. S. E. (Ed.): *The Behaviour of Domestic Animals.* London, Bailliere, Tindall & Cassell Ltd., 1962.

Dilger, W. C.: The behavoir of Lovebirds. *Sci. Amer., 206*:88–98, 1962.

Dobzhansky, T. H.: Of flies and men. *Amer. Psychol.*, 22:41–48, 1967.

Elston, R. C., and Campbell, M. A.: Schizophrenia: Evidence for the major gene hypothesis. *Behavior Genetics, 1*:3–10, 1970.

Falconer, D. S.: *Introduction to Quantitative Genetics.* Edinburgh and London, Oliver & Boyd Ltd., 1960.

Fisher, A. E.: The effects of differential early treatment on the social and exploratory behavior of puppies. Ph.D. Dissertation, Pennsylvania State University, 1955.

Freedman, D. G.: *Human Infancy in Evolutionary Prospective.* New York, Basic Books, Inc., Publishers, 1971.

Freedman, D. G., and Freedman, N. C.: Differences in behavior between Chinese American and European American newborns. *Nature, 224*:1227, 1969.

Fuller, J. L.: Measurement of alcohol preference in genetic experiments. *J. Comp. Physiol. Psychol.*, 57:85–88, 1964.

Fuller, J. L., Easler, C., and Smith, M. E.: Inheritance of audiogenic seizure susceptibility in the mouse. *Genetics, 35*:622–632, 1950.

Ginsburg, B. E.: Genetics as a tool in the study of behavior. *Perspect. Biol. Med., 1*:397–424, 1958.

Ginsburg, B. E.: Causal mechanisms in audiogenic seizures. *In Psychophysiologie Neuropharmacologie et Biochimie de la Crise Audiogene. Colloques Internationaux du Centre National de la Recherche Scientifique*, No. 112, pp. 227–240, 1963.

Ginsburg, B. E.: All mice are not created

equal: Recent findings on genes and behavior. *Social Service Review, 40*:121–134, 1966.

Ginsburg, B. E.: Genetic parameters in behavioral research. *In* Hirsch, J. (Ed.): *Behavior-Genetic Analysis,* New York, Mc Graw-Hill Book Company, 1967.

Ginsburg, B. E.: Breeding structure and social behavior of mammals: A servo-mechanism for the avoidance of panmixia. *In* Glass, D. C. (Ed.): *Genetics and the Study of Intelligence and Personality.* New York, Rockefeller University Press and Russell Sage Foundation, 1968.

Ginsburg, B. E.: The role of genic activity in the determination of sensitive periods in the development of aggressive behavior. *In* Faucett, J. (Ed.): *Violence and Aggression.* AMA-APA Symposium, 1970.

Ginsburg, B. E.: *In* Cancro, R. (Ed.): *Intelligence: Genetic and Environmental Influences.* New York, Grune & Stratton, Inc., 1971.

Ginsburg, B. E.: Developmental genetics of behavioral capacities: The nature-nurture problem re-evaluated. *Merrill-Palmer Quarterly, 17*:187–202, 1971.

Ginsburg, B. E., and Laughlin, W. S.: The multiple bases of human adaptability and achievement: A species point of view. *Eugen. Quart., 13*:240–257, 1966.

Ginsburg, B. E., Cowen, J. S., Maxson, S. C., and Sze, P. Y.: Neurochemical effects of gene mutations associated with audiogenic seizures. *Progress in Neuro-Genetics, 1*: 695–701, 1967.

Ginsburg, B. E., and Laughlin, W. S.: The distribution of genetic differences in behavioral potential in the human species. *In* Mead, M., et al. (Eds.): *Science and the Concept of Race,* New York, Columbia University Press, 1968.

Goldschmidt, E. (Ed.): *The Genetics of Migrant and Isolate Populations.* New York, The Williams & Wilkins Co., 1963.

Gottesman, I. I.: *Heritability of Personality, a Demonstration. Psychol. Monogr., 77,* 1963, 21 pp.

Gottesman, I. I., and Shields, J.: A polygenic theory of schizophrenia. *Proc. Nat. Acad. Sci. U.S.A., 58*:199–205, 1967.

Gruneberg, H.: *Animal Genetics and Medicine.* New York, Hoeber Medical Division, Harper & Row, Publishers, 1947.

Henry, K. R.: Audiogenic seizure susceptibility induced in C57BL/6 mice by prior auditory exposure. *Science, 158*:938–940, 1967.

Henry, K. R., and Bowman, R. E.: Acoustic priming. *In* Welch, B. L., and Welch, A. S. (Eds.): *Physiological Effects of Noise.* New York, Plenum Publishing Corporation, 1970.

Hinde, R. A.: Behavior and speciation in birds and lower vertebrates. *Biol. Rev., 34*:85–128, 1959.

Hirsch, J.: Studies in experimental behavior genetics. II. Individual differences in geotaxis as a function of chromosome variations in synthesized *Drosophila* populations. *J. Comp. Physiol. Psychol., 52*:304–308, 1959.

Hirsch, J.: Behavior-genetic analysis at the chromosome level of organization. *In* Hirsch, J. (Ed.): *Behavior-Genetic Analysis,* New York, McGraw-Hill Book Company, 1967.

Hirsch, J.: *In* Cancro, R. (Ed.): *Intelligence: Genetic and Environmental Influences.* New York, Grune & Stratton, Inc., 1971.

Ikeda, K., and Kaplan, W. D.: Patterned neural activity of a Mutant *Drosophila melanogaster. Proc. Nat. Acad. Sci., U.S.A., 66*: 765–772, 1970.

Jensen, A. R.: How much can we boost IQ and scholastic achievement? *Harvard Educational Review, 39*:1–123, 1969.

Jumonville, J. E.: Influence of genotype-treatment interactions in studies of emotionality in mice. Ph.D. Dissertation, University of Chicago, 1968.

Kallman, F. J.: *The Genetics of Schizophrenia.* New York, J. J. Augustin, Inc.—Publisher, 1938.

Kallman, F. J.: The genetic theory of schizophrenia: An analysis of 691 schizophrenic twin index families. *Amer. J. Psychiat., 103*:309–322, 1946.

Kempthorne, O.: *An Introduction to Genetic Statistics.* New York, John Wiley & Sons, Inc., 1957.

Lejeune, J., Turpin, R., and Gautier, M.: Le mongolisme. Premier exemple d'aberration autosomique humaine. *Ann. Genet., 1*:41–49, 1959.

Lerner, I. M.: *Genetic Homeostasis.* New York, John Wiley & Sons, Inc., 1954.

Lerner, I. M.: *The Genetic Basis of Selection.* New York, John Wiley & Sons, Inc., 1958.

Li, C. C.: *Population Genetics.* Chicago, University of Chicago Press, 1955.

Li, C. C.: *In* Cancro, R. (Ed.): *Intelligence: Genetic and Environmental Influences.* New York, Grune & Stratton, Inc., 1971.

Lindzey, G.: Emotionality and audiogenic seizure susceptibility in five inbred strains of mice. *J. Comp. Physiol. Psychol., 44*:389–394, 1951.

Manning, A.: The sexual isolation between *Drosophila melanogaster* and *Drosophila simulans, Anim. Behav., 7*:60–65, 1959.

Manning, A.: Genes and the evolution of insect behavior. *In* Hirsch, J. (Ed.): *Behavior-Genetic Analysis,* New York, McGraw-Hill Book Company, 1967.

Maxson, S. C.: The effect of genotype on brain mechanisms involved in audiogenic seizure susceptibility. Ph.D.. Dissertation, University of Chicago, 1966.

McClearn, G. E.: Genotype and mouse activity. *J. Comp. Physiol. Psychol., 54*:674–676, 1961.

McKusick, V. A.: *Mendelian Inheritance in*

Man: Catalogs of Autosomal Recessives and X-Linked Phenotypes. Baltimore, The Johns Hopkins Press, 1966.

Razavi, L.: Sex chromosomes, hand-prints and sexual behavior. *In* Erwin, F. (Ed.): *The Biology of Sociology and Violence,* A.A.A.S. Symposium, 1971.

Roberts, E.: Synaptic neurochemistry: A projection. *In* Hirsch, J. (Ed.): *Behavior-Genetic Analysis.* New York, McGraw-Hill Book Company, 1967.

Roderick, T. H.: Selection for cholinesterase activity in the cerebral cortex of the rat. *Genetics, 45*:1123–1140, 1960.

Rosenthal, D.: The offspring of schizophrenic couples. *J. Psychiat. Res., 4*:169–188, 1966.

Scott, J. P.: Genetic differences in the social behavior of inbred strains of mice. *J. Hered., 33*:11–15, 1942.

Shields, J.: *Monozygotic Twins.* London, Oxford University Press, 1962.

Sidman, R. L., Green, M. C., and Appel, S. H.: *Catalog of the Neurological Mutants of the Mouse.* Harvard University Press, Cambridge, Massachusetts, 1965.

Stern, C.: *Principles of Human Genetics.* San Francisco, W. H. Freeman and Co. Publishers, 1960.

Sze, P.: Neurochemical factors in the development of genetically determined susceptibility to audiogenic seizures in the mouse. Ph.D. Dissertation, University of Chicago, 1969.

Sze, P. Y.: Neurochemical factors in auditory stimulation and development of susceptibility to audiogenic seizures. *In* Welch, B. L., and Welch, A. S. (Eds.): *Physiological Effects of Noise.* Plenum Publishing Corporation, 1970.

Thiessen, D., and Nealey, V.: Adrenocortical activity, stress response and behavioral reactivity in five inbred mouse strains. *Endocrinology, 71*:227–232, 1962.

Tryon, R. C.: The genetics of learning ability in rats. *Univ. Calif. Publ. Psychol., 4*:71–89, 1929.

Vandenberg, S. G.: *Methods and Goals in Human Behavior Genetics.* New York, Academic Press, Inc., 1965.

Vandenberg, S. G.: *In* Cancro, R. (Ed.): *Intelligence: Genetic and Environmental Influences.* New York, Grune & Stratton, Inc., 1971. In press.

Walter, R. O., and Hamilton, J. B.: Supermales (YY sex chromosomes) and androgen-treated XY males: Competition for mating with female killifish *Oryzias latipes. Anim. Behav., 18*:128–131, 1970.

Wimer, R. E., Wimer, C. A., and Roderick, T. H.: Genetic variability in forebrain structures between inbred strains of mice. *Brain Res., 16*:257–264, 1969.

Wright, S.: *Statistical Genetics in Relation to Evolution.* Paris, Hermann, 1939.

Wright, S.: *Evolution and the Genetics of Populations. Vol. 1: Genetic and Biometric Foundations.* Chicago, University of Chicago Press, 1968.

6 PSYCHOLOGICAL ASSESSMENT

Regina Yando

The state of the art in psychology is to a certain extent comparable to the practice of medicine 50 years ago, when the physician still lacked many critical pieces of information, and intuition and "common sense" played a much larger role than they do now. Today the adequate treatment of human behavior problems requires more scientific rigor and more understanding than is available from even the most advanced behavioral science research. Stated simply, psychology is a young science. But certainly this is no cause for embarrassment. What is, however, most unfortunate and embarrassing is the fact that the popular conception of psychology centers more on the dramatic, often unwarranted, assertions that find their way to newspapers and magazines, rather than on the well-defined, though incomplete, body of scientific knowledge that *is* currently available. As can be seen throughout this book, the available knowledge is of the utmost utility and importance. Accordingly, it is the purpose of this chapter to clarify the scientific nature of the work of the practicing psychologist, to explain his role *vis-à-vis* the physician, and to describe the tools at his disposal to aid him in the formal discipline of psychological assessment.

THE NATURE OF PSYCHOLOGICAL ASSESSMENT

Assessment is not, of course, the exclusive domain of the psychologist. Viewed simply as the process of trying to understand people, assessment is something we all practice daily. In essence, psychological assessment is nothing more than a formalized attempt at understanding, which utilizes specialized knowledge, tools and techniques in order to aid the psychologist in making decisions. This basically simple idea, however, has been subject to a variety of interpretations.

The model of psychological assessment that the physician was, and to a great extent still is, most apt to encounter is that of psychodiagnosis. Essentially, the "psychodiagnostician" attempts to elucidate the underlying etiology of the psychological problems of "patients," thereby contributing to the determination of prognosis and to the selection of optimal treatment. Clearly the psychodiagnostic model is similar to the model of differential diagnosis used in medicine.

Recently, however, this traditional model of assessment has been influenced by a number of changes in professional attitudes. Among these are a general acceptance of the limitations of the psychiatric classification system and an increased awareness of the difficulties inherent in conceptualizing psychological problems as disease entities. Accordingly, the emphasis in current psychodiagnosis has shifted from a description of symptomatology to such problems as the study of the "total person," including an individual's potential strengths as they may relate to treatment.

In addition to the modifications of the psychodiagnostic model, however, a variety of social problems, such as juvenile delinquency, racial conflict and economic deprivation, have also obtruded into our conception of assessment. Because these social influences, like public health problems, must often be dealt with outside the clinical setting, they have revealed the need for models of assessment entirely different from those of psychodiagnosis.

To meet this need, several alternative models of assessment have in fact arisen. To cite only one example, the "behavioral model" utilizes the language and structure of learning theory, and has gained wide acceptance in schools and, more recently, in hospital settings. The assessment in this instance attempts not only to delineate patterns of behavior that require change, but also to identify those environmental factors which control the behavior and which may be manipulated to produce desired changes. The emphasis is on the direct application of assessment information, for the purpose of treatment, by persons other than highly specialized professionals. There are, in addition, several other important alternative models of assessment which we cannot discuss here, each of them having a different view of our simple idea of "understanding people."[1]

Clearly, then, the model of assessment the psychologist employs is going to vary, depending on his theoretical and personal values. It should, however, be stressed that whatever his underlying orientation, the basic approach he uses in assessment will follow the pattern of scientific inquiry: (1) a systematic collection of data concerning a person's behavior, followed by (2) the organization and (3) the interpretation of the behavior observed. All models of assessment thus represent an attempt at the exact analysis of an individual's behavior through the use of standardized procedures. They stress an organized and intentional manner of communication which has derived in large part from experimental research, and are in this way fundamentally different from our casual "everyday" attempts at understanding others.[2]

THE PHYSICIAN AND THE PSYCHOLOGIST

The importance of psychological factors in medicine has long been recognized. (An excellent survey of the area is provided by Lief et al., 1963.) On the other hand, the potential application of psychological knowledge in medicine has been

[1]Various other models of assessment have been proposed; among the important ones are the so-called experimental, decision-making and operations research models. A further discussion of these can be found in Arthur (1969).

[2]The connection between assessment and experimental work hinges on the word *behavior*. Behavior constitutes directly observable data amenable to scientific investigation. Such constructs as emotion, drive, need and thought are *inferences* and must be treated as such.

recognized only recently. Any number of current medical journals, such as *Pediatrics* and *Developmental Medicine and Child Neurology*, do, however, reveal a growing interest in the development of collaborative psychological and medical research. It is somewhat surprising, then, to discover that this same literature reveals a dearth of information regarding the ways in which the physician and psychologist involved in practice should work together.

Physicians are becoming increasingly involved with problems that are of social and behavioral, as well as of somatic, etiology. Referring to the new "family physician," Alpert (1968, p. 663) has stated:

> He can be a marriage counselor, can recognize and advise regarding learning disorders, and use his relationship with his patients to manage chronic diseases and plan rehabilitation. He is more of a psychiatrist and more of a social scientist and less of a specialist in unusual disease. He is an expert in the technique of obtaining a consultation and knows how to select and use his consultants.

As Alpert's statement points out, it is a relatively new kind of physician who has a knowledge of social science and an expertise in using consultations. And yet just what use the physician should make of a psychological consultant remains largely an unexplored and undocumented area. Not all patients need to be seen by a psychologist, so what should be the criteria for referral? How should the problem be defined? There are no rigid answers to these questions. It is up to the physician to recognize (1) the limits of his competency and (2) the potential utility of psychological assessment in the diagnosis, treatment and rehabilitation of his patients.[3]

[3]The contribution of psychological factors to medical problems is the subject of Chapter 1 and of numerous other works. It is a topic that will not be discussed at length in this chapter.

Assuming the physician does see the need for an assessment, the decision to seek a consultation raises many pragmatic questions, particularly for the physician who is not affiliated with a clinic having a staff psychologist. Where does one make a referral? What kind of psychologist should be contacted? What are the requirements of a referral request? How should the resulting assessment be interpreted?

In general there are three types of psychological specialists who, as part of their professional work, engage in assessment: the clinician, the counselor and the school psychologist. All of them may be found either in private practice (independently or in association with other professionals such as psychiatrists) or in various institutional settings such as schools, mental health clinics and courts of law.

Although there is an extensive overlap in the functions of these psychologists, certain types of problems are usually brought to the attention of different specialists. The clinician is most apt to be involved with problems of severe maladjustment to the total life setting; the counselor is primarily concerned with vocational adjustment; and the school psychologist works mostly with learning disabilities and social problems.

The appropriate assessor having been chosen, the formal referral request from the physician will be important in determining the nature of the assessment. Although various agencies have, with the wisdom inherent in all bureaucracies, created a myriad of referral forms, all referrals do ask for a statement of the problem. The physician should consider the following guidelines in stating the problem:

(1) What behaviors of the person in question define his problem? Note that this is not quite the same as specifying the symptoms which char-

acterize a disease, since our interpretation of "normal" will at best be rather arbitrary.

(2) In what situations does such behavior occur? (Only at home? Only at school?)

(3) What is the frequency and intensity of the behavior in question?

Much of this information can be obtained only with difficulty, but the time spent in gathering it prior to referral will prevent needless confusion and repeated patient visits to both the physician and the psychologist.

In addition to this information, the physician should add his own inferences regarding the problem, and how he arrived at them. This should be followed by the specific questions he wants answered. Such a referral request may appear to be a large order, but many of the communication problems among professionals result simply from the substitution of ambiguous unstated expectations for explicit questions.

Any hope we have of true interdisciplinary cooperation between physicians and psychologists hinges on this problem of communication. Professionals in both fields are uniquely equipped to discern particular kinds of information about children, but unless this information is exchanged in *both* directions, the whole concept of consultation becomes a meaningless exercise.

A psychologist who cannot discover why a child with a normal IQ and good interpersonal relationships is failing in school and who therefore recommends a physical examination must tell the physician everything he knows about the case. A family physician who refers a child with epilepsy must tell the psychologist everything that is relevant about the child and his family. It seems obvious that this should be done, but all too frequently the interdisciplinary communication is via confused, misled or uncomprehending parents. "Take your child for a checkup" or "You might want to see about a psychologist for your son" is simply no substitute for articulate communication between professionals in complementary fields. Both the physician and the psychologist are looking at the same child, and together they may hold enough information to solve an otherwise intractable problem.

METHODS OF ASSESSMENT

Numerous methods can be used to gather assessment data. They include interviews and observations, both structured and unstructured; tests; the examination of personal documents; and the judgment of others. With these data, the assessor, utilizing his knowledge of psychological research and theory, actually formulates a microcosmic theory about a particular person and is responsible for evaluating it, deducing its consequences, communicating it to others and implementing procedures for the control of the behavior it describes.

Although several methods of assessment have been enumerated, this section will be concerned primarily with testing. The reason for limiting ourselves in this way is simple: testing represents the best standardized and best quantified method of assessment.

All psychologists, of course, must use such methods as interviewing and observation in gathering assessment data, but even if structured, these methods are highly dependent on subjective interpretation by the psychologist. The goals and techniques of an interview, for the most part, are dictated by the theoretical orientation of the interviewer, and behavior that is observed must be subjectively analyzed for its content.

Most of the work done in the systematization and quantification of methods other than testing is still largely in the realm of experimental research and is not readily available for general use. A great deal of excellent research (Weick, 1968), for example, has been done on observation techniques, including an attempt at the development of procedural rules for obtaining time samples of behavior in natural settings (Barker, 1963). Similarly, there has been a fair amount of research on the content analysis of interviews (Marsden, 1965). Unfortunately, the research still does not typify the day-to-day practical use of observation and interviews. Observation turns more on the acuity of the observer than on any formal regimen of procedure, and the interview can as often produce a wasteland of verbiage as it can a series of useful insights. Certainly the physician, who faces the enormously complex tasks of the medical diagnostic interview, already recognizes the general demands and limitations of the interview technique.

There is little more that can be said of these methods without further immersing ourselves in current research or attempting to instruct in a subject best taught by experience. Recognizing that observation and interview, though often not amenable to exact analysis, remain essential tools for collecting data necessary for a good assessment, we wish now to turn our attention to the more highly standardized area of testing.

Testing data are sufficiently objective to permit the physician himself to become a competent judge of psychological reports. Furthermore, the competent judge of tests becomes more capable of evaluating the less standardized parts of an assessment and of judging the use that the psychologist has made of them. The following discussion, then, is designed to provide the physician with sufficient basic information to enable him to judge the significance and limitations of psychological tests.

Testing: Basic Concepts

A test is defined as a tool that elicits some specific sample of a subject's behavior under carefully controlled conditions. A good test is designed to provide its user with a standard method with which to compare two or more individuals.

What constitutes a "good" test, however, is a complex question. Does a test actually measure what it claims to measure? Are individual test scores comparable to scores obtained on a variety of similar tests? Is the test reliable? Are the norms representative of the population for whom the test was intended? The problems are numberless, and though we will touch on many of them at some length, a complete definition of a "good" test lies outside the scope of this chapter.

Literally hundreds of tests are published yearly; they have been constructed to sample almost every conceivable attribute of man. Nonetheless, they can be classified into the following three general categories: (1) tests of general intellectual development, (2) tests of specific abilities such as achievement and aptitude and (3) tests of personality, including attitudes, values and interests. The format of most of these tests may be either objective or projective, depending on the type of response desired. The objective test presents the subject with a limited set of responses from which to select an answer (as on multiple choice tests), whereas projective tests present some type of ambiguous stimulus (like the classic inkblot) which requires the subject to provide a creative response. The latter gives the subject the opportunity to interpret the stimulus on the basis of his own personal experiences and feelings. Most tests, both objective and projective, may be administered either on an individual basis or to groups.

The range of decisions that are influenced by these tests is, of course, enormous. Still, as the mother weeping over her child's low IQ score so well demonstrates, there is a lack of knowledge as to the precise meaning of test scores. In order to avoid incorrect assumptions about the meaning of these scores, it is important for those who will use them to have a working knowledge of how tests are constructed and the criteria upon which they should be judged.

Perhaps the first thing to point out is that the title of a test often tells you nothing at all about what the test measures. In fact, discerning just what a test does measure is one of the most complex issues facing the test constructor. What does an IQ test measure? (This is an appallingly complex question which we shall discuss at length later.) Does a mechanical aptitude test measure potential mechanical ability or simply the subject's interest or lack of interest in the field? In searching for the answers to such questions, test designers must really assume the role of experimental epistemologists. Fortunately, however, they have some well-defined techniques to aid them—and those who use their tests— in determing what test scores mean.

Test Scores. The familiar theoretical normal curve, or "gaussian probability distribution," is a mathematical mode, the properties of which are well defined and very useful in many areas of science. In general, any random variable X that is influenced cumulatively by a large number of factors, each of which, by itself, contributes only a small effect, can be described by a normal distribu-

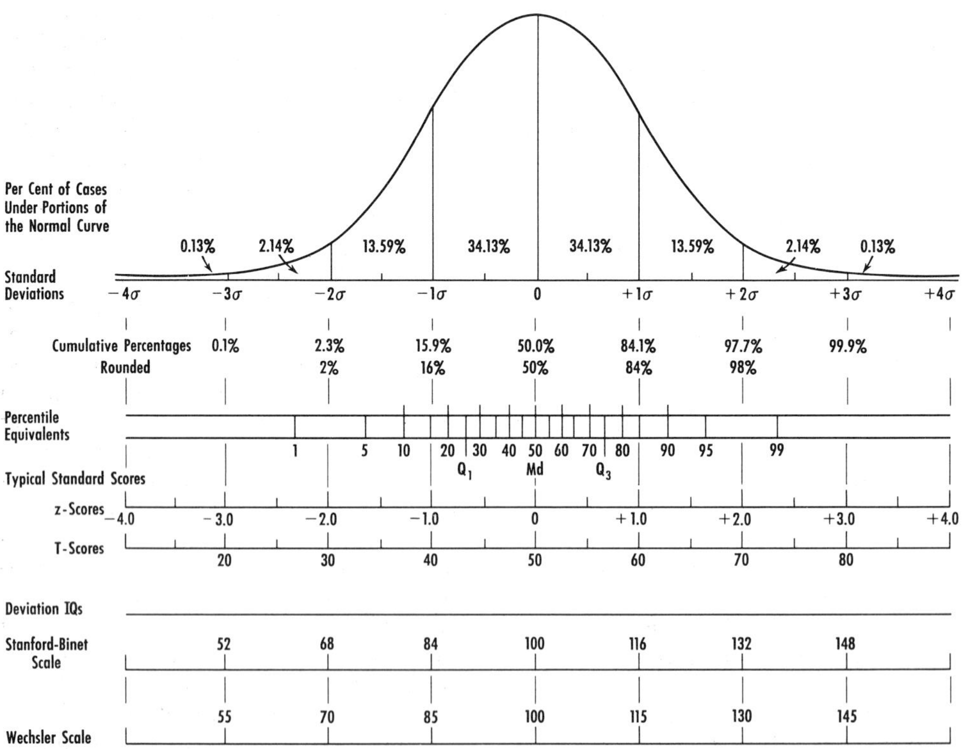

Figure 6–1 A normal distribution curve. This curve shows the per cent of cases under segments of the curve (marked off in terms of sigma) and also percentiles and standard scores. (*From* Munn, N. L.: *Psychology*. Boston, Houghton Mifflin Company, 1961, p. 747.)

tion.[4] Accordingly, as Galton first observed, the distribution of most complexly determined human characteristics from weight to anxiety approximates this normal density function. It is important to us here because it provides the basis for a variety of statistical analyses, and for understanding the relationship between different types of test scores. (See Fig. 6–1).

There are two major characteristics associated with any distribution: the central tendency and the variability. The central tendency can be measured in three ways: by the familiar arithmetic mean (μ), which divides the sum of all scores (Σ X) by the number of scores (N): $\mu = \frac{\Sigma X}{N}$; by the median, which is simply the middle score; and by the mode, which is the score that appears most frequently. In a normal distribution all three coincide; but in practice, where the ideal

[4]The idea of the normal curve had its origins in the measurement of errors. The empirical observation was made that erroneous measurements tended to be symmetrical about the apparent true value, becoming consistently less frequent as the absolute value of the deviation from the true value increased. The simplest equation embodying these observations is: $f(X) = Ke^{-X^2/2}$ where e is the base of the natural logarithms and K is some constant. Given some mean (μ) and standard deviation (σ) as parameters, the normal curve is then given by:

$$f(X) = \frac{1}{\sqrt{2\pi\sigma^2}} e^{-(X-\mu)^2/2\sigma^2}$$

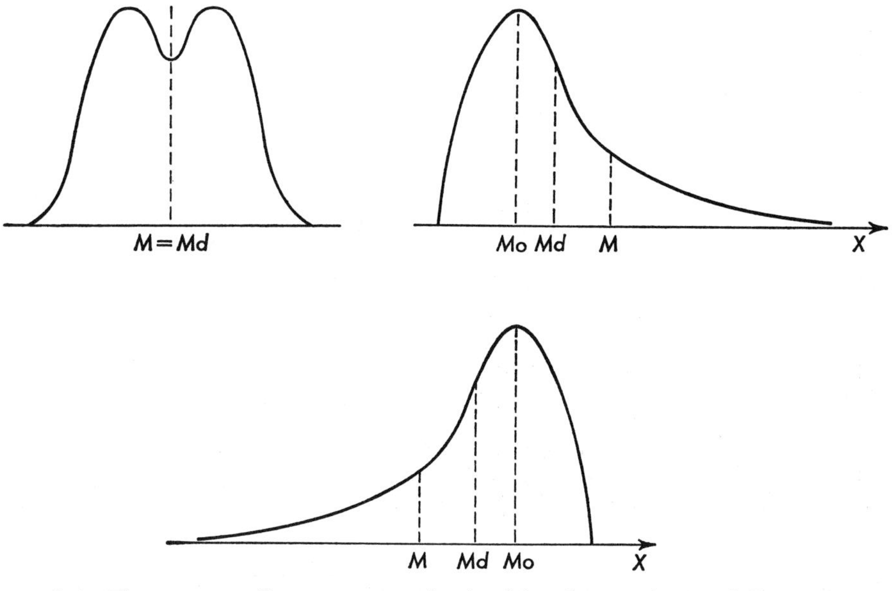

Figure 6–2 These curves illustrate various kinds of distributions having different means (M), medians (Md) and modes (Mo). (*From* Hays, W. L.: *Statistics for Psychologists.* New York, Holt, Rinehart & Winston, Inc., 1966, p. 174.)

distribution is only approximated, the three do differ and are not interchangeable. The more they vary, the poorer is our approximation of the normal density function. (See Fig. 6–2.)

Measures of variability indicate the spread of the scores. A rough way to measure variability is simply to examine the range of the scores, but by far the most precise and satisfactory method is the standard deviation (σ). This measure is calculated by obtaining the deviation of each score from the mean ($D = X - \mu$), squaring each deviation (D^2), finding the sum of the squares (ΣD^2), dividing by the number of cases, and taking the square root of the quotient: $\sigma = \sqrt{\frac{\Sigma D^2}{N}}$ (though if N is small [$N < 60$], it is necessary to divide by $N - 1$). The standard deviation, when applied to a normal curve, gives us a precise method of specifying the variation in scores. Between $\pm 1\sigma$ will fall approximately 68 per cent of all scores; between $\pm 2\sigma$, 95 per cent; and between $\pm 3\sigma$, 99 per cent. It is apparent that if σ is large, there is a wide variation in scores; whereas a small σ implies that the scores tend to pile up at the mean and that a result slightly above or below the mean is exceptional. (See Fig. 6–3.)

Most tests yield a raw score, which is simply a numerical statement of a person's performance—the number of items he answered correctly, the amount of time spent on a task or some similar measure. A raw score in and of itself is meaningless. In order to be interpreted, a raw score must be compared to some normative group. The norms of a particular test refer to the test performance of the group of people upon which the test is standardized. That is, after a test is constructed it is administered to a representative sample of the people for whom it was designed (e.g., a test of fifth grade arithmetic skills would demand a representative sample of fifth graders). The quantitative description of the distribution of their scores on the test, including the mean

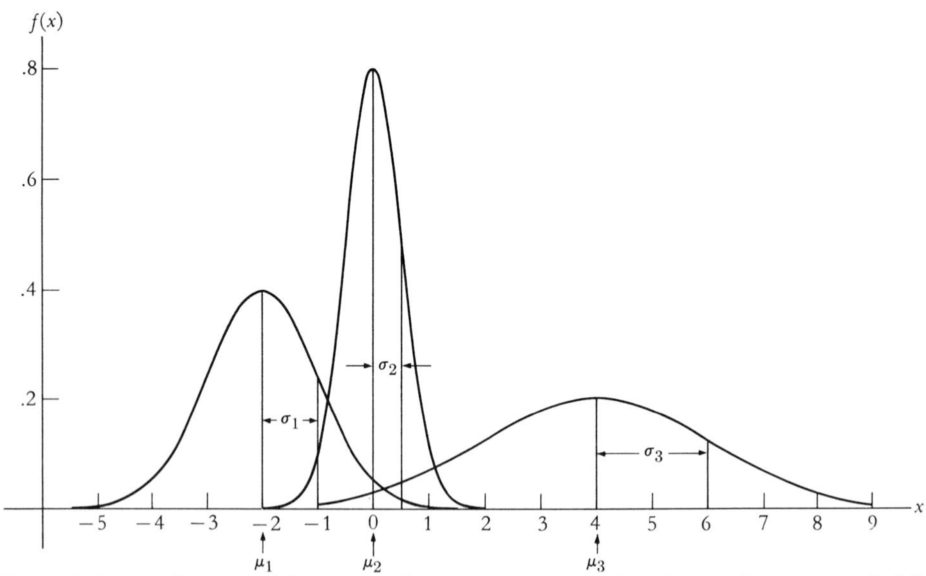

Figure 6–3 A collection of three normal or gaussian probability density functions with differing means and differing standard deviations: $\mu_1 = -2$, $\sigma_1 = 1$; $\mu_2 = 0$, $\sigma = 0.5$; $\mu_3 = 4$, $\sigma_3 = 2$. (*From* Mosteller, F., and Tuckey, J. W.: Data analysis, including statistics. *In* Lindzey, G., and Aronson, E.: *The Handbook of Social Psychology*, 2nd ed. Reading, Massachusetts, Addison-Wesley Publishing Co., Inc., 1968, Vol. II, p. 87.)

and the standard deviation, constitutes the norms for that test.

In order to evaluate the scores either within or between tests, however, raw scores must be converted into derived scores—for example, *percentiles* or *standard scores.*

A percentile score indicates what percentage of persons in the norm group falls below a given raw score. If, for example, 40 per cent of the norm group obtains fewer than 20 items correct on an analogy test, then a raw score of 20 corresponds to the 40th percentile. It is important to note that percentile scores (or any other score) *cannot* be compared unless the norm groups on which they are based are comparable.

The importance of knowing the norms becomes clear if you consider this example: Mike Doe, a college senior at Orange University, obtained a raw score of 125 on an analogies test consisting of 200 items. He did as well as or better than:

1. 99% of sixth graders in Orange Elementary School.
2. 80% of seniors in Orange Junior High School.
3. 50% of college freshmen at Orange University.
4. 60% of college seniors at Orange University.
5. 10% of medical students at Orange University.

Obviously, specification of the norm group determines his proper percentile rank.

Another standard score, the z-score, enables us to determine the relative status of any given score in a distribution. To say that Harry Doe received a score of 110 is really quite meaningless unless we are given a good deal of additional information. A score of 110 is excellent when the mean *for the group upon which the test was standardized is 90 with a standard deviation of 10;* it is only fair when the mean is 115 with a standard deviation of 25.

The standard score clarifies the situation by expressing the raw score in terms of its deviation from the mean:[5]

$$z = \frac{X - \mu}{\sigma}$$

Under different conditions Harry's score yields quite different z-scores:

$$z_1 = \frac{110 - 90}{10} =$$

2 (the 98th percentile)

$$z_2 = \frac{110 - 115}{25} =$$

−0.2 (about the 45th percentile)

Note that everything depends on the mean and the standard deviation established by the normative group. For comparable normative groups, however, any set of test scores that approximate a normal distribution can be transformed into exactly comparable sets of z-scores, and therein lies the usefulness of the standard score.

A second score, the T-score, is used simply to eliminate the need for decimals and negative numbers in z-scores. The T-score arbitrarily uses a mean of 50 (or sometimes 500) and a standard deviation of 10 (or 100) according to the rule $T = 50 + 10z$. On a test where the mean is 60 and the standard deviation 10, a score of 45 corresponds to a z-score of $\frac{45 - 60}{10}$, or −1.5; and to a T-score of 50 + 10 (1.5), or 35. (Again, see Fig. 6–1.)

A recent important adaptation of standard scores is the concept of deviation IQ. Where the old IQ score

---

[5]If we transform normally distributed raw scores to z-scores, thereby setting $\mu = 0$ and $\sigma = 1$, then substitution into the general equation for the normal distribution yields a simple standard rule given by:

$$f(X) = \frac{1}{\sqrt{2\pi}} e^{-Z^2}/2$$

This equation describes the standard normal distribution.

was given by $100 \times \frac{\text{mental age}}{\text{chronological age}}$, the deviation IQ's are actually standard scores with a mean of 100 and a standard deviation approximating 16. The Wechsler intelligence scales (mean 100, SD 15), the 1960 revision of the Stanford-Binet (mean 100, SD 16) and many newly developed tests, have scores expressed as deviation IQ's. Figure 6–1 summarizes the relationships among the types of scores that have been discussed relative to the normal distribution.

It must be emphatically pointed out that a direct comparison of scores from different tests cannot be made unless two conditions are met:

1. There must be a normal distribution (or a mathematically "normalized" distribution) of scores.
2. Those taking the tests must be comparable to the normative groups upon which the tests were standardized.

Validity. Technically, what a test measures or the extent to which a test accomplishes its goals determines its *validity.* The American Psychological Association's pamphlet *Standards for Educational and Psychological Tests and Manuals* defines three types of validity: content validity, criterion-related validity, and construct validity. (See Table 6–1.)

CONTENT VALIDITY. A primary goal of many tests is to determine an individual's performance in an area, using only a sample of the possible situations or problems pertinent to that area. With such a goal in mind, it is important to determine how well a specific test samples the topic or "content" that it intends to measure, since only a rather small number of the possible items can be included on any one test. How well the content of the test samples the subject matter under consideration determines the *content validity* of the test. The achievement and proficiency tests employed in schools are the principal examples of tests for which this form of validity is especially important. Content validity is determined by a subjective evaluation of the manner in which the sample of items was developed and how typical this sample is of the total universe of items. For example, a test of achievement in a physics course would seem to be valid, by definition, if it consisted of physics problems as opposed to chemistry problems. However, it should be pointed out that sampling of content (or the definition of the subject area under consideration) can be more difficult than it initially seems to be. (What if the physics problems were of a type not seen on any homework assignments?) Several empirical techniques can be used to help in this subjective judgment of content. If possible, for example, parallel forms of the test should be administered before and after a course of study to determine whether there is an improvement in scores.

CRITERION-RELATED VALIDITY. The goal of many tests is to provide either a current estimate or a prediction of an individual's performance in some area. Validity in these instances demands the use of an external criterion with which to compare the results of the test. If a relationship between the external criterion and the test results exists, the test is said to have *criterion-related validity.* In a further refinement of terminology, two forms of criterion-related validity are recognized: *concurrent validity* and *predictive validity.* The former is concerned with the assessment of present status. Is John Doe a good doctor? A test designed to answer this question must show agreement with, for example, the evaluation provided by a team of senior physicians. Similarly, predictive validity is concerned with the estimation of future performance. Will Fred Doe be a good doctor? Here we must

*Table 6–1 Three Types of Validation**

Question Asked	Procedure	Principally Applied To	Example
		Criterion-Related	
How do measures of some valued performance (criterion) relate to the test scores?	Give test. Collect data on the criterion, ordinarily after the person has spent some time in training, on a job, or in therapy. There may be different treatments for different groups. Examine the correspondence of criterion scores to test scores.	(a) Tests used in selecting employees and students.	(a) Admission test for law students is checked against later marks.
		(b) Tests used in deciding what treatment should be given a patient or student.	(b) To find out what sort of persons respond well to an antidepressant drug, the drug is given to people with different personality test scores.
		(c) A test intended to substitute for a more cumbersome assessment procedure.	(c) Diagnosis of brain damage from Block Design performance is compared with a neurological examination.
		Content	
Do the observations truly sample the universe of tasks or the situations they are claimed to represent?	Examine the test items and the responses called for. Compare with a full description of the universe the test is supposed to represent.	(d) Tests used to evaluate educational programs.	(d) Content of a test of shorthand ability is compared with content of office correspondence.
		(e) Observation procedures in research on typical behavior.	(e) A schedule for observing what questions children put to their teachers is checked for representation of types of lesson, time of day, etc.
		Construct	
How can scores on the test be explained psychologically? Does the test measure the attribute it is said to measure?	Set up hypotheses regarding the meaning of test scores, stating how high scorers and low scorers are expected to differ, or what influences are expected to alter scores. Test the hypotheses one by one.	(f) Tests interpreted as measuring mental processes or personality traits. Includes tests used to describe the individual in diagnosis or guidance. Includes outcome measures in scientific research and educational evaluation.	(f) A test of art aptitude is studied to determine how largely scores depend on art training, on experience in Western culture, on mental set to be unconventional, etc. A measure of "suggestibility" is studied experimentally to see if scores are influenced by (e.g.) previous relations with the tester.

*Table 5–1 (pp. 124–5) "Questions asked in validation research" in *Essentials of Psychological Testing,* 3rd Edition, by Lee J. Cronbach (Harper & Row, 1969).

await the outcome in order to ascertain whether the test affords a good prediction. Ultimately this is determined either by a subjective evaluation or by a test for physicians which has demonstrated concurrent validity. The criteria most often used in tests of predictive validity are academic achievement and on-the-job performance.

CONSTRUCT VALIDITY. Although criterion-related validity is usually cited in test manuals as indicative of what a test measures, the problem of what a test *actually* measures hinges on the concept of *construct validity.* The reader should question why it is assumed that "intelligence," for example, is a trait on which judgments of brightness and dullness in school are based. If a person is dull in school, is he necessarily unintelligent? Such questions ask whether the test actually measures the trait, quality or, to be most accurate, the hypothetical construct it purports to measure. The evaluation of construct validity requires an investigation of the hypothesis or theory underlying what is being tested. This demands, however, that the investigator specify *operationally* what is to be called a measure of the construct in which he is interested. This often leads us back to a measure of criterion-related validity.

If we were, for example, to question the criterion-related validity of a new intelligence test, it could be compared immediately with other well-recognized intelligence tests such as the Stanford-Binet, or it could be used to predict the college performance of high school students. But note that neither of these tests of validity tells us anything definitive about "intelligence." Clearly, there is no one criterion equivalent to the construct under study. At best it is possible to find criteria which, though not equivalent to the construct, do seem to be intimately related to it. "Anxiety," for example, can be related to a variety of physiological indicators such as palm sweating, increased pulse rate and a patient's subjective reports of tension. Although none of these observable behaviors is in and of itself equivalent to anxiety, the existence of a relationship between these variables and the "anxiety scores" of a specific test increases our confidence that the instrument is measuring the trait under consideration.

It is apparent, then, that the demonstration of construct validity involves a complex process analogous to that used in the development and verification of a theory. It requires precise operational definitions, an extensive accumulation of data from diverse sources and constant retesting to reflect new hypotheses concerning the trait we are attempting to understand.

Reliability. In addition to questions of validity, the designer of tests must worry about the reliability of the instrument; that is, the accuracy and consistency of test results. Tests are subject to numerous potential sources of error in both design and administration. Instructions may be unclear or ambiguous; the test may be uninteresting; or a person may be distracted during testing. These and other chance factors induce a variability in test results which, if too large, lessens the confidence we can place in those results.

There are two basic methods of measuring reliability. The first is concerned with the problem of response variability or the *stability* of the instrument; the second, with test variability or test *equivalence.* Stability is generally measured by a test-retest method: after an initial testing, the same test or a test composed of similar items is given again to the same subjects in order to discover how much the scores vary with time. Equivalence is measured by testing two groups with comparable forms of a test; often a test is divided in half, and the results of the two halves are compared (split-half reliability).

Standard Error of Measurement. The concept of reliability underlies the computation of the standard error of measurement. This is a particularly useful measure in the interpretation of individual test scores, and it can readily be understood in the following way. If a single child, John, were given an IQ test, say, 100 times, we would find that any number of chance circumstances would cause his scores to vary somewhat. These deviations would fall in a normal distribution around John's mean score, which we can interpret as his true score. One standard deviation ($+1\ \sigma$) of this distribution is defined as the standard error of measurement. If John's mean score on the tests were 100 and the standard error 5, this means that he has a 68 per cent (or two to one) chance of scoring between 95 and 105 if tested again.

If many children are repeatedly given a test, we can easily compute the standard error of measurement of the instrument by using the following formula:

$$\text{s.e.} = \sigma\sqrt{1 - r}$$

Here, σ is the standard deviation of the test scores, and r is the test-retest reliability coefficient (which is explained later). The smaller the standard error of measurement, the more assurance we can have that the score of a child on any test will not vary appreciably from scores obtained at any other time.

Correlation. In discussing reliability and validity, we have frequently mentioned the comparison of test scores, both those obtained with the same instrument and those obtained from different tests. To understand the data relating to these comparisons, it is necessary to discuss briefly the measurement involved in studying relationships.

A coefficient of correlation (denoted by r) is a quantitative statement of the degree of relationship between two sets of scores (variables). While it is unnecessary to explain the mathematical derivation of a correlation coefficient, it is necessary to know what it stands for, since statements of reliability and validity are given in this mathematical form.[6] Coefficients range from $4 = +1.00$ to $r = -1.00$. Plus 1.00 indicates a perfect linear relationship between two variables; that is, given one, you know exactly what the other is. In mathematical terms, $y = Cx$ for *all* measured values of x and y, and some constant C. The coefficient -1.00 also indicates a perfect linear relationship of the form $y = -Cx$. Zero correlation ($r = 0.00$) indicates a random distribution or no relationship at all; one value of x can correspond to any value of y. Intermediate values of r indicate varying degrees of linear dependence of y on x, as can be judged from the relative "fatness" of the scatter diagrams in Figure 6–4.

If you know that two tests correlate perfectly, you obviously need not test on the second, since x has perfect predictive value. Equally obvious is the fact that such perfection does not exist. Since measurement errors alone dictate that no two tests will correlate perfectly, we must constantly deal with correlation coefficients of intermediate value, where the predictive power of x is only approximate. These correlations can be deceptive. A correlation of 0.60 does not imply a 60 per cent relationship or that $x = Cy$ in 60 per cent of all cases. To understand the actual meaning of a coefficient, it is necessary to square it. The value r_{xy}

[6]There are several methods of calculating a coefficient of correlation. The most widely used is the *product-moment* method given by the formula:

$$r = \frac{\Sigma\, xy}{N\, \sigma_x\, \sigma_y}$$

Here, σ_x and σ_y are the standard deviations of the x and y distributions.

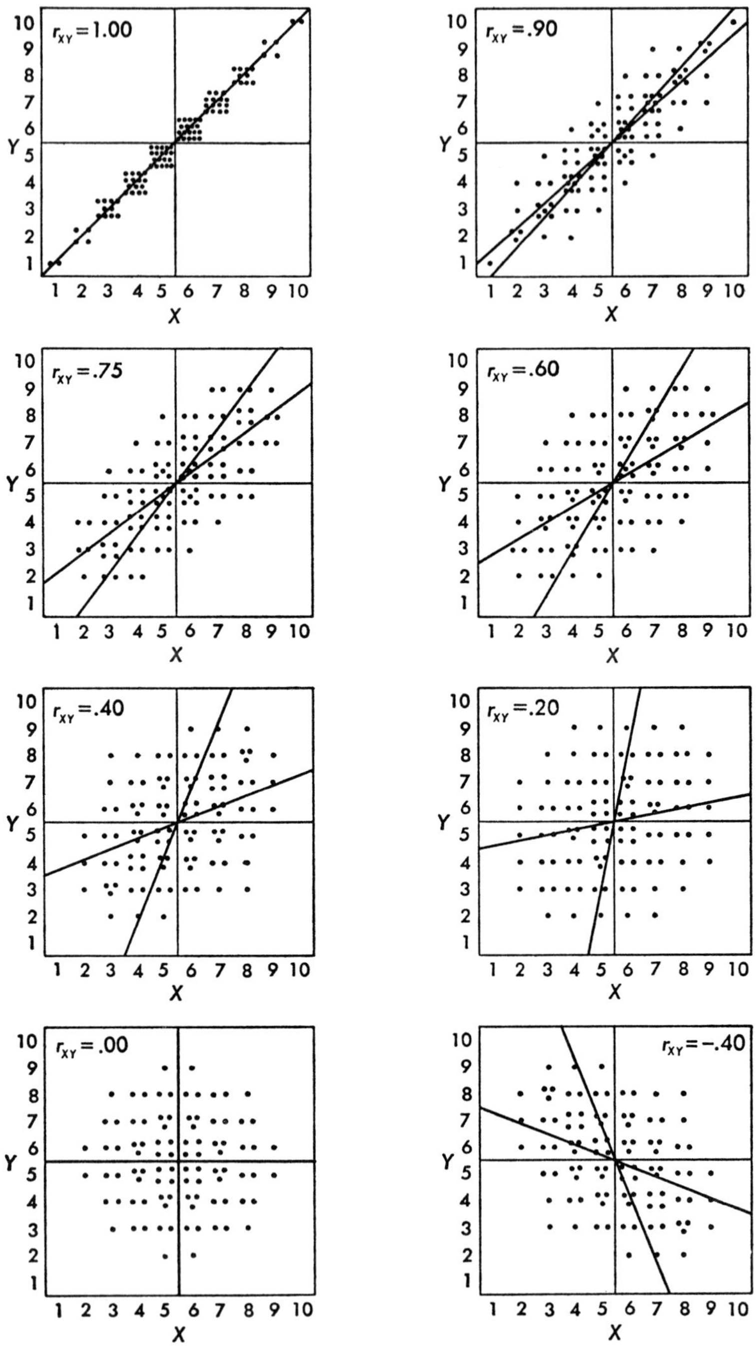

Figure 6–4 Scatter diagrams yielding correlations of various sizes. (*From* Cronbach, 1960, p. 114.)

*Table 6–2 Comparisons of Results Obtained From Kuhlmann-Anderson Seventh Edition Tests, the Revised Stanford-Binet Intelligence Scales, and the Wechsler Intelligence Scale for Children**

K-A Booklet	Group	N	Range	Mean	S.D.	Other Test	Range	Mean	S.D.	r
K	Kdgn	108	67–170	118.6	19.10	S-B, L	79–142	116.0	14.7	.70
K	Kdgn	75	85–171	115.7	16.0	S-B, L-M	66–155	115.7	17.0	.56
B	Grades 2 and 3	31	62–109	80.6	13.0	S-B, L, L-M	65–108	84.4	11.8	.65
CD	Special Class	34	52–91	68.8	9.6	WISC	54–93	71.1	10.0	.69

*This is an illustration of the statistics of validity. The Kuhlmann-Anderson, a group intelligence test, is shown to have concurrent validity with reference to the WISC and the Stanford-Binet at the .56 to .70 level. (From *Technical Manual for Booklets K, A B, and CD, Kuhlmann-Anderson Test,* 7th ed. Princeton, New Jersey; Personnel Press, 1963, Table 6, p. 19.)

= 0.60 actually implies that 0.36 or 36 per cent of the total variability of y can be attributed to a linear dependence on x. Another way of expressing it is that the error of prediction (as indicated by the "fatness" of the scatter diagram) is only about 100 per cent − 36 per cent or 64 per cent of what it would be had we paired values of x and y in a completely random fashion. This may not sound particularly impressive, but in fact it is indicative of a rather good linear relationship. In general, a psychologist views a correlation of 0.60 as high. (See Table 6–2.)

This discussion has mentioned only the fundamentals, and much has been left unexplained; it is entirely possible, for example, that a small correlation in some circumstances is exceedingly good, while a high correlation that was reached by using an unrepresentative or a very small sample is totally insignificant. The point most in need of emphasis here is that while a correlation implies a linear relationship, it does not imply that x causes y. Someone has found that the number of illegitimate births in New York City has correlated over many years with the price of rum in Havana. If a causal link exists, it is certainly an obscure one; the correlation is spurious, since, in fact, it just happens that both indices are on the rise.

In summary, correlation forms the basis for determining the validity and reliability of tests which seek to measure the same quantity; we should expect the scores of different IQ tests to intercorrelate highly. We should, however, treat with a good deal of suspicion any correlations which are based on small or biased samples, or which purport to measure the "relatedness" of tests measuring two entirely different quantities.

Sources of Information

Since the foregoing discussion merely introduces the topic of methods of assessment, the reader is referred to other sources for a more comprehensive treatment of the problem. Obviously, the primary source of information concerning a test is the test manual. For the person who is only indirectly involved with testing, however, manuals are usually unavailable. Besides, manuals are designed to *sell* the test and are seldom sufficiently self-critical. The most indispensable set of references are the various editions of Buros' *Mental Measurements Yearbook* (1938–1965). These volumes not only list tests, authors and publishers, but they also contain one or more independent critical reviews of each instrument. Such reviews usually cover both the test manuals and the pertinent research publications. Two valuable texts which also deal with this material are Anastasi's *Psychological Testing* (1968) and Cronbach's *Essentials of Psychological Testing* (1969).

AREAS OF TESTING

Having covered the basic concepts associated with assessment, we wish now to introduce the reader to some specific areas of testing. These areas —intelligence, personality and infant study—are delineated in order to illustrate several of the many diverse constructs which underlie various approaches to measurement. Since the scope and variety are enormous, only a limited number of tests can be presented here. The tests selected for inclusion are representative of those the physician will probably encounter most frequently. The theoretical and methodological information discussed in this section should, however, enable the physician to evaluate the materials given for any test in the Buros yearbooks. The most common tests in current use are listed in Table 6–3. Though many are not covered in the following text, most will become familiar to any frequent reader of psychological reports.

Intelligence

Before moving to a discussion of particular tests, we must first deal with the issue of intelligence. It is a subject we approach with some degree of temerity, for it is a concept whose impact on society has had few parallels. Intelligence is a ubiquitous term, and not many people are unconcerned about this facet of their personality. In the aftermath of early Soviet space achievements and a sudden awareness of the sophisticated technological foundations of our era, "intelligence" has become a major civic concern verging on a national hang-up.

But what is intelligence? This question has precipitated some of the most heated arguments in psychology, yet the only certainty that remains is the lack of agreement on an answer. Within the framework of this chapter, then, we can only hope to provide some insight into the reasons for this current state of affairs. We wish to say something about the nature of the controversies, about what "intelligence" is *not* and about those misconceptions of intelligence which must be avoided.

The "problem of intelligence" can, perhaps, be most easily understood in terms of the difference between *content* and *process* (Zigler, 1967; Tuddenham, 1966). The distinction is a fundamental one and can be illustrated using a medical analogy. The physician who practiced in the era before the advent of bacteriology and virology, for example, could measure various physiologic signs—body temperature, pulse rate, depth of respiration—and use his measurements to *classify* a disease; i.e., to reach a diagnosis. But none of the signs he measured, despite the ease with which they could be compared to the norms of functioning, revealed anything about the underlying disease *process* under observation. Consumption was as likely the act of God as it was the onslaught of a bacillus. Furthermore, early signs of abnormality in body functioning could often lead to any of several disease outcomes—death, debility or cure. The medical analogy will prove to be an imperfect one when applied to psychology (where, for one thing, intelligence is not a disease, and the "norms" of mental functioning are ambiguous), but hopefully this point is clear: the *content* of measurement does not necessarily reveal anything about the *process* which determined those measurements, nor does the content necessarily predict the ultimate outcome of a situation governed by a process which is imperfectly understood (though the accumulation of signs does lead to a more accurate prognosis).

To apply this argument to the issue of intelligence we must briefly examine the evolutionary history of the concept. Early in the development of formal psychology, "intelligence" was the province of those investigators interested either in the construction of tests or in the application of mathematical techniques to the analysis and understanding of test results. Those in the former group were little concerned with the theoretical underpinning of their work; their major efforts focused on solving such pragmatic problems as educational classification in a new era of universal schooling. Most of the early "intelligence" tests were thus clearly empirical devices designed to meet specific social needs. This is not to stay that early test constructors did not define intelligence; the designer had to have some definition, either implicit or explicit, in order to select test items. However, the numerous definitions posited by this *ad hoc* method were usually simple omnibus statements emphasizing such qualities as the ability to reason, to learn, to solve problems or to adapt to new situations.

None of this, however, tells us what intelligence "is." (Is it all of these qualities? Some? A weighted average? None?) We now know something of how test items were selected but still nothing of the process which will determine *all* the outcomes, not just, for example, that of school grade placement. All we have, really, is a rubric, a term operationally defined by a test. We have in this approach nothing that tells us very much about the general nature of cognitive functioning.

The first "theoretical" attempt to explain intelligence derived from the mathematical analysis of test scores. In 1904, Charles Spearman, applying the technique of factor analysis[7] to a number of different tests, proposed that all intellectual activities were comprised of two components: a general factor (the well-known "g" factor of his equations), which was common to all intellectual abilities, and a series of specific ("s") factors, which were to be found only in particular kinds of abilities. Spearman's two-factor (or two-component) theory marks the beginning of the factor-analytic approach to intelligence. As a school of thought today, factor analysis is divided on the global *versus* the specific nature of intelligence. This is, however, less a philosophical than a technical controversy, since the demonstration of a general factor depends largely on which of the many available factorial techniques is used in the analysis.

But again, the factorialists, although having made important contributions to the understanding of the extent and relatedness of human differences, have approached the nature of intelligence in a contextual manner. They have examined the tests used to measure intelligence in order to arrive at the meaning of a concept which simply is not delimited by those tests.

As one might expect, the factor-analytic technique leads us directly to the heredity-environment (or "nature-nurture") controversy. Spearman tentatively identified his "g" factor as "mental energy," an atomistic, irreducible psychic entity. Could this not be a hereditary factor? The controversy, of course, did not develop in this simplistic fashion, but the issue is clear. Are tests valid

[7]Factor analysis is a complex mathematical technique which reduces a large set of intercorrelated test scores to smaller subsets of test scores, thus enabling the researcher to answer the question of how many different basic variables account for the variation in the performance on a variety of tests.

Table 6–3 Tests Commonly Used in Assessment

NAME OF TEST	AGE RANGE	TYPE OF TEST
Arthur Point Scale of Performance Tests	5 to 15 years	Nonlanguage performance test of general ability (I)*
Bayley Infant Scales of Development	2 to 30 months	Infants' general ability (I)
Blacky Pictures	5 years and over	Projective technique (I)
Bender Visual-Motor Gestalt Test	Children and adults	Diagnostic: intellectual impairment associated with organicity (I)
Cattell Infant Intelligence Scale	3 to 30 months	Infants' general ability (I)
Children's Apperception Test	3 to 10 years	Projective technique (a downward extension of the TAT) (I)
Culture Fair Intelligence Test (Cattell)	4 years to adult	Nonculture test of general ability; not dependent on language ability (G)**
Durrell Analysis of Reading Difficulty	Grades 1 to 6	Achievement test: comprehension of oral and silent reading, rate, word recognition and analysis (I)
Gates-McKillop Reading Diagnostic Tests	Grades 3 to 10	Diagnostic: reading disabilities (I)
Gesell Developmental Schedules	4 weeks to 6 years	Infant behavior development (I)
Goldstein-Scheerer Tests of Abstract and Concrete Thinking	Children and adults	Diagnostic: intellectual impairment (I)
Goodenough-Harris Drawing Test	5 to 15 years	Nonverbal general mental ability (G)
Illinois Test of Psycholinguistic Abilities	4 to 10 years	Abilities and disabilities associated with communication (I)
Interim Hayes-Binet Test for the Blind	3 years to adolescent	Special test for the blind: general mental ability (I)
Kuder Preference Record—Vocational	Grades 9 to 12; adults	Vocational interests (G)
Leiter International Performance Scale	2 to 18 years	Nonculture test for foreign-born and deaf children (I)
Lincoln-Oseretsky Motor Development Scale	6 to 14 years	Motor development: coordination and motor speed (I)

*I = Individually administered tests.
**G = Group administered tests.

Table 6–3 Continued

Name of Test	Age Range	Type of Test
Machover Draw-a-Person Test	Children and adults	Projective technique (I)
Make A Picture Story Test (MAPS)	6 years and older	Projective technique (I)
Merrill-Palmer Scale of Mental Tests	18 months to 6 years	Nonverbal mental ability (I)
Minnesota Multiphasic Personality Inventory (MMPI)	Older adolescents and adults	Self-report personality inventory (G)
Porteus Maze Test	3 years to adult	Nonlanguage test of mental ability (I)
Progressive Matrices (Raven's)	8 years to adult	Nonverbal general ability (I,G)
Rorschach	Children and adults	Projective technique (I)
Rosenzweig Picture Frustration Test	4 years to adult	Projective technique (I)
Rotter Incomplete Sentences Blank	Adolescents and adults	Projective technique (I)
Stanford-Binet Scale (Revised): 1937–Terman and Merril–Forms L and M; 1960–Form L-M	2 years to adult (not standardized for older adults)	General ability (intelligence) (I)
Thematic Apperception Test (TAT)	Children and adults	Projective technique (I)
Vineland Social Maturity Scale	Birth to maturity–especially children	Social maturity (I)
Wechsler Adult Intelligence Scale (WAIS)	16 years to adult	General ability (intelligence), verbal and performance scales (I)
Wechsler-Bellevue Intelligence Scale Forms I and II	10 years to adult	General ability (intelligence), verbal and performance scales (I)
Wechsler Intelligence Scale for Children (WISC)	5 to 15 years	General ability (intelligence), verbal and performance scales (I)
Wechsler Pre-School and Primary Scale of Intelligence (WPPSI)	4 to 6½ years; bright 3, dull 7 and over	General ability (intelligence), verbal and performance scales (I)
Wide-Range Achievement Test	Kindergarten to college	Achievement in reading, spelling and arithmetic (I,G)

measures of intelligence? Is the IQ constant? Is heredity the primary determinant of intelligence? Needless to say, the "facts" have accumulated in support of both sides of the issue, and to attempt an adjudication lies far beyond the scope of our intentions.

At present, in fact, the controversy has subsided—or at least metamorphosed—somewhat. Intelligence is generally conceded to be a hypothetical construct and is also viewed as the product of some unspecified interaction between heredity and environmental factors. Nevertheless, albeit in a more sophisticated form, the controversy still manages to re-emerge—witness the recent furor stimulated by Jensen's (1969) consideration of the genetic contribution to the intelligence of various racial groups.

To return to our content-process distinction, the wide acceptance of the study of cognition (for which psychologists are indebted to the work of Jean Piaget) indicates that active and exciting attempts are underway to understand the processes involved in intellectual functioning. More important for the area with which this chapter is concerned, researchers are beginning to construct assessment techniques based upon this new knowledge (Laurendeau and Pinard, 1968; Tuddenham, 1970).

However, as the Jensen debate indicates, the new concern with the analysis of process has not entirely replaced the prior concern with content. But for the most part there has been a shift of emphasis. Theoreticians no longer deal with the issue of whether cognitive or intellectual development is due to genetic or environmental factors alone, "but rather with the central question of the exact degree of malleability of the cognitive structure and the related question of how particular environmental inputs affect particular aspects of cognitive development" (Zigler and Butterfield, 1967, p. 2). Malleability is the key word; the search for the *extent* to which the environment may usefully be manipulated has now superseded the search for the *absolute* potential of the infant or child.

This discussion is not intended to discourage the reader utterly, but rather to point out that "intelligence," which forms the basis for so many crucial decisions, should not be accepted glibly on the basis of misconception, the popular notion of intelligence or the social need to transform every child into a genius.

Obviously we should not throw out the baby with the bath water; tests do serve the useful classificatory purposes for which they were designed. But extreme caution should be exercised in the use of IQ test information. The intelligence test yields an IQ score, which is nothing more than an indication of a person's ability level at a given time as compared to a normative age group. It is a measure of the present ability of the child regarding knowledge which is associated with academic institutions and is practically useful as a predictor of the child's ability to profit from instruction. On the other hand, it does not define a child's ability to learn new skills or acquire new knowledge, nor does it define the manner in which he might do this.

In conclusion, we would like to cite one description of what an adequate theory of intelligence should be:

> It should provide a rational basis for the construction of single-score and multi-score tests of intelligence and aptitude; it must account for the empirically known relationships among them—and between them and the usual criteria of educational and vocational success. . . . It must provide an explanation of the curve of change in ability throughout the entire life span from earliest infancy to senescence, and allow for the fact that performances involving different test content wax and wane at different rates and shift

in their differentiation from one another at different life stages. It must take into account the influences of brain damage and disease, sensory and motor impairment, infection, and drugs of various kinds. It must comprehend the facts on family resemblance in level and organization of abilities, accumulated in fifty years of research on the role of heredity in human differences. At the same time it must account for the demonstrated influence of education and training in altering test performance, including data on differences associated with schooling, class level, ethnic group membership, language, generation, etc. And lastly, it should be at least congruent with psychological theories of learning and motivation and theories on other levels of investigation and description, e.g., neurophysiology, biochemistry, genetics, etc.[8]

Obviously, psychology has a long way to go.

Stanford-Binet Scale. It is appropriate that our discussion of individual tests begin with one of the oldest and most successful of psychological instruments. In 1904 Alfred Binet and his coworkers, working under the auspices of the Ministry of Education in Paris, began to study methods which might identify those children attending public school who could not profit from such education. The 1905 Binet-Simon Scale was constructed to meet this practical demand. The test was composed of 30 items designed to elicit information pertinent to a variety of functions which Binet regarded as essential components of intelligence. Judgment, reasoning and comprehension were given highest consideration. The 30 items, arranged in ascending order of difficulty, had been standardized on both a group of approximately 50 normal children, ages 3 to 11, and an unspecified group of retarded children.

The initial success of the instrument led Binet to revise and improve his scale in 1908. The major change in this revision was a grouping of tests into age levels. All the tests that the "normal" 3-year-old could pass were identified and placed together, and an identical procedure was followed for each year to age 13. This revision meant that the child's test score could now be expressed in terms of a "mental age." A child who could do the five-year tests, but none of those at the six-year level was given a mental age (MA) of 5. The child with a chronological age (CA) of 5 and a MA of 5 was considered average. A second revision in 1911 merely extended the scale to the adult level. Since then, the Binet has been translated into English and has undergone three subsequent revisions: in 1916; in 1937, when Forms L and M were created; and in 1960, when the present Form L-M was published. These revisions were made under the direction of L. M. Terman at Stanford University, and the tests are now called the Stanford-Binet.

Terman's 1916 revision of the Binet was so extensive that it created virtually a new test. Over one-third of the items were new, and many former items were changed or discarded. This scale was standardized on an American population of approximately 1000 children and 400 adults. Included for the first time also was the concept of IQ, which had originally been developed by William Stern. The IQ was simply the ratio of a child's mental age to his chronological age, multiplied by 100 to eliminate the decimal point. For example, the child with an MA of 9 and a CA of 8 has an IQ of $9/8 \times 100$ or 113. The IQ, then, expresses a child's mental growth up to the time of testing, revealing how far ahead or behind he is relative to a peer group of the same chronological age.

The second Stanford revision (1937) consisted of two equivalent

---

[8]Tuddenham, R. D.: The nature and measurement of intelligence. *In* Postman, L. (Ed.): *Psychology in the Making.* New York, © Alfred A. Knopf, Inc., 1966, pp. 516–517.

forms, L and M. These were restandardized on another American population of 3184 subjects. There were approximately 100 children at each half-year interval from age 1½ to 5½, 200 at each one-year interval from age 6 to 14 and 100 at each one-year interval from age 15 to 18. Geographical distribution was taken into consideration, and testing was conducted in 17 communities located in 11 widely separated states. An attempt was also made to include a representative sample of the various socioeconomic levels, but the sample was somewhat higher in socioeconomic status than was the general population. In addition, all the subjects were white.

The final 1960 revision was designed to incorporate the best aspects of Forms L and M. The result was a new and single form, L-M. The selection of items for Form L-M was based on the performance of approximately 4498 subjects ranging in age from 2½ to 18 years, who had taken either Form L or Form M between the years 1950 and 1954. Obsolete items were eliminated. However, the test was not restandardized, and consequently it reflects the ethnic and socioeconomic biases of the 1937 Forms.[9] In addition, the conventional ratio IQ was replaced by the deviation IQ.

The tests on the 1960 Stanford-Binet are grouped into age levels ranging from 2 years to Superior Adult. Between the ages of 2 and 5 the test levels correspond to half-year intervals; between the ages of 5 and 14 the test levels correspond to yearly intervals. The remaining four tests are called Average Adult, and Superior Adult I, II and III. There are six tests for every test level with the exception of the Average Adult level, which contains eight tests. An alternate test is provided for each level. (The test can also be adminis-

[9]It should be noted that there have been various attempts at the standardization of the Stanford-Binet on ethnic groups. See, for example, Kennedy (1963).

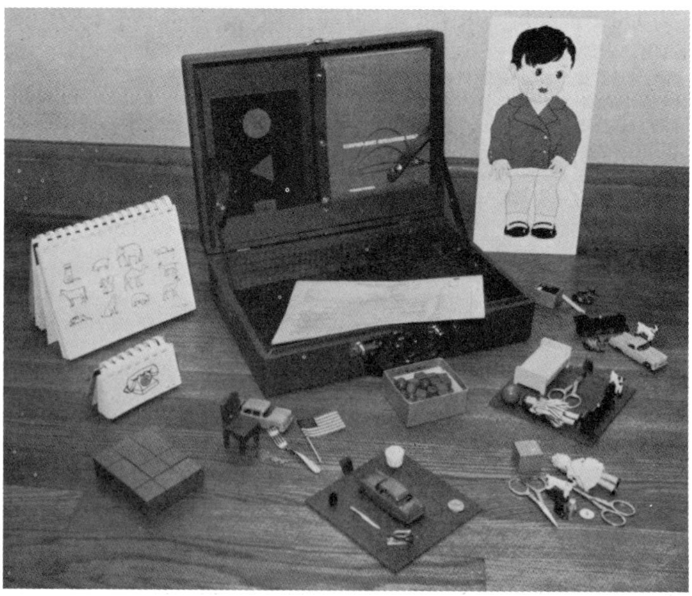

Figure 6–5 Test materials employed in administering the Stanford-Binet. (*From* Anastasi, A., 1968, p. 193. Courtesy Houghton Mifflin Company.)

tered in an abbreviated form, which includes only four of the six tests at each level.) Figure 6–5 shows the test kit and materials included in the Stanford-Binet. As can be seen, most of the items in the picture are those used with younger children. The various items on the Stanford-Binet range from simple manipulative tasks to tests of abstract reasoning. Test items at the younger age levels involve manipulation of objects (such as block building—year 2), identification of objects (identifying things according to their use—years 2 to 6) and various tests of eye-hand coordination (copying a circle—year 2, copying a square—year 5 and copying a diamond—year 7). Tests of upper age levels employ primarily verbal items involving sentence completion, analogies, and vocabulary, though it should be noted that similar items do appear in lower level tests.

The Stanford-Binet is administered individually and must be given by a trained examiner. When giving the test, the examiner first establishes rapport with the subject. The first items administered are below the level expected of the child. This is done in order to establish the *basal age*—the scale level at which the child passes all tests. The tests for higher levels are then given in order until the child fails *all* tests at some level (the ceiling level).

For example, if a child is 9 years 8 months and appears to be approximately normal, he is given items for year 9. Assuming that he passes all items at level 9, he is next given items for level 10. Should he pass all but one item in level 10, items in level 11 are given. Here perhaps he passes only four items. At year 12 he succeeds in completing three items. Let us assume at year 13 he fails all items. The test terminates at this point. The child's MA is calculated as follows:

Year		*Score in Months*
9	All tests passed	108 (basal age)
10	Five tests passed	10
11	Four tests passed	8
12	Three tests passed	6
13	All tests failed	0
		132 = 11 years 0 months

Using the 1960 revision and the deviation IQ, the child's MA would be 11-0. This combined with the CA 9 years 8 months yields a deviation IQ of 110. The examiner is not, however, interested only in IQ; for diagnostic purposes he will analyze the test record carefully for any information (such as strengths or weaknesses in functioning) which will contribute to the overall assessment of the child.

In general the Stanford-Binet is considered to be one of the most reliable standardized intelligence tests. Reported reliability coefficients for the various ages and IQ levels of the Binet are all in the 0.90 range. The error of measurement is approximately 5 IQ points, indicating a two to one probability that the IQ attained by a child in one testing differs from his true Stanford-Binet IQ score by 5 or less points. Chances are 99 to 1 that the score varies by no more than 13 points. It should be noted that the test is more reliable for older than for younger (i.e., below 6 years) children and also for lower than for higher IQ's. The Stanford-Binet should not be used for adults or for brighter subjects over the age of 15. Obviously, it stresses verbal abilities, and its validity with bilingual, disadvantaged and dyslexic subjects is questionable.

Numerous concurrent and predictive validity studies have been conducted, most of them utilizing academic achievement as the criterion. Validity coefficients usually fall between 0.40 and 0.75 with, as would be expected, higher coefficients for highly verbal criteria. In general, the Stanford-Binet is one of the best instruments of its kind.

Wechsler Scales. Although designed to be administered on an individual basis and for many of the same purposes as the Stanford-Binet, the Wechsler Scales differ from the earlier test in several ways. In terms of organization, the Wechsler groups similar items of a given type into subtests arranged in increasing order of difficulty, while the Stanford-Binet groups dissimilar items into discrete age-level tests. Further, the Wechsler is designed to yield both a *performance* and a *verbal* IQ, and the subtests are arranged accordingly. Wechsler intended his scales to provide not only a measure of intelligence but also assessment information relevant to a psychiatric diagnosis. As it turned out, the tests have proved most useful as measures of general intelligence.

The first form of the Wechsler scales was published in 1939 as the Wechsler-Bellevue Intelligence Scale. Its purpose was to provide an adequate IQ test for adults. Although quite similar to the Bellevue, the Wechsler Adult Intelligence Scale (WAIS), published in 1955, was designed to alleviate the technical shortcomings of the former scale, particularly with regard to the reliability of various subtests and to the size and representativeness of the normative sample. Standardization of the WAIS used 1700 individuals—an equal number of men and women distributed over seven age levels between 16 and 64 years. Geographical location, urban-rural residence, race, education and occupational level were representative of the 1950 United States Census.

The WAIS is composed of 11 subtests: six comprise the verbal scale, and the other 5 make up the performance scale. The verbal scale tests include information, comprehension, arithmetic, similarities, digit span and vocabulary. The performance scale subtests are digit symbol, picture completion, block design, picture arrangement and object assembly. Performance tests take into consideration both speed and accuracy. Each subtest yields a standard score with a mean of 100 and a standard deviation of 3. Verbal, performance and full scale scores are expressed as a total of the scaled scores, which in turn, through appropriate tables, are converted into deviation IQ's with a mean of 100 and a standard deviation of 15. The errors of measurement reported for the WAIS are 3 points for the verbal subtests, 4 points for the performance subtests and 2.60 for the full scale. These values compare favorably with the Stanford-Binet error of measurement of 5 points.

Frequent correlations have been run between the WAIS and the Stanford-Binet. With random adult samples, the validity coefficients cluster around 0.80, whereas lower correlations are reported for more selected samples such as college students. The highest correlations are found between the Stanford-Binet and the WAIS verbal scale, whereas the correlations between the Stanford-Binet and the performance scale are relatively low. In general, older and duller subjects tend to attain higher IQ's on the WAIS than on the Stanford-Binet. Although much of research pertaining to the WAIS has been reported (Guertin, et al., 1966), more systematic validity data are needed. Despite this fact, the WAIS has proved to be an extremely useful general measure of adult intelligence.

Apart from its use as an intelligence scale, the WAIS has been extensively studied as a diagnostic instrument. Through a variety of analyses applied to an individual's subtest scores, numerous systems of clinical interpretation have been proposed (Rapaport, 1945). As yet, however, investigations have offered little empirical support for such

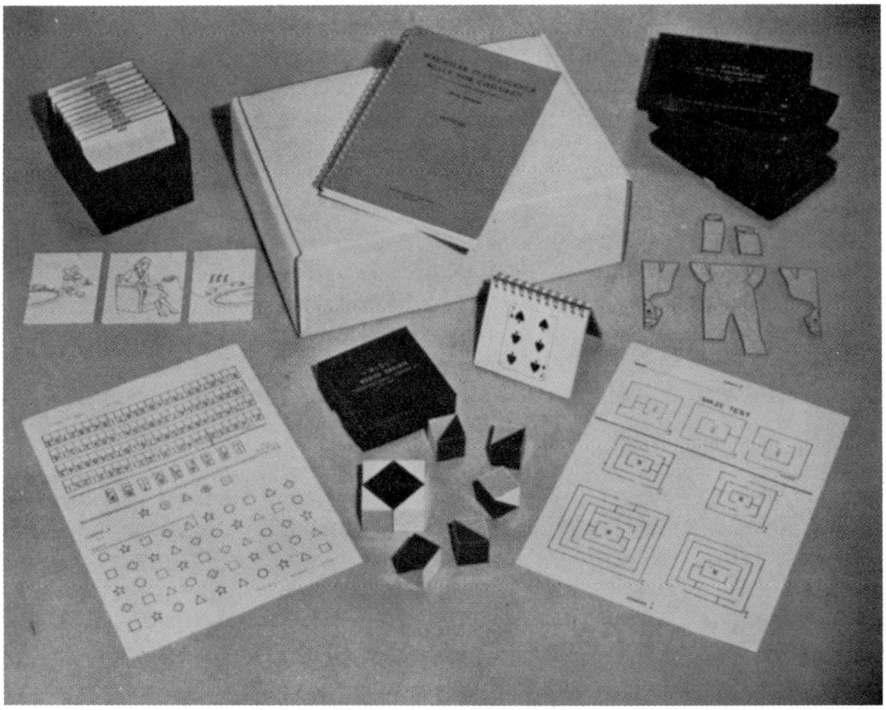

Figure 6–6 Materials used with the Wechsler Intelligence Scale for Children. (*From* Anastasi, A., 1968, p. 283. Courtesy the Psychological Corporation.)

procedures. Still, the WAIS can yield a wealth of qualitative data which can often suggest new hypotheses to the clinician.

The Wechsler Intelligence Scale for Children (WISC), published in 1949, is very similar in organization to the WAIS. It consists of 12 subtests, two of which are used as alternate or supplementary tests. (See Fig. 6–6.) The subtests are also grouped into verbal and performance scales. The standardization sample included 100 boys and 100 girls at each age level from 5 to 15 years, totaling 2200 individuals. A small, institutionalized, mentally retarded sample was included. The children were taken from 85 communities in 11 states; geographical area, urban-rural residence and parental occupation are representative of population distributions in the 1940 United States Census. All of the children were white. Again, the overall reliability coefficients are high (0.86 and above), and the standard errors of measurement range from 3.00 to 5.61 IQ points. Subtest reliabilities, however, are lower, and interpretation using subtest scores should take this into consideration. Comparisons of the WISC with the Stanford-Binet are for the most part 0.80 and above, but it should be noted that the Stanford-Binet yields higher scores than the WISC for brighter and younger subjects, while the WISC yields a significantly higher IQ for the mentally retarded. As with the WAIS, more validity data are needed, though in general the WISC compares favorably with other scales of intelligence. Although most clinicians find the WISC valuable as a diagnostic instrument, it should be cautioned that the clinical interpretation systems developed for the WAIS are in no way applicable to the younger WISC sample.

The most recent Wechsler scale, published in 1967, is the Wechsler Pre-School and Primary Scale of Intelligence (WPPSI) for children 4 to 6½ years of age. Of 11 subtests, eight are downward extensions of WISC subtests; three are newly constructed. The verbal and performance subtests are administered alternately. They include information, vocabulary, arithmetic, similarities, comprehension, animal houses, picture completions, mazes, geometric designs, block designs and a supplementary memory test. Standardization included 100 boys and 100 girls in each of six, one-half year age groups from 4 to 6½—1200 children in all. Using 1960 United States census data, geographical area, father's occupation, urban-rural residence and ethnic group were taken into consideration in the selection of the standardization sample. Reliabilities for both subtests and overall scales are reported to be in the 0.80 to 0.90 range. According to the manual, for a group of 98 children ages 5 to 6 years, the correlation coefficient with the Stanford-Binet is 0.75. Unfortunately, the recency of publication precludes any statement concerning the validity and usefulness of the WPPSI.

Personality

As was necessary in the case of intelligence, our discussion of personality assessment must be introduced with a few words concerning the construct which underlies the instruments. However, since much of this material is presented in Chapter 7, our comments will be quite brief. We may begin with what is perhaps the most conventional definition of personality; namely, that of Allport: "Personality is the dynamic organization within the individual of those psychophysical systems that determine his unique adjustments to his environment" (1937, p. 48). However, as Nevitt Sanford has pointed out, eminent psychologists engaged in the study of personality do not agree about "what the elements of personality are, how they are organized, what the boundaries of personality are, and how personality interacts with other phenomena" (1968, p. 587).

Given that the conceptual systems developed to explain personality have emanated from such diverse sources as clinical practice, experimental psychology and social anthropology, it is hardly surprising that a great diversity of opinion exists. Despite disagreements, however, the current literature dealing with personality indicates that there is fairly good agreement as to what the problems are, and a healthy questioning of traditional assumptions is increasing. The reader is referred to Sanford (1963) and Hunt (1965) for a further discussion of the issues involved, and to Zigler and Child (1968) for an attempt to synthesize the data and theory from the many relevant fields of study.

To some extent the issues in personality parallel those which characterize the construct of intelligence. For example, the nature-nurture controversy takes the form of intrinsically *versus* extrinsically motivated behaviors. (Is behavior dependent primarily upon factors within a person or upon the external circumstances which obtain in any given situation?) As with intelligence, resolution of the issue requires an interactionist outlook. Similarly, the content-process distinction in the measurement of intelligence is applicable to the measurement of personality. Interestingly, current literature also is beginning to stress the role and importance of cognitive processes in the development of personality. Clearly, Tuddenham's criteria for an adequate theory of intelligence, cited earlier, are also applicable to any presumptive theory of personality.

Despite the similar problems involved in defining the constructs of personality and intelligence, however, the measurement of personality affords considerably less precision and predictive power than does intelligence testing. Hopefully, the reasons for this will become clear in the discussion which follows. For the present we wish only to emphasize that "personality" must be approached with the same objectivity that one applies to any ambiguously defined set of ideas.

Projective Techniques. Projective techniques are only one type of "personality test"; other instruments, such as the self-report inventories—notably the Minnesota Multiphasic Personality Inventory (MMPI)—and some interest tests, are also included under this rubric. In general, personality tests are those instruments used in the measurement of motivational, interpersonal, attitudinal and emotional characteristics, as opposed to abilities, which are measured by the intelligence, achievement and aptitude tests. Structured personality tests like the MMPI differ from the unstructured or projective techniques primarily in the freedom of response permitted the subject. Structured tests require the subject to choose among a limited number of responses (e.g., True? False? Cannot say?), while projective techniques give the subject complete freedom to form his own response.

Projective techniques are currently in wide use in clinical assessment, especially with children. Despite widespread usage, however, psychometric standards like validity and reliability are not conventionally applied to projective tests as they are to structured tests. Accordingly, anyone using projective measures should know as much as possible about them. At the same time it must be stressed that *both* kinds of personality tests require clinical interpretation before any prediction can be made.

An example of the rationale underlying the use of projective techniques in assessment is given in the following statement by Frank (1939, pp. 402–403):

> We may approach the personality and induce the individual to reveal his way of organizing experience by giving him a field (objects, materials, experiences) with relatively little structure and cultural patterning so that the personality can project upon that plastic field his way of seeing life, his meaning, significance, patterns, and especially his feelings. Thus, we elicit a projection of the individual personality's *private world* because he has to organize the field, interpret the material and react affectively to it.

Whether one should accept the assumptions implicit in this and other similar approaches to the measurement of personality (e.g., a response to an ambiguous stimulus reflects the personality of the subject) is at present an unanswered research question. That it is not an easily answered question is revealed by the voluminous experimental literature on projective techniques (Zubin et al., 1965; Megargee, 1966). The methodological approaches devised to ascertain reliability and validity are beset with difficulties. The major problem is in the search for reliable external criteria against which to validate the tests. With tests of intelligence, for example, objective criteria, such as academic grades, are relatively easy to define. Criteria for projective tests (such as the frequently used psychiatric diagnostic classification) are often as badly in need of validation as the technique itself. Among the many problems which further complicate validation and plague the test constructor are the meaning of a subject's response, the manner in which it should be classified and interpreted and, above all, what determines it.

Why should research continue in so murky and recalcitrant an area of clinical study? We can only offer the explanation given by one team of researchers: "Some of the claims and clinical hunches which the experimentalists now disdain may become cornerstones of new, objective findings when the more powerful tools of the future become available" (Zubin et al., 1965, p. 611).

Again, the ambiguity in the area of personality testing is not presented to confuse but rather to emphasize the care which should be utilized when considering psychological reports that deal with the interpretation of projective techniques. At present, such tests can best be considered clinical tools which contribute to the formation of the hypotheses used by the qualified clinician.

Rorschach. One of the most widely known and provocative projective tests is the Rorschach. In this test the subject is asked to relate what he sees in a series of 10 inkblots. The blots (see Fig. 6–7), because of their irregular and ambiguous forms and colors, lend themselves to a wide variety of interpretations. The technique was devised by Hermann Rorschach, a Swiss psychiatrist who initially used the blots in an experimental study of the form perception of various groups of psychiatric patients. His scoring system was published in 1921 and was elaborated and revised by subsequent investigators, notably Beck (1945, 1952), and Klopfer et al. (1954).

During the administration of the Rorschach, the examiner keeps a verbatim record of the subject's responses, carefully noting his behavior and his emotional and verbal expressions. Systematic questioning of the subject with regard to each of his responses is undertaken after the 10 cards are presented.

Interpretation of the Rorschach can be based on fairly objective systematic scoring systems. Although various schemes have been developed, the most common categories of scores are location, determinants, content and popularity. Location scores indicate, for example, whether the subject responds to the whole blot, commonly perceived subdivisions or unusual details in the blot. Determinant scores are concerned with whether the subject takes into account such elements as form, color, shading and "movement" of the blot. The content scores are based primarily upon the general class of the thing seen—persons, animals, anatomical features and so forth. Finally, a popularity score is determined by comparing the subject's response with what are known to be the most frequent responses to a particular card. For example, Card V is popularly referred to as a bat flying, but it might also, with some creativity, be described as a ballet dancer, arms outstretched and outfitted with wings for her portrayal of a butterfly.

Although the scoring of the Rorschach utilizes systematic procedures, the interpretative process is highly elaborate and not a subject for the neophyte. In general, originality and number of responses have been associated with the subject's intelligence and productivity. Location scores are most often associated with intellectual orientation and variations in conceptual ability. With regard to the determinant scores, color responses are related to emotionality and to a subject's reactivity to his environment; form responses, to intellectual objectivity; movement responses, to spontaneity and imagination; and shading responses to such diffuse emotional states as anxiety. Frequent responses in specific categories—such as parts of the anatomy—may indicate a particular type of concern or difficulty, but the interpretation of content scores is always considered subordinate, though integrally related, to determinant factors.

Some examples of Rorschach responses may help to clarify how a

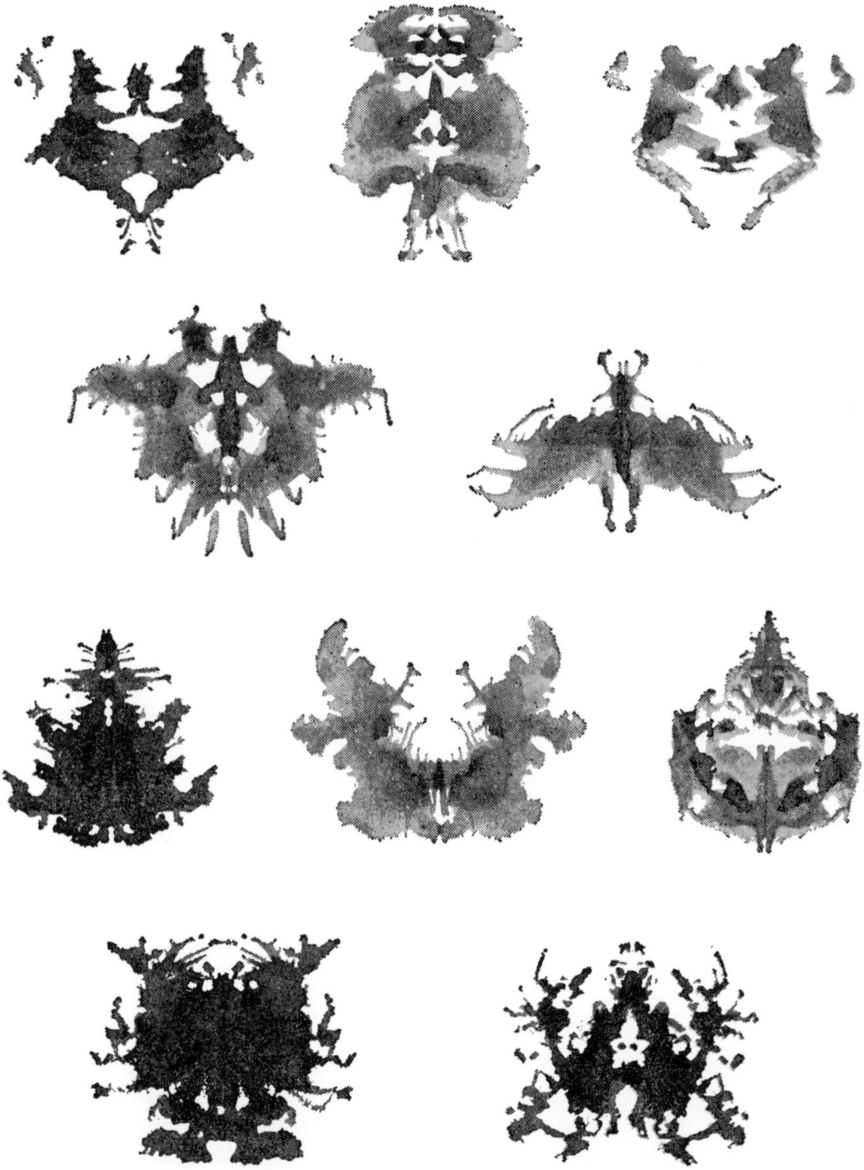

Figure 6–7 Rorschach inkblots. When the test is administered, each blot is presented on a separate card. (Reproduced with permission from Kleinmuntz: Personality Measurement. Homewood, Illinois, the Dorsey Press, 1967 c., p. 269.)

response is scored and also the difference between a normal and pathological response. In general, pathological thinking is characterized by excessive concreteness or looseness in a subject's perception of the blot. For example, Card I is frequently seen as a butterfly. Such a response would be scored as a whole response, appropriate form, animal content, and popular. Looseness and shifting of perceptual boundaries and an extreme affective elaboration of the central portion of Card I characterizes the following response: "A baby being born . . . no—going to be delivered because he's still under the skin . . . it's trying hard to come out . . . it has hands and feet . . . it's like an x-ray of the stomach . . . yes—it's the mother . . . I'm not sure who the hands and feet belong to."

Another sign of pathology, particularly in adults, is the confabulation of whole responses. Such as response generally reflects an accurate perception of some part of the blot with concomitant distortion of the remaining area. The following response to Card III (generally perceived as two human figures) exemplifies confabulation:

Answer: "It's a girl dressed up for Sunday school."
Examiner inquiry: "A girl? Could you show me?"
Answer: "Right here, this is her bow."
Inquiry: "Can you tell me any more about it?"
Answer: "No—her bow—makes her going to Sunday school."

Another pathological response (in an adult) can be seen in this response to Card IX, which incorporates a type of primitive logic. Referring to the lower central portion of the blot, the response was: "The South Pole—because it's at the bottom."

One last illustration should be included to give the reader an idea of the type of response often obtained from a "normal," highly intelligent subject. For Card III consider this whole response, which is human and has good form and movement. "Here we have two dancing girls swinging about some type of gymnastic equipment . . . their dresses are flying out and their hats have fallen off as they whirl about."

It must be emphasized, however, that clinical hypotheses are the result of looking at the total body of responses and not at a single response such as has been given in the examples. A single poor form response is meaningless, whereas numerous such responses would suggest to the clinician a variety of hypotheses regarding the person's ability to deal with reality. These hypotheses would, in turn, be strengthened or weakened by other characteristics of the protocol (e.g., content scores) and ultimately by all of the other data accumulated in the assessment.

Although the Rorschach may be used with children, the normative data was derived mostly from an adult population. Ames (1952, 1954, 1959) has published norms on children between the ages of 2 and 10 and on adolescents from age 10 to 16. However, interpretation of children's Rorschach results should be extremely guarded. Children are just as likely to react to momentary emotional states or to last night's Chiller Theater as they are to reveal significant personality characteristics. Furthermore, developmental differences among children must also be given careful consideration.

The validity and reliability of the Rorschach have long been matters of contention (Holzberg, 1960). Studies indicate that the Rorschach is neither reliable nor valid in terms of traditional test criteria. It is at best, therefore, a clinical tool which can provide suggestive and corroborative data in the hands of a skilled clinician.

Thematic Apperception Test. Another well-known and widely used projective technique is the Thematic Apperception Test (TAT), developed by H. A. Murray and his colleagues at the Harvard Psychological Clinic. In contrast to the Rorschach, the TAT employs rather highly structured stimuli (Fig. 6–8) and requires a subject to answer in a more meaningfully organized manner.

The test materials presented to any one subject consist of 19 black and white pictures and one black card, which are administered in two one-hour sessions (10 cards each). There are actually 31 TAT cards available. From these, a selection is made of 20 of the most pertinent cards for boys, girls, males over 14 and females over 14 (i.e., there are four overlapping

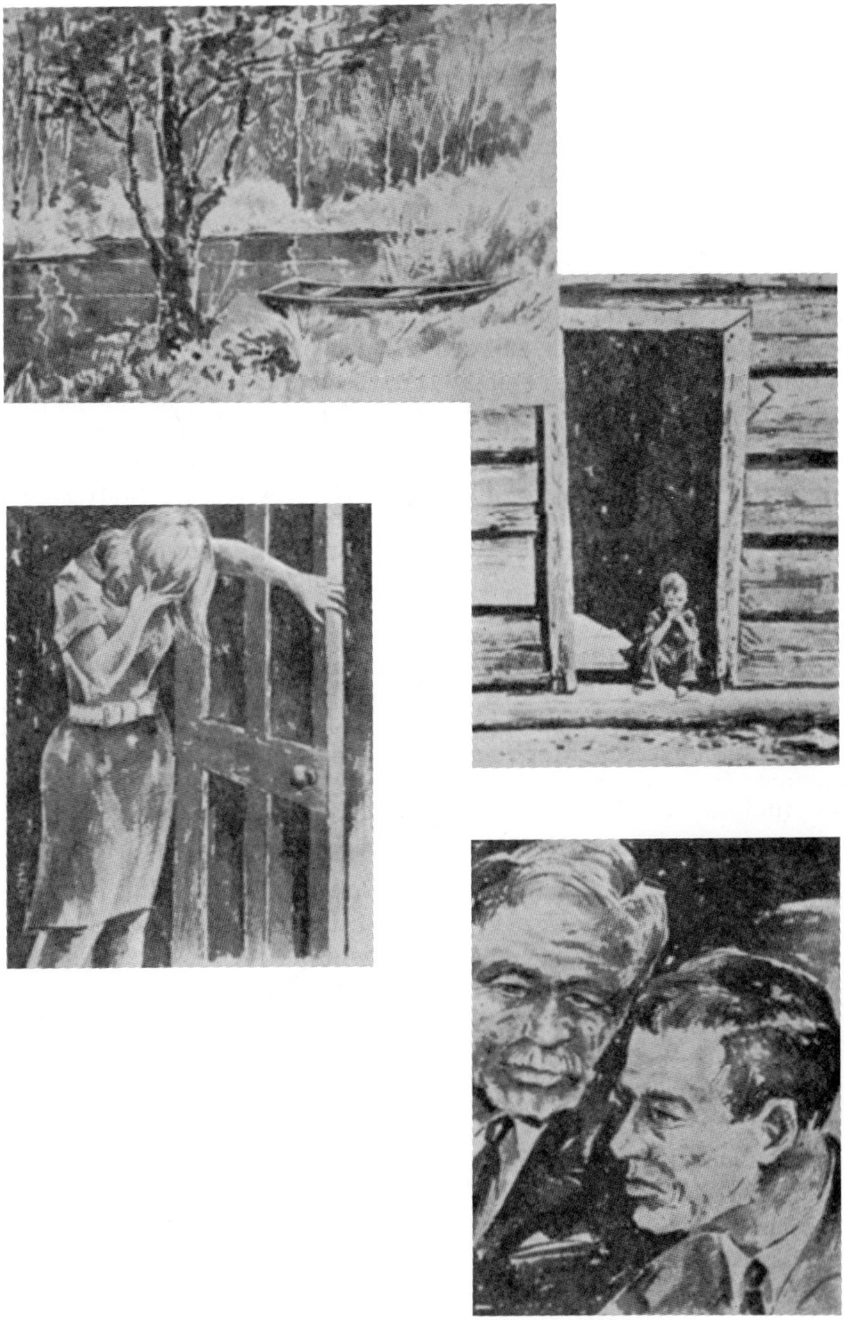

Figure 6–8 Several illustrations of scenes that appear on the TAT cards. (Reproduced with permission from Kleinmuntz: *Personality Measurement.* Homewood, Illinois, The Dorsey Press, 1967 c., p. 269.)

sets of 20 cards each). Each card is administered individually. The subject is directed to interpret the pictures by telling a story about what is happening in the picture, what events led to the scene portrayed, what the characters are thinking and feeling and the eventual outcome of the story related.

Interpretation of the TAT is based upon the assumption that a person, in relating his story, will identify in the central character ("hero") of his story those attributes which are or have been significant components of his own personality. Further, it is assumed that other characters in the story will be likened to such people as the person's parents or siblings and that the plot will be created from actual or fantasied events which have been of major significance in the development of the person's personality. In general, the analysis of the content of the stories is based upon the motivational determinants of personality suggested by Murray's theory of needs and presses. Needs are those motivational variables which emanate from within the person; they include, among over 20 others, the needs of nurturance, achievement and aggression. Presses are those forces from the environment which interfere with or facilitate the satisfaction of an individual's needs. Being praised or criticized by another person, being loved or being faced with a physical danger such as an angry dog are illustrations of presses. The frequency, intensity, duration and uniqueness of the need and press themes in the stories are used to assess the relative strength of needs and presses in the subject.

While the Rorschach has only two or three popularly accepted scoring systems, numerous methods of scoring have been devised for the TAT. Few of these, however, have achieved widespread use in the clinical setting. This is equally true with regard to normative data. Although normative information has been published on various aspects of the TAT responses, such as speed of response, themes developed, emotional tones expressed and roles of characters, clinicians generally use such data as a framework for interpretation rather than as rigid guidelines. This is probably due to the fact that the highly structured stimulus of the TAT readily lends itself to the creation of subjective, idiosyncratic systems of interpretation based upon a clinician's "personal" collection of "normative" data. A much greater dependence on norms is required by the ambiguous projective methods.

Although it is not possible to present and analyze a variety of TAT responses, a consideration of several of the factors to which clinicians attend in interpretation may help clarify the use of the TAT. For example, the card which depicts a young woman standing with her head down and her face covered with her hand (see Fig. 6–8) is generally interpreted as conveying a negative emotional quality. It should therefore elicit a theme which deals with the causes of the woman's emotional state and tells what she should do about it. For the most part, a theme conveying a happy emotional quality is not a "normal" response to this picture. Referring back to needs and presses, the reader can easily see how such a picture would elicit information pertaining to the person's dependency and nurturance needs and the type of environmental presses which would foster such needs. Who or what, for example, has caused her problem? How can she or someone else solve her problem?

Again, it must be emphasized that the formation of clinical hypotheses from the TAT, as with the Rorschach, is possible only in the context of the total body of information derived from the assessment. Similarly, the questionable reliability and validity of this instrument classifies it chiefly as a clinical tool, not a psychometric instrument.

Bender Visual-Motor Gestalt Test. The Bender Visual-Motor Gestalt Test may appear to be a somewhat anomalous inclusion in this section on personality tests. It was developed as a test of visual perception to study children and adults with psychological disorders, and it is widely employed as a projective technique. Of late, however, it has gained popularity as an informal test of neurological impairment. It is probably this latter use of the Bender as a test of organic disorder that physicians will encounter more frequently.

Based upon figures employed by Wertheimer in his studies of Gestalt principles, the Bender consists of nine designs, which the subject is instructed to copy (Fig. 6–9). Each design is presented as a black line drawing on a three inch by five inch card. The Bender is most commonly administered on an individual basis, each card remaining in the subject's view while he reproduces it. Reproduction from memory is the most common variation on this basic format.

Although subjective interpretation is perhaps most common, several objective scoring systems have been devised for both adults (Pascal and Suttel, 1951) and children (Koppitz, 1964). Koppitz' work includes norms for children between the ages of 5 and 10 years; for children between 6

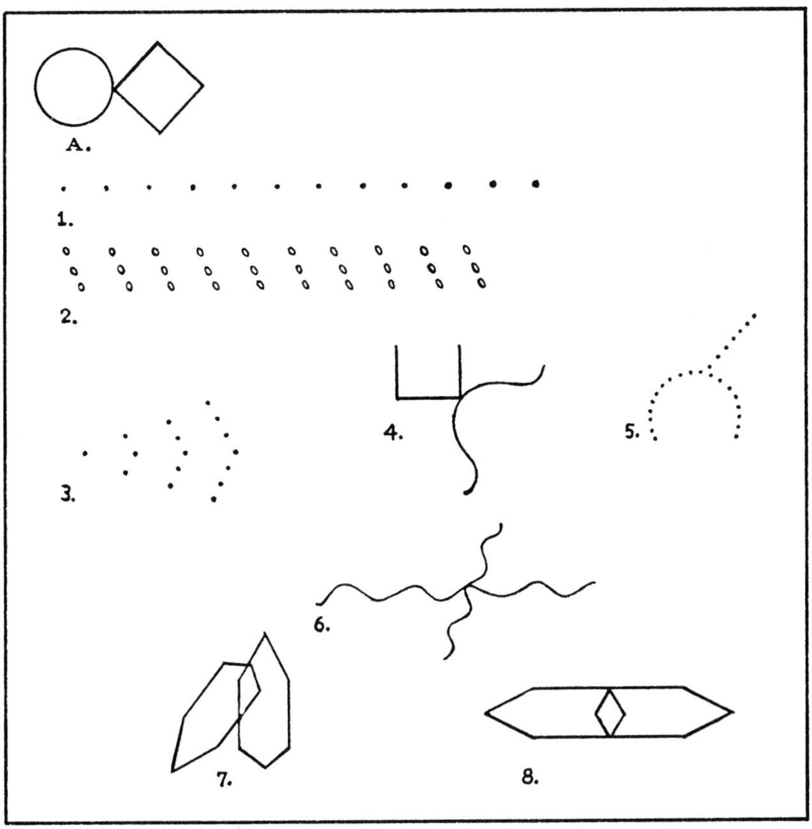

Figure 6–9 The figures for the Bender Visual-Motor Gestalt Test. (Copyright, The American Orthopsychiatric Association, Inc. Reproduced by permission.)

and 12 years, normative data have been presented by Armstrong and Hauck (1960). For a summary and evaluation of the numerous ways in which the Bender Visual-Motor Gestalt Test has been administered, evaluated and "validated," the reader is referred to Tolor and Schulberg (1963). While some satisfactory reliability data are reported for various scoring systems, however, validation studies are for the most part inconclusive (Billingslea, 1963).

Interpretation of the test is associated with various misrepresentations of the original designs. For example, evidence for neurological impairment is associated with such test signs as the production of angles for curves, rotation of the figure through an angle greater than 45 degrees, perseverations and disproportioned figures. Test signs for psychopathology include the association of heavy lines with hostility, of exact replication with obsessive-compulsive behavior and of overlapping figures with thought disorganization. It should be pointed out, however, that interpretation of the Bender is deceptively easy. Because it is simple to administer and does not have the inherent ambiguity of tests like the Rorschach, it is subject to much use and misuse by untrained persons. It is advisable to be particularly aware of the limitations of this test when reading reports based upon it.

Clinically, the test is most useful as an aid in the diagnosis of organic pathology in groups like the mentally retarded and the senescent, in the determination of readiness for reading and in assessing perceptual-motoric immaturity. Unfortunately, in younger children the signs of organic disorder, emotional disturbance and immaturity are difficult to differentiate. Needless to say, brain injury does not reveal itself as a single set of behavioral patterns, and the many complicating factors, such as developmental status, extent of injury and locus of injury, are just beginning to be investigated. A great deal of research is yet required if we are to understand the precise behavioral correlates of a given physiological disorder.

Infant Study

Within the field of psychology, certainly the past 10 years have belonged to the infant. In that time the infant has emerged from the role of a somewhat passively reactive organism to that of an active participant in his environment, capable of initiating behavior and, in his own manner, solving problems. Not only has the past decade been characterized by an increase in the sheer volume of infant research, but it has also seen a significant growth in methodological sophistication. These developments, coupled with the modification of psychology's previous conception of intelligence, have led to important changes in our approach to infant assessment.[10]

To date, however, most attempts to demonstrate the usefulness of infant tests in predicting future intellectual development have met with little success. Repeated studies (Anderson, 1940; Bayley, 1955; Cavanaugh et al., 1957) have supported the conclusion that "mental tests" administered during the first year of a child's life are of little value in predicting later intelligence. Although this generalization has been challenged (Knobloch and Pasamanick, 1960), an adjudication of the evidence suggests that most current infant "tests" should be considered as useful appraisers of the health and developmental status of an infant rather than as instruments of prediction. They provide the examiner with the means

[10]For an excellent critique and review of the history, development and content of infant tests, see Stott and Ball (1965); also, Thomas (1970).

to obtain objective and quantifiable data concerning current behavioral functioning and, with the exception of extreme cases of retardation or precocity, may be seriously misleading concerning the future.

The physician, however, should be aware of the fact that poor predictive validity is hardly the only criticism leveled at most current infant scales. Limited norms, inadequate manuals and lack of theoretical rationale have been cited as limitations. The utmost caution should therefore be exercised in the use and interpretation of infant tests.

Such criticisms, of course, do not preclude the possibility of developing infant tests with predictive validity. Several investigators (Uzgiris and Hunt, 1966; Escalona and Corman, 1967) are currently engaged in the construction of infant scales based on Piaget's theory of intelligence.[11] Although more research is needed to evaluate such approaches, they are indicative of attempts being made to meet the limitations of previous scales. They are statistically more sophisticated, and they show an increasing concern with the establishment of a relationship between tests and theories of development.

In light of the criticism which has been leveled at all currently available infant scales, the following brief review of several of the most common "tests" will concern itself primarily with content rather than with questions of reliability or validity.

Gesell Developmental Schedules. The first attempt to evaluate the behavioral development of infants began in 1919 when Gesell and his associates embarked upon a series of longitudinal studies to collect normative data. Although the total normative sample included 107 infants, only small portions of this sample were seen at any one time for the repeated observations required of a longitudinal study. Also, only middle-class, white, American-born infants were used. The Gesell Developmental Schedules, then, can best be described as a standardized procedure for evaluating and observing the behavioral development of a child.

The Schedules are designed to assess four areas of behavioral development: motor, adaptive, language and personal-social. The data collected are based upon direct observation, the child's response to standard stimulus objects and supplementary information reported by the mother. The manual provides detailed descriptions (verbal and pictorial) of the behavior typical of different age levels from 4 weeks to 6 years. Although it is primarily qualitative in nature, the Gesell Schedules have had an immeasurable influence on infant testing. Items from the Gesell Schedules have been incorporated in almost all subsequent infant scales.

Cattell Infant Intelligence Scale. The Cattell Scale is a widely used test, developed as a downward extension of the 1937 Stanford-Binet Form L. The scale, which groups items into age levels, extends from ages 3 to 30 months and yields mental age and IQ scores. A combination of Stanford-Binet, Gesell and original items is employed. The standardization sample consisted of 274 white, middle-class children, with varying numbers of these children being retested at 3, 6, 9, 12, 18, 24, 30 and 36 months.

Test items at the youngest age levels, similar to the Gesell, are largely perceptual in nature (e.g., following a dangling ring with the eyes); an attempt was made, however, to restrict the use of motor items which might depend largely on home training. Complex manipulatory tasks (e.g., pegboards) and verbal tasks (following oral instructions) are introduced as the age of the child increases.

The Cattell is less difficult to administer and is shorter in length than the Gesell. In general, it is also considered to have a more objective scoring system than the Gesell.

Bayley Infant Scales of Development. The Bayley Infant Scales represent one of the best standardized instruments of its kind. Released in 1968 after several years in research form, the Scales are a revision and standardization of the California First-Year Scale, which was developed for use in the Berkeley Growth Study (Bayley, 1968). Test items are drawn from Gesell, Cattell and newly developed materials. The Scales, which yield a Mental Development and a Psychomotor Development Index, present standard score norms for each of 14 age groups from 2 to 30 months. An Infant Behavior Record is also provided for rating the qualitative (interpersonal and affective) aspects of behavior.

The Bayley Scales were standardized on a sample of more than 1200 infants and children. The sample was controlled for age, sex, urban-rural residence, parental education and race. Considering the care and research which has gone into the construction of these scales, they should prove to be an extremely useful instrument for those involved in the evaluation of infants.

INTERPRETATION AND COMMUNICATION OF ASSESSMENT INFORMATION

It is appropriate that the concluding section of this chapter focus on the issues involved in the interpretation and communication of assessment information. Although we have dealt briefly with these topics throughout the chapter, it remains necessary to emphasize their significance in the context of the total process of assessment.

The written psychological report sent to a referring agency is not a simple compendium of test findings, but rather an interpretative statement of psychological data obtained from observations, interviews and tests. The reasons for this synthetic approach are numerous. Test findings can be misinterpreted, misunderstood and misused by someone who is unaware of the limitations and significances of test results. (For an example, the reader is referred to Gilbert's [1966] report on the banning of group intelligence tests by the New York City Board of Education in 1964.) Stated simply, test scores must be interpreted in light of the myriad of factors that may influence them. To illustrate our meaning, we can use the following "molecular" example. The Year VII section on the Stanford-Binet begins with a test item called Picture Absurdities. One of the pictures is of a man and a woman sitting in the rain. The child is presented with the picture and asked, "What's funny about that picture?" Let us assume that the child either doesn't answer, or says, "I don't know" or "Nothing." Since this is an "intelligence test" item we might be led to conclude that the child simply is not "smart" enough to answer the question. He doesn't know the answer.

Such a conclusion is, of course, unwarranted. The child's statement does not directly reveal whether he can understand the absurdity. To understand clearly why this is so, consider the following questions which are raised by this one incorrect response and which must be evaluated in the light of the implications they hold for the results of the test as a whole:

1. Can the child see the picture? (Is his vision normal? Is the room well lighted?)

2. Can he visually organize the picture? (What is his visual perceptual ability? Is he familiar with the objects in the picture?)
3. Can he hear the instructions? (Is his hearing normal? Are there distracting noises?)
4. Can he understand the instructions? (Does he have difficulty with auditory perception? Can he understand the meaning of the words?)
5. Can he indicate what is wrong with the picture? (Can he express himself verbally?)
6. Will he indicate what is wrong with the picture? (Is he anxious? Is he afraid? Is he bored?)
7. Has anyone ever told him to come in out of the rain?

Obviously, the child may be dull, but one or several of these factors, or other factors not mentioned, could be responsible for his incorrect response. Accordingly, a test score which is a composite of many molecular items cannot be reported as a number alone. A test is a measure of behavior, and the measure itself must be interpreted. The interpretation of tests depends upon the user's knowledge of human behavior and his skill as a clinician.

However desirable it might be to eliminate the need for such subjective interpretation, it remains an essential feature of assessment at all levels. This can be summarized in the following way. The psychologist must (1) interpret the meaning of the referral request (see p. 278) in order to choose appropriate test materials and to formulate meaningful questions and hypotheses, (2) interpret the observational, interview and test data obtained, (3) interpret how these data interrelate and how they correlate to data from other sources and (4) interpret the meaning of the treatment in order to define the possible effects of alternative solutions to the problem in question. Because the interpretation of a test score does not exist in a vacuum, and because final interpretation of assessment data must be made relevant to the questions to be answered and the decisions to be made, it is evident that the psychologist and the physician must work closely together. As Levine, referring to the psychologist in the role of a consultant, has stated (1968, p. 560):

> You cannot be of any service to the person making the referral unless you can specify what decision he is facing, what alternatives are available to him, what the utility or value of these alternatives is, and finally, what relevance test data and observation have in terms of specifying outcomes for each of the alternatives once they are adopted.

If the psychologist is to be a useful consultant to a physician (and vice versa), these needs must be met.

SUMMARY

In retrospect, a more appropriate title for this chapter might have been "Assessment in Transition." The rigid traditional model of assessment has undergone a rather radical change, and several more plastic and sophisticated models have emerged. Major constructs, such as intelligence and personality, are also being revised in the light of both new research findings and an increase in our understanding of human behavior. Obviously this will continue to have an important effect on both the construction and the interpretation of tests.

This chapter has attempted to reflect these trends and to present the physician with some of the information necessary to evaluate the present and future utility of assessment in his work with patients. Hopefully, it will help enable him to consult wisely.

Above all, we have stressed the need for enhancing the communication between the psychologist and the physician. How these professionals can work together to their mutual satisfaction and the greater benefit of the patient is clearly a question still open to research.

ACKNOWLEDGMENTS

Preparation of this article was facilitated in part by the U.S. Children's Bureau, PHS Grant Number CB-12HSP-906. The author would like to thank Jerome Kagan, Susan Litzinger, Steven Reiss, Abby Sheldon, Ann Sandor and Bruce Smith for their critical reading of the manuscript. Also, thanks are due to Maureen Tedesco, Ellen Scott, Ellen Barreto, Rosalind Schultz, Sylvia Goldstein and Mary Selvey for their help in typing various parts of the manuscript.

REFERENCES

Allport, G. W.: *Personality: A Psychological Interpretation.* New York, Holt, Rinehart & Winston, 1937.

Alpert, Joel J.: The function of the family physician. *Conn. Med., 32*:663–666, 1968.

American Psychological Association: *Standards for Educational and Psychological Tests and Manuals.* Washington, D.C., 1966.

Ames, L. B., Learned, J., Metraux, R. W., and Walker, R. N.: *Child Rorschach Responses: Developmental Trends from Two to Ten Years.* New York, Hoeber Medical Division, Harper & Row, Publishers, 1952.

Ames, L. B., Learned, J., Metraux, R. W., and Walker, R. N.: *Rorschach Responses in Old Age.* New York, Hoeber Medical Division, Harper & Row, Publishers, 1954.

Ames, L. B., Learned, J., Metraux, R. W., and Walker, R. N.: *Adolescent Rorschach Responses: Developmental Trends from Ten to Sixteen Years.* New York, Hoeber Medical Division, Harper & Row, Publishers, 1959.

Anastasi, Anne: *Psychological Testing,* 3rd ed. New York, The Macmillan Company, 1968.

Anderson, J. E.: The prediction of terminal intelligence from infant and preschool tests. *39th Yearbook of the National Society for Studies in Education,* 1940, Part I, pp. 385–403.

Armstrong, R. G., and Hauck, P. A.: Correlates of the Bender-Gestalt scores in children. *J. Clin. Psychol., 11*:153–158, 1960.

Arthur, A. Z.: Diagnostic testing and the new alternatives. *Psychol. Bull.,* 72:183–192, 1969.

Barker, R. G. (ed.): *The Stream of Behavior: Explorations of its Structure and Content.* New York, Appleton-Century-Crofts, 1963.

Bayley, Nancy: On the growth of intelligence. *Amer. Psychol., 10*:805–818, 1955.

Bayley, Nancy: Behavior correlates of mental growth: Birth to thirty-six years. *Amer. Psychol., 23*:110–117, 1968.

Beck, S. J.: *Rorschach's Test. A Variety of Personality Pictures.* New York, Grune & Stratton, Inc., Vol. II, 1945.

Beck, S. J.: *Rorschach's Test. Advances in Interpretation.* New York, Grune & Stratton, Inc., Vol. III, 1952.

Billingslea, F. Y.: The Bender Gestalt: A review and a perspective. *Psychol. Bull., 60*: 233–251, 1963.

Buros, O. K. (ed.): *Mental Measurements Yearbooks.* Highland Park, New Jersey, Gryphon Press, 1938–1965.

Buros, O. K. (ed.): *Reading Tests and Reviews.* Highland Park, New Jersey, Gryphon Press, 1968.

Buros, O. K. (ed.): *Personality Tests and Reviews.* Highland Park, New Jersey, Gryphon Press, 1969.

Cavanaugh, M. C., Cohen, I., Dunphy, D., Ringwell, E. A., and Goldberg, I. D.: Prediction from Cattell Infant Intelligence scale. *J. Consult. Psychol., 21*:33–37, 1957.

Cronbach, L. J.: *Essentials of Psychological Testing,* 3rd ed. New York, Harper & Row, Publishers, 1969.

Escalona, Sibylle K., and Corman, H. H.: The validation of Piaget's hypothesis concerning the development of sensori-motor intelligence: methodological issues. *Presented at the Society for Research in Child Development.* New York City, March, 1967.

Flavell, J. H.: *The Developmental Psychology of Jean Piaget.* Princeton, New Jersey, Van Nostrand Reinhold Company, 1963.

Frank, L. K.: Projective methods for the study of personality. *J. Psychol., 8*:389–413, 1939.

Gilbert, H. B.: On the IQ ban. *Teachers College Record,* 67:282–285, 1966.

Guertin, W. H., et al.: Research with the Wechsler Intelligence Scales for Adults: 1960–1965. *Psychol. Bull., 66*:385–409, 1966.

Holzberg, J. D.: Reliability re-examined. *In* Rickers-Ovsiankina, Maria A. (ed.): *Rorschach Psychology.* New York, John Wiley & Sons, Inc., 1960, p. 361–379.

Hunt, J. M.: The traditional personality theory in the light of recent evidence. *Amer. Sci., 53*:80–96, 1965.

Jensen, A. R.: How much can we boost IQ and scholastic achievement? *Harvard Educational Review, 39*:1–123, 1969.

Kennedy, W. A., Van De Reit, V., and White, J. C.: A normative sample of intelligence and achievement in Negro elementary school children in the southeastern United States. *Monogr. Soc. Res. Child. Develop.,* 1963, Vol. XXVIII, No. 6.

Klopfer, B., Ainsworth, Mary D., Klopfer, W. G., and Holt, R. R.: *Developments in the Rorschach Technique. Technique and Theory.* New York, World Publishing Company, Vol. I, 1954.

Knobloch, H., and Pasamanick, B.: An evaluation of the consistency and predictive value of the 40 Week Gesell Development Schedule. *Psychiat. Res. Rep. Amer. Psychiat. Ass., 13*:10–41, 1960.

Koppitz, E. M.: *The Bender-Gestalt Test for Young Children.* New York, Grune & Stratton, Inc., 1964.

Laurendeau, M., and Pinard, A.: *Les Premieres Notions Spatiales de L'enfant.* Neuchâtel, Switzerland, Delachaux & Niestle, 1968.

Levine, D.: Why and when to test: Social context of psychological testing in projective techniques. *In* Rabin, A. I. (ed.): *Personality Assessment.* New York, Springer Publishing Co., Inc., 1968. pp. 553–580..

Lief, H. I., Lief, V. F., and Lief, N. R. (eds.): *The Psychological Basis of Medical Practice.* New York, Hoeber Medical Division, Harper & Row, Publishers, 1963.

Marsden, G.: Content-analysis studies of therapeutic interviews: 1954–1964. *Psychol. Bull., 63*:298–321.

Megargee, I. (ed.): *Research in Clinical Assessment.* New York, Harper & Row, Publishers, 1966.

Pascal, G. R., and Suttell, Barbara J.: *The Bender-Gestalt Test: Quantification and Validity for Adults.* New York, Grune & Stratton, Inc., 1951.

Rapaport, D., et al.: *Diagnostic Psychological Testing.* Chicago, Year Book Medical Publishers, Inc., Vol. I, 1945; Vol. II, 1946.

Sanford, N.: Personality: Its place in Psychology. *In* Koch, S. (ed.): *Psychology: A Study of a Science.* New York, McGraw-Hill Book Company, 1963, Vol. V, pp. 488–592.

Sanford, N.: Personality: The Field. *In* Sills, D. L. (ed.): *International Encyclopedia of the Social Sciences,* New York, The Free Press, 1968, Vol. II, pp. 587–606.

Stott, L. H., and Ball, R. S.: Infant and preschool mental tests: Review and Evaluation. *Monogr. Soc. Res. Child Develop.,* 1965, Vol. XXX, No. 3.

Thomas, Hoben: Psychological assessment instruments for use with infants. Merrill-Palmer Quarterly, *16*:179–223, 1970.

Tolor, A., and Schulberg, H. C.: *An Evaluation of the Bender-Gestalt Test.* Springfield, Illinois, Charles C Thomas, Publisher, 1963.

Tuddenham, R. D.: The nature and measurement of intelligence. *In* Postman, L. (ed.): *Psychology in the Making.* New York, Alfred A. Knopf, Inc., 1966, pp. 469–525.

Tuddenham, R. D.: Psychometrizing Piaget's *méthode clinique. In* Athey, I., and Rubadeau, D. (Eds.): *Educational Implications of Piaget's Theory.* Waltham, Massachusetts, Ginn/Blaisdell, 1970, pp. 317–324.

Uzgiris, Ina C., and Hunt, J. McV.: An instrument for assessing infant psychological development. Unpublished manuscript. February, 1966.

Weick, C. E.: Systematic observational methods. *In* Lindzey, G., and Aronson, E. (eds.): *The Handbook of Social Psychology.* Reading, Massachusetts, Addison-Wesley Publishing Co., Inc., 1968, Vol. II, pp. 357–451.

Zigler, E.: Mental retardation: Current issues and approaches. *In* Hoffman, M. L., and Hoffman, L. W. (eds.): *Review of Child Development Research.* New York, Russell Sage Foundation, Vol. II, 1967.

Zigler, E., and Butterfield, E. C.: Motivational factors and IQ changes in culturally deprived children attending nursery school. Unpublished manuscript, 1967.

Zigler, E., and Child, I. L.: Socialization. *In* Lindzey, G., and Aronson, E. (eds.): *The Handbook of Social Psychology,* 2nd ed. Reading, Massachusetts, Addison-Wesley, Publishing Co., Inc., 1968, Vol. III, Chap. 24.

Zubin, J., Eron, L. D., and Schumer, F.: *An Experimental Approach to Projective Techniques.* New York, John Wiley & Sons, Inc., 1965.

7 PERSONALITY DEVELOPMENT

Jerome Kagan

The phenomena of human growth fall into two patterns: enlargement or change. The leaf expands as it grows but never alters its essential shape. The butterfly passes through dramatically different stages from egg, to larva, to the flying creature that emerges from the chrysalis.

Man illustrates both kinds of development. Bone and muscle become larger and heavier but retain essentially the same structure throughout life. The establishment of adult personality characteristics, however, is subject to major changes during the first 12 years of life. Personality is a murky word that refers to the dimensions of differences among people that are presumed to be relatively permanent. We do not regard eating three meals a day as a personality trait in our culture because most American adults behave this way. But we do regard shyness as a personality attribute because some people are shy and others are bold. A personality trait is a psychological characteristic that is non-normative and theoretically significant. The totality of an individual's personality involves the relation among the actions, motives, beliefs and feelings that differentiate one person from another and display continuity over time. A theory of personality development must trace the connections between the personality of the child and that of the adult in order to understand how the adult organization derived from that of the child. If we understood how an adult personality developed, we could better understand how it functions in adulthood.

Consider two women, similar in temperament, both of whom decided to be professional biologists. One woman is the daughter of a scientist who encouraged her to become a biologist ever since she was in elementary school. Her father spent many evenings reading to her and persuaded her that if she became a scholar he would be very pleased. She was highly motivated to succeed in graduate school because she wanted her father's approval. A second woman initially wanted to be a physicist because a teacher suggested, early in her adolescence, that she had talent in physics. Her parents were neither pleased nor displeased with this choice. After two years of college she decided that physics was too difficult and shifted her interest to biology because it held some interest for her and allowed her to capitalize on her background in science. These two histories supply valuable information for predicting the adult behavior of the two women. The first should persist more strongly in the face of hardship than the second because the choice was closely linked to her family relationships.

A second reason for inquiring into personality development is practical. Behaviors learned in early childhood guide the adoption of future behaviors. It is often of practical importance to be able to predict occupational choice, grades in college or future pathology from behavior displayed during the early school years. Moreover, most of the psychological ills that plague man and society are difficult to modify in the adult. Schizophrenia, suicidal depression, drug addiction and criminality are the result of a long history of specific experiences. If we knew the childhood prodromal signs of these adult symptoms, we might be able to effect prophylactic measures before these tendencies develop.

Sensitive Periods in Development

Many developmental theorists assume that the structures learned in childhood direct the adoption of future behavior and provide a thread of continuity to human development. It is also assumed that there are sensitive periods in development, and experiences during these periods predispose the adult to various psychological structures. The sensitive period notion implies that specific psychological processes are developing rapidly during particular periods of development, and that intrusion during the sensitive period is likely to alter the course of the behavior or structure developing at that time. The term sensitive period refers to those eras when an event has its most dramatic influence on a specific psychological process.

An example of a sensitive period in a child's physical growth is the first three years of life, which constitute the period of most rapid growth in stature. This is also the time when the quality of diet exerts its maximal effect on the adult's final height. There is a relation between the time in which stature is developing most rapidly and the time when it is most vulnerable to environmental deficiency.

Sensitive period phenomena are not as easy to demonstrate in human psychological development as they are in human physical growth or animal development. However, many psychologists regard the first few years of life as a sensitive period for the establishment of a trusting attachment to adults. One can view psychological development as a series of curves, with each curve representing a different psychological process. (See Fig. 7–1.) The sensitive

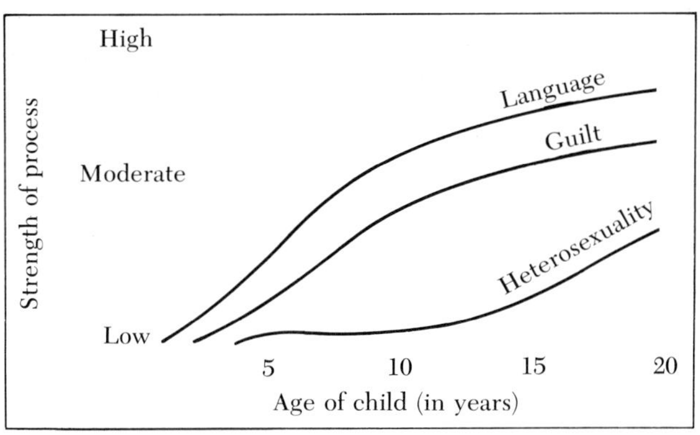

Figure 7–1 Relation of growth of response processes to the age of a child.

period concept assumes that the period during which the slope of each of the curves is maximal will differ according to the psychological process developing at that time.

CONTRASTING CONCEPTIONS OF DEVELOPMENT

Among psychologists there are basic philosophical differences regarding the fundamental nature of the child and his growth. One dimension of controversy involves the degree to which the child is viewed as active or passive in response to his setting. John Locke is the founder of the English empiricist tradition which sees the child as passive in the hands of environmental forces. The child's behavior is molded by experience. The continental tradition, represented by Rousseau, regards the child as actively manipulating and engaging his environment, trying to mold it to his skills and attempting to understand it in terms of his existing knowledge. Behaviorism and psychoanalysis regard the child as passive; while Piagetian theory views him as active.

A second controversy pivots on the degree of continuity to be expected in psychological development. Does the child's behavior progress continually, by gradual accretions and without sudden dramatic shifts, or is the course of developmental progress step-like and segmented into stages. The term stage in psychological theory has no explanatory value but implies that the organization of psychological structures or behaviors is different during the different stages. Most stage theories assume that the child must pass through successive stages in a fixed order. Psychoanalytic theory states that there is a fixed sequence of psychosexual developments, beginning with the oral stage and progressing through the anal, phallic and genital stages. Piaget's theory states that the child passes from the sensory motor stage through the concrete operational stage to the final stage of formal operations. Most stage theories in psychology are descriptive rather than explanatory, for they lack an explicit set of rules that states the mechanisms by which a child progresses from one stage to the next. Behaviorism, which does not make use of a stage concept, is concerned with the processes that produce changes in behavior.

The third controversy turns on whether development proceeds toward an idealized goal, in contrast to an open-ended program like biological evolution, where no special terminal state defines the goal of growth. Freud and Piaget are both idealists. Freud suggested that at psychological maturity the adult would have invested his libidinal energy in a love object and anxiety over sexuality would be minimal. Piaget argues that the capacity for logical reasoning is the goal of development. When the adolescent can solve problems in a systematic and hypothesis-testing manner, he has reached the final stage of formal operations. Behaviorism and modern cognitive theory, by contrast, do not conceptualize development as proceeding in a specific direction. The child is acquiring beliefs and responses, but there is no specifically defined end point that is fundamentally more mature or desirable than another, independent of the culture in which the child is growing. Most psychologists take a position on each of these dimensions that is often implicit rather than explicit. This chapter is dominated by the view that the child is active rather than passive, that there are stages in development, but that there is no idealized goal toward which man is developing, independent of the needs and pressures of his environment.

THEORIES OF HUMAN DEVELOPMENT

Theories of human development have been neither logically rigorous nor successful in accounting for both motivational and intellectual phenomena. The two major approaches to the development of the child's personality have been psychoanalytic theory on the one hand, and social learning theory on the other. The two great theorists of mental development have been Jean Piaget and Heinz Werner.

Personality Theory

There are two critical differences between the conceptions of psychoanalytic theory and of social learning theory with respect to the establishment of individual differences in children. Psychoanalytic theory assumes that there is an ideal state toward which the child is developing. The child passes through a series of stages culminating in an idealized adult state characterized by low anxiety, capacity for sexual satisfaction, effective defenses and an ability for love and work. One of the major concepts of psychoanalytic theory states that the source of fundamental drive energy changes with development. Thus, during the first year of life drive excitation rises in the oral region of the body and the infant seeks gratification through reduction of that excitation. As a result, this period is called the oral stage of development. During the second year of life, the source of excitation shifts to the anal area, and the objects and behaviors that bring gratification change during this anal stage. During the preschool years, the source of excitation shifts to the genitals, and Freud regards this as the phallic period of development. During the final genital stage of development, gratification is sought in a love relationship with another. A second important principle states that although the id is constantly seeking gratification of the major drives of the organism, the ego and superego set limits on this process. As the child grows, the reality principle gradually controls the pleasure principle. Development is primarily concerned with the growth of the ego, which is responsible for the acquisition of behaviors, beliefs and controls that channel the discharge of fundamental drives through thought and defense mechanisms.

Social learning theory takes a more relativistic and arbitrary stance with respect to idealized states of adult maturity. Social learning theory is concerned with the mechanisms that will explain differences in behavior, motives and values among children. The major principles involve the effects of external reward and punishment as administered by parents, teachers and peers, on the child's tendency to adopt the behaviors and values of others.

These two theories also differ with respect to their primary focus. Psychoanalytic theory is concerned with the internal processes surrounding motives, fears and defenses, and only secondarily with behavior. Social learning theory is primarily concerned with overt actions of the child rather than with internal aspects of thought. As a result, the principles and concepts of these theories are different, but they are complementary rather than contradictory.

Theories of Intellectual Development

Piaget and Werner, the two great theorists of intellectual development, both postulate ideal states toward which the child progresses. Piaget's theory is the more detailed and rests on the fundamental notion that the child's mental development passes through stages until he arrives at a stage of thinking that resembles that of the Western adult. The five stages are (1) the sensory motor stage from birth to 18 months, (2) the intuitive stage from 18 months to 3 years, (3) the preoperational stage from 3 to 7 years, (4) the concrete operational stage from 7 to 12 years and (5) the stage of formal operations that characterizes the adolescent and adult.

Most of the research and theoretical concerns have been focused on the last three stages. Prior to the concrete operational stage the child seems unable to reason about several important classes of problems, even though he has adequate language to do so. The first of these problems is the ability to represent a series of actions mentally. Thus, the concrete operational child can have a mental representation of a route he might take to a friend's house. Second, the concrete operational child shows the ability to conserve. He believes that liquids and solids do not change their amount or quantity merely because their external shape changes. Third, the concrete operational child understands relational terms such as darker, bigger and larger, and ceases to think about them in absolute ways. The child is able to reason simultaneously about a part of the whole and the whole. If the 5 year old child is shown eight yellow candies and four brown candies and asked, "Are there more yellow candies or more candies?" he is likely to say, "More yellow candies," because he cannot reason about a part and a whole simultaneously. But the child in the stage of concrete operations answers this question correctly. The fourth characteristic of the operational child is his ability to organize objects along a quantified dimension, called serialization.

The final stage, formal operations, begins at age 12 and is characterized by the adolescent's ability to think about hypothetical problems that are not necessarily in accord with his experience. He is willing to think about possibilities. The adolescent generates all the possible solution hypotheses to a particular problem. Consider the following question, "A man was found in the back seat of a car which had hit a telephone pole. What happened?" A child in the stage of concrete operations might think up a reasonable answer that satisfied him and state it. The older child would generate all the possible ways this event might have happened and then select the most logical. The adolescent's thought is self-consciously deductive and resembles that of a scientist. The stage of formal operations is basically an orientation toward problem solving, the tendency to isolate the elements of the problem and to systematically explore all the possible solution hypotheses regardless of their hypothetical quality. Formal thought is rational and systematic. Finally, the adolescent often broods about his own thought and is self-conscious about his introspections.

Werner's influence has been considerably less than that of Piaget, and will be given briefer mention. His basic principle is that development proceeds from a state of relative globability and lack of differentiation to a state of increasing articulation, differentiation and integration. Although this idea makes intuitive sense, recent research indicates that the young infant is more differentiated than Werner believed. Differentiation refers to a differentiation of functions. According to Werner, all parts of the organism initially operate in a similar way, and only gradually does each assume different functions. Werner believes that the child's thought becomes more discrete, more analytic and more flexible as he matures. Werner believes that the same objective solution to a problem can be brought about by different functions, in contrast to Piaget who posits only one principle of solution to certain problems.

Werner emphasizes how the child generates hypotheses and remains flexible, while Piaget emphasizes the gradual attainment of a single hypothesis. Finally, Werner has been more concerned with language than Piaget, and sees it as a more vital part of the child's mental life.

DEVELOPMENT DURING INFANCY: ATTACHMENT

From the moment a baby is born, he acts. Some of these actions are spontaneous; others are reactions to biological needs. Some of the actions are necessary for survival; others are not. The baby spontaneously scans the environment, listens to sounds, vocalizes, sucks, smiles, thrashes and cries. As he approaches the third month of life, he begins to cling to people and objects, and he manipulates his fingers, his mother's hair, his blanket and his toys.

What is the role of the caretaker, particularly the mother, in this complex set of actions? Since the mother is an interesting stimulus object to look at, listen to and manipulate, the infant typically spends long periods of time scanning her face, babbling when she speaks and smiling when she smiles. The nursing infant also makes sucking responses to the mother and assumes a definite posture during feeding. Even when the child is bottle feeding, he is usually cradled in the mother's arms, and the relaxed posture is associated with the person feeding him.

Crying is an important response that the infant is capable of expressing from the first hours of life. If the infant is separated from his mother by a few feet or more, the crying response acts as an effective signal to the mother to retrieve or to attend to her baby. There is every reason to believe that the squeal of a young puppy performs the same function as the infant's cry. This cry guarantees that the infant will not be in distress for too long a time. When the caretaker comes to relieve the distress, the infant typically relaxes his muscles and, when held upright, rests his head on the mother's shoulder and holds her.

Thus, most reactions of the young infant that occur spontaneously (looking, babbling, smiling, crying, sucking, clinging) are directed to the adult caretaker rather than to a rattle, the crib or a bottle. As a result the infant becomes attached to the caretaker, whether the location is a city apartment, a suburban home or a hut in the mountains of Guatemala. Attachment is defined here as *the degree to which the infant is predisposed, to initiate reactions toward the caretaker when he is alerted, afraid or in a state of depression or distress.*

Experiments with infant monkeys raised with artificial mothers constructed of wire mesh or wire mesh covered with terry cloth reveal that when the monkeys were given the choice of going to either mother, regardless of which one had fed them, they usually close the terry cloth mother and spent more time clinging to it than to the wire mesh mother. This preference for the cloth mother persisted for many months. Even if the bottle were only attached to the wire mother and the infant could never feed from the terry cloth mother, the monkey would still spend much more time on the terry cloth mother than on the wire mesh mother. The infant monkey would go to the wire mother only when hungry; it would feed until satisfied and then return to the terry cloth mother for most of the day.

The terry cloth mother more effectively reduced the infant monkey's fear. When a fear-provoking stimulus (such as the large wooden model of a spider) was placed with the monkey, its initial reaction was to run to the terry cloth mother rather than to the wire mesh mother. After a while, if the terry cloth mother was present, the young monkey was likely to venture out to explore the fear-arousing stimulus. However, if only the wire mesh mother was present, the monkey remained fearful and was less likely to explore the open space around the strange stimulus. (Harlow and Zimmermann, 1959; Harlow and Harlow, 1966).

Other studies suggest the following conclusions. If the young monkey is to develop normally, it must have some interaction with an object to which it can cling during the opening months of life. Another monkey is best as a caretaker, but a terry cloth surrogate allows the infant to cling and is, therefore, better than a wire surrogate. The clinging response is as natural to the monkey as perhaps scanning and vocalizing are to human infants. In time of stress the monkey runs to the object to which it normally clings.

The opportunity to cling and grasp, a behavior that young monkeys normally display at birth, seems to be important to the development of the infant monkey's attachment to the mother and to the mother's power to allay fear and distress. There appears to be a strong similarity between this clinging behavior in the monkey and that of a one-year-old human child who runs to his mother and hides his face in her skirts if a strange person enters the house or if an unexpected noise is heard.

The present conception of attachment is based on the hypothesis that each organism is provided with a special set of responses that it can emit at birth or soon after. These responses are like complex reflexes. The infant emits these responses to the first appropriate stimulus that the environment supplies; this object is likely to become the target of attachment.

In the natural context of the jungle the young monkey clings to the hairy undersurface of his mother for several months after birth. Because nature has supplied the infant monkey with a strong grasping reflex, the monkey becomes attached to those objects that allow it to display this response. The mother is the most effective stimulus for this reaction. Upon hatching, the duck or chicken typically follows a moving object; under natural conditions the mother is the first moving object the young bird encounters. The chick becomes attached to the mother because the mother allows the natural response of following to occur.

The human infant scans, smiles, babbles, sucks, manipulates and holds, among other things. The mother is often the stimulus that elicits these responses. She talks and stimulates the baby to babble; she moves her face and stimulates the child to scan; she allows the baby to play with her hair and fingers and permits the manipulative responses to appear. As a result, the baby gradually becomes attached to the mother.

If, in addition to allowing these responses to occur, the mother provides food, alleviates pain and supplies pleasant tactile stimulation, then we have *three* mechanisms that will lead the child to value a human adult: the reduction of discomfort due to hunger, thirst or pain; the receipt of pleasant sensations; and the attachment process, in which the adult becomes the stimulus object for the infant's early behaviors.

Consequences of Attachment

There are two important consequences of these early experiences of attachment and pleasure with the caretaker. First, the responses that the infant makes to the caretaker will generalize to other people. Second, the infant will develop the fairly articulated schema for the caretaker's face, form and voice that is necessary for separation anxiety to occur. Let us consider each of these consequences in detail.

Generalization of Responses

The principle of generalization states that if the infant makes a set of responses to one class of objects, he is likely to make them to similar objects, but not to objects that are very dissimilar to the original. Perhaps the best support for this principle comes from a study of monkeys that were raised under a variety of conditions (Sackett et al., 1965).

One group was initially reared by a human for three weeks, and then each monkey in the group was placed in a wire cage with no physical contact with any other monkeys until it was one year old. The monkeys in a second group were reared by their natural mothers until one year of age. Each of the monkeys in a third group was placed in isolation at birth and could neither see nor touch humans or other monkeys until it was 6 months old; then they were each put in wire cages until one year of age. During the second year of life, all the monkeys lived in wire cages but had daily opportunities to play with other monkeys.

When the monkeys were between 2 and 3 years of age, each was placed in a circular chamber with a human on one side and a monkey on the other. The monkey could approach either side or stay in the center and approach neither the human nor the monkey. The monkeys who were reared by a human for the first three weeks and then isolated in wire cages for the rest of the first year spent more time with the human than did any other group. The early experience with the human apparently led to a preference for a human. The monkeys reared by their mothers spent most of their time approaching another monkey. The monkeys reared in complete isolation for the first six months spent most of the time in the center of the chamber, approaching neither monkey nor human.

This generalization of approach responses from the earliest object of attachment to a similar object is also true for the human infant. Rheingold (1965) has demonstrated the generalization of an infant's social responses from a mother substitute to other people in a rigorous experimental study. The investigator selected 16, 6-month-old infants who were living in an institution in which many volunteers cared for each child. For eight of these infants (the experimental babies) the investigator herself played the role of mother eight hours a day, five days a week, for eight consecutive weeks. During this time she bathed and diapered them, played with them, smiled at them and generally tried to be as good a substitute mother as possible. The other eight infants (the control babies) were cared for in the typical institutional fashion, with several women performing the motherly duties for each child in a routine fashion. Moreover, the experimental babies received more nurturance than the control babies during the eight week period. Thus, the experimental babies differed from the control babies in two ways: They had one person care for them consistently, and they received more care during the eight week period.

All infants were tested each week during the eight-week experimental period and for four weeks following the termination of the experimental treatment. The tests administered included tests of social responsiveness to three kinds of people—the experimenter, an examiner who administered the tests and at the end of the eight-week period, a stranger. The eight experimental infants who had been cared for by the surrogate mother showed more social responsiveness to her and to the examiner than did the control children. These results support the notion that social acts learned in response to a nurturing and socially stimulating caretaker will generalize to other people.

The Relation Between Attachment and Anxiety

Continued experience with an object establishes a schema for that object. As a result, the infant becomes vulnerable to the experience of fear when he encounters an event discrepant from his schema. The infant is subject to many instances of fear, but two major classes of anxiety seem to grow out of a close attachment to an adult. One is called *stranger anxiety*; the other, *separation anxiety.*

Anxiety as a Reaction to Discrepancy. One of the early causes of distress in the infant is encounter with a stimulus that involves a moderate discrepancy from a schema that the infant has already established. The anxiety caused by a strange human face is a clear example of this phenomenon. The child of 8 months is sitting in his high chair, playing with his cereal. A strange woman enters the kitchen and stands facing the baby. The infant studies the stranger for 10 seconds; his face tightens, and suddenly he begins to cry. It is clear that the stranger has elicited the cry, for if the stranger leaves the child becomes happy again. If the stranger reappears it is likely that the child will cry again. We call this event *stranger anxiety*, and in American children it is typically seen first at about 6 months of age, shows peak frequency at 8 months and then gradually vanishes by the time the child is 12 to 15 months old. Moreover, the infant is likely to show less fear to the stranger if he is sitting on his mother's lap rather than sitting a few feet from her—much as Harlow's monkeys were less fearful if they were holding the terry cloth mother than if they were separated from it. Apparently, proximity to the mother inhibits the fear, as if the child felt more secure when held by her.

This display of fear to an object that partially resembles one for which a schema has been formed can also be seen in kittens. In one study, 5-week-old kittens were given one of three treatments. One group of kittens was handled and played with by a different person five days a week for four weeks. A second group was given the same handling for the same length of time, but was handled by only one experimenter. The third group of kittens was given no handling at all. At the end of each five-day period during the four weeks of handling, a stranger test was given each kitten. Each kitten was handled by a stranger who did not know to which group a particular kitten belonged. Each week a different stranger was used. The kittens who were either handled by only one experimenter or who were not handled at all showed the most fear; they made many attempts to escape or they froze or retreated when called. Apparently the kittens who were exposed to several different people were able to adapt more easily to the stranger because being handled by a stranger was not a *discrepant* experience. The kittens handled by one person showed little fear of the person to whom they had become accustomed, but they, as well as those handled by no one, showed fear to all other strangers—a feline form of stranger anxiety—because the strangers were discrepant stimuli (Collard, 1967).

The sequence of infant smiling in response to a familiar schema at four months, and anxiety to a strange face at eight months resembles the imprinting sequence in ducks. Ducks approach a moving object for the first 13 hours of life, but avoid it after that time.

The infant—human or bird—initially shows approach responses to the object encountered most regularly. After a firm schema for that object has developed, they may show some temporary fear to stimuli that resemble the original object. Why is there this temporary period of fear? Mental development consists, in large measure, of the development of schemata for objects and events. As schemata become established more firmly, the infant encounters stimuli that are a bit discrepant but yet bear a partial resemblance to his particular schema. It is reasonable to guess that the infant's reaction to the discrepant event will depend on whether he has some response to make to it—some way of interpreting or acting upon it. If the infant has a reaction, he is not likely to become anxious and cry. In fact, he may signify his ability to deal with the strange event by smiling or laughing.

The emergence of stranger anxiety is interpreted as indicating that by six to eight months, most infants have developed such a good schema for their mother's face that the stranger is a discrepancy. The infant is alerted. But he is too immature to make a constructive response to this discrepant stimulus. He cannot deal with the strange person, and as a result he cries. Five months later he is more mature and is able to do something. He can ask, "Who is that, Mommy?" he can run to his mother; or he will have been exposed to so many strange faces that his schema for a face will be more generalized. A new face becomes a less discrepant event than it was five months earlier.

Separation Anxiety. A second form of anxiety makes its appearance in American infants at about 10 months of age, and begins to vanish by the time the child is 18 months of age. The event that elicits the fear is different from the one that causes stranger anxiety. The child is playing in the living room with some toys; he sees his mother go to the front door and leave. As the door closes he begins to cry. A 6-month-old American infant would typically not cry in this situation. Why then does the one year old? On the surface, this fear does not seem similar to stranger anxiety. The child has seen the mother leave the house many times and, therefore, this event should not be discrepant from an acquired schema. Before considering various interpretations, let us compare the experiences of a typical middle class American infant with those of an infant from another culture.

The American infant spends most of his time in a crib in a room separate from the mother. During at least half his waking hours he is alone scanning the room, playing with his crib, watching the curtains. The mother comes to her baby primarily when he cries, when she thinks he is hungry or when she thinks he needs a diaper changed. The single human being he comes to know better than any other is his mother. However, because his mother is not always near him, he also learns to make responses to objects, such as pieces of blanket and stuffed animals in his crib. Many American infants become intimately attached to their furry animals or their blankets.

Let us now look at a baby raised in a different stiuation—a small hut in Uganda. Uganda babies are typically nursed until they are 2 years old. Most American infants are either not nursed or are weaned from the breast before they are 5 months old. A Uganda mother is usually available to her child, and the infant is often fed on demand. Toilet training is begun early and is initiated by the mother, who holds the baby in a squatting position with the mother supporting him and the baby holding onto the mother. Thus the infant makes clinging responses to the mother early in the first year while he is being bowel trained. The American mother usually lets her baby soil his diapers during the first year, and the baby lies passively in the crib while he is being changed. Also, the Uganda mother carries her baby with her most of the day—either straddled across her hip or held in place on her back by a sling of cotton cloth. The baby goes with the mother most of the day and does not experience the mother's leaving the room or the hut, an event the American baby experiences many times each day. In sum, the American baby spends most of his first six months in a crib alone; the Uganda baby spends most of his time being held by someone (Ainsworth, 1967).

The Uganda baby shows anxiety to separation from the mother as early as 6 months of age, which is two to four months before a typical middle class American infant shows this reaction. There are several possible interpretations. One involves the earlier notion that a discrepancy from a schema elicits anxiety. As the Uganda infant is usually with his mother, the perception of the mother leaving him is an obviously discrepant event. If he has no other response to make, he will cry.

Because the American infant is not with his mother continually, he requires more time to develop a schema in which the mother is an essential stimulus element of his immediate situation. That is, the infant has some schema for his immediate context, and when he is very young the mother is not an essential part of this schema. However, as he matures and the mother becomes a more distinctive object, it becomes more likely that if she is in the room where he is playing she will be an essential part of his schema for the "room." It is reasonable to assume that the more regular the presence of the mother, the earlier the infant will reach the point where he includes the mother as part of his schema. The Uganda baby is with his mother almost continually, so we would expect him to regard the mother as an essential part of every situation. Her absence presents a discrepancy that elicits anxiety. The American infant does not reach this stage until 10 or 11 months of age.

The above interpretation of separation anxiety rests in part on the same fundamental principle that was used to explain stranger anxiety, even though these two fears do not seem to be similar on the surface.

This interpretation of separation anxiety implies that the closer the attachment of the baby to the mother, the more frequent and intense the separation anxiety. The Uganda baby, we infer, is more closely attached to its mother than the American baby, and this inference fits with the fact that he has many more opportunities to scan, cling, hold, manipulate and play with his mother than does an American baby of the same age.

The opportunity to make a response that might bring the infant into closer contact with the mother seems to allay the infant's fear. In a series of studies, Rheingold placed 10-month-old children in a strange room under one of four conditions: with the mother, with a stranger, with toys or completely alone. As long as the mother was in the room the infant did not cry. But the infants who were not with their mothers were likely to cry within one minute of being placed in the room; the presence of toys or a stranger did not help. These observations suggest that the strangeness of the room (an event that is discrepant from the child's schema) produced the fear. But the presence of the mother protected the child from anxiety. The critical importance of the availability of a response that brought the child into visual or physical contact with the mother is illustrated in the following observations. The 10-month-old infant was placed with the mother in a room which had an open door that led to the same strange empty room that had made most of the other infants cry. The infants in this situation often crawled into the empty room but *did not cry when they arrived there.* The infant would look around and then crawl back to his mother in the adjoining room. For a short period of time the infant was alone in the same strange room that had made the other infants cry. The difference was that these babies could do something effective if they became apprehensive—they could crawl back to their mother. The infants who cried in the earlier observations could do nothing.

In sum, it appears that separation anxiety involves two components—the discrepancy that is produced by being separated from the mother in a strange context, and the inability to make any relevant response that brings him to his mother. Separation anxiety should vanish when the mother's absence is no longer a discrepant event or when the child can do something about the mother's absence. Both of these changes occur with age. As the child grows, he experiences more frequent separations from his mother, and with maturity he is able to interpret her absence and reassure himself of her return.

Lack of a Primary Caretaker: The Institutionalized Child

A child who does not have a primary adult devoted to his care should not become attached to an adult. He should be less likely to show stranger and separation anxiety and he should be less socially responsive than family reared children. He should be less likely to smile, vocalize, laugh or approach adults, and he should be retarded in language.

We know that absence of any relation with a living object has grave consequences for the infant monkey. If a monkey is placed in isolation for the first six months of his life, he shows extremely abnormal behavior when he is removed from isolation. He avoids all social contact, appears very fearful, clutches at himself and crouches. If the period of isolation is less than six months, the monkey begins to approach normal behavior after a while and usually recovers. But if the isolation lasts longer than six months or over a year, the social and sexual behavior of the monkey is abnormal indeed. Often these monkeys do not recover and never interact appropriately with others. They show extreme fear and occasional aggression.

Even the monkeys who were raised with the terry cloth mothers described earlier, and who seemed secure with them, were initially fearful with other monkeys and did not show normal social or sexual behavior when they grew up. After a year of living with other monkeys, they gradually recovered, but the absence of a living mother with whom the infant monkey could interact seriously affected its social behavior. We do not know the critical actions that a live mother performs that produce normal psychological growth. Movement is probably one of these critical factors. Monkeys raised with a terry cloth mother who was attached to a motor (the terry cloth mother moved irregularly in the cage) were less fearful and socially more responsive than monkeys raised with stationary terry cloth mothers.

No human child is raised in total isolation, but the effects of lack of a caretaker can be studied in infants raised in an institution. A child raised in an institutional environment, even a clean and conscientiously administered one, has dramatically less opportunity to become attached to an adult. Hence, he should show less anxiety when an adult leaves, develop less well-articulated schema of an adult face and be less likely to develop stranger anxiety. As the infant does not have the opportunity to engage in face-to-face vocalization, he should be less vocal, and because his crying rarely brings anyone, the frequency of his crying or protesting should decrease gradually.

Provence and Lipton observed 75 babies living in an institutional environment in the United States where nutrition and care were adequate and the infants were not physically ill. The description of the institutional environment will help the reader appreciate the conditions under which these infants lived.

> The younger group of infants (age 4 days to 8 months) occupied cribs placed singularly in glass partitioned cubicles. The room was clean, cheerful and light with adequate heat and ventilation. The infants were fed in their cribs with bottle propped. When cereals, fruits and vegetables were added to the diet they were also given in a propped bottle with a large holed nipple rather than given by spoon. . . . Sometimes a stuffed toy was placed in the crib for the baby to look at. After about 4 months of age, simple rattles, beads and so on, were placed on a string suspended across the crib sides and the single playpen which contained other age appropriate toys. . . . Each infant in this group shared the time and attention of the attendant with 7 to 9 other infants in the same age range for the 8 hour period of the day when she was present. For the remaining 16 hours of the day, there was no person in the nursery except at feeding time when an attendant who also had similar duties in other nurseries heated formulas, propped bottles, and changed diapers.[1]

Not only were the infants fed without the presence of an adult, but there was minimal variability in their experience. There were no vocalizations from other people, no reciprocal play, no close relationship between a child's crying and the reaction of someone else.

In contrasting how these babies were different from those raised in families, it should be noted, first, that there were no major differences between normal and institutionalized babies prior to 3 or 4 months of age. It was only after four months that the differences became evident. The institutionalized babies vocalized very little, they neither cooed nor babbled and they cried infrequently. Moreover, they did not adapt their postures to the arms of an adult: "They felt something like sawdust dolls; they moved, they bent easily at the proper joints, but they felt stiff and wooden."

These infants were not picked up very often and, therefore, one would not expect them to make the kinds of postural adjustments that babies ordinarily make. By 8 months of age most of these infants were markedly less interested in grasping or approaching toys, and they began to lose interest in their external environment. During the second half of the first year, body rocking became very common and was more frequent than would be observed among family reared babies. Stranger anxiety was rare, and the infants' facial expressions were bland and clearly not so expressive as those of family reared infants. If they were frustrated they would cry passively or turn away; rarely would they make an attempt to conquer a frustration. Finally, language was delayed. There were no words at all at one year of age, and vocalization and language were the behaviors that were most seriously depressed. The following is a description of one of these babies at 45 weeks of age:

> Outstanding were his soberness—his forlorn appearance, and lack of animation. The interest that he showed in the toys was mainly for holding, inspecting and rarely mouthing. When he was unhappy he now had a cry that sounded neither demanding nor angry—just miserable—and it was usually accompanied by his beginning to rock. The capacity for protest which he had earlier was much diminished. He did not turn to adults to

[1]Provence, S., and Lipton, R.: *Infants in Institutions*. New York, International Universities Press, 1962, p. 133.

relieve his distress or to involve them in a playful or pleasurable interchange. He made no demands. The active approach to the world, which had been one of the happier aspects of his earlier development, vanished. As one made active and persistent efforts at a social interchange he became somewhat more responsive, animated and motorically active, but lapsed into his depressed and energyless appearance when the adult became less active with him.[2]

There were two descriptive comments by observers that seemed to convey the impression Teddy made at this time: One was, "The light in Teddy has gone out." The other was, "If you crank his motor you can get him to go a little; he can't start on his own."

All of the behaviors that were most likely to be learned as a result of interaction with an adult (i.e., clinging, crying to distress, approaching adults for play and vocalization) were most clearly retarded or absent in the institutionalized children.

BEHAVIORAL DIFFERENCES AMONG INFANTS

During the 30 years between 1920 and 1950, most psychologists assumed that all healthy infants were basically similar in temperament and ability and that the differences observable at age 5 were the product of differential experience. However, in the past 10 years careful study of the human infant has revealed that these immature organisms differ dramatically along several dimensions. It is possible that these differences, real as they are during the first six months, are short-lived and exert minimal influence on behavior during the preschool or early school years. The answers to this issue must be left to the research of the decades to come. There is value, nevertheless, in noting some of the behavioral patterns that differentiate infants during the first six months, for it may be that these patterns help shape important developmental processes.

Vigor of Activity

The intensity of motor activity is one of the most striking characteristics that differentiates young infants. Some infants move their arms and legs with great force; others move with minimal vigor. Some vocalize lustily; the babbling of others is soft. Some bang toys or strike their cribs with much energy; others are more placid. It is tempting to speculate that these vigorous infants will be more energetic or lively when they are 10 years old than their placid counterparts. What evidence we have is congruent with this expectation, but there is not yet enough information for complete confidence in it.

Irritability

A second obvious difference among infants refers to the ease with which they cry and fret and the amount of effort required to placate them. Some infants become irritable at slight or no external provocation, whereas others do not cry unless pain and discomfort are relatively high. Moreover, some infants appear to possess an inhibiting mechanism that brakes the spiraling character of irritability. These infants typically will fret for half a minute and then stop spontaneously with no external interference, behaving as though they possessed mechanisms that inhibited the buildup of extreme upset. In other infants, crying increases rapidly in intensity until it reaches a maximum and either the mother placates the infant or he falls off to sleep, exhausted. These infants seem to lack

[2]Provence, S., and Lipton, R.: *Infants in Institutions.* New York, International Universities Press, 1962, pp. 134–135.

the capacity to inhibit the growth of a tantrum; when fretting begins, the reaction goes to completion.

It is easy to imagine the differential impact of these two types of infants on a mother. The hyperirritable infant is more likely to vex and puzzle a parent. Initially, this infant will elicit care from the mother as she attempts to placate her crying baby. However, if the mother's attention is not effective in quieting her child, his irritability may begin to provoke anger and lead to less maternal affection. The extremely irritable baby therefore experiences patterns of maternal reactions different from those the more contented child experiences, even though the basic personality of the mother is the same.

Stimulus Satiability

Although most normal infants begin to show habituation when they are 3 months of age, there are some quite dramatic differences among children of the same age in the *rate* at which they become bored with—or habituate to—a particular pattern. Often, children who are vigorous in their movements show faster rates of habituation than do more placid infants, and large, chubby boys show slower rates of habituation than do small, wiry boys.

Infant boys who show a rapid rate of habituation tend to invest short periods of sustained attention to a particular toy or activity. They will put blocks in a pail for 10 seconds and then quickly skip to another activity for 10 to 15 seconds. Boys who show a slow rate of habituation are likely to spend a minute or two putting blocks in a pail before shifting to another activity. Thus, the speed with which an infant becomes bored with a visual stimulus during the opening months of life seems to be associated with a faster tempo of play during the latter half of the first year.

Evidence from other investigations suggests that behavioral tempo continues to be relatively stable from the preschool period to the school years. School-age children differ markedly in their tendency to make decisions quickly, as opposed to brooding a long time before deciding to act, and in their tendency to skip restlessly from activity to activity, in contrast to investing long periods of time on a particular task. It is possible that these differences in 6-year-olds are related to the differences in rate of habituation and tempo of play observed during the first year.

Threshold for Attention Change

Infants also differ in the intensity of stimulus energy and in the uniqueness of a stimulus necessary to attract their attention. Some babies orient to minimal changes in visual or auditory input and appear to be alerted by slight changes in their surroundings. Others require more perceptible changes before their attention is elicited. This threshold of attention variable has been called "perceptual sensitivity."

Social Responsivity

It is not clear whether social responsivity is biologically based or is developed entirely through experiences in the early weeks of life. It is clear, however, that by 16 weeks of age there are dramatic differences among infants in the degree to which they elicit positive, affectionate, socially responsive overtures from adults. The socially attractive child smiles, babbles frequently and becomes very responsive (laughing, cooing) when an adult talks to him, tickles him or picks him up. The socially unresponsive infant is generally quiet, is less likely to smile or babble when adults look at or talk to him and tends to fret or stiffen when someone picks him up.

Obviously, these two types of babies will elicit different degrees of social stimulation from adults. The responsive baby should become even more responsive as a result of increasingly frequent interaction with others, whereas the initially unresponsive baby is likely to become even more withdrawn and quiet, since adults will be less inclined to play with him.

These five attributes are some of the most obvious differences observed among young infants. It is not yet possible to state the relationship among the manifestations of these attributes, or their power to predict a personality in later years. It may even be that dispositions less obvious to an observer are more critical for future development than the ones outlined above.

How Behavioral Dispositions in the Infant Influence Personality Development

On the basis of knowledge, it is reasonable to suggest that there are some unlearned behavioral dispositions present at birth. Some of these dispositions are stable over time and may facilitate or impede the acquisition of particular motives, anxieties and instrumental acts either directly or indirectly as a result of the special reactions these dispositions evoke in the caretaker. There are two complementary ways by which temperamental dispositions of the infant might influence the later personality of the child.

The simplest mechanism operates under the assumption that a particular temperamental trait—vigor, let us say—leads the infant to behave in ways that predispose him to learn special reactions and to encounter special experiences. A vigorous one-year-old is likely to lash out and knock down physical obstacles when frustrated. As a result, he may learn how to deal with obstacles early. The vigorous infant also may encounter frequent parental punishments and pressures because he gets into more "mischief" than a less vigorous infant. The rationale for these predictions rests on the assumption that the vigor (or any disposition in the infant) is a more or less fixed entity that has certain constant consequences in the environment (a vigorous infant will attack obstacles and will encounter restriction). This general and rather simplistic point of view is partially responsible for the belief that inactive infants will become shy and pensive 10-year-olds and that active infants will become sociable and active 10-year-olds.

A second and more plausible mechanism by which infant temperament might influence later personality development engages a subtle set of interactions; it operates under the assumption that the parent categorizes the infant along selected dimensions. These categorizations are determined in part by the infant's actual characteristics. The parent's pattern of reactions toward the infant then corresponds to some extent with the label or category applied to the child.

Take, for example, two mothers, each of whom has a highly irritable baby. Both babies cry incessantly, cannot be satisfied easily and do not respond positively to affection. One mother interprets this behavior as indicative of the infant's dislike for her. She feels threatened by her inability to placate the infant, and she begins to treat him as a hostile and irritating child. The other mother interprets the irritability as a sign of illness (colic, perhaps) and nurtures the infant more than she would a less irritable child. Since she views her infant as fragile and sensitive, her behavioral reaction is increased solicitousness. These different reactions to infants with identical behavioral attributes derive from the mother's different interpretations of these attributes.

One important attribute that influences a parent's categorizing process is the sex of the child. There is some evidence that mothers react differently to boys and girls as early as 12 weeks of age. For instance, a mother is more likely to let her son cry longer than her daughter. She may rationalize this behavior by asserting that she does not want to "baby" her son: "He has to learn to take stress," she may say. A mother is more likely to imitate the vocalizations of her daughter than of her son, but more likely to stimulate and amuse her son than her daughter through flexing and manipulating his muscles and touching him (Moss, 1967). Some of the differential handling is, of course, a result of different behaviors in the infants. But some of it is due to the mother's automatic reactions that result from the implicit labeling of the sex of her child. The mother-infant relationship is a sensitively tuned interaction in which the mother's unconscious image of the ideal adolescent boy or girl directs her caretaking actions.

Thus, we should not expect any constant personality structure to develop from specific infant characteristics alone. Mothers differ in their interpretations of a given infant attribute, and maternal reactions are based in part on that interpretive label. The child's emerging behaviors will be shaped in accordance with the interaction between these maternal reactions and his particular, early behavioral dispositions.

EARLY SOCIALIZATION

Socialization is the process by which the child acquires the dominant beliefs, values, motives and behaviors of his culture and gradually becomes more similar to other members of a particular cultural, ethnic or religious group. The acquisition of culturally appropriate behaviors, beliefs and values involves recognition of the ideal traits a person should possess, as well as the undesirable traits he should be free of or should inhibit.

What Behaviors and Values are Socialized?

The major psychological entities that are socialized include the following:

1. Acquisition of desired behaviors, such as the skills of reading, arithmetic, cooking, social poise and talking to a large group without being anxious.
2. Inhibition of undesirable behaviors such as aggression, destruction, dependency, crying, tantrums and spontaneous urination or defecation.
3. Acquisition of culturally approved values such as sincerity, altruism, cleanliness, honesty, conscientiousness, dominance and ambition.
4. Suppression of undesirable values such as hate, narcissism, idleness and sexual infidelity.

Because socialization of behaviors and values is a dynamic and constantly changing process, the child alters both values and actions as he grows. For example, the 2-year-old boy has not yet learned that it is inappropriate to cry for help when he has a problem; the 10-year-old boy, on the other hand, believes strongly that it is childish and inappropriate to ask for help with problems, and he will inhibit crying and request aid when faced with a difficult task.

The specific behaviors and values that are regarded as desirable or undesirable will differ across cultural groups. The Mayan Indian peasant boy in Guatemala is taught that he must learn to help his father with the coffee plantation, remain close to his family and contribute to their financial stability. The son of a Chicago lawyer is taught to do well in school and to become independent of his family. Although the content of what is socialized differs across cultures, psychologists believe that the mechanisms of socialization are the same for all cultures.

Mechanisms of Socialization

Socialization is accomplished through four basic mechanisms: (1) the desire to obtain the affection, regard, acceptance and recognition of others, (2) the motive to avoid the unpleasant feelings generated by punishment or rejection by others, (3) the desire to be similar to particular people the child has grown to respect, love and admire (a process called identification), and (4) a general tendency to imitate the actions of others. Acquisition or inhibition of overt actions is most readily accomplished through social rewards and punishments, supplemented by observations of the behavior of others. Acquisition or suppression of values and beliefs is less likely to be facilitated by watching others behave, and more likely to be the product of identification with a desirable model.

Each of these four mechanisms—desire for reward, fear of punishment, identification and imitation—is strongest at different periods of development and facilitates different aspects of the socialization process.

First Steps in Socialization

During the second and third years of life the child's joint desires for parental acceptance and for avoidance of punishment are the major mechanisms in socialization. The child is too young to identify with his parents or other adults, and although the 2-year-old child does observe others and imitate some of their actions, observational learning is not a major basis for socialization during the second year of life.

This discussion will be restricted to the behaviors and values that are typically socialized in *Western* society during this age period, because social scientists have acquired the most valid information about our own culture. These behaviors and values include learning to inhibit spontaneous bowel and bladder evacuation, regressive crying, destruction of property and open aggression to others. All four classes involve *inhibition of a behavior that is relatively strong in the child's repertoire.* American parents generally do not regard the child as mature enough to learn positive values like honesty, sincerity, persistence and altruism, or behavioral skills like reading, painting or tying shoelaces. In most American homes the first socialization attempts are directed at stamping out undesirable behaviors. The primary instruments used for this task are reward for successful inhibition, and punishment for failure to inhibit the prohibited actions.

Toilet Training: An Example of Early Socialization

The socialization of toilet training is discussed in detail below not because it is the most important response that is socialized but because (1) most cultures socialize this behavior, (2) it provides a good example of the inhibitory mechanisms that are involved in early socialization and (3) there is more research on toilet training than on other aspects of socialization during this early period. It should be noted, however, that aggression, destruction of property or regressive crying could just as well have been chosen to illustrate the process of socialization.

Inhibition Learning

The essential characteristic of toilet training is the learning of an inhibition—that of spontaneous evacuation. The degree to which anxiety over punishment, observation and imitation of others, or reward dominates the learning of this inhibition depends on the age when the toilet training is initiated. If a parent waits until the child is 3 years old, anxiety is less important than if training is started at 12 to 15 months of age. Let us consider, first, the role of anxiety in motivating the inhibition of spontaneous evacuation in a child under 18 months.

Anxiety as an Inhibitory Mechanism. The mother is able to elicit anxiety in the child through (1) physical punishment of the prohibited response and (2) gestures or communications that symbolize loss of nurturance. The hypothetical analysis of this sequence, using defecation as the response to be inhibited, is found at the bottom of the page (**1**). These events occur in close temporal succession. For the inhibition response to take place, the anxiety must gradually move forward in the temporal sequence, so that it is eventually elicited by the stimulus that signals defecation. In that case the prevailing response to anxiety will be temporary inhibition of the response originally elicited by the stimulus. This sequence is shown at the bottom of the page (**2**).

In short, if the anxiety that was originally based on punishment moves forward in the temporal sequence, so that it occurs in response to the stimulus for defecation, the normal sequence of stimulus → defecation will be interrupted. The child might signal to his mother to indicate that he has to defecate (using postural or language signs), or he might go to the bathroom himself (assuming he is able to walk and has learned the connection between defecation and that particular room).

If the anxiety elicited by the urge to defecate was originally based solely on painful physical punishment, no additional assumptions are required to explain the learning of correct toilet habits. But if the anxiety was based primarily on the caretaker's gestures of disapproval that symbolized a possible withdrawal of acceptance, then an extra cognitive component must have been established prior to the socialization training. The child must have had a set of experiences that made the caretaker a valued person and led the child to anticipate anxiety if the caretaker gave signs of possible disapproval or withdrawal of nurturance.

It is reasonable to assume that the 18-month-old is conceptually mature enough to have learned the value of an affectionate relationship with another person, primarily the mother. A mother can manipulate her relationship with her child to produce the desired toilet training, because

(**1**)

Internal stimulus for defecation	→ (ELICITS)	Response of defecation	→	Imposition of punishment (or potential loss of nurturance)	→	Experience of anxiety (with its distinct noxious properties)

(**2**)

Internal stimulus for defecation	→	Experience of anxiety	→	Inhibition of response of defecation

anxiety over loss of maternal acceptance of nurturance, like anxiety over punishment, can become anticipatory, disrupt the automatic defecation sequence and lead to inhibition of the defecatory reflex. The greater the child's awareness of the response desired by the mother, the easier the inhibition training will proceed.

To sum up: (1) If there is a nurturant relationship between caretaker and child, so that anxiety over anticipation of loss of nurturance can be an incentive to learning, (2) if the child is given instructions about the proper responses and the appropriate place to evacuate and (3) if the child is sufficiently mature to be aware of what behavior is required of him, then relevant cognitive links will occur simultaneously with the arousal of anxiety over defecation, and will facilitate successful inhibition.

Other Mechanisms for Learning Inhibition. Although anxiety learned because of punishment, disapproval and anticipated loss of nurturance seems to be the primary incentive for learning to inhibit spontaneous evacuation in the child under 2 years of age, it is theoretically possible that the mechanisms of identification, observation and imitation, and simple reward can mediate the learning of this inhibition. For example, as a consequence of his desire to strengthen his identification with his parents, the child might learn proper toilet habits. However, identification with a parent is not strong during the second year of life; it generally does not begin to grow until the child is 3 to 4 years of age.

The child might spontaneously watch and imitate the habits of his parents or of an older sibling, as he does when he picks up his father's pipe or applies his mother's lipstick. But if imitation is to mediate toilet training, the child must have the opportunity to see the action that is to be copied; the stimuli he experiences when he has the urge to evacuate must be associated with the actual behavior of a model. However, inhibiting spontaneous defecation is not a public response, for most adults close the bathroom door behind them. Although the child can observe where he is to go to evacuate, he cannot observe the private act of inhibition of evacuation. For the most part, the learning of toilet habits by the 12-month-old through observation and imitation alone is not very likely.

Finally, it is possible for a child, who understands language and has been given verbal instructions on what to do when he feels he must defecate, to become trained through consistent reward of inhibition every time he goes to the proper toileting place. In practice, however, most parents find it extremely difficult to refrain from a punitive statement or punishing action when the child has an accident. It is likely, therefore, that in most cases, anxiety over physical punishment or parental disapproval, in differing intensities, is involved in the acquisition of appropriate toilet habits.

Basically, the child learns to inhibit unrestrained exploration of his environment and "destruction" of household property in a manner similar to the learning of inhibition of spontaneous evacuation. For example, when the parent punishes the child for tearing a new curtain, the child learns to inhibit his urge to pull on it. The major difference between the inhibition of evacuation and that of property destruction or exploration lies in the distinctiveness of the stimuli with which the anxiety becomes associated. The stimuli for evacuation are internal, intense and relatively distinct. The stimuli that incite the child to explore something (curtains, drawers, vases, pots) are external and relatively indistinct. If the child is punished for pulling pots from the kitchen cabinet, it is unlikely that an inhibition resulting from this punishment will immediately generate to the sight of clothes in a bedroom closet. A new set of punishments must be administered if the child is to learn to inhibit exploration in this new situation.

Thus, the learning of inhibitions over exploration requires more time than does the inhibition of evacuation—and is more tedious. The urge to defecate occurs only three or four times daily, whereas the child's urge to explore attractive objects can be aroused a hundred times a day, depending on the variety of attractive objects in his environment. Since the parent cannot be present to punish each "dangerous" exploration, the child has many opportunities to extinguish the anxiety reaction to exploration and potential property destruction.

Consequences of Overly Severe Toilet Training

Overly severe training refers to the use of excessive punitive procedures that generate strong anxiety. Five of the consequences of overly severe toilet training during the second and third year of life that can have lasting effects on the child's personality are (1) hostility toward and fear of the training agent (usually the mother), often accompanied by excessive resistance to any limitation on autonomy, (2) anxiety over sexual thoughts and behavior and over the body's anal and genital areas, (3) anxiety over dirt and disarray, (4) conception of the self as dirty and bad and (5) inhibition of spontaneity. Each of these consequences is discussed in the following text.

Hostility Toward and Fear of the Mother. A mother who is excessively punitive or threatening in her training can become a source of anxiety arousal in the child. Excessive punishment of toilet accidents may generate urges to resist maternal coercion and perhaps result in aggressive behavior toward the parent in the form of kicking, pushing, biting and, if language is available, verbal attacks. These violent discharges are not like the aimless rage of an 8-month-old but instead are directed attacks on a specific person.

A more impersonal method of expressing hostility is resistance to the training itself. This resistance is apt to be expressed by refusal to evacuate while sitting in the bathroom. Often the mother will sit with the child for half an hour and finally, in exasperation, remove him, only to encounter immediate evacuation on the floor. When the mother displays her obvious upset at this event, she provides the child with gratification for his hostile motives. The parent who displays extreme upset in similar situations rewards the child's resistant disposition and lays the foundation for a personality that resists any curbing of autonomy.

Anxiety over Sexuality. The 3-year-old does not clearly differentiate among the acts of evacuation, the organs involved and the products. He tends to apply the same simple word or phrase to the three referents, maximizing the similarity among them. The close proximity of the external genitals, the urethra, and the anus makes it likely that anxiety over evacuation will generalize to sexual functioning when the 7-year-old learns words for the unique stimulation derived from the genitals. If the strong anxiety linked to the genitals persists into adolescence, the young adult is likely to experience conflict in sexual behavior.

The close semantic link between bowel and bladder functioning and the genital-sexual complex is supported by data from an intensive interview study with middle-class American mothers. These mothers could not keep the topics of sex training and toilet training separate. The interview questions kept the topics separate, but the mother's answers did not. "When we were discussing the modesty standards [actually referring to sex and nudity], mothers would describe their efforts to train their children not to urinate outdoors" (Sears et al., 1957, pp. 107–108). In the minds of many mothers, and in the minds of children, there is an intimate association between urination and defecation on the one hand and exposure of genitals and sex modesty training on the other. It is not surprising that the separate anxieties associated with each of these areas support one another.

Anxiety over Dirt and Disarray. If the mother tells the child "you are dirty" every time he soils, and accompanies these statements with punishment, anxiety will become attached to the word "dirty" and in time will extend to the child's environment—to dirty fingers, dirty rooms, dirty floors. One defensive response the child may adopt that attenuates the anxiety is to remove and avoid dirt compulsively and to maintain an aversive posture to any kind of disarray. Of course, a child also learns to avoid being dirty as a result of direct punishment for dirty fingers or clothes.

Anxiety over the Self-Concept. The stigma "you are dirty" or "you are bad" applied by parents to the child each time he soils, eventually may affect the child's self-concept. The parents' reactions to the child and their verbal evaluations of him are basic sources of his attitudes toward himself, for the child views the parents as omniscient and is prone to believe that their evaluations are accurate.

Inhibition of Spontaneous Responding. Inhibition of a response to a particular stimulus or situation is a major component of socialization, and our culture regards appropriate inhibition as characteristic of maturity. But undesirable consequences may arise if a tendency to inhibit behavior gains too much strength too quickly. It is possible that the association of an urge to act and strong anxiety, as experienced in toilet training, may lead to the tendency to "inhibit responding" *whenever* anxiety is experienced.

For example, the inhibition of the urge to explore a new toy is a possible consequence of excessively fearful punishments surrounding toilet training. Similarly, the inhibition of an aggressive outburst in response to the mixed stimuli of anger and anxiety, or the inhibition of sexual behavior in response to erotic excitement and apprehension, might result from severe toilet training. The generalization of inhibition to actions other than those involved in the original toilet training is suggested by clinical observations and is theoretically reasonable.

The Importance of Rules for the Child

Socialization is the acquisition of the rules of social living. This process is important not only because it provides for a more harmonious society—the reason for which parents generally believe they socialize their children—but also because it gives the child *rules* to reduce the uncertainty of each day. Children, as well as adults, become apprehensive when they are not certain of what is permitted and what is prohibited. Rules provide that certainty.

Consider these observations made in the home of a 27-month-old boy. The boy had put some freshly ironed clothes into the toilet bowl. When his mother discovered this violation, she became upset and spanked him hard for several minutes. He cried for a long time and was clearly both afraid and in pain. His mother was often inconsistent in her punishments of rule violations. Sometimes she would punish an act with vigor, but on other occasions she would ignore it. The next day the boy put a new set of freshly ironed clothes into the toilet, walked into the kitchen, announced to his mother what he had done and then stiffened his body as if to prepare himself for a spanking.

Why did he commit an act that he knew would bring painful punishment? One explanation is that he had a stronger desire to be certain of his punishment than he did to avoid being punished. By committing that violation, he was controlling when a punishment would be administered. He would not be in the uncomfortable state of not knowing "when the knife would fall." The learning of rules for appropriate beliefs and behaviors fills an important human need for certainty and structure.

Anxiety as an Affect

It has been suggested that anxiety over possible punishment or parental rejection is one important force in socialization. As discussed previously, fear of the unfamiliar is a common experience during the first year of life. Two of the child's frequent responses to the emotion of fear or anxiety are crying and withdrawal. Let us consider more directly the relation between crying or withdrawal on the one hand, and the emotion of fear or anxiety on the other. Before delving into this issue we must first examine the meaning of the word *emotion*, or, as it is termed in psychology, *affect*.

Characteristics of Affects

The concept of affect defies precise definition. The popular and traditional view assumes that there are some basic internal physiological changes—such as increased heart rate, motor discharge or sweating—that either accompany or cause the emotional states that we label anger, excitement, fear and so forth. These internal physiological states are presumed to have consistency within an individual and, perhaps, universality throughout mankind.

Recent research developments suggest the need for some modification of this traditional view. An affect is now thought to involve an interpretation of a combination of three sets of conditions: (1) perception of internal bodily sensations, called visceral afferent stimulation (referring to perceived change in the level of stimulation coming from heart, intestine, stomach, muscles, skin and other internal organs), (2) the immediate external situation or context of the individual (home, beach, office or classroom) and (3) the thoughts and images the individual is having at the time. Sadness, fear, happiness, anger and other affects are names for combinations of these three sets of conditions.

During most of the child's waking day he is acting, thinking and imagining in a variety of environmental and interpersonal situations or contexts, such as playing with a sibling, talking with a parent or fighting with a playmate. These contexts are not regarded as affect situations until one necessary ingredient is present: The child must perceive a change in the quality or intensity of the internal sensations originating in his muscles, stomach, intestines, heart, skin and so forth. When he feels different from the way he usually feels, he is in an "emotional" situation.

Thus, an affect is experienced when a person recognizes a discrepancy between the intensity or quality of the internal stimulation he feels and the intensity which is normal for him. Some affects are marked by a perception of internal sensations that are very strong or intense, and therefore noticeable, to the person. Excitement, rage, joy and fear belong to this class. Other affects are characterized by bodily sensations less intense than a person's normal sensations. Sadness, apathy and lassitude are included in this class.

Generalized Excitement in Infants versus Specific Affects in Older Children

When the older child or adult experiences a change in the quality or intensity of his internal feelings, he *interprets* the change. The immediate context and his thoughts are used as the basis for explaining why he feels different. The interpretation specifies the affect.

This interpretation is influenced by (1) the direction of the discrepancy the individual notices (that is, higher or lower intensity of stimulation), (2) the content of his images and thoughts, (3) his immediate context and (4) the language labels available to him. For instance, a perception of decreased arousal level combined with thoughts about missing one's family while in a strange hotel room is likely to be labeled depression or loneliness. The same level of decreased arousal combined with thoughts about the hard day at the office while on the late bus home at 7:30 P.M. is likely to be labeled fatigue.

Because the infant has no language ability, he cannot interpret and label his discrepant feelings. When he experiences changes in sensations, he usually exhibits only states of generalized excitement. He cries, laughs or thrashes to external events or internal sensations directly, not as a consequence of interpretation. The 6-month-old infant who sees his mother smile and feels her tickle may laugh; when he feels a cramp or sees a strange face, he may cry. But six years later the child's laughter or crying is marbled with meaning and is more closely linked to certain contexts. The 6-year-old has learned to evaluate his feelings; the infant has not. An infant does not experience disgust, pride, joy or guilt, in the adult sense of these words, for he does not have the thoughts about himself and other persons that are an integral part of these adult emotions.

Role of the Social Environment in Development of Affects

The *context* of the social environment has been found to have a definite effect on how a person interprets the visceral afferent stimulation and associated cognitions that accompany the context. Empirical support for this view has come from experiments conducted by Schachter and his colleagues (Schachter and Singer, 1962; Schachter and Wheeler, 1962). They found that adults with the same induced state of bodily feelings reacted differently depending on the context in which they were placed and whether they had an explanation for their visceral sensations. The subjects were injected with adrenalin, which led to perceived bodily changes in heart rate and tactile sensations. Subjects who watched a funny movie reacted to these bodily changes by labeling their feelings as "humor" and "joy." Subjects who watched a sad movie reacted by labeling their feelings as "depression." In both instances the subjects were aroused by the adrenalin and were aware of a discrepancy from their normal state of feeling.

These experiments indicate that the richness and appropriateness of an emotion are governed as much by the person's labeling of his feelings according to the context, as by the raw feelings themselves. In an adult or older child there is an increased tendency for behavior to reflect the affect interpretation that is applied. This is in contrast to the infant and the very young child, whose behavior is more directly controlled by, or conditioned to, the visceral afferent stimuli. Thus, the cry of a 15-month-old is likely to be a direct reaction to the pain of being spanked or to the experience of the unfamiliar. The cry of the 3-year-old could be a direct reaction to visceral afferent stimulation, but it is just as likely to be a reaction to the expectation of being sent to his room, or a strategy of obtaining sympathy when he feels "persecuted" by restrictive parents.

The Nature of Anxiety

Anxiety is an affect because it always has a cognitive aspect. Anxiety is present when the child experiences unpleasant visceral sensations in a context in which he anticipates that something painful or uncomfortable might occur. Thus, the 3-year-old who cringes from his mother when she warns him of his father's reaction to a toilet accident is probably experiencing the affect of anxiety. The response of cowering or crying in this particular context is the result of anxiety. On the other hand, the crying of the 5-month-old to a strange face is probably not a reaction to anxiety. The infant of this age is too immature to interpret his visceral sensations. The crying is a direct reaction to a discrepant event, not to the anticipation of some painful experience.

The condition that is most likely to produce the affect of anxiety in a child 3 years or older is uncertainty about a future event. Major sources of uncertainty are possible loss of nurturance or affection, anticipation of physical harm and lack of congruence between a rule or socialization standard the child has learned and his evaluation of his current beliefs or behaviors. Refinements, elaborations and subtle combinations of these sources of anxiety give rise to such unpleasant affects as helplessness, depression, guilt and shame, which appear during the later preschool and the early school years.

Although psychologists agree that anxiety is an important affect in childhood, there is no agreement as to how to measure it or how to distinguish among the specific sources of anxiety. There has been no lack of effort in this direction; psychologists have tried interviews, questionnaires, inkblot tests and measures of palmar sweating and heart rate, but none of these is a completely satisfactory means of measurement. The concept of anxiety continues to be discussed because it is believed to be an essential idea; hopefully, social scientists will eventually devise an exact method for measuring its presence and intensity.

THE CONCEPT OF IDENTIFICATION

A 5-year-old boy feels proud as he watches his father defeat a rival in tennis or sees his brother hit a tie-breaking home run. A young girl feels the elation of being "grown up" as she puts on her mother's apron and attempts to bake a pie. A young boy feels ashamed when authorities arrest his father or commit his mother to a mental institution. In each of these cases the child behaves as if he possessed some of the characteristics of another person to whom he feels similar. The proud 5-year-old boy feels as if he, and not his father, had won the tennis match. The girl who prepares to bake a pie behaves as though she had her mother's culinary skills. The boy suffers as if he, not his parent, had been arrested or institutionalized. The concept of identification is used to explain the phenomenon of vicarious sharing in the emotional states of others.

Identification is, in part, the belief of a person that some attributes of a model (for example, parent, siblings, relatives, peers and fictional figures) are also possessed by the person. A boy who realizes that he and his father share the same name, who notes that they have similar facial features and who is told that they both have lively tempers develops a belief that he is similar to his father. *When this belief in similarity is accompanied by vicarious emotional experiences in the child that are appropriate to the model, we say that the child has an identification with the model.*

How Identification Is Established and Strengthened.

Children do not develop strong identifications with everyone to whom they are similar, but they do develop identifications with more than one model. The conditions that determine the strength of the identification are therefore important. Four related processes must be examined in order to obtain an understanding of how identification works.

Process 1. The person (*P*) believes that he and a model (*M*) share particular physical or psychological attributes. *P* believes that some of the characteristics of *M* also belong to him. The more distinctive these shared attributes are, the stronger is *P*'s belief.

There are three major ways that the child may perceive similarity to the model: (1) by adoption of the model's attributes, (2) by believing others who tell him that he shares similarities with the model and (3) by initially recognizing some fundamental similarities, including surname, basic affective states (such as anger, joy and disgust) and physical characteristics (genitals, special skin markings, color of eyes or hair). As a result of these accumulated similarities the typical 6-year-old believes that he is more similar to his parent, specifically the parent of the same sex, than he is to any other adult he knows.

Process 2. *P* experiences vicarious affective reactions that are appropriate to events that *M* is experiencing. The identification is present when *P* feels as though events that happen to *M* are happening to him. He often behaves as if the world will react to him as he believes it will react to *M*.

The assumption that a child vicariously experiences the affect that he believes the identification model would feel has not been proved, but it has been demonstrated in the laboratory. One such attempt was made in a study by Kagan and Phillips (1964). Boys and girls (age 5½ to 8½) were brought to a laboratory with either the father (for boys) or the mother (for girls). Each child was told he was going to watch a contest between his parent and an adult stranger of the same sex. The contest involved the identification of blurred pictures projected on a screen. Both the parent and the stranger had been prerehearsed to fail or pass specific pictures on the test. It was expected that the child would show greater elation when his parent was successful or the stranger failed than when the parent failed or the stranger succeeded. These results would indicate greater vicarious emotional involvement with the parent than with the stranger.

After the child was told how the contest worked and after electrodes for measuring his heart rate were attached, all communications were directed toward the two adults and the child was ignored. His overt behavior and his heart rate reactions were studied while the adults were trying to solve the problem and after the examiner announced whether the adults had passed or failed the item. It was found that the child smiled much more following parent success or stranger failure than after parent failure or stranger success. The child behaved as if he were elated by his parent's success. Moreover, he showed the greatest excitement, as measured by increase in heart rate, following parent success and stranger failure than after the other conditions. Although there are several ways to interpret the results, they are consonant with the suggestion that children are likely to share vicariously in the affective states of the models with whom they perceive basic similarities.

Process 3. *P* wants to acquire the attributes of *M* that he perceives to be desirable; *P* wishes to have access to the positive goal states that he believes *M* to possess.

The child perceives that adults, especially his parents, are stronger, more powerful and wiser than he is, and that they have special privileges and easy access to desirable goals. The child wants these privileges and goals for himself. For instance, he wants to be strong, to be able to order other people around, to decide what and when to eat and where and when to go to bed, to drive a car, to swim in deep water, to pick up heavy things. In short, the child would like to possess the skills and privileges of adults.

The attractiveness of an identification model seems to be based both on the model's nurturance of the child and the degree to which the model seems to possess desirable attributes, especially power over the child and over other adults, competence at tasks the child considers important, receipt of affection from the parent of the opposite sex and acceptance by others.

Process 4. *P* adopts and practices attitudes and behaviors that *M* displays, because he believes that by increasing his similarity to *M* he might command *M*'s desirable attributes.

The child assumes that since he possesses some of the tangible, external characteristics of the model, he might also possess the model's desirable psychological properties—power, affection from others and instrumental competencies. In effect, the child seems to believe that objects appearing alike on the outside have similar internal properties. Thus, the greater the overlap of external similarities between himself and the model, the greater he considers the possibility that he will possess the model's power, affection and competence—the intangible psychological qualities he wishes to command. The desire for those qualities leads him to adopt and practice the model's characteristics.

The Interrelation of the Four Processes. These four processes combine to yield two causal sequences. The first two processes, whereby the child believes that he shares unique and distinctive attributes with the model and, therefore, experiences vicarious emotional reactions appropriate to events the model experiences, lead to the establishment of an identification. Their joint occurrence defines identification.

The second causal sequence involves the last two processes. As the child adopts additional attributes of a model, in the service of a desire to possess the model's goals, he will perceive that he, in fact, shares more attributes with the model. Consequently, he will experience even more intense vicarious emotional reactions and a stronger identification.

The four processes are thus interrelated because each time the child imitates the behavior of the model or adopts an attitude of the model, he perceives an increased similarity to the latter. This perception strengthens his belief that he must also possess the model's covert characteristics and allows him to share vicariously more of the positive affects of the model. The more desirable the model (Process 3), the greater the degree to which the child will strive to adopt the model's attributes (Process 4). The adoption of these behaviors leads the child to perceive increased similarity to the model (Process 1), which promotes more intensive vicarious affective reactions in the child (Process 2).

The Effect of Identification on Behavioral Development

The processes surrounding identification with and imitation of a model are as influential in determining behavioral differences among children as are differential reward and punishment of specific acts. Consider, for example, the lower-class child whose teachers reward him for studying and punish him for poor school performance, but whose parents do not display any personal interest in the acquisition of knowledge. This child is not as motivated to master school tasks as is the child whose parents display an active interest in his education. A child places special value on those behaviors practiced by desirable models.

Aggressive, dependent and sexual behaviors also assume different strengths in the child's behavioral repertoire, according to the extent that these behaviors are displayed by the models with whom the child has chosen to identify. When the pattern of adult reward and punishment agrees with the model's overt behavior, the child is most likely to practice that action. For example, a girl whose mother rewards dependent responses and is herself dependent on her husband is likely to become strongly dependent on her parents and friends. Prediction of the child's behavior is less certain, however, if these two conditions act antagonistically. For instance, if a father rewards his son's aggression toward others but is rarely aggressive himself, the frequency and style of aggressive behavior in the son is difficult to predict. However, consistency between the pattern of reward and the model's behavior is more likely than inconsistency, because parents are likely to reward explicitly those behaviors they themselves manifest most frequently.

The Effect of Identification on Self-Labels

Identification is not only important for the sculpting of overt behavior; it is also critical for the development of the ambiguous process of self-definition, which is sometimes called a *self-concept.* The child's self-concept consists, in part, of his evaluation of the degree to which his attributes match those that the culture has designated as desirable. The critical dimensions for Western culture include virtue, honesty, strength, size, attractiveness, intelligence, autonomy, wealth and power. To some extent the child's evaluation is determined by his social experiences. For instance, his self-conception of his power is based to some extent on his ability to defeat a rival, demonstrate his strength on an athletic field or achieve good grades. But the child also tends to label himself on the basis of his identification with a model. The boy who has developed an identification with an intelligent father begins to regard himself as intelligent. A girl who is identified with a beautiful mother views herself as more attractive than she would if her parent were not beautiful.

Negative self-evaluations can be established in a similar manner if a model's attributes are undesirable. One critical antecedent of psychopathology is the child's belief that he shares basic similarities with a negatively valued parent. Intensive interviews with seriously disturbed adults, including those with schizophrenic reactions, have provided evidence that many of these people feel unworthy, incompetent or basically evil because they believe that they are fundamentally similar to a parent whom they regard as unworthy, incompetent or unloving. The severely disturbed and unhappy person does not want to possess these undesirable traits, but the identification that has taken place has caused these beliefs.

A 5-year-old confronted with the fact that he is more similar to his parents than to any other adult he knows (because they share the same surname, body build and often the same features) inevitably develops some minimal identification with them. This minimal identification develops regardless of how undesirable or how unattractive the parents may be. As the child begins to recognize the negative qualities of the parental model, he also begins to believe that some of these qualities are part of his own set of personal characteristics.

Further Implications of Identification

The development of beliefs, motives and behaviors that reflect the dominant or expected standards of a culture are easier to explain than those that deviate from the norms. In most instances it is possible to explain normative behaviors without resorting to the concept of identification. The child sits in school, runs on the playground, talks at the school lunch table. These behaviors are appropriate in those contexts and do not require the concept of identification to explain them. Neither does the child's conscientious making of his bed each morning necessarily involve identification. More likely than not the child is motivated to perform this task in order to avoid parental punishment. Most of the behaviors that the child displays during the day either are habitual responses to a particular context or are motivated by a desire for positive reward or a desire to avoid punishment.

These mechanisms will not, however, explain why a child whose parents praise good grades and punish poor school performance obtains poor grades, why a 10-year-old boy who is told his grandfather won a Nobel Prize suddenly shows a spurt of motivation, or why a 30-year-old woman whose mother became psychotic at age 31 becomes tense and apprehensive as if she believed that she too were about to become psychotic. These behaviors are not appropriate to any particular context, nor do they bring praise or postpone social punishment. Many of these actions are derived from beliefs about one's attributes established as a result of perceived similarity to a model. Others are attempts to strengthen a beginning identification. The child will imitate the parent of the same sex in order to maximize similarity to him, and thereby increase his identification with that parent. The child is predisposed to imitate the parent of the same sex because he initially perceives more similarity to that parent than to the parent of the opposite sex.

During the years 3 to 6 the child identifies primarily with his parents, for they are the adults whom he knows best and whom he respects and admires. As he grows older, his parents' power and competence wane as he becomes aware of other adults who possess qualities and skills that surpass those of his parents. He meets local heroes or heroines; he hears about great athletes, astronauts and scientists. Often the extreme motivation that is required to work on a scientific discovery or a novel requires either an identification with a model who has played this role or an attempt to maximize similarity to such a model. One reason for the relative paucity of outstanding women scientists and artists is the lack of available role models for young girls. The child is more likely to believe he can command power, glory or greatness if someone of his own sex, ethnic, religious or racial group has done so in the past. The perception of similarity, which is one of the necessary conditions for identification, facilitates attempts to imitate the model.

The adolescent and young adult

establish identifications with groups (clubs, colleges) and with ideas (liberal attitudes, civil rights beliefs, philosophical positions). As he grows, he develops partial identifications with many different people. Some of these identifications are strong, and some are weak. Each identification contributes to his image of himself. The test for the presence of identification is relatively simple. If a person experiences positive feelings (joy or elation) when good things happen to the model, and negative feelings (sadness or shame) when bad things happen to the model, an identification is present. The beliefs about the self are derived, to some extent, from the models with whom the person has developed identifications.

The Importance of Perceived Similarity

A major issue in identification and imitation involves the emphasis placed upon the child's initial perception of similarity to the model. This similarity can be based on concrete physical attributes (short hair, trousers, dresses) or merely on the fact that the model and the child are called by the same categorical name (such as boys, men, ladies, Christians). The child wants consistency and order in his world. All objects or people with the same name should have the same characteristics. Once he learns what he is called—be it boy, Quaker or Negro—he acts to elaborate that definition.

Many theorists acknowledge the relevance of the model's power over the child in governing the degree of identification or imitation of the model. But some do not place heavy stress on whether the child believes in some initial basis of similarity to the model. However, it does seem reasonable to expect that if the child felt that he shared neither attributes nor categorical similarities with the model, he would doubt his ability to share vicariously in the model's goals. As a result, he would not strive to increase behavioral similarity to that model.

The relevance of perceived similarity to imitation has been demonstrated in several experiments. In one study, young children who were normally impulsive in their behavior were taught to become more reflective (Kagan et al., 1966). One group of first graders was taught to be reflective by a warm and friendly trainer (a woman for the girls and a man for the boys) using normal tutoring conditions. A second group was trained under identical conditions, except that prior to training the trainer took time to persuade each child that he or she shared basic attributes with the child. For example, the trainer would ask the child how many siblings he had and would then comment that he had the same number as the child. Questions about interest and favorite animals were answered first by the child, followed by the trainer noting the similarity between the child's choices and his own. The actual training to make the children more thoughtful and reflective was identical in both groups, and for both groups the trainers announced that they were thoughtful when they solved problems and that they valued this trait.

If the child's desire to maximize similarity to a model is enhanced by an initial perception of similarity to the model, then the children trained by the adult who emphasized similarity to the child should have become more reflective after training than the children in the other group. This prediction was confirmed for the girls, but not for the boys. There was no difference between the boys trained under the two conditions. However, although the boys in this study were trained by a male adult, they were tested by a female; whereas the girls were both trained and tested by a female adult. Thus, one would expect the tested effects of training to be more striking for the girls.

Perceived similarity to the model also facilitates imitation in older children. Young adolescent boys were told that they would be given a game-like task to solve after they watched a boy in a film work on the same task. Some of the subjects were led to believe they were similar to the model boy portrayed in the film; others were led to believe they were different from the model. After viewing the film each boy was allowed to work on the task for seven minutes. The boys who believed they were similar to the film model imitated many more actions of the film model than did the other group of boys (Rosenkrans, 1967).

A perception of similarity can increase feelings of empathy. Boys and girls in the first grade were shown a series of slide sequences depicting 7-year-olds in different emotional situations. Some of them involved happy events (a birthday party, winning a television contest); other slides displayed sadness (a lost dog, social rejection), fear (a lost child, a frightened dog) and the emotion of anger (a false accusation). After the child was shown the slide, a short narration was read so that he would understand clearly what the picture was about. Some children saw girls depicted in the slide sequences, and other children saw boys. Immediately following each slide sequence the child was asked simply to state how he felt. The boys were much more empathic when they were observing boys in the pictured situations, whereas the girls were more empathic when they were observing girls. Thus, a perception of similarity, in this case similarity in sex, facilitated empathic responses (Feshbach and Roe, 1968).

A perception of similarity to a model has also been found to increase the probability that the child will attend closely to what the model says or does. This conclusion has important implications for learning and school performance. It is supported by an experiment on the relation between perceived similarity and attention in two groups of college women who had been previously classified as highly involved either in obtaining good grades or in leading a social life (Chang, 1965). The women were told that they were to judge the creativitity of a pair of poems that two other female students had written. Each of the two hypothetical poets was described as being concerned with either good grades or an active social life. Thus, the subjects who were motivated to obtain good grades perceived themselves as resembling one poet; the socially motivated subjects perceived themselves as similar to the other poet.

The subjects heard the poems read on tape and then, instead of being asked to comment on the creativity shown in the poems, were asked to recall as much as they could of both poems. Since they had not expected to be asked to recall the poems, differences in the amount recalled should reflect differential attention to the two models. The subjects who were concerned with grades recalled more of the poem read by the model described as academically motivated, whereas the socially motivated girls recalled more of the poem read by the model who was more concerned with social life. It seems that perceived similarity to a model oriented the women to attend more closely to that model.

Further support for the central role of perceived similarity comes from the fact that children do not imitate the behavior of every person to whom they are exposed or identify with every model who has power. Psychiatric reports suggest that sons with excessively powerful and competent fathers often fail to identify with them. One possible explanation of this failure is that the boy may perceive no major bases of similarity to the father (that is, they may differ in body build, in frequency and intensity of affective states, in occurrence of failure at tasks). When the child cannot perceive some basis of similarity to the parent, he may be discouraged from attempting to establish an identification and consequently may not strive to adopt the model's characteristics.

In the current civil rights struggle, the Negro leaders recognize that the Negro child has a difficult time perceiving similarity to the white majority and, thus, identifying with the white culture. It is reasonable that they would request to have a totally Negro community, which would make the Negro child's task of identifying with appropriate Negro models easier than if he were in an integrated community. A Negro child is apt to feel less regret when a powerful Caucasian boy in his class is hurt than if the same misfortune befalls a less privileged Negro peer 100 miles away. The phenomenon of vicarious sharing in the affective states of a model appears to require a perception of similarity to another.

The Role of Identification in Acquisition of Standards

One of Freud's most significant statements was that "the superego is the heir of the Oedipus complex." Freud meant that the child's major defense against the anxiety created by the Oedipal conflict is identification with the parent of the same sex. The primary consequence of this identification is the adoption of the parents' standards regarding those behaviors and wishes that the society values.

Socialization of standards in the child under 3 years rests on the desire for affection from the parents and the need to avoid their punishment or rejection. During the preschool and early school years, a new motivational force supplements the purely external goals of social reward or avoidance of punishment. The 5-year-old realizes that certain standards of behavior and thought characterize "grown-up" children and adults, especially the adult model that is represented by the parent. Since the child wants to be like the adult models he has selected, he begins to adopt their behavior, attitudes and values.

Thus, the acquisition of standards is based not only on fear of external punishment, but also on the belief that these standards are appropriate for the child to possess. If the father is kind to other people and if the child wishes someday to be like his father, then he should come to believe that kindness is an appropriate characteristic to display. It should be one of his defining characteristics, just as his eyes, arms and legs are part of his anatomical attributes.

Consequences of Deviation from Standards

Standards are similar to schemata for objects. Once a child acquires a schema for a face an encounter with a discrepancy from that face elicits fear and a sense of discomfort. Similarly, once a 5-year-old believes that kindness is an appropriate characteristic for him to possess, he will experience discomfort if he recognizes that he deviates from this standard—if he sees a discrepancy between the standard and his behavior. Consider the 4-year-old who has been exposed repeatedly, 20 times a week for several years, to exhortations from his parents as to how he should behave if he is going to be grown up! He hears again and again such commands as "Wash your hands," "Do not yell at your mother," "Be kind to your sister." A point will come when these statements will harden cognitively and become accepted as the appropriate way for him to act. Behavior or thoughts that are discrepant from a standard are liable to provoke guilt or shame.

Differences Between Guilt and Shame. At a superficial level, guilt and shame seem similar, for both are characterized by an unpleasant feeling that results from violating a standard. At a somewhat deeper level, however, one finds that there are means of differentiating the two. The *behavioral manifestations* of shame and guilt are one means of differentiation. Shame is commonly, although not always, accompanied by blushing or lowering of the head and eyes. Guilt does not typically lead to any characteristic set of behaviors that are quite so public.

The *conditions* that elicit guilt and shame provide another basis for differentiation. The unpleasant feelings called shame are elicited by an expectation that *other people* will be disappointed in the fact that a standard has been violated. The unpleasant feelings called guilt are caused by expectations that the *self* will disapprove. The child is likely to feel shame when he believes he has violated a standard that someone has held for him. Shame is therefore tied to anticipation of disapproval from others for violation of a standard that the child accepts. Guilt, on the other hand, is more independent of the expectation of disapproval from another person. The child experiences guilt when he anticipates reprisal from his own conscience for violation of a standard he has set for himself, rather than of a standard he believes other people have set for him.

Shame typically occurs before guilt in the developmental process, for the learning of standards is fostered by the exchange of social acceptance because of one's practice of appropriate actions. Initially, many standards are set by other people. Although the child is aware of the standard and accepts it as appropriate for himself, he has not necessarily decided that it should be one of his defining attributes. The role of judge still resides in the external world. However, when the child himself eventually becomes the judge, the punishment is meted out by the self, and guilt is experienced.

This subtle distinction between shame and guilt can be appreciated by considering the following question: Does the child believe he has a choice with respect to initiating a certain act? There are some responses for which society gives the child little freedom of choice. He feels a pressure to behave in a particular manner because his family and friends expect it. It is as if society demands this behavior and he has no choice but to obey. Under these conditions, if the child does not behave in accordance with these standards he feels ashamed. He anticipates disapproval from parents, friends or teachers because he has violated their expectations of how he should behave. If the child believes he has a choice regarding a particular action, he perceives that the expectations of his social environment are not explicit. Under these conditions, he is more likely to experience guilt if he violates a standard. Guilt is a reprimand to the self for a mistake, for selecting the wrong alternative.

Let us consider some specific behavioral examples to illustrate this point. If a child's parents expect him to help his younger brother in a crisis, the standard "help your brother" is fully defined and allows no choice. The child would then feel shame if he did not aid his brother. If, on the other hand, the child felt that he had a choice, if he felt that his parents might not punish him for not being helpful, he would probably experience guilt for not coming to his brother's aid.

For the standard of nurturance, as indeed for most standards of conduct, the cultural requirements seem to be clearer and more commanding for girls and women than for boys and men. A girl typically orients to her parents, to her boyfriend, to her husband and to the wider social community for guidelines as to how to behave. As a result, she is more likely to feel shame than guilt when she violates a standard. In her view of the world she has no choice. The boy is more likely to feel guilt over violation of a standard because as he matures he comes to see that the source of authority for moral judgments must be himself. He is more likely to recognize that he has a choice. It is in a moral situation where choice exists that the conditions for guilt—that is, self-reprimand—are bred.

What Standards Are Established

Dependence, aggression, sexuality and task competence are some of the major behavioral areas around which standards develop during the period from 3 to 6 years of age. The order in which these specific standards are established during these years is not known in detail, and depends in part on the child's family background.

A primary determinant of the rate of establishment of standards is the frequency with which specific behaviors and their associated affects are given unambiguous verbal descriptions. It is likely that hostile feelings and resentful and angry thoughts will be frequently labeled as such by persons in the social environment. Aggressive postures, words and behaviors are public. American parents, for example, often label the child's pouting face, foot stamping or verbal barbs by remarking, "Don't be angry," or "Stop being so mad." In addition, parents display signs of anger that are appropriately labeled by others. The child's sexual excitement, urges for mastery or feelings of dependence or helplessness, on the other hand, are not as frequently and unambiguously labeled by the adult community. It follows, therefore, that standards concerning aggression and anger should emerge earlier than standards dealing with dependency, sexuality or task mastery.

An important standard adopted during the latter part of the preschool period involves task competence. The 5-year-old may cry when he loses a competitive game, smash his fist on the parts of a puzzle that he cannot fit together successfully or withdraw sheepishly from a rope he cannot climb. These signs of disappointment, anger and shame are consequences of the child's recognition that he has deviated from the standard that represented what he felt was the appropriate level of quality of performance.

The articulation of this standard is one reason that children become increasingly inhibited in school and reluctant to risk a guess or to offer an answer of which they are unsure. The 2-year-old, in contrast, is still innocent of a well-defined standard of competence and as a result feels free to try anything and to ask any question, regardless of how silly it might seem. As a child gradually accepts the burden of the standard that says he is "supposed to be correct and knowledgeable," he avoids placing himself in situations where that standard might be violated. If at the same time a child is aware of what is incorrect and believes that incorrectness is a violation of a standard, then he is driven to protect himself from exposure—and from possible shame and guilt.

Although cultures differ in the degree to which they promote standards of aggression, dependency and sexual modesty, all cultures promote different standards for males and females in certain psychological areas. Most of the psychological differences between adult men and women are the result of these different standards for the sexes. In our culture, men are supposed to be aggressive and women are supposed to be dependent when attacked or frustrated. Men are expected to inhibit signs of strong fear, emotion and weakness; women are expected to cry if stress is intense and to display their emotions overtly. Men should be interested in athletics, mechanics, science and mathematics; women should favor the arts, cooking, gardening and literature. These arbitrary assumptions about the appropriate behaviors for men and women in our culture are called sex role standards and are impressed upon the growing child through the process of *sex typing.*

This process refers to the tendency for each culture to promote the adoption of different behaviors for boys and girls and to establish different attributes as desirable for the respective sexes. The child generally learns these values between 3 and 10 years of age. Although the effects of sex typing are most apparent during the school years, the process commences during the preschool period.

The concept of sex typing and the related concepts of sex role standard and sex role identity have achieved much prominence among psychologists during the last decade. It is surprising, however, that this prominence has been so late in coming, for the behavioral differences between the sexes are public and have an ancient and transcultural heritage. Sociology and anthropology have not been neglectful of these concepts; more than a quarter of a century ago Linton (1936) wrote, "The division and ascription of statuses with relation to sex seems to be basic in all social systems. All societies prescribe different attitudes and activities to men and women."

The process of sex typing first requires the learning of behavioral standards that are different for boys and girls.

The Sex Role Standard

A standard is a belief about the appropriateness of a characteristic—be it an attitude, a motive, an affect, an external attribute or a response. Children attempt to develop and maintain a belief system about the self that coincides with those attributes they have learned to regard as "good," and to renounce and avoid attributes regarded as "bad." The bases for the evaluations of "good" or "bad" are culturally derived; they include for the Western community the belief that a person should be valued by and attractive to others, should develop the necessary instrumental skills and competencies to deal with selected problems, should possess the attributes and skills that the majority of the culture judge to be appropriate for his sex, should be rational, coherent, independent and responsible and should not engage in behaviors or become preoccupied with thoughts prohibited by the primary reference group (such as violence, aggression, disobedience, dishonesty, selfishness and open sexuality).

Thus, the Western middle-class child believes he should tell the truth, speak and think coherently and behave in a way appropriate to his sex role. Many standards are of approximately equal importance for boys and girls. But the standard that is called a "sex role standard" sets different values on a particular attribute depending on whether the child is male or female.

The child's learning of the content of a sex role standard resembles his learning of the meaning of any concept. He learns that a glass is clear, has a cylindrical shape and is used to hold liquid. A ball is round, made of rubber and bounces. Similarly, the child learns the definitions for boy and girl by noting what boys and girls do and how they look, and by listening to what adults and such sources as television tell him are the respective critical attributes of the words "boys" *versus* "girls," "men" *versus* "women," "fathers" *versus* "mothers."

The early discrimination of persons into these distinct classes is facilitated by the presence of a variety of clearly discriminable cues that include dress, bodily form and proportion, strength, distribution of hair, depth of voice, posture at the toilet, typical interactive behavior with another person and characteristic behavior in the kitchen, the garage or the backyard. The definition of the words "boy" and "girl," "male" and "female" compose what is known as the sex role standard, and these standards dictate the adoption and practice of motives, attitudes and behaviors that are appropriate for the respective sexes.

Females are supposed to inhibit aggression and open display of sexual urges, be passive with men, be nurturant to others, cultivate attractiveness and maintain an emotional, socially posed and friendly posture with others. Males are urged to be aggressive in the face of attack, independent in problem situations, sexually aggressive, instrumentally competent, in control of regressive urges and suppressive of strong emotion, especially anxiety. Parsons' (1948) dichotomy of masculine and feminine roles into instrumental *versus* expressive is consistent with the above attributes assigned to those roles. Instrumental roles require skills at solving environmental problems; expressive roles require skills in dealing with people.

This list of masculine and feminine attributes may strike readers as unrealistically traditional and not representative of contemporary values. However, existing data indicate that despite a common adult assumption that sex role standards are changing at a rapid rate, children continue to believe that aggression, dominance and independence are more appropriate for males and that passivity, nurturance and the ability to get along with others are more appropriate for females (Parsons, 1948; Hartley, 1960).

Sex Role Identity

A sex role standard has been defined as a belief shared by the members of the culture regarding the characteristics that are appropriate for males and females. But the abstracted concept of the ideal male or female as viewed by the culture is to be distinguished from a particular individual's conceptualization of his own degree of masculinity or femininity. The degree to which an individual regards himself as being masculine or feminine determines his sex role identity. Although this identity is but one component of a complex, interlocking set of beliefs that makes up his complete self-concept or self-identity, it is mandatory that the individual assign himself a value on the dimension of masculinity *versus* femininity. Although a person can be indifferent to some specialized attributes that might make up a self-identity (for example, a knowledge of photography or an ability to prune trees), he cannot be indifferent to his sex role identity.

How can a person determine how masculine or feminine he is? The degree of match or mismatch between the culture's sex role standards and the individual's assessment of his own overt and covert attributes provides him with a partial answer to this question. It is a partial answer because the belief system that is labeled sex role identity is not completely conscious. There is an imperfect correlation between possession of accepted sex role attributes and the integrity of one's sex role identity. A man who possesses many masculine traits might not necessarily regard himself as highly masculine. But it is unlikely for a man who possesses none of the culturally approved sex typed attributes to regard himself as highly masculine. Possession of some sex typed traits is necessary, but not necessarily sufficient, for a firm sex role identity.

The Significance of the Child's Sex Role Identity

The child' continuing desire for a stable and firm sex role identity is central to his development, for this desire imposes strong constraints on future behavior choices. The sex role identity has special significance for two psychological developments that occur in the preschool and early school years: (1) stability of behavior over time and (2) differential mastery of academic skills.

The effect of sex role identity on stability of behavior touches an issue of both practical and theoretical significance. Knowledge of that period of development during which an intimation of future behavior can be obtained is important for teachers, psychiatrists and psychologists as well as for other practitioners who wish to initiate preventive or early treatment procedures, whether the situation requiring attention is delinquency, excessive fears or academic problems. It is generally acknowledged that asocial behavior, sexual deviations and academic retardation in a 14-year-old are often resistant to conventional psychiatric treatment. Knowledge of the period during which these behaviors are being established would justify initiation of procedures at that time to prevent the early forms of personality disorder from becoming firmly entrenched. This knowledge would also be theoretically useful in pinpointing the developmental period during which investigations into the learning of deviant responses would be most profitable.

A study of the longterm stability of behavior from birth to adulthood in a group of middle-class subjects from the Fels Research Institute's longitudinal population suggested some important conclusions regarding the relation of sex role identity to behavioral stability (Kagan and Moss, 1962). Briefly, the procedure involved study of the relation between two independent sets of data on the same individuals: (1) ratings of adult behavior based on interviews when the subjects were between 20 and 30 years of age and (2) independent ratings of their behavior during the four developmental periods from birth to age 3, from 3 to 6, from 6 to 10 and from 10 to 14. The childhood ratings were based on behavioral observations in the home, nursery school, day camp, public school and interviews at the Institute. The major behavioral variables studies included aggression, dependency, passivity, intellectual achievement, anxiety over social interaction, heterosexual behavior and sex typed activities.

There was a strong association between the occurrence of a certain class of behaviors during age 6 to 10 and the occurrence of a similar behavior during young adulthood. The strongest correlation held for behaviors that matched sex role standards (see Fig. 7–2). If a sex role standard required inhibition of a behavior, the continuity from childhood (age 6 to 10) to adulthood was minimal. To illustrate: According to what we know of sex role standards, childhood passivity and dependence in stress situations should correlate with passivity and dependence for adult women but not for men. Since these

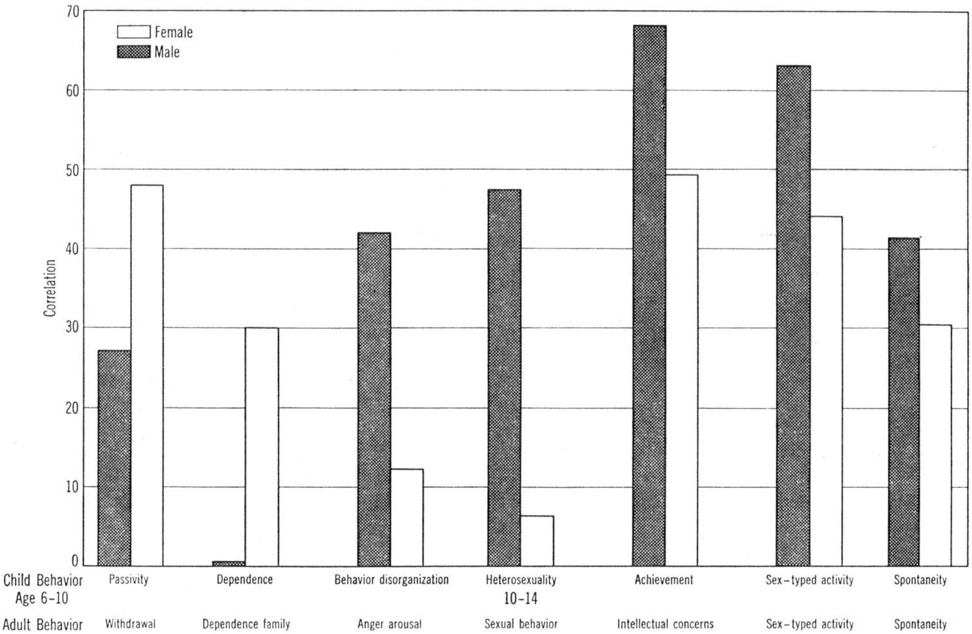

Figure 7–2 Summary of correlations between selected child behaviors and similar adult behaviors. (Adapted from Kagan, J., and Moss, H. A.: *Birth to Maturity: A Study in Psychological Development.* New York, John Wiley & Sons., Inc., 1962.)

traits violate masculine sex role standards, a passive or dependent boy would experience considerable pressure both from his parent and from the outside environment to inhibit overt passive behavior. For instance, one subject in this investigation showed a marked shift from dependence to independence during late childhood. His father placed an unusually high value on autonomy of action, and as the boy approached early adolescence he experienced strong family pressure to inhibit dependent behavior. The change in his behavior can be traced in his case history.

At 2½ years of age the subject (*S*) was described as unusually passive and cautious: *S* spent an unhappy week at nursery school. He cried a great deal and looked ready to cry even when he was not actually doing it. He drew away when other children approached him, and he seemed afraid of them. Usually he stood around and looked lost.

At 4½ years of age, passivity was still a characteristic response for the boy. This was one of the group's most isolated members. He was noncompetitive, unassertive and sedentary. He shrank from actual physical contact with others, and his relationship with his peers was a long distance verbal one. When he was verbally rebuffed he smiled weakly and put his hands behind his back. *S* was the most eclipsed member of the group because of his apprehension, shyness and inhibition.

By age 8, some shift toward independent behavior had occurred. There was a forced independence and swagger, and *S* had learned to use his intellectual skills as a weapon of power over others. He lectured and bragged to his peers; the fear that was manifest at age 4 was more disguised. He became less dependent on his family and more committed to hard work in school.

As a late adolescent the conflict over being passive had swelled in intensity and his standard did not permit retreat from potential failure stituations. At age 16, for example, he realized that he was still afraid of dating girls and decided that there was only one effective way to conquer this fear. He invited to a dance the most popular girl in the school, even though he had never been out with her before. He admitted that the primary reason for inviting her was to test his ability to conquer his fears. When he was asked if he ever went to his parents for advice, he replied, "My father was not approachable and I didn't go to him for advice. In fact, he used to tell me to solve my own problems by myself and I felt uneasy about going to him for help. My mother wouldn't know what to tell me anyway."

The expression of aggression and the initiation of sexual behavior, unlike passivity and dependency, are acceptable responses for males but not for females. The data from the longitudinal population revealed that aggression toward adults and heterosexual behavior during childhood was related to frequency of anger arousal and sexual behavior in adulthood for men but not for women.

An intense concern with good grades in school and mastery of intellectual skills is appropriate and encouraged for both sexes among the middle class; sex role standards do not dictate strong inhibition of intellectual mastery for either sex. As a result, concern with intellectual skills should be relatively stable for both sexes. The results of the study affirm this expectation with the degree of continuity slightly higher for males than for females.

Finally, the child's tendency to practice sex typed behaviors is highly stable from early childhood to adulthood. The correlations between practice of sex appropriate activities during the period from 6 to 10 and adulthood were 0.63 for men and 0.44 for women. This finding is supported by data from the Oakland Growth Study (Mussen, 1961, 1962), which revealed a moderately high relation between degree of masculine interest in males during adolescence and during adulthood.

In sum, childhood behaviors that are congruent with sex role standards are likely to remain strong and display continuity from childhood through adulthood. Behavior that deviates markedly from sex role standards will be inhibited as a result of the child's desire to avoid social rejection and to model himself after culturally approved role models.

The Effect on Intellectual Mastery

Although competence in intellectual and academic tasks is not as clearly a consequence of sex role identity as is the expression of aggression or dependency, it appears that the degree of involvement in challenging intellectual problems is greater for adolescent and adult males than for females. Particularly well documented is the fact that mastery of problems requiring analysis and reasoning (primarily those involving spatial and mechanical reasoning, science and mathematics) is viewed as more appropriate for boys than for girls. When adolescent or adult subjects were presented with problems involving primarily mathematical or geometric reasoning, males consistently obtained higher scores than females. Moreover, there was a low positive relationship between interest in culturally approved masculine activities (athletics and mechanics) and the quality of problem solving scores for both sexes.

The female who rejected traditional feminine interests performed better on mathematical and geometric problems than did the girl who had adopted traditional feminine behaviors. On problems dealing with feminine interests such as cooking and gardening materials the females scored better than on problems dealing with guns, money and geometric designs, even though the logical steps and computations were identical. It seems that the typical female believes that the ability to solve problems involving geometry, physics, logic or arithmetic is a uniquely masculine skill, and her motivation to attack such problems is low. This decreased involvement may reflect the fact that the girl's self-esteem is not at stake in such problems. Or she may feel threatened by the possibility that she might perform with unusual competence on such tasks, for excellence on such tasks might be equated with a lack of femininity.

Although an intense involvement in academic mastery is more characteristic of the adolescent and adult male than of his female counterpart, this is not the case in the primary grades. From kindergarten through grade four girls typically outperform boys in all areas, and the ratio of boys to girls with reading problems ranges from 3 to 1 to 6 to 1 (Tyler, 1947; Bentzen, 1963). Why is there a developmental shift between the ages of 6 and 17? One reason has been mentioned above: among late adolescent boys, academic proficiency becomes linked to vocational success, and their motivation is stronger than it was during the early years of school. Moreover, the girl's motivation toward mastery decreases with age as a result of anxiety over feeling intellectually more competent than the boy. She also may experience conflict over excessive intellectual competitiveness. It is not uncommon for an adolescent to view competitive intellectual striving as an aggressive behavior. Since the typical female acquires stronger anxiety over aggressive and competitive behavior than the male, she experiences greater conflict over intellectual competition (Buss, 1961; Kagan and Moss, 1962). This conflict can lead to inhibition of intense strivings for academic excellence.

Another reason boys gradually increase in academic superiority is that their perception of the sex typed character of school and academic work changes. The average American boy perceives the primary school atmosphere as excessively feminine: His introduction into school is conducted by female teachers, who usually initiate the activities of painting, coloring and singing. Moreover, most teachers place a premium on obedience, decorum and inhibition of aggressive and restless behavior—values that are clearly more appropriate for girls than for boys.

Recent studies with second graders confirm the suggestion that the school situation is viewed as more feminine than masculine. The children were taught different nonsense syllables to stand for maleness and femaleness. They were then shown pictures of school-related objects, such as a blackboard, a page of arithmetic, a book, a school desk and a library, as well as nonacademic stimuli such as a lion, a bird and a cup, and were asked to label them with one of the "masculine" or "feminine" nonsense syllables. The results indicated that the second graders were more likely to label the school objects feminine than masculine (Kagan, 1964). This tendency diminished with age, especially for boys. The labeling of the nonacademic objects was as expected—that is, the children called a cup feminine and a lion masculine.

Since the typical 7-year-old American boy perceives the school atmosphere as "feminine," he is likely to resist complete involvement in its activities and should be expected to fall behind in academic areas. As mentioned earlier, more boys than girls in American schools are classified as seriously retarded in reading ability. However, if this argument has merit, then in a community with a large proportion of male teachers there should not be a larger proportion of boys than girls with serious reading problems. The island of Hokkaido in northern Japan is such a community. In grades one and two close to 60 per cent of teachers are men and 40 per cent are women. The occurrence of reading difficulties is not more frequent among boys than girls. In fact, the percentages are equal—about 9 per cent of each sex are considered to have problems with reading.[3]

Thus, it seems that during the opening years of school, the boy's motivation to master academic skills is partly dependent on his view of its appropriateness for his sex role identity. However, during the adolescent years a more sophisticated differentiation of academic work occurs. This differentiation turns on the schism between the sciences and the humanities. The adolescent begins to classify knowledge on three related dimensions: Is it practical or impractical? Does it have an important effect upon the world, or is it unrelated to instrumental changes in the environment? Does it deal with machines or words? Since a pragmatic, instrumental and mechanical orientation to nature is important in the sex role standard for males (Parsons 1948), some adolescent boys are highly motivated to master the sciences but poorly motivated to master "impractical" subjects that involve only words and ideas, such as language or history. Similarly, the girl who has chosen a masculine career, such as law, medicine or science, may experience anxiety over exerting effort in an activity that is not traditionally feminine. There is an implicit association between subject matter and sex role standards.

It appears that for most adult members of Western culture there are strong semantic associations between the words "masculinity" or "femininity" and specific areas of knowledge. This is an unfortunate connection, for one would hope that knowledge would retain neutrality amid the warring factions of the mind. There is, however, cause for some optimism. American elementary and secondary schools—long the exclusive domain of female faculty—now contain a larger proportion of male teachers, especially in the high schools.

MOTIVATIONAL DEVELOPMENT

All children acquire ideas about goals they would like to attain. These ideas are called motives, and they undergo lawful changes with development. The concept of motive is distinct from the concept of biological drive. A drive is a state of deprivation or discomfort caused by a disturbance in the physiology of the organism. Hunger, thirst, cold and pain are biological drives. Each drive leads to the activation of certain structures in the central nervous system and often produces sensations that are unpleasant. However, these drives are to be distinguished from motives. In simplest form a motive is a wish, a set of images or thoughts that represent events the individual desires to experience or to possess. Motives are cognitive and have no necessary relation to overt action. The child may have wished for many years to be able to fly but may have taken no steps toward attaining that goal. Motives have two states, potential and active, just as energy has a potential and kinetic state. Most of

[3]These data were supplied by Dr. Kuzuo Miyake.

the time the child is not experiencing a motive related to a desired goal and, at these times, the motive is in a potential state. Motives are transformed from a potential to an active state when some event arouses the motive. The arousing event is called an incentive. Children differ in the ease with which an incentive can evoke a motive. Some are easily provoked to the wish to have their mothers hug them; others rarely have such thoughts. Some respond to the slightest frustration with hostile motives; others require excessive frustration before they experience hostility. The easier it is for a particular incentive to elicit a motive, the stronger that motive. The child's motives exist in a hierarchy. That is to say, at any one stage of development some motives are stronger than others and dominate the child's psychological experience. At 2 years of age the motive for a close relationship with the parent dominates most other motives, while at 15 years of age this motive is much weaker in comparison with the motive for a satisfying heterosexual relationship.

Since motives have no necessary link to overt action, we must understand the factors that determine whether a motive will prompt the child to attempt to gratify it. The child must first have learned responses that effectively gratify the motive. A 6-year-old who has a strong desire to control his older brother may not have learned how to effect this control and, therefore, will not evidence signs of this motive in his everyday behavior. A second factor governing the probability of a motive leading to a behavior is the child's expectancy that the action will be successful in obtaining the goal. The 5-year-old who has been in three foster homes, none of which responded to his requests for affection and help, is likely to stop displaying such requests and become sullen and withdrawn. The lower the child's expectancy of gratifying a motive, the less likely he will be to direct his behavior toward attainment of that goal. Anxiety over displaying the goal-related behavior is a third factor that controls the link between motive and action. A motive in a 2-year-old is likely to lead to behavior aimed at gratification because young children have not learned to delay or inhibit attempts at gratifying their strong motives. The 7-year-old, by contrast, has learned that he must delay many of his desires and inhibit certain actions because of guilt or fear of parental rejection. The fourth and final determinant of goal-directed behavior is the immediate situation in which the child becomes aroused. The child who feels strong hostility toward his mother is not likely to behave in a relevant way if he is sitting in a classroom, although he would be much more likely to express this motive if he were at home. In general, the social environment reacts to and classifies the child primarily on the basis of his actions, rather than his motives, and it is through his behavior that other people initially come to know him. Society generally cares more about whether a child hits other children than about his hostile thoughts; cares more about his overt sexual behavior than the quality of his sexual fantasies.

Why We Need the Word "Motive"

The major reason for requiring the concept of motive for the description and understanding of human behavior rests with the faith that some of our actions are influenced by anticipations of the future. We cannot account for all of a person's behaviors unless we invent a word to explain why someone suddenly changes his action without provocation from the external environment. Imagine a quiet library containing 15 people.

One persons rises from his chair, leaves the room and returns 10 minutes later. We ask him why he left, and he tells us that he had to make a telephone call to arrange a dinner date. He had a future goal in mind and acted in a way to insure attainment of the goal. We need a concept to explain why people display behavior that is not appropriate or expected in a certain situation. A person stops one sequence of behavior and begins another. If there is no obvious, external cause for the change in action, it is likely to be in the person's mind. When that cause is the idea of a future goal, we say the person is motivated.

Motives also help to explain why a person may resist performing a request, or believing what he is told. Since it is easier to conform that to resist, there must be a reason for the nonconformity, and the reason may lie within the person. He must prefer to do what he is doing or to think what he is thinking. He must have an idea of what he prefers to do or believe, and we need a word to describe this typically human state.

Not all behaviors are motivated. In fact, most behaviors are the result not of a motive, but of the immediate situation. A person sits in an auditorium because that is the expected action. The person may have been motivated when he initially purchased a ticket for the concert, but his sitting behavior in the auditorium is governed by the situation. We have to view behavior as composed of paragraphs. The first action, like the first sentence of a new paragraph, is generated from within. But once the first action has been taken, there is a restriction on the next one. Once you start a sentence of greeting to someone, the rest of the sentence is governed partially by the initial utterance. The situation demands a certain kind of completeness. If we could tell when a person was beginning a new paragraph in his behavior, in contrast to when he was merely acting in the middle of one, we would be better able to understand his motives.

The concept of motive was originally introduced into psychology to bear the burden of the idea of *cause*, which was popular in physics and chemistry. The view of nature during the past few centuries has been dominated by the physical sciences, which have insisted until recently that every event in nature has a cause. Contemporary social scientists were influenced by this faith and believed that the task of science was to find the causes of behavior. Sigmund Freud was strongly influenced by this view of human nature and made it an essential theme in his psychological theory. The basic human motives, which Freud called the id impulses, were viewed as the causes of behavior and of symptoms. If the motives were obvious to neither the person nor the observer, then they must be unconscious. But there had to be a motive for all behavior. Current conceptions of human action are not so uncritically wedded to the idea that all action has a motive, which is not equivalent to saying actions have no cause. Some actions are the product of unlearned, rather automatic reflexes such as sneezing and coughing. These behaviors are caused, but the cause is not a motive. Other actions are habitual to certain subtle feeling states. A professor talking to a small group of students suddenly rises from his chair and walks around a few moments before sitting down again. It is not necessary to assume that he wanted to stand up, that there was any specific goal to be attained. He stood up because this action had become a habitual response to a certain quality of excitement, much like the babbling of a 4-month-old infant to a smiling face. The babbling of the baby reflects the excitement generated by studying the face. The infant does not want to babble, nor is it necessarily gratified by making this noise.

The most important examples of specific behaviors which are not motivational are the many learned reactions to particular situations. An American child sits in a chair to eat, the Japanese child kneels on a pillow, a New York commuter in La Guardia airport stands at a counter. The specific postures of sitting, kneeling or standing are not motivated. These postures are appropriate for the context in which the person is dining. The presence of a chair invites sitting, a pillow invites kneeling, a counter invites standing. The reader may reply that it is not the specific posute displayed that is motivated, but the act of eating. Yet we know that a person often eats breakfast at 8:00 A.M., lunch at noon and dinner at 7:00 not because he has any desire for food, but because it is the appropriate time to eat. The context of the family sitting at the breakfast table at 8:00 A.M. invites the action. The total situation that encompasses waking in the morning and seeing the table set with bacon and eggs calls for the act of sitting down for breakfast. Many actions are learned rituals to particular contexts, and are not necessarily the product of a motive.

There are, on the other hand, many behaviors that are the result of motives, and we shall consider how they develop and influence action.

Elaboration of the Meaning of Motives

Although a motive is an idea about a goal, it is not always fully conscious and well detailed. It is not always like the state we experience when we instruct ourselves, "I must go to the post office, then to the barber and be back at the office by 1:30." A motive can be a verbalized reminder, a fleeting image or a fragmented version of either. More often it is a mental state that can best be described as an *abstract mental set.*

A mental set can be likened to the tuning of a radio or television set. When you move a dial to a particular setting the television amplifier becomes maximally receptive to one set of signals and minimally receptive to all others. Similarly, when a person switches a channel from a news broadcast to a replay of a Gary Cooper movie, he sets himself to receive certain sounds and sights. As he turns the channel he is mentally preparing himself for a particular set of events. This preparation is the set we call motive. It may be an image of what he is about to see, but it need not be. It is more likely to be an abstract psychological state that is difficult to specify further.

A particularly good illustration of the meaning of motive as set involves the simple behavior of driving home after a day at work. An executive leaves his office at 6 P.M. briefly reminding himself where he is going. The self-instruction takes less than a second. His mind then turns to other matters—the evening's work, the problems of the next day, the unsolved crises in the laboratory. He gets in his car, starts the ignition, leaves the parking lot and automatically makes the correct set of turns without ever thinking about the goal toward which he is driving. He arrives home without really thinking about what he is doing. Had he decided, as he left the office, that he was going to a restaurant on the opposite side of the city, he would have made a different set of correct turns and also arrived at his goal. There was a brief moment when a representation of a goal set the executive to select a group of action routines that ran off automatically. The motive was the brief representation of the goal.

A motive limits both perception as well as action, for it acts like a governor on a motor or a program in a computer. The mind can be likened to a large collection of routines with an executive deciding which routine should be activated. The motive instructs the executive to focus more selectively on one set of routines, and to ignore others.

Sensory Motives: The First Motives

The first motives acquired by the young child are wishes to experience a small set of pleasant feelings—fullness when hungry, cessation of pain, warmth when cold, genital stimulation, physical contact. Although it is obvious that the child wishes to repeat events that are physically pleasant—one 4-year-old calls his penis "happiness"—the conditions that determine pleasantness are not always that clear. The desirability of the feelings produced by genital stimulation, a sweet taste or warmth are obvious, and we shall call them *sensory motives.* A second set of sensory motives includes reduced stress, pain and similar unpleasant feeling states.

It is important to appreciate the fact that most of the motives of the older child, in contrast to the younger child, are directed at attaining thoughts and interpretations of experience. The motives of the younger child, are more often directed at specific external events. The 3-year-old wants his mother; the 4-year-old wants a tricycle. The desired goal in each case is an external object. The lonely 10-year-old wants reassurance or a sign that he is valued by his parents. The specific external events desired by the older child are idiosyncratic equivalences for symbolic goals he requires.

The Motive To Control Uncertainty

One of the basic motives characteristic of all phases of development is the desire to control uncertainty. There are three major classes of uncertainty. In the first, an event is discrepant from a schema. The event can be in the outside world—a strange animal or a friend's failure to smile—or can originate within the body—an odd feeling in the chest or an intermittent throbbing in the forearm. These events alert the person and generate uncertainty. If these odd experiences cannot be explained, fear occurs.

A second cause of uncertainty arises when there is lack of congruence between two ideas or between an idea and behavior. The child who believes in God is told by a friend that this idea is silly. A child who believes his father to be wise and beloved overhears a relative criticize the father's competence and virtue. Now the child has two beliefs that are inconsistent, and he is uncertain as to which he should believe. He cannot hold both, and he must do something to resolve the uncertainty. Two ideas claim the same source of legitimacy, and the executive must decide which one is the fraud. Usually the conflict is resolved by changing both ideas and then accepting each as partially valid. Uncertainty is also generated when there is inconsistency between behavior and belief. The child feels he is honest and has just told a lie. He believes he is brave but has just crossed the street to avoid running into a bully. His actions cast doubt on his belief about himself. His faith is shattered and uncertainty follows. If the child can resolve the uncertainty, no fear will occur. If he cannot rationalize the inconsistency, he will become upset.

Unsureness about the future is the final source of uncertainty, especially if the doubt hovers over unpleasant events. The child wonders if he will be punished, hit, fail or be rejected. The state of not knowing when psychological catastrophe will strike is one of man's most discomforting states. If he cannot ignore the doubt or reassure himself, fear or anxiety will mount, often to an intensity that prevents any productive action or thought.

Each of these sources of uncertainty leads to the primary motive to gain control of or reduce in some way the ensuing uncertainty. But there are many ways to accomplish this goal. Some children will have learned that staying close to a parent alleviates uncertainty; we say these children have a dependency motive. Others try to get adult praise for a painting, a report card or a clean room, and we say that these children have a motive for recognition. Others may bully a weaker child in the service of a motive for dominance or hostility. Each of these desires grows out of the motive to control uncertainty: we call them *secondary motives.* Since children are raised by human beings rather than by machines, and since most adults are capable of helping the child reduce uncertainty, many children want a close, reassuring relationship with adults. This is one reason why we often view dependent children as uncertain, anxious or insecure. But some children learn to withdraw from adults when they are anxiously uncertain because they have not had the experience of an adult's helping them to control uncertainty and fear. The central dynamic sequence leading to secondary motives starts with discrepancy alerting the individual. If he can not interpret, modify or act upon it, he becomes upset and is motivated to attain goals that he believes will give him control. Hence, most of the popular motives ascribed to people can be derivatives of a primary motive to control uncertainty and subsequent emotional distress.

However, if the person can act upon the initial discrepancy, the primary motive will not be activated. If the child can ignore or modify the discrepancy, the primary motive will not grow. This aborting of uncertainty can be seen in many situations.

A one-year-old watches his mother leave him alone in a strange room. If he is not actively engaged in any activity, he is more likely to become afraid and cry than if his attention is absorbed in some activity. Uncertainty elicits fear only when there are no available reactions that either cope with it or detract attention from it.

Many social institutions are conveniently organized ways to provide action routines to deal with uncertainty. Religion, work, school and even sex are complex ritualized involvements that bind attention and turn the person's mind from preoccupation with discrepancies and inconsistencies that cannot be easily interpreted or acted upon.

To summarize, *psychological uncertainty is evoked when events discrepant from established schema, or inconsistencies between thoughts alert a child who has no coping response available.* He becomes anxious, and is motivated to alleviate both the uncertainty and anxiety. Each child learns a set of specific goal-directed routines to be used under these conditions. These secondary motives represent the child's solution to his problem.

Let us now turn to a second set of motives and emotions: namely, anger, hostility and aggression.

ANGER AND THE MOTIVE OF HOSTILITY

The relation between anger and hostility parallels the relation between anxiety and uncertainty. Let us consider first the conditions that elicit the emotion of anger.

Interruption of a Response Routine

Any interruption of a chain or a sequence of behavior that is directed toward a goal can provoke anger. The child is building a tower of blocks and his brother knocks them down. The mosiac of internal sensations created by this event is one component of anger. The second component involves the child's evaluation of the cause of the interruption. Most of the time the evaluation of cause centers on the immediately present source of the frustration and involves a wish to hurt, physically or psychologically, the person that caused the interruption. This mental representation of harm delivered to the frustrating person defines the motive of hostility. Consider the parallel with uncertainty and anxiety. A discrepant event that can not be handled provokes anxiety; blocking of a sequence of action provokes anger. The emotion of anxiety often leads to a motive to reduce uncertainty; the emotion of anger often provokes the motive of hostility. Hostility is a primary motive, as is the wish for control of uncertainty, that is likely to be learned when the child is angry. We say "likely to be learned" because it is not necessary that the child learn to wish harm to someone whenever he feels angry. If a person does not know what force interrupted his behavior—what caused the tower to fall—he is not likely to have a hostile wish. In fact, under these circumstances he is likely to become afraid rather than angry. Consider the common experience of a stuck door. Anger develops if one believes that someone locked it from the other side. Anger, perhaps at the self, develops if one believes that the door is warped because he failed to oil it before winter began. But if one is sure that the door is neither locked nor warped, yet unsure as to why it will not open, anxiety is likely to occur. The stuck door has now become a discrepant event that cannot be explained.

Anxiety or anger can arise in the same external situation depending on personal interpretation. Anxiety occurs when there is no immediate explanation for an event that is discrepant or blocks a response routine. Anger occurs when one believes he knows the cause of the unwanted event. There are some intriguing predictions that follow from this analysis. If an event is unusual, people who do not reflect upon possible explanations are apt to become angry; those who pause to analyze the situation rationally are more likely to become anxious. The national unrest in America prior to the 1968 presidential elections made many academic intellectuals anxious because they realized that no one person or group was to blame for the strife that tore at the nation's spirit. The "conditions and the times" were held responsible, but one could not become angry with an entity as abstract as "the conditions and the times." Other segments of the population became angry at the hippies, the Blacks, the college students or all three, because they believed these persons were the cause of the unrest. Many voted for George Wallace out of anger and hostility to those who wanted Humphrey or McCarthy elected. They wanted to hurt those who had frustrated them. The more knowledge one has about a situation that *has* no clear or simple cause, the less likely will anger be a dominant reaction. But the more knowledge one has about situations that *have* clear causes, the more likely one will become angry, especially if the cause is human.

One therefore expects a child to pass through several developmental phases during which the balance of anger and anxiety will change. During the first three years, when the child has very few explanations for unusual human actions, he is likely to become frightened at discrepant human behavior. As he approaches school age and develops some fixed ideas as to cause, the balance shifts toward anger as the more common reaction. The 8-year-old boy is angered by his failure to obtain a position on the neighborhood baseball team because he blames a peer or an adult for this frustration. The younger child of 3, by contrast, is not likely to become angry at being excluded from a peer activity. The blaming by the 8-year-old effectively transforms anxiety to anger by placing the source of discomfort in the external world. A child's mood can easily be transformed from anxiety to anger as he realizes, or persuades himself, that the odd event that he could not understand was a trick perpetrated by someone. When the initially frightened child realizes the human source of his fear he complains angrily "why did you scare me"?

A Second Occasion for Anger: Threat

A threat or challenge to one's standards also provokes anger. Name calling is the classic example. Why does a 10-year-old become angry if she is called stupid, homely or afraid? One interpretation assumes that a threat to a standard is similar to the blocking of a response routine. A person's actions flow from his standards, and a threat to the standard leaves behavior without a rational foundation. A child would not study if he believed he were stupid and could not master the subject. An adolescent would not try to establish a relationship with a girl if he were sure he would not be attractive to her. The undermining of standards is an obstacle to initiating action. Each person's actions must be in some degree of harmony with his beliefs, for beliefs give direction to behavior. Thus, if we imply a child is unintelligent, we suggest that his diligence is foolish because he can never attain competence. This threat is a direct block to future perseverance. All name calling implies that the negative trait in the "slur" makes it impossible for the person to behave in any other way. Anger is generated when a response routine is directly or potentially interrupted.

The emotion of anger must be differentiated from the motive of hostility. Hostility is a wish to cause pain, distress or anxiety to another person or to a surrogate for that person. The person to whom the hostility is directed is the one who is believed to be the thwarting agent or the one who threatens the child's standards. Although anger and hostility often occur together, they can occur separately. The 5-year-old who cannot open the screen door to enter the house becomes angry and may stamp his foot, but he may not have hostile wishes toward anyone at that moment. The situations that arouse anger change with development. During the first two years of life, restriction of the child's natural tendency to explore the environment is a major cause of anger. The parents' tendency to force the child to sleep, to stay within fenced areas and to keep away from attractive but fragile objects often elicits anger. During the preschool years, when the child is given more freedom, deprivation or postponement of specific goals elicits anger. During the school years, when even more freedom is granted to the child, he usually becomes angered by events that threaten standards regarding sex role, passivity, autonomy or acceptance. These values are threatened when someone implies that the child has an undesirable set of characteristics, or when the child encounters a salient person who holds values different from those held by the child.

Although it is usually assumed that all aggressive behavior is derived from hostility, this is not the case.

Some behaviors that hurt people are not in the service of anger or hostility. Aggression, therefore, is best defined as any action that causes pain, anxiety or distress to another, and is also in the service of a hostile motive or the emotion of anger. The advantage of this definition is that it allows us to reject actions that unintentionally hurt others, but to include acts that, on the surface, appear to be culturally valued but that intentionally cause distress to another person.

The Motive for Mastery

The motive to master or perfect a skill—called effectance by Robert White (1959)—is related to, but not identical with, the motive to control uncertainty. The first difference is that this motive does not have a distinctive feeling state that precedes the motive. A 4-year-old sees a pile of blocks in the corner and quietly sits down and builds an elaborate house. Although deeply involved, it is unlikely he experienced any strong feeling as he walked toward the blocks, or even as he began working. Second, the desire to perfect a skill, finish a task or conquer a challenging problem can arise from secondary motives based on uncertainty and hostility. A child may work at school to prevent criticism from teacher or parent, and hence reduce uncertainty over adult acceptance. A boy may practice baseball to obtain a position that a rival wanted. James Watson's lively description of the competitive mood that motivated him and Sir Frances Crick to discover the structure of DNA illustrates the capture of mastery through hostile wishes. But the motive for effectance also seems to have its own primary foundations. These are based on three related factors: the desire to match behavior to a standard, to predict and control environmental events and to define the self.

The Desire To Match Behavior To a Standard

The child is continually acquiring ideas about the world. As he establishes these representations, he comes to believe in them and tries to maintain them. Some of these representations are experienced directly; he knows that pudding is eaten with a spoon and that handkerchiefs are put in pockets. Other rules he has heard about but not experienced: bobsledding is exhilarating, marijuana is relaxing. These rules are like compasses that guide behavior and reasoning. Jonathan Richardson noted over 250 years ago, "For it is a certain maxim, no man sees what things are, that knows not what they ought to be."

Each person attempts to simulate, by construction or imitation, these idealized rules. The 4-year-old builds a house of blocks because he has an idea of what a house of blocks should look like, and the blocks are available. Man climbs mountains because he has a representation of the scene at the top, and because a mountain is available. There is, however, an additional factor that limits the evocation of this motive. It is foolish to expect that any time a child sees some blocks he will stop and build a house. There has to be, in addition, some uncertainty about attaining the idealized state. If the child is perfectly certain he can build a house of blocks, or certain he can not, he will not build it. He has to be a little unsure. Hence, *one basis for the mastery motive is possession of a representation of an idealized state of affairs, coupled with some uncertainty about the ability to match behavior to that standard.* This uncertainty is usually not accompanied by the unpleasant feelings of anxiety. Rather, the affect state accompanying mastery is more subtle and pleasant, and invites the term *excitement.* Whether excitement or anxiety is generated by uncertainty often depends, first, on whether the person can deal with the discrepancy and, second, on whether he created it or whether it was imposed from without. Anxiety is more likely to occur when the course of the uncertainty is imposed and/or when the individual has no reaction to cope with it. Excitement occurs when the child generates the uncertainty and/or he has a relevant coping action. The person seeks uncertainty when he believes he can deal with it; he avoids uncertainty when he believes he can not.

The Desire To Predict and To Control

A second related basis for mastery involves the wish to predict and to control future events. We spend some of each day estimating the weather, or the traffic conditions at 6:00 P.M. The ability to predict permits the feeling of control. The attraction to new experience often derives from the desire to predict the self's reaction in a novel context. One force behind the youth's initial experimentation with mescaline, marijuana or LSD is the wish to know if the self "can take" the strong feelings and emotions produced by the drug. The continued use derives, in part, from the desire to become adept at predicting one's feelings and thoughts in the drugged state. When prediction becomes accurate the person may stop this activity. Affect is most intense while predictive control is being gained, not when it has been attained. Animals, too, seem most aroused when they are mastering a new habit, not after the habit has been learned (Fischer, 1970). Man typically selects tasks to master that have some uncertainty and for which he has some initial set of responses appropriate to the venture. Uncertain challenges that do not engage any behavioral implementation are shunned. This dynamic leads to the third basis for mastery, the desire for self-definition.

The Desire To Define the Self

Each individual wants to know the quality and uniqueness of his psychological characteristics; those attributes that define the *self-as-object* to the *self-as-person.* The attributes viewed as salient depend on the culture's prejudices, and the child turns toward the culture to discover the characteristics he should try to master. But even after he learns them he often requires others to help him evaluate how well he is doing. Society tells the girl to be beautiful, but she can only know her attractiveness by comparing herself with women who define the total range of beauty, and by deciphering the sincerity of flattering men.

Only a few adults have such a firm conceptualization of the self that decisions about skill, beauty or value can be made without social display or comparison. Children are clearly not capable of this autonomous decision, but each child wants to know his assets and limitations, and is motivated to mastery in order to obtain this information. The child's identity is composed, in part, of his profile of talents, and he must master some tasks if he is to develop an identity. One of the critical requirements is the uniqueness of the valued skill. There is minimal psychological advantage in acquiring a normative talent. The ability to walk, hold a fork or open a door adds little to self-definition. Children and adults are driven to acquire a few valued routines that others do not have, or to develop an extraordinary competence in a normative one. The more unique the profile of unusual competencies, the better delineated the identity.

Mastery, therefore, can serve several more basic motives: the desire to reduce uncertainty, to gain predictive control and to define the self. The motive for mastery can be gratified in almost any behavioral context one can imagine, from backyard to battlefield. The criminal robs a bank, the young wife prepares a bouillabaisse, the sergeant drills his platoon, the student plans a protest march. Psychologists have narrowed their attention too narrowly on instances of this motive in intellectual domains. Man likes to test himself throughout the total range of his capacities, and a healthy society provides a variety of arenas in which self-examination can thrive. When there are too few choices for test, many lose the vitality that is so distinctly human.

Sexual Motivation

It may seem odd that sexual motivation is the fourth rather than the first motive to be discussed, considering the fact that Freud gave so much emphasis to this motive. Sexual motivation is important in childhood, but we do not believe it is as critical as the desire for certainty, hostility or mastery. However, the most important distinction between sexuality and the other motives is that sexuality is primarily a sensory motive; the others are not. The primary goal of sexual motivation is the sensation derived from genital stimulation. The primary goal for the other motives is not a sensory state but a cognitive state. Of course, mental representations of goals soon become associated with this sensory motive. The child experiences sexual excitement when he sees someone of the opposite sex undressed, when he hears a sexual joke, when someone brushes against him. Any one of a wide variety of events can become linked with the feelings of sexual excitement, and each of these events can serve as goals for secondary sexual motives.

It is important to realize that the primary sexual motive is not the same as the desire to appear masculine or feminine, nor the same as the motive for dating, marriage or promiscuity. Each of these actions can serve the primary sexual motive, but they need not. They can serve other motives, as indicated earlier.

Although the primary sexual motive, which is a sensory motive, does not undergo much change with development, the secondary motives do. During the first few years the primary sensory motive dominates the less salient secondary ones. During the preschool and early school years many children have developed such affectionate relations with the parent of the opposite sex that secondary motives to see that parent nude or a desire for strong, intense, physical affection become ascendant. During the early adolescent years the dominant secondary motive is to establish heterosexual relationships. This motive dominates almost all other motives during the adolescent period.

There has been unusually severe anxiety surrounding sexual motivation in children and adults in the United States and in many parts of Western Europe. The conflict has become painfully clear in the excessive preoccupation with sexuality in Western culture. Hunger, thirst and fatigue are as salient sensory motives as sexuality, but there is no fetishistic and obsessive concern with these motives.

In one sense, sexual motivation is easier to understand than nonsensory motives. We begin with a relatively distinct set of pleasant sensations that become conditioned to a variety of people and objects. If sexual behavior and motives were not so heavily and consistently punished, they would not have to go underground and would not become psychologically attached to so many substitute stimuli.

Sexual motivation plays two roles

in the psychological development of the child in Western society. During the preschool and early school years it is an important ingredient of the affectionate bond between the child and the parent of the opposite sex, and makes the child more receptive to adopting the values of that parent. However, the anxiety generated by sexual motives toward the parent is influential. Conscious sexual motives and self-stimulating behavior represent violations of a standard (discrepancy between two beliefs or between a belief and a behavior) and, as indicated earlier, generate anxiety and an accompanying strong desire to alleviate that distress. The child expects punishment for these motives and his preferred reaction is to behave in a way that will make parental punishment less likely. The strategy is to become obedient to parental requests, to do well in school, to become responsible, honest, trustworthy and virtuous—if these are the traits the parent promotes. If the parents encourage a different set of characteristics, the child will adopt them. There is only one danger in this dynamic. If the anxiety over sexual motivation is unusually intense and the accompanying guilt pervasive, the child may deprecate himself and come to the conclusion that he can not do anything well. Further, excessive guilt over sexual motives can provoke the child to seek punishment for them. Such children often misbehave in unusual and inexplicable ways. They become irritatingly mischievous or annoying, and their behavior often puzzles the parents. This behavior can be the child's way of inviting punishment as an atonement for his sexual motives and actions.

In sum, the preschool and early school years are witness to the growth of several motive and behavioral systems. By the time the child is ready for school, motives for affiliation, genital stimulation, instrumental help, affection, effectance and hostility are components of his personality. Several factors determine whether any of these motives will lead to actual attempts at gratification. The possession of behaviors that can gratify a motive, the degree of anxiety associated with gratification and the expectancy of gratification all influence the child's goal-directed behavior. Finally, a behavior that seems intended to gratify a specific motive may be aimed at gratifying a quite different motive. It is difficult to make absolute statements about the meaning of particular goal-oriented behaviors or to predict what behavior will result from a motive. Each child possesses his private code, and more must be learned about the way he thinks if the aims of his actions are to be interpreted correctly.

THE PEER GROUP

The peer group fosters rebellion against the socialization demands of the adult community, promotes discussion of sexuality and sexual exploration and gives license for aggressive play and for venting of hostility. The child feels safe discussing and expressing prohibitive actions with peers. Friends function as mutual psychotherapists. A child who suffers intense anxiety over his resentment toward his parents may feel less guilt when he hears that his friends also experience strong hostility toward their families.

A second reason the peer group is so influential is that it can communicate its evaluation—positive or negative—of the child by giving or withholding group acceptance. Evaluation by parents functions in the same manner, but the child seems to prefer the group's positive evaluation and constant signs of acceptance. Why is parental acceptance insufficient? The child trusts the group's evaluation and often mistrusts that of adults. The child may feel that parents and teachers are either overly accepting of his undesirable qualities or overly critical of him and thus are not capable of an accurate evaluation of his attributes. The child behaves as if he believed in the greater validity and inherent wisdom of peer evaluation.

The child needs other children his age to evaluate his degree of competence at diverse skills and his attractiveness to others. The typical 10-year-old does not have absolute measuring rods to help him evaluate how bright, handsome, wise, honest, capable or likeable he is. There are no absolute definitions for these qualities, as there are for height, weight or skin color. The child naturally and spontaneously uses his immediate peer group as the reference for the qualities he wants to measure. His evaluation is partially dependent on the size and psychological quality of the reference group and is thus highly relative. Specifically, the larger the peer group, the less likely will the child be to conclude that he is high in the rank order and therefore the less likely to decide that he is unusually smart, handsome or capable of leadership.

Astronauts are chosen partly for their self-confidence and capacity to tolerate stress. Although almost half our population lives in three large urban areas, the vast majority of the astronaut candidates grew up in rural or semiurban areas. These men were able to perceive themselves in childhood as more skilled, coolheaded and inventive than most of their peers because they grew up in small towns where few boys were as talented as they. If one of these astronauts had grown up in Chicago, for example, he would have encountered many boys as brilliant as or more brilliant than he, and he might not have developed the belief that he was exceptional. The child's evaluation of his intelligence is less a function of his absolute IQ than of his perceived rank relative to his peers.

A third factor in peer group influence is the provision of role models for identification. Some peers are respected and command power positions, so that the child is predisposed to adopt the leader's standards and behaviors in the hope of eventually commanding the same power and competencies.

Finally, peers teach the child a role to play in a group. Unlike the typical small family with two adults and two or three children of different ages and sexes, the same-sex peer group has no obvious differentiation by age and sex. But it is natural for members of a group to organize and to differentiate. The differentiation in the peer group involves assignation of different roles to various members. The children who are cast in these roles take them seriously and behave in a manner dictated by the role given to them. One reason for adopting the behavior appropriate to the role is that the group gives acceptance and even distinction to the child who plays the role properly.

The peer group, then, acts as a psychotherapist, helps the child evaluate himself on critical attributes, provides him with role models with whom he may identify and gives him a role to play. The peer group exerts major control over the child because it represents important resources that the preadolescent requires.

SIBLINGS

The psychological influence of siblings on the child's personality development is felt most keenly when the child is between 3 and 9 years of age. The arrival of a sibling at this time represents the greatest threat to the first-born's relationship with his mother. For the second-born it is the time when the older sibling is perceived as an omnipotent and invulnerable competitor, with special status and privileges. Thus, each position in the family has its own set of advantages and disadvantages. Perhaps the best way to systematize the developmental correlates of birth order is to specify some of the unique experiences associated with a particular position and the behavioral consequences of these experiences.

Differential Characteristics of First-Born and Later-Born Children

The critical experiences associated with being a first-born child are (1) the tendency to orient to the parents for values and to identify with parental rather than peer models, (2) anxiety over loss of parental nurturance when the second-born child arrives and (3) a perception of the privilege that parents usually accord the first-born because of his status and age. These experiences are likely to lead to certain psychological outcomes, described in the following text.

Standards. First-born children have higher standards than later-born children about competencies and attributes that are positively valued by the parent. Occasionally these standards are likely to be excessively high. The child must discover for himself the standard of how "good" he is supposed to be at a task. The first-born is forced to use his parents as a reference for the level of competence he should try to attain. The later-born child, however, is exposed to less competent performance, since he looks to his older siblings as well as to his parents for guidance in setting a standard of excellence. The later-born child generally has more realistic standards because his reference includes the performance of adults *and* children.

Identification. Because the first-born has only adult models available to him, he is prone to identify primarily with them and, as he grows older, to choose them as models. Since adults, in fact, have more power and competence than children, the first-born is likely to pass through a period of more intense identification than is the later-born child. The fact that the later-born child has an older child as an available model dilutes the younger child's motivation to identify with adult models.

Orientation to the World. The first-born is more likely to experience an orderly world, for he can usually obtain from his parents coherent and orderly answers to his questions about events that puzzle him. Moreover, his parents do not impulsively snatch his toys or irrationally interfere with his play. Consider, however, the situation of a typical second-born child. When he is playing with a toy, his older brother may suddenly race toward him and grab the toy without explanation. If he asks his older brother why it is raining, he may receive one answer the first time and a different answer the next. The world should appear less orderly, less predictable and less rational for the later-born child. In the extreme case a later-born child may develop a picture of a predatory world in which one must vigilantly protect one's possessions against the onslaughts of the unpredictable older sibling.

Anxiety over Loss of Affection. The three attributes just listed are usually regarded as "advantages" of being the first-born child. There are some consequences of this status, however, that might be viewed as disadvantageous. The first-born is subjected to anxiety over loss of parental affection in a more traumatic way than is the later-born child. The first-born becomes accustomed to the exclusive affection of his parents; since he is not required to share this resource, he comes to expect a certain amount of intense attention. The inevitable attenuation of attention that must occur when the next child is born represents a dramatic loss of parental nurturance, over which the first-born is likely to become highly anxious. Furthermore, since he normally received nurturance from adults, he tends to continue to turn to them for help when he is anxious. In short, he is likely to be overtly dependent in time of stress if an adult is around. The later-born child is not so severely affected by potential loss of affection because he enters a world in which he is always sharing his parents with his older siblings; he grows up expecting and accepting this situation.

Guilt. The first-born child is predisposed to experience more guilt, especially over hostility, than is the later-born child. This expectation is based on the assumption that the first-born is naturally jealous of the new baby and his special status but has no way to rationalize his hostility. Because he knows and is told repeatedly that babies are entitled to extra attention, he perceives that his hostility is not appropriate and cannot be justified. The inability to justify his resentment leads to guilt (for he has violated a standard) and self-derogation. The later-born child is better able to justify any hostility toward his older sibling, because the first-born is, in fact, aggressive toward him and does enjoy privileges he does not possess. Being able to rationalize his resentment makes him less likely to experience strong guilt over these hostile thoughts.

Sense of Inadequacy. A unique attribute of the later-born child is the sense of inadequacy he may feel when he compares himself with his older sibling, especially if the age differential between the two is small —say, two to four years. The later-born child typically sees himself as physically weaker, intellectually less competent and socially more awkward. He does not excuse these inadequacies by acknowledging the obvious age differential between himself and his older sibling. Because he compares himself to the older sibling as if they were the same age, he can only conclude that he is less adequate.

Conclusions on Sibling Differences Based on Order of Birth

The set of attributes just ascribed to first- and later-born children is conjectural but consistent with existing theory and data (Altus, 1966; Warren, 1966). If these hypotheses are generally correct, several conclusions can be drawn. First-borns, in contrast to later-born siblings of the same sex, should be more concerned with social acceptance and rejection, less likely to break the rules imposed by authority, more ambitious and hard-working, more cooperative, more prone to guilt and anxiety and less openly aggressive. First-borns should view the world as an orderly and essentially knowable place rather than as a chaotic jungle where social predators lie waiting at every turn.

Research findings suggest that first-born children are more likely to be anxious over potential rejection from adult figures, to choose adult models as figures for identification, to view events that happen to them as the product of their own actions, to be willing to cooperate with adults conducting psychological experiments and to be more anxious and more dependent on others in time of stress. This greater anxiety among first-borns is indicated by evidence that first-borns respond with more fear to the prospect of physical harm (Helmreich and Collins, 1967) and report an electric shock to be more painful than do later-borns (Nisbett and Schachter, 1966). First-born college men are less likely than later-borns to participate in dangerous sports like football, soccer and rugby, but are just as likely to participate in less dangerous sports like crew (Nisbett, 1968). One hundred adult men and women who were staying in a New York hotel during a power blackout in November 1965 were asked the question, "How nervous or uneasy did you feel during this experience?" The first-borns admitted to slightly greater anxiety than did the later-borns (Zucker et al., 1968).

First-born children of parents who value school success adopt and practice this value with greater vigor than do later-born children, as indicated by the disproportionately high percentage of eminent men who are first-born or only children. First-borns, for example, are predominant among Rhodes scholars (Apperly, 1939), listings in *Who's Who* (Jones, 1954) and distinguished scientists (Roe, 1953). There seems to be a disproportionate number of first-born children who attain very high scores on intelligence and aptitude tests and who matriculate at colleges with high admission standards (Altus, 1966). Moreover, middle-class first-born and middle-class only children are subjected to more restrictiveness, greater pressure to achieve and more intense induction of guilt over violations of standards than are later-born children.

First-born children, in contrast to later-born children, tend to adopt more idealistic philosophical positions and prefer single unifying principles in moral codes or in science to schemes that are expedient or that have many qualifications. In a recent study (Stein, 1966), 54 Harvard freshmen were interviewed; 27 were older sons with a younger brother, and 27 were younger sons with an older brother. Each student was presented with a series of philosophical statements that either condoned or criticized three points of view:

1. The search for truth is good and, regardless of the consequences, should be pursued, in contrast to the point of view that one must take into account the outcome of an inquiry.

2. Man is essentially good, in contrast to the point of view that man is essentially bad.

3. The role of science is synthesis in contrast to analysis.

Each student had to state his understanding of each philosophical statement and to indicate his degree of agreement or disagreement with it. The difference between first- and second-born sons held only for those 16 freshmen who admired and felt similar to their fathers—that is, for the young men who seemed to have identified with their fathers. Among this group, the nine first-borns were more likely to value man and his creative works, to endorse the importance of human freedom, to regard the formulation of a general and unitary theory as the most important aim of science and to favor a morality that is based on principles rather than on expediency. For example, the statement that produced the greatest difference between the first- and second-borns was this:

> In striving toward ends that he finds morally acceptable, man must not resort to methods that violate other acceptable principles. Arguments of "expediency" are invalid and cannot obscure the fact that an immoral act is immoral regardless of whether it is used to achieve a final state that is just or one that is unjust.

None of the first-borns disagreed with this item; whereas more than 40 per cent of the later-born group did. This commitment to moral standards and reluctance to sway from principles on the part of the first-born agrees with our theoretical description of the different relationship first- and second-born children have with their parents.

Interacting Effects of Sex, Birth Order and Spacing of Siblings

The most comprehensive empirical study of the effect of siblings on personality development has been reported by Koch (1965a, 1956b), who studied sex, birth order and spacing of siblings in 384 families. The four types of sibling combinations (older boy; younger girl, older girl; younger boy, two sisters, two brothers) were equally represented, and there were groups of siblings separated by one to two years, two to four years and four to six years. The teachers of these children observed and rated them on a variety of behaviors. The results indicated that all the major variables —sex, birth order and spacing—interacted in producing differences in the children's behavior.

The sex of the older sibling was found to be an important determinant of the adoption of sex typed behavior by the younger child. Girls with older brothers, as compared to those with older sisters, were more masculine in their behavior (that is, they were more ambitious and aggressive and performed better on tests of intellectual ability). Boys with older sisters were less masculine (less aggressive, less dominant) than were boys with older brothers. These results support the hypothesis that the younger child identifies to some degree with the older sibling and imitates his behavior because the older child is perceived to possess desirable attributes and resources.

When birth order alone was considered, Koch found that the first-born children generally had stronger and more consistent standards regarding honesty, responsibility and aggression than did the second-born children. However, the effect of birth order was dependent on both the sex of the siblings and spacing. When the siblings were of the same sex and separated by less than two years, there were few behavioral differences between them. When the spacing increased to four years and the siblings were of different sexes, behavioral differences were most marked. Koch concluded that a two to four year age difference between siblings provided the most threatening situation to the older child. If the first-born was 3 years old when the new baby arrived, he was very likely to become anxious over possible withdrawal of nurturance. If the first-born was only a year old, on the other hand, his self-image was still diffuse enough so that he probably did not regard the baby as a major threat to his bond with his mother and, therefore, not a competitor for his mother's affection. If the older child was 8 when the sibling arrived, he was already on the road to independence from his parents and was less threatened by the newcomer. In general, it is difficult to speak of the influence of birth order without acknowledging the effect of the other two variables, sex and spacing.

It appears that sibling position is an important psychological variable because it presents a microcosm of the significant social experiences of adolescence and adulthood. To be first or second, to be dominant or submissive, to side with authority or to rebel against it, to feel guilt over hostility or to be able to "place the blame" are tendencies that begin to be differentially strengthened during early childhood as a result of the child's sibling position.

The consistent personality correlates of sibling position serve to remind us that despite the importance of parental rewards and punishments, the mere existence of a younger or older sibling in the family can be an active force in the psychological development of a child. Every child and adult lives in a social structure and perceives his position in that structure. That perception molds his attitudes about himself, his vulnerability to anxiety and his beliefs about others.

THE ROLE OF THE FAMILY

A child is influenced by his parents, siblings, peers, teachers and the public media. Parents and siblings have their major effect during the first six years; peers and teachers during the preadolescent period; the public media during early adolescence. Parents can mold the behavior of the child through reward, punishment and instruction, and as a consequence of their position as models for the child. If parental acceptance and praise are valued, each can be used to establish and maintain selected behavior in the child. Punishment also produces changes in behavior, whether the punishment be spanking, threat of rejection or deprivation of goals. The anxiety generated by anticipated punishment leads to inhibition of the undesirable response and substitution through instruction and through modeling, which facilitates imitation and identification.

Two important dimensions of parental behavior are affection-hostility and control-autonomy. The affectionate parent is accepting, approving and understanding. The hostile parent is excessively punitive, and critical and holds a negative view of the child. The dimension of control-permissive is defined by the degree to which the parent restricts the child and enforces demands in the areas of sexuality, hostility, manners, neatness, orderliness, care for household goods and obedience. A child can live with one of four types of parents: (1) affectionate and permissive, (2) affectionate and controlling, (3) hostile and controlling or (4) hostile and permissive. Some psychologists believe that each of these four types is associated with different kinds of child personalities. The affectionate-permissive parent produces a friendly, dominant and high self-esteem child. The affectionate-restrictive parent produces a more dependent, less friendly, less creative and more hostile child. The hostile and restrictive parent produces a child with high guilt and a disposition to shyness and social withdrawal. The hostile-permissive parent produces an aggressive child with poor control over his behavior.

Consider some examples of apparent maternal rejection that illustrate the difficulties in inferring rejection from overt parental behavior.

1. Mothers in the isolated areas of northern Norway rarely ask their children to move when they find them blocking a doorway. The mothers simply pick them up silently and move them out of the way with an indifference that is characteristic of the treatment shown a pair of shoes that are out of place. An American psychologist would be prone to label such "aloof" behavior as rejecting if it were observed in a middle-class mother in Chicago. But this behavior in the rural Norwegian setting is normative and does not necessarily reflect an attitude of rejection.

2. An uneducated, unwed mother slaps her 4-year-old boy across the face when he does not come to the dinner table on time. The intensity of the mother's act tempts an observer to conclude that the mother hates or at best does not like her child. However, during an interview conducted by the observer, the mother says that she cares about her child and only wants to ensure that he does not grow up to be a delinquent. She believes firmly that physical punishment is the most effective way to socialize him. In this case her behavior seems motivated more by love than hate.

3. A 20-year-old girl from a blue-collar family talks feelingly about the severe restriction and punishment she experienced as a child but adds that she now appreciates her parents, for they helped her develop the char-

acter she has today. In another part of the city, the 20-year-old daughter of a free-lance writer evidences hatred for her parents, who she claims were too permissive. She is convinced that their laissez faire attitude reflected a lack of concern for her welfare. Can we say for certain which set of parents was rejecting?

These examples convey the conceptual problems surrounding the word "rejection"; it should be clear that there are three different meanings of the word. It can be defined in terms of the parent's behavior, the parent's attitude or as a belief held by the child. Let us examine the last two meanings.

The Parental Attitude

A parental attitude of rejection is defined as one of dislike for and resentment of the child. However, it is not obvious which specific behaviors are most likely to reflect that attitude at various ages. Neglect of the child's needs for food, warmth and comfort; open and direct criticism; and expressions of rage at the child are popular and even reasonable indexes of a rejecting attitude. Both mothers with a rejecting attitude may not exhibit these behaviors overtly, and there is no general agreement on what might constitute more subtle behavioral indexes of a rejecting attitude. Moreover, a mother who was not generally rejecting but who had high standards for her child might display signs of rejection if the child violated these standards.

It is generally assumed that an attitude of rejection is one end of a dimension, the other end of which is usually labeled acceptance. As with rejection, acceptance is an attitude that may find varied expressions in different mothers. Psychologists often assume that physical affection is the obvious expression of maternal acceptance, but there is some reason to question the validity of this assumption. Mothers who are aware of their hostile feelings toward the infant may display intense physical affection to reduce their guilt and to attentuate the anxiety elicited by recognition of their basic resentment. Some mothers may not initiate close physical contact with their children because they believe it is not good for them or because of anxiety over the sexual associations that affectionate behavior arouses. Middle-class mothers in certain parts of the Netherlands, for example, put their young infants in an unheated room, away from the heated rooms in which they work, and do not go to their babies until they decide it is time for them to be fed, regardless of how intensely the babies may cry. Although these mothers value and love their infants, they believe that aloof treatment is good for young babies.[4]

It is not easy, therefore, to tell whether a mother loves her baby by noting how often she displays a particular set of behaviors toward the baby. As mentioned earlier, mothers of different cultural and subcultural groups express their accepting or rejecting attitude in different actions, and a mother's behavior is not always an accurate reflection of her attitude.

In spite of these difficulties, there has been considerable study of behavioral indexes of parental rejection and acceptance. Schaefer (1959) studied the variables used in many independent investigations of maternal behavior and found the results remarkably similar. He concluded that a fundamental characteristic of maternal behavior is the rejection-acceptance continuum. It is possible, however, that the conceptual heritage of Western trained psychologists demanded this result. For example, Western prose and poetry, as well as

[4]Personal communication from Dr. Freda Rebelsky (1968).

empirical work in the social sciences, deify the dimension of love-hate. These attributes are typically the first ones evaluated when a parent is observed. Moreover, since Western thought dictates that a loving mother never treats her child harshly, an American psychologist generally *expects* to find the two variables of acceptance and rejection at opposite end of a continuum.

The common belief that attitudes of rejection or acceptance can be identified by objectively watching the mother perform certain acts is in need of revision. Moreover, there is a second and much different definition of rejection that originates with the child's perception of his value.

The Child's Concept

The child's view of acceptance is based on the degree to which he believes the parents value him. The child arrives at this conclusion on the basis of the quality and frequency of the parents' sacrifices for him and of his perception of the enjoyment they derive from being with him. The child of 9 is fully aware of the resources that a parent can give with no hardship and those that he is reluctant to share with the child. If the parents have little money, a gift of a one dollar toy is viewed by the child as a sign of great affection, for he realizes he has been given a scarce resource. However, the wealthy executive who brings home a five dollar toy after each four day business trip may not be credited by the child with a great deal of affection. On the other hand, a long walk on Sunday morning by the executive father and his son, an event the child rarely experiences, probably has the value of the dollar toy given to the less privileged child.

Thus, the child's feeling of being valued or accepted must take into account his idiosyncratic perceptions of the value of various gifts. The resources that he evaluates as scarce are the major tokens of affection, and these evaluations may vary from child to child. This situation is not, however, completely relative. Most parents, regardless of their finances, are unwilling to make the sacrifices of very expensive gifts, long periods of uninterrupted attention and reciprocal friendship either because of sincere efforts to avoid spoiling their children or because of their own narcissistic needs. Thus, many children come to regard the same resources—such as uninterrupted attention and extravagant gifts—as symbolic of love and positive evaluation.

The psychologist's task is first to assess the range of resources that the parent commands and then to measure the child's differential evaluation of each of these resources. This information permits categorization of the degree of rejection or acceptance felt by the child and, by inference, the rejecting or accepting quality of the parent's behavior. This concept of rejection and acceptance is relative, not absolute, for it rules out the possibility of deciding that any particular parental reaction *always* is viewed as rejection by the child.

Of course, the child's belief concerning his value has no validity for the infant; it is true only for the child 3 or 4 years of age or older. It takes several years to develop the conceptual maturity necessary for a child to evaluate his worth in the eyes of another; the definition of rejection based on the child's concept is appropriate only for the child who thinks symbolically.

In short, then, in considering the behavioral dimension of rejection and acceptance it is necessary to distinguish the following three meanings of these words: (1) the quality and frequency of particular acts that are presumed to reflect rejection or acceptance, (2) the parent's attitude toward the child and (3) the child's assessment of his value in the eyes of the parent. Since a particular set of behaviors does not always reflect a rejecting parental attitude for all caretakers, whoever they may be, and is not always perceived as rejecting by the child, the term rejection takes on a relativistic definition.

Maternal Restriction and Autonomy

The dimension of restriction and autonomy concerns the mother's tendency to control or restrict her child, as opposed to following permissive, laissez-faire practices. The restriction-permissiveness continuum conforms more to specific maternal behaviors than does the acceptance-hostility continuum and thus presents fewer methodological problems. A controlling mother punishes deviations from her standards, prevents the child's explorations of new areas and punishes excessive independence of action. The mother who gives relative autonomy allows the child more freedom to express some of his idiosyncratic tendencies. She does not punish all the child's explorations, and she allows some assertion of independence.

Although a mother's restriction and autonomy conform more to specific behaviors, the degree to which she is restrictive or permissive with her child shows less stability over the first 10 years than does the degree to which she is affectionate or hostile toward him. That is, an American mother who behaves as if she loved her one-year-old child is likely to remain affectionate through the first decade of the child's life. However, a mother who is overly permissive with her infant may be either highly permissive or highly restrictive when the child is 10 years old. This difference seems to be due to the fact that the degree to which a mother restricts or grants freedom to her child is a function of the degree to which she feels he *requires* control.

The mother of a 6-year-old boy who has suddenly become unruly may increase her degree of restrictiveness in order to control her son. The mother who has been so overcontrolling that her 9-year-old daughter has become excessively shy may become concerned and ease her restrictions. The typical parent adjusts the tightness of control to match the child's behavior. As a result, the degree of restriction and permissiveness is not very stable over the first 10 to 12 years.

This intimate and reciprocal relationship between mother and child can be seen even during the opening weeks of life. Moss (1967) has observed mothers and infants when the latter were 3 and 12 weeks of age in the natural setting of the home. The infant's crying was a major determinant of the mother's behavior. If the infant cried a lot, the mother spent a lot of time with the child, holding him, picking him up and talking to him. If the child was unusually quiet and nonirritable, the mother was likely to spend much less time near him and playing with him. The infant's behavior was a major determinant of the degree to which the mother demonstrated nurturant acts toward him. In effect, the infant was partly shaping the mother's behavior. This causal chain tends to contradict the popular myth that the degree to which a mother cares for her child is entirely a function of her internal motives and conflicts.

Research on the Rejection-Acceptance and Restriction-Autonomy Continuums

Numerous studies have attempted to relate maternal affection, hostility, permissiveness and control to the child's behavior. Most of these investigations have been cross-sectional, have used children between 3 and 15 years of age and have implicitly assumed that the mother's attitude or behavior caused the child's behavior. This implicit assumption may, however, be fallacious. The mother's attitude toward her child, as we have noted, can be a reaction to his behavior at that time or during the previous months, rather than an antecedent of the behavior he is displaying. Moreover, many studies have used parental interviews to assess maternal acceptance or restriction and rarely supplement these data with direct observations of the mother to determine the validity of the mother's verbal report.

Schaefer (1959) has suggested that the rejection-acceptance and restriction-autonomy continuums are independent of each other and that mothers should be categorized into one of four major types: accepting and controlling, accepting and permissive, rejecting and controlling or rejecting and permissive. Schaefer further suggests that each of these four maternal types is linked to a specific syndrome in the child.

The antisocial child who displays his aggression directly is hypothetically linked to a mother who is both rejecting and permissive. This linking implies that the rejection creates strong hostile feelings in the child and reduces his motivation to inhibit his asocial behavior, which is not punished because of the mother's permissiveness. However, it is possible that the child's aggression led the mother to become hostile to her child. The accepting and permissive mother presumably produces a child who is confident and relatively uninhibited.

The combination of acceptance and control in a mother supposedly causes signs in the child of excessive guilt, phobias ties, obsessive thoughts, academic problems or ulcerative colitis. However, acceptance and moderate control, especially a control that demands independent and responsible behavior, seem to produce mature, self-reliant children. In a study by Baumrind and Black (1967), more than 100 preschool children were observed in nursery school in order to arrive at descriptions of their personalities. During the same period, the behavior of the children and their parents was observed in the home, and each parent was interviewed separately. Approving and affectionate parents were found to have the most autonomous boys. In addition, parents who made demands for maturity and self-reliance and were approving had children who were independent and responsible in the nursery school.

The psychotic child is assumed to be the product of maternal rejection and excessive control acting on the child's deviant biological dispositions. The rejection presumably creates feelings in the child of self-hatred and strong hosility toward the mother. However, the mother's control prevents the child from expressing his feelings and leads to fear of prohibited behaviors. The combination of a negative self-image, extreme guilt and failure to learn how to retaliate can lead to serious and persistent withdrawal, which can lead to psychosis in the biologically predisposed child.

This scheme is admittedly oversimplified, for it omits the influence of the father and does not consider the biological variables that might make the child susceptible to particular pathological syndromes, but it is an initial attempt to classify parental actions and should not be rejected out of hand.

Other Maternal Variables

Maternal variables other than acceptance, rejection, restrictiveness and permissiveness may affect the child's behavior. One such factor is the degree of consistency the parents display in their behavior toward the child. Rejecting mothers are, of necessity, inconsistent in their ministration of comfort and affection. Perhaps it is this inconsistency that contributes to those behaviors in the child that have been regarded as a consequence of a rejecting atmosphere.

The degree of verbal discipline and the regularity with which a rationale for discipline is offered are variables that might affect a child's behavior. A mother who is arbitrary in her restrictiveness is apt to confuse the child and generate strong hostility, in contrast to the mother who sets limits in a context in which her actions are explained. The coherent and rational quality of the mother's communications to the child is another dimension that needs further study.

The period of infancy, when the child is most dependent on the nurturance of the mother, provides a setting for another variable—the delay between the onset of need in the child, as evidenced by his crying, and the administration of some nurturance that will satisfy the need.

The parent's behavior as a model represents still another variable. Since the parent is a model, the attitudes and acts he or she exhibits are likely to be adopted by the child. When the parent's behavior matches the content of a parental socialization demand, the child is faced with a consistent socialization situation. However, the child is confronted with an inconsistent situation when the parent speaks aggressively to the spouse, strikes the child and insults friends but consistently punishes all such displays of aggression in the child. It is likely that the effect of the parent as a model for aggression in this situation is a critical for the child's behavioral pattern as is the degree of punishment of aggressive behavior (Sears et al., 1957).

Cause and Effect Sequences in the Mother-Child Interaction

Maternal actions toward a child do not always have an immediate effect on the child's behavior; some maternal behaviors display a "sleeper" effect. For example, a mother's attempt to accelerate her child's intellectual skills at age 5 may have a profound influence on his level of intellectual mastery at age 10. The Fels Institute longitudinal investigation gives evidence that sleeper effects can occur (Kagan and Moss, 1962). A hostile and overly critical maternal attitude toward daughters during the first three years of life, for example, was predictive of adult mastery in the daughters, whereas a hostile or a critical maternal attitude during the preschool or early school years showed a negligible relation to the daughters' adult mastery behavior. Similarly, maternal protection and nurturance of daughters during the first three years predicted a tendency toward withdrawal from stressful situations in adulthood; maternal protection during the preschool years showed no relation to adult passivity in time of stress.

These results give credence to the assumption that the reciprocal nature of the mother-child interaction changes with time. Not only does the mother's effect on the child vary at different ages, but the child's ability to provoke relatively permanent changes in specific maternal reactions increases with age. The 6-year-old is more likely to produce a major alteration in the mother's characteristic behavior toward him than is the 2-year-old.

The mother typically has expectations as to what the child's conduct should be like, or to what standards his behavior should conform. The greater the discrepancy between her expectations and her evaluation of the child, the greater is the likelihood that she will either modify her expectations or modify her behavior, and exert pressure on the child in an attempt to direct him according to her expectations. Because the infant's personality is relatively amorphous, the discrepancy between the mother's standards and what she perceives in the infant is necessarily small; the mother sees the infant as she would like to see him, as an object primarily to be acted upon. The form and content of maternal behaviors toward her child, therefore, are not as contaminated by the effects of the infant's behavior as they are by the behaviors of the more complex 10-year-old.

A mother's concern with the intellectual development of her 2-year-old is more likely to be an index of her own basic needs and values than is her degree of concern with the performance of her 10-year-old daughter who is failing in school. Mothers change their expectations and values as the child develops, and the lack of concern with the 10-year-old's school grades could be merely a defensive maneuver the mother recently required to protect herself from excessive disappointment. Similarly, encouragement of independence, a critical attitude, or overprotection toward a 10-year-old may be lately developed reactions to the child's excessive dependence, rebelliousness, or fragile defenses.

It is possible, therefore, that certain maternal practices—such as nurturance, restrictiveness and hostility—that are manifested during the first three years provide the most sensitive index of the mother's basic attitudes toward the child and, perhaps, of her lasting effect on his future behavior. The further elucidation of cause and effect sequences in development may require longitudinal study of parent and child. For example, a cross-sectional investigation of the relation between maternal protection and passivity in a 10-year-old might yield a negligible association between these variables, but if the maternal behavior had been assessed when the child was 3 years old, a strong positive relation with the child's behavior when he was 10 might have emerged.

Certain parent-child interactions are particularly vulnerable to the sleeper effect. Maternal behaviors that are apt to change in frequency and intensity over the first decade, such as kissing, reward of dependency and physical punishment, are more likely to show this phenomenon than are relatively stable attitudes (for instance, about sexuality or about the appropriateness of traditional sex typed traits). Furthermore, maternal reactions that are unique to the child's behavior during the school years, such as concern with grades or punishment of overt aggression, may produce misleading correlations between contemporaneous assessments of maternal and child behavior.

Factors Controlling Maternal Reactions: The Child's Attitudes and the Mother's Temperament

There is a danger in inferring cause and effect sequences—especially the effect of a maternal practice on a response of the child—merely from an association between a particular type of parental attitude or behavior and the child's personality. Close observation of the mother-infant and mother-child interaction indicates that the mother's reactions are governed to some extent both by the child's attributes and by her own temperament. If the child is irritable, she reacts with more anger than if he is content; if he is vigorous, she treats him with either more or less restriction than if he is quiet. Even in the opening weeks of life, the mother's behavior is governed by the characteristics of the baby. Irritable babies tend to receive more nurturance than quiet, placid, happy ones. Boys, being generally more irritable than girls, tend to elicit more maternal handling (Moss, 1967).

The mother's reactions to her child's behavior are also affected by her own temperament. Some of the mothers in the study by Moss (1967b) had been interviewed prior to the birth of their infants, at which time their dispositions to be affectionate and nurturant to the infant were assessed. The mothers who were regarded then as more nurturant were indeed more responsive to their infants at 3 weeks and 3 months of age than were those who were regarded as more hostile to the unborn baby. Thus, it is not surprising that the most frequent interaction will occur between the irritable child and the basically affectionate and nurturant mother, and that the placid child with a non-nurturant mother will receive the least handling.

The Mother's Interpretations. The mother's behavior toward her child is governed to some extent by her *interpretation* of the child's attributes. The mother typically pins a label on the child, based initially on his sex, activity level, vigor, size, health and irritability, and she reacts to this label. As a result of the initial labeling, mothers usually will let 16-week-old infant boys cry longer than girls of the same age, for they feel boys have to learn to take stress. They are generally more protective of small, light babies, because they feel these infants require more care. As the child approaches preschool age, his attributes become more complex, and his parents often must revise the labels they give him. At this stage the labels are based on the child's intellectual competence, attractiveness and popularity; favorable and unfavorable labels will elicit different maternal reactions to the child.

The child's sex is a major determinant of a mother's reactions. Rothbart and Maccoby (1966) describe an experiment in which mothers and fathers listened to the tape-recorded voice of a 4-year-old whose voice could have been perceived as either male or female. Some parents were told the voice was a boy's; others were told it belonged to a girl. After the experimenter described a typical family situation, the parents heard the taped voice make such remarks as, "Daddy, come look at my puzzle," "Help me," "I don't like this game—I'm gonna break it." After each statement the experimenter stopped the tape, and the parents wrote down what they would say or do in response to the statement. Mothers were more permissive for the boy's voice and fathers were more permissive for the girl's voice. Moreover, fathers allowed more aggression toward the parent from the girl than from the boy; mothers allowed more aggression from the boy than from the girl.

Mothers do not assign the same labels and do not react uniformly to the same set of attributes. One mother may regard her son's motor vigor and resistance to sleep as a sign of autonomy and high spirits and be pleased that he will probably develop into an active, masculine boy. Another mother, with a different value system and a different set of conflicts, may consider that these same attributes are indicative of future violence and delinquency and should be punished. Two mothers might interpret extreme irritability in their daughters in different ways: one as a sign of the child's artistic sensitivity, the other as a sign of her own incompetence. In the latter case the irritability would be threatening to the mother, causing her to withdraw from involvement with her daughter.

The child's basic characteristics, therefore, rarely evoke a constant or invariant response in a mother. The child's attributes are cryptic messages that the mother decodes and acts upon. If she misreads the message, she may take the wrong action. Since mothers have different standards, motives and conflicts, they use different criteria to decode the infant's behavior. As a result, similar child behaviors may evoke dramatically different interpretations and reactions.

The Mother's Expectations. Mothers have an initial set of expectations about how their children will grow, and they typically act on the basis of these predictions. A mother who decides that her infant will probably not perform well in school may not read to him when he approaches preschool age. A mother who believes her daughter will be propular will arrange to surround her with friends as she grows up.

There are striking differences among mothers in the nature of the expectations they have for their children. Some of these differences are attributable to social class, others to the sex of the child, still others to the mother's unique conflicts and motives. As part of a continuing study of a large group of parents and infants, mothers of 16-week-old babies were asked to predict what their children would be like when they were 10 years old. Some mothers in the group had never graduated from high school, some were high school graduates and the others had either attended or graduated from college.

For some traits, such as popularity, there were no important differences among the mothers of the three educational levels or between mothers of sons and mothers of daughters. However, traits such as cautiousness, responsibility and stubbornness produced interesting differences. The poorly educated mother was more likely than the better-educated mother to say that her daughter would be stubborn, cautious, not very interested in music and poor at arithmetic. Among mothers of sons, the less well-educated parent was more likely to predict that her child would be athletic, not cautious, not responsible and likely to jump from one activity to another.

Lower-class parents predicted more independence for their daughters than for their sons, but upper middle-class mothers in general expected more independence from both sons and daughters than did lower-class mothers. Similarly, the upper middle-class mother expected more responsibility from her son than did the lower-class parent.

These expectations closely match reality. For example, 10-year-old sons of parents with little education are, in fact, less responsible than are 10-year-old sons of college educated parents. And lower-class boys are less cautious and more impulsive than are middle-class boys. It is likely that the mothers' expectations played an important role in shaping the final outcome of these aspects of their children's personalities.

SUMMARY

This chapter has attempted to introduce some of the major concepts and themes that bring order to the first decade of human development. Most of the discussion has necessarily been hypothetical, for unfortunately there is little proven information on the mechanisms of development, or on the ways in which experience influences the organization of motives, standards, beliefs and behaviors.

One of the major themes of the chapter has been that the establishment of the various components of a psychological system such as motives, standards, expectancies, emotions, sources of anxiety and behaviors, occurs at different periods in development. However this approach is necessarily descriptive, rather than theoretical. This approach resembles Piaget's scheme for intellectual development; Piaget outlines the stages of cognitive functioning that allow one to predict that a 9-year-old will show signs of conservation and will be able to deal with some hypothetical problem situations, while the younger child will not. Similarly, this chapter states that a child is unlikely to show the capacity for guilt before he shows anxiety over loss of love. However, both Piaget and the personality developmentalist have been unable to provide statements explaining how a child passes from one stage to the next or how environmental experiences facilitate or obstruct his growth. Those who study personality development have not been able to detail the mechanisms that will explain how a particular maternal action or sibling organization influences the psychological development of the child. Theories of psychological development lack the tight net of interlocking propositions that permit satisfactory explanation and powerful prediction.

The concepts of identification, discrepancy from schemata, anxiety, motives and standards assume a heavy burden of explanation in this chapter. Empirical work in the future must determine the wisdom of these particular choices and the utility of their implications. Nonetheless, it appears that it is reasonable to believe that the organization of motives and anxieties changes as the child matures and, as a result, the meaning of the child's overt behaviors becomes increasingly ambiguous. The task that faces developmental psychologists is to map the child's overt behavior on the mosiac of dynamic internal processes that function to continuously adapt the child to environmental demands and to help him make sense of his rich and varied experiences.

REFERENCES

Ainsworth, M. D. S.: *Infancy in Uganda.* Baltimore, The Johns Hopkins Press, 1967.

Altus, W. D.: Birth order and its sequellae. *Science, 151*:44–49, 1966.

Apperly, F. L.: A study of America's Rhodes scholars. *J. Hered., 30*:494–495, 1939.

Baumrind, D., and Black, A. E.: Socialization practices associated with dimensions of competence in preschool boys and girls. *Child Develop., 38*:291–328, 1967.

Bentzen, F.: Sex ratios in learning and behavior disorders. *Amer. J. Orthopsychiat., 33*:92–98, 1963.

Buss, A. H.: *The Psychology of Aggression.* New York, John Wiley & Sons, Inc., 1961.

Chang, B.: The relation between identification with a model and attentiveness to verbal information from the model. Unpublished Senior Honors Thesis, Harvard University, 1965.

Collard, R. R.: Fear of strangers and play behavior in kittens with varied social experience. *Child Develop., 38*:877–891, 1967.

Feshbach, N. D., and Roe, K.: Empathy in six and seven year olds. *Child Develop., 39*: 133–145, 1968.

Fischer, K. W.: Unpublished Doctoral Dissertation: "Structure and development of sensory-motor actions." Harvard University, 1970.

Harlow, H., and Harlow, M. H.: Learning to love. *Amer. Sci., 54*:244–272, 1966.

Harlow, H. F., and Zimmermann, R. R.: Affectional responses in the infant monkey. *Science, 130*:421–432, 1959.

Hartley, R. D.: Children's concepts of male and female roles. *Merrill-Palmer Quarterly, 6(a)*:83–91, 1960.

Helmreich, R. L., and Collins, B. E.: Situational determinants of affiliative preference under stress. *J. Personality Soc. Psychol.,* 6:79–85, 1967.

Jones, H. E.: The environment and mental development. *In* Carmichael, L. (Ed.): *Manual of Child Psychology.* New York, John Wiley & Sons, Inc., 1954, pp. 631–696.

Kagan, J.: The child's sex role classification of school objects. *Child Develop., 35*:1051–1056, 1964.

Kagan, J., and Moss, H. A.: *Birth to maturity: A Study in Psychological Development.* New York, John Wiley & Sons, Inc., 1962.

Kagan, J., Pearson, L., and Welch, L.: The modifiability of an impulsive tempo. *J. Educ. Psychol., 57*:359–365, 1966.

Kagan, J., and Phillips, W.: The measurement of identification. *J. Abnorm. Soc. Psychol., 69*:442–443, 1964.

Koch, H. L.: Attitudes of children toward their peers as related to certain characteristics of their siblings. *Psychol. Monogr., 70,* No. 426, 1956(a).

Koch, H. L.: Some emotional attitudes of the young child in relation to characteristics of his siblings. *Child Develop., 27*:393–426, 1956(b).

Linton, R.: Status and role. *In* Linton, R.: *The Study of Man: An Introduction.* New York, Appleton-Century-Crofts, 1936, pp. 113–131.
Moss, H. A.: Maternal influences and early social visual behavior. Presented at the annual meeting of the American Orthopsychiatric Association, 1967(a).
Moss, H. A.: Sex, age, and state as determinants of mother-infant interaction. *Merrill-Palmer Quarterly, 13*:19–36, 1967(b).
Mussen, P. H.: Some antecedents and consequents of masculine sex-typing in adolescent boys. *Psychol. Monogr., 75,* Whole No. 506, 1961.
Mussen, P. H.: Long-term consequents of masculinity of interests in adolescence. *J. Consult. Psychol., 26*:435–440, 1962.
Nisbett, R. E.: Birth order and participation in dangerous sports. *J. Personality Soc. Psychol., 8*:351–353, 1968.
Nisbett, R. E., and Schachter, S. S.: Cognitive manipulation of pain. *J. Exp. Soc. Psychol., 2*:227–236, 1966.
Parsons, T.: Age and sex in the social structure of the United States. *In* Kluckhohn, C., and Murray, H. A. (Eds.): *Personality in Nature, Society, and Culture.* New York, Alfred A. Knopf, Inc., 1948, pp. 269–281.
Provence, S., and Lipton, R. C.: *Infants in Institutions.* New York, International Universities Press, 1962.
Rheingold, H. L.: The modification of social responsiveness in institutional babies. *Monogr. Soc. Res. Child Develop., 21*:(No. 2, Serial No. 63), 1956.
Roe, A.: A psychological study of eminent psychologists and anthropologists, and a comparison with biological and physical scientists. *Psychol. Monogr., 67,* No. 2, 1953.
Rosenkrans, M. A.: Imitation in children as a function of perceived similarity to a social model and vicarious reinforcement. *J. Personality Soc. Psychol., 7*:307–315, 1967.
Rothbart, M. K., and Maccoby, E. E.: Parents' differential reactions to sons and daughters. *J. Personality Soc. Psychol., 4*:237–243, 1966.
Sackett, G. Porter, M., and Holmes, H.: Choice behavior in rhesus monkeys. *Science, 147*: 304–306, 1965.
Schachter, S. S., and Singer, J. E.: Cognitive, social, and physiological determinants of emotional state. *Psychol. Rev., 69*:379–399, 1962.
Schachter, S. S., and Wheeler, L.: Epinephrine, chlorpromazine, and amusement. *J. Abnorm. Soc. Psychol., 65*:121–128, 1962.
Schaefer, E. S.: A circumplex model for maternal behavior. *J. Abnorm. Soc. Psychol., 59*: 226–235, 1959.
Sears, R. R., Maccoby, E. E., and Levin, H.: *Patterns of Child Rearing.* New York, Harper & Row, Publishers, 1957.
Stein, R.: The effects of ordinal position and identification on philosophy of life, occupational choice, and reflectiveness-impulsivity. Unpublished Senior Honors Thesis, Harvard University, 1966.
Tyler, L. E.: *The Psychology of Human Differences.* New York, Appleton-Century-Crofts, 1947.
Warren, J. R.: Birth order and social behavior. *Psychol. Bull., 65*:38–49, 1966.
White, R. W.: Motivation reconsidered: The concept of competence. *Psychol. Rev., 66*: 297–333, 1959.
Zucker, R. A., Manosevitz, M., and Lanyon, R. I.: Birth order, anxiety, and affiliation during a crisis. *J. Personality Soc. Psychol., 8*:354–359, 1968.

8 CHILDHOOD ACCIDENTS AND INJURIES

Ross A. McFarland and
Roland C. Moore

The purpose of this chapter is to identify the major causes of accidental injury to children and to outline preventive measures. First, a statistical treatment of the frequency of deaths and injuries in the United States will be given, including relevant information on age, sex and the most frequent types of accidents. This will be followed by an analysis of injuries and their causes as related to the interactions between children and their physical and social environments. Emphasis will be placed on the more recent epidemiological approaches, which have proved to be so successful in the control of diseases. Attention will also be given to the design of products and equipment used by children in terms of human engineering and of children's behavioral characteristics.

The major areas in which most injuries and deaths of children occur will then be reviewed. Some of the most important areas include motor vehicle accidents, poisonings, burn injuries and recreational mishaps (e.g., those involving bicycles, toys and playgrounds and backyard pools).

The remainder of the chapter will concern itself with the issue of the unusually accident-susceptible child, and with the role of social influences in the occurrence of injuries among children. The emotional factors in family life will also be given special attention.

ACCIDENTAL DEATHS AMONG CHILDREN

Frequency of Accidental Deaths

In the United States, accidents now exceed any disease category as cause of death among persons between the ages of 1 and 37 years. Among infants less than one year old, deaths from accidents rank sixth, after, respectively, deaths from immaturity, postnatal asphyxia, congenital malformations, pneumonia and birth injuries. Above age 37, deaths from accidents rank third, those from heart disease and cancer taking the first and second places.

Of the 115,000 accidental deaths that are estimated by The National Safety Council to have occurred in 1968, approximately 15,700, or about 14 per cent of the total accidental deaths, involved children under age 15 (1969a). Death rates from disease in children have decreased markedly over the past three decades due to advances in medicine. However, those from accidents have improved but slightly, with a fairly consistent number of about 15,000 deaths occurring annually in this age group.

The distribution by age and sex of accidental deaths, and the death rates among children is shown in Table 8–1, which is based on the most recent official data.

The preponderance of male deaths over female deaths is significant at all the ages shown, with the disparity between the sexes becoming more pronounced at the preadolescent and adolescent ages.

The foregoing discussion refers only to deaths. Accidents result in injuries of varying degrees of severity far more frequently than they cause deaths. Permanent disabilities in children have far-reaching consequences in individual adjustments and in adult productivity which may exceed those following disabling accidents to older persons. Various limited studies have estimated that serious injuries outnumber deaths from children's accidents by as much as 100 to 150, to 1. Although the extent to which head injuries occur in children at early ages is not known, neurosurgeons are becoming increasingly aware of their sequelae.

Perhaps the most reliable estimate of the prevalence of nonfatal injury among children comes from the National Health Survey conducted by the U.S. Public Health Service. The latest data (1967) suggest that in one year, 8,922,000 children under the age of 6 suffer accidental injuries which result in one or more days of restricted activity or require medical attention, or both. This indicates that 38 of each 100 children under 6 years of age are injured to this extent per year. Among those 6 to 10 years of age, the number receiving injuries was estimated at 13,168,000, or 30.1 per 100 per year. In this latter group, the injuries accounted for an estimated 9.8 million days lost from school (National Center for Health Statistics, 1967).

Major Classes of Accidents Resulting in Death

It should come as no surprise that the patterns of accidental death and injury among children vary with age, sex and level of physical and social development. Infancy has hazards

Table 8–1** Accidental Deaths and Death Rates from Accidents Among Persons Under 20 Years of Age in the U. S., 1967*

	Deaths			Death Rates per 100,000		
Age	Total	Male	Female	Both Sexes	Male	Female
Under 1	2751	1552	1199	77.7	85.9	69.2
1– 2	1559	874	685	32.4 (ages 1–5)	38.1 (ages 1–5)	26.5 (ages 1–5)
2– 3	1342	798	544			
3– 4	1184	765	419			
4– 5	989	609	380			
Under 5	7825	4598	3227			
5– 9	4010	2649	1361	19.2	24.9	13.3
10–14	3864	2849	1015	19.4	28.2	10.4
15–19	11,036	8628	2408	62.4	98.6	27.4

*Selected data from *Vital Statistics of the U.S., 1967*. Vol. II: *Mortality*, Part A.

particular to that phase, as do all the succeeding stages throughout childhood. As one author has aptly stated, "Children, like nearly all animals, are strongly inclined toward locomotion, and like all primates, are chronically bent on manipulation. They tend to explore the environment and to investigate the possibilities of objects. They get about and they pry into things. . . . Some places, some objects, and some events in the environment are dangerous. Hence children necessarily and unavoidably come close to certain kinds of danger" (Gibson, 1961).

The kinds of "dangers" which are the leading causes of accidental death among infants, children and young adolescents are shown in Table 8–2, which represents United States statistics for the year 1967. In the official data, year-by-year figures are available only below age 5; those for children above age 5 are given in five-year groupings.

There are several features of interest in Table 8–2, apart from the relative numbers of deaths associated with the different kinds of accidents. It is evident that more boys than girls are fatally injured. In most types of accidents, this difference is slight during the first year of life but tends to become progressively greater as the children get older. The data also indicate that different types of accidents result in peak fatalities at different stages of the age distribution, and show variations in trends

Table 8–2 Fatalities from Leading Types of Accidents in the U. S., Classified by Age and Sex, 1967*

	Age (One-Year Grouping)					Age (Five-Year Grouping)			
Type of Accident	Under 1 Year	1	2	3	4	Under 5 Years	5–9	10–14	15–19
Motor Vehicle									
Total	321	367	484	464	431	2067	2079	1766	7889
Male	159	201	275	293	258	1186	1306	1177	5942
Female	162	166	209	171	173	881	773	589	1947
Fires and Explosions									
Total	189	242	244	258	199	1132	474	181	146
Male	92	129	136	155	107	619	258	113	86
Female	97	113	108	103	92	513	216	68	60
Drowning									
Total	68	252	215	174	130	839	638	733	976
Male	39	147	160	131	99	576	504	586	913
Female	29	105	55	43	31	263	134	147	83
Inhalation or Ingestion of Food or Objects									
Total	620	104	38	25	15	802	41	21	42
Male	366	67	22	18	6	479	27	14	24
Female	254	37	16	7	9	323	14	7	18
Falls									
Total	163	136	86	53	40	478	96	84	163
Male	93	78	48	39	24	282	66	61	132
Female	70	58	38	14	16	196	30	23	31
Poisoning by Solids and Liquids									
Total	45	151	73	36	20	325	17	14	133
Male	25	83	34	21	12	175	6	9	104
Female	20	68	39	15	8	150	11	5	29

*Selected data from *Vital Statistics of the U.S., 1967.*

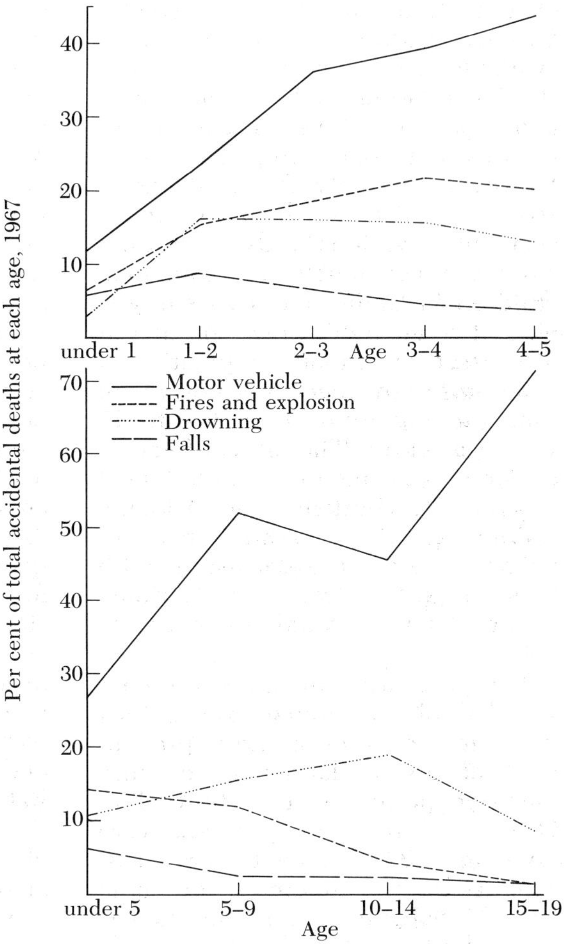

Figure 8–1 The percentage of total accidental deaths among children in 1967 resulting from four major categories of accidents.

The curves in the top part of the figure show the variation in children under 5 years of age by single years of age. In the lower figure, the data have been grouped in five-year intervals, covering the range from under one year of age through 19 years of age. (Based on data from *Vital Statistics of the U.S., 1967.*)

across the age span covered. For example, there were more deaths among infants under one year of age from the inhalation or ingestion of food or other objects than from any of the other causes listed.[1] In children between the ages of one and two this category has dropped to the lowest rank, a position then maintained consistently across the older age ranges. Deaths from poisoning are most frequent at ages 1 and 2, thereafter decreasing through the childhood range. These trends, and the relative importance of the various types of accidents, are shown graphically in Figure 8–1. The curves are based on the percentage of the total number of accidental deaths, at each age, resulting from the leading accident classes.

[1]The National Safety Council indicates "mechanical suffocation" as the leading cause of accidental deaths in infants during the first year of life. In the *U. S. Vital Statistics,* "Mechanical Suffocation" is listed under location of accident, but without age data. This category has become suspect in recent years, however, and it is now believed that many of the fatalities included have resulted from acute overwhelming infections (Wheatley, 1956).

NONFATAL INJURIES AMONG CHILDREN

A brief indication was given earlier on the general prevalence of nonfatal injuries among children on the basis of data from the National Health Survey. Additional information is available from a number of recent studies relating to home accidents and to particular types of accidents or injuries, e.g., poisonings and burns. However, probably the most extensive set of data on the spectrum of accidents of various kinds comes from a study of accidental injuries among children in California. This study is of particular significance in that it was based on a total "population at risk," with coverage over periods of time ranging from at least 4 to 15 years per child. Though confined to children residing in a limited geographic area (Berkeley and Oakland, California), the overall rates developed were quite consistent with those reported from the National Health Survey (Manheimer et al., 1966).

The population in this study consisted of 8874 children whose families were members of a large prepaid medical service plan for one or more four-year periods of the child's life. Of the children, 51.5 per cent were boys and 48.5 per cent were girls. This coverage amounted to some 53,448 "child years," and the analysis of accidents was based on the records of more than 13,000 medically attended injuries. Injuries were categorized as severe (resulting in hospitalization or requiring three or more outpatient visits) or as minor. Analysis was made in terms of injury rates for the population as a whole, and for subgroups by age, sex, race and sibling order. Also included were type of injury, part of body injured and major classes of accidents.

The overall frequency rate was 2.46 per 1000 children per year, or one accident per child in each four-year period. At all ages, rates for boys were higher than for girls (see Table 8–3). Accident rates for boys increased with age, especially for the "severe" injuries. Among girls, frequency rates were highest in the first four years of life, then declined steadily. Girls' severity rates, after an increase at the 8 to 11 age level, dropped sharply at the 12 to 15 age level. The rates for white children were higher than among Negroes, and those for Orientals were lowest. Rates were also highest among children whose fathers' occupations were classed as professional, and lowest among those whose fathers were semiskilled or unskilled workers.

It was also of interest that in chil-

Table 8–3 Nonfatal Injuries Classified by Sex and Age: Annual Rates per 1000 Children*

Age and Sex	Rate of All Injuries	Rate of Severe Injuries	Number of Children Injured
0– 3 Years			
Boys	287.8	30.8	1648
Girls	212.5	27.5	1488
4– 7 Years			
Boys	288.7	40.9	2307
Girls	192.9	25.9	2098
8–11 Years			
Boys	302.5	53.0	2082
Girls	187.0	31.2	1901
12–15 Years			
Boys	328.6	69.4	948
Girls	146.6	21.3	890

**From* Manheimer, D. I., et al.: 50,000 child-years of accidental injuries. *Public Health Rep.*, *81*: 522, 1966.

dren with older siblings, rates were lower in the preschool years and higher in the teens than among children without older siblings. The variation in individual frequencies of injury may be noted from the fact that in the largest subclass of children (white boys, ages 4 to 7) about 35 per cent had no record of injury, 30 per cent one injury and 19 per cent two injuries. The range was from zero to nine or more injuries in the four-year period.

The frequency distribution of specific injuries is shown in Table 8–4. The highest rate for any single type of injury was in the category laceration, but fracture was the most frequent class of severe injury. Age was a strong influence in the distribution of types of injury. Burn rates for both boys and girls decreased sharply after age 4, and poisoning rates decreased even more so. The frequency of laceration remained relatively constant through age 8 and then decreased sharply. Fracture rates at ages 12 to 15 were four times as great as in the first 4 years, and sprains and strains were some 7 times as frequent in the oldest age range. On the other hand, little difference in injury type between the sexes was apparent. About one injury in seven was severe; fractures were severe three times out of four, but they were only sixth in frequency.

With regard to part of body injured, the head was most frequently involved in all injuries and ranked second in the severity rates; arms were severely injured most frequently. Hand injuries were second in frequency, followed by injuries to legs, feet and arms, in that order.

Age variations in regard to part of body injured were also observed. The rate of head injuries dropped sharply between ages 4 and 12. Internal injuries (mostly from poisoning) decreased, especially after the first 4 years. Leg, foot, hand and arm injuries increased with age. Rates for injuries to the lower part of the body increased among the older boys.

Data in relation to type of accident are shown in Table 8–5. Accident types showing a decrease in frequency with increasing age included falls, suffocation and contact with hot objects. An increase in rate was noted for collisions, contact with sharp objects and being struck. Bicycle accidents and dog bites were most frequent between ages 4 and 11.

It might be expected that studies similar to the foregoing would manifest some deviations from the distributions shown if carried out in other geographic areas of the country or on populations not limited to membership in a health service plan. For example, the finding of lower rates of nonfatal injury among Negro children

*Table 8–4 Nonfatal Injury Rates Classified by Type of Injury, per 1000 Children**

Type of Injury	Rate of All Injuries	Rate of Severe Injuries	Per Cent of Severe Injuries
Laceration	63.8	9.2	14.5
Contusion	45.5	4.7	10.4
Sprain, Strain	30.8	2.6	8.4
Abrasion	27.9	3.1	11.2
Perforation	21.6	0.8	3.9
Fracture	21.4	15.7	73.5
Burn	9.5	2.6	27.3
Poisoning	4.8	0.5	9.4
Concussion	2.2	0.9	40.3

**From* Manheimer, D. I., et al.: 50,000 child-years of accidental injuries. *Public Health Rep.*, *81*:526, 1966.

*Table 8–5 Injury Rates Classified by Type of Accident, per 1000 Children**

Accident Type	Rate of All Injuries	Rate of Severe Injuries	Per Cent of Severe Injuries
Fall	56.8	11.9	21.0
Contact with sharp or rough object	29.2	2.6	8.8
Collision with person or object (except moving vehicle)	22.7	3.6	16.0
Dog bite	13.4	0.6	4.8
Struck by falling, flying, thrown objects	10.2	2.1	20.2
Bicycle or pedal vehicle	9.5	2.7	28.7
Caught in, pinched, crushed	8.2	1.3	15.2
Contact with hot object or substance	6.7	2.0	29.8
Motor vehicle	6.2	1.2	19.5
Occupant	4.4	0.7	15.9
Pedestrian	1.8	0.5	28.6
Poisoning	6.2	0.5	7.3
Suffocation	5.8	0.4	6.6

**From* Manheimer, D. I., et al.: 50,000 child-years of accidental injuries. *Public Health Rep., 81*: 528, 1966.

compared to white children appears contradictory to reports from numerous other studies, which have shown higher fatality rates among Negro children. Analysis of the data, however, did not indicate a difference in readiness between white and Negro families to seek medical attention for injury. Thus, a question remains whether a socioeconomic bias related to participation in a health service plan influenced the finding in the California study.

In general, other information relating to the prevalence and distribution of nonfatal accidental injuries among children comes from studies of home accidents (Hemphill, 1952; Hemphill and Velz, 1953; California State Department of Public Health, 1957; Mac Queen, 1960; Stallones and Corsa, 1961), local surveys of children's accidents (Rice et al. 1956; Fowler, 1958; Stallones and Corsa, 1961) and a variety of studies on particular types of accidents or injuries. Earlier studies have been chiefly concerned with accident data found in hospital and other medical records, without much reference to a defined population "at risk." Attempts have been made in more recent investigations to overcome this difficulty through such procedures as the systematic sampling of households in a given geographic area, in relation to home accidents; or by including all children within a given area who were born within a certain time interval (Rowntree, 1950; Baltimore and Meyer, 1969).

ANALYSIS OF CAUSES OF ACCIDENTAL INJURIES

In a classic paper, Gordon proposed that the methods used in analyzing the distribution and causation of disease were applicable to understanding the causation of accidental injuries and would result in better information as a basis for their prevention (Gordon, 1949). This proposal was accompanied by the demonstration that when distribution of accidental injuries was analyzed in terms of the age and sex of the victims and in reference to types of accidents and the mechanisms of injury, characteristic variations were found that were similar to those relating to diseases. At that time, epidemiology was primarily the study of factors influencing the distribution of infectious diseases. Thus, applied to accidents, it was suggested that the causes of accidental injuries reside in interactions between a susceptible "host," an injuring "agent" and facilitating environmental circumstances.

A first step in this approach involved a study of the distributions of accidents and injuries in terms of who the affected persons were, and when, where and how accidents and injuries occurred; and also in regard to different classes of accidents and the specific agencies and mechanisms of injury involved.

This "descriptive" epidemiological approach has been important in assessing the overall magnitude and scope of the problem and in indicating the relative significance of various accident classes or circumstances in contributing to the total number of accidents. As well, it has aided in identifying the segments of the population experiencing a disproportionately high incidence of accidents, and the segments in which specific types of accidents are especially important. Such data have also served as a starting point for more analytical approaches; for example, postulation of causal hypotheses to explain associations observed in the data, and design of studies to test such hypotheses and the influence of preventive measures. An interdisciplinary approach is essential. Application of the epidemiological approach to the study and control of accidents involves the contributions of epidemiologists, biostatisticians and a variety of other disciplines including medicine and the biological sciences, especially psychology and the behavioral sciences (MacMahon et al., 1960). Also, various fields of the physical sciences and engineering have an important role in design of equipment and in understanding the causative factors in injuries (McFarland and Moore, 1961).

In the application of epidemiological methods to the field of accidents, one approach has been the analysis of various medical records or official health statistics. However, classifications used in such records are not necessarily suited for causal analysis. For example, primarily "manifestational" classification of injuries is employed in the International Classification of Diseases; e.g., "skull fracture," "lacerations," "contusions." This type of classification is treatment-oriented, and although useful for planning emergency medical services, therapy and rehabilitation, it generally has limited value for understanding causes and for development of prevention. A further limitation of the information on accidents contained in official health statistics is that often they include only fatalities. Accidents which result in a large number of deaths are not necessarily those in which there is a high frequency of nonfatal injuries.

Of greater usefulness is the "supplementary Classification of External Cause of Injury" (E802–E998), which classifies according to the kinds of accident sequence that victims have experienced. This "experiential" classification includes two general types of information: one which emphasizes exposure to a particular object without reference to the mechanism or "contingency" (e.g., railway accident, motor vehicle accident), and one which emphasizes the "contingency" without reference to the objects involved (e.g., a fall on the same level). For research purposes, such classifications have provided too little detail, and the development of alternative ways of grouping accidents has frequently been necessary. For example, in one extensive study of home accidents, fully 25 per cent could not be classified under the international system, except as "other." By developing a two-dimensional code consisting of 34 accident contingencies (e.g., fall from, bitten by) in combination with 100 specific objects, it was possible to classify all but one per cent of the accidents, and to identify in a manner satisfactory for meaningful analysis 200 kinds of accidents occurring in the home (California State Department of Public Health, 1957).

Another method used to study accidents has been termed "investigative epidemiology." Rather than the analysis of data taken on large samples of the population, this involves the intensive investigation of individual cases, usually a relatively small number and in reference to injuries in a specific type of accident. This approach is currently exemplified by injury-surveillance teams of the Public Health Service. By monitoring the occurrence of medically attended injuries in particular communities, types of accidents which occur with unusual frequency (e.g., an increase in scald burns in children) or new and unusual accidents can be identified and the individual cases subjected to detailed analysis of all the circumstances involved (Marland and Burg, 1969).

Some problems in interpreting the results of research result from variations in the definition of what constitutes an accident in different studies, and in failure to adequately measure exposure in a given population. Accident research in general has also been characterized by numerous methodological deficiencies such as inadequate sampling in time or numbers, inappropriate study design or statistical treatment, analysis of variables out of context and overgeneralization of findings. There has been considerable improvement in these areas in recent years, however. While much remains to be accomplished, a considerable amount of valid information accumulated from epidemiological studies has increased the understanding of accident causation and in some cases has led to the development of more effective prevention. (Suchman, 1961; McFarland, 1963; Haddon et al., 1964). The significant findings relating to the accidents and injuries among children will be discussed in the remainder of this chapter.

SOURCES AND PREVENTION OF INJURY IN CHILDREN'S ACCIDENTS

Preventing children's accidents requires a knowledge of the frequencies with which various agents produce accidental injury, and relating this information to circumstances of the children and the environmental situation. For example, the substances ingested by children in accidental poisonings vary with age and sex of the child, geographical area and socioeconomic circumstances of the family. Injuries to young infants frequently involve falls to the floor from surfaces where they have been placed. In the suburbs, dressing tables, Bathinettes and cribs are more frequently implicated; in less privileged areas the infants roll off table tops, beds and other adult furniture. Falls are the leading cause of nonfatal injury up to age 14, most frequently as a result of tripping or slipping. Drownings among boys are far more frequent than among girls and often involve such activities as playing on thin ice and on the banks of rivers, creeks and canals. Girls' accidents more often occur indoors, involving falls (as on stairs) or contact with hot objects (Wheatley, 1951; McFarland, 1955).

Thus, effective preventive measures against injuries among children will show a shifting emphasis with age and sex. Initially, protecting children against accidents is the only possible procedure. As the child acquires locomotion, rudimentary skills and simple language, training and supervised experience in situations of hazard become increasingly important. At later stages, constant protection becomes less possible and probably less desirable. Education in safety then becomes the chief procedure for the control of behavioral factors and consequent prevention of accidents (Armstrong and Cole, 1949; Dietrich, 1952). The importance of cooperation between various health and community agencies has also been emphasized (McFarland, 1956).

Sources of Energy as "Agents" of Injury

An important aspect of the prevention of injury among both children and adults relates to methods of control of the "agents" involved, and to preventing harmful interactions between "host" and "agent." While it has been customary in epidemiological studies to consider the environmental objects causing injury in accidents as the "agents," a more basic concept involves the fact that all injuries result from abnormal exchanges of energy between persons and the physical environment (King, 1949; Gibson, 1961). Accidental injuries result from (1) the application of various forms of energy to the human body in amounts exceeding the tolerance thresholds of its various parts and (2) interference with the normal exchanges of energy between the body and its environment (e.g., in drowning). The forms of energy producing accidental injuries of all types include thermal energy, electrical energy, ionizing radiation, mechanical energy and chemical energy (Haddon, 1967).

The concept of energy as the cause of injury presents a close analogy to the agent that causes a disease. Each form of energy produces specific kinds of injury. For example, thermal energy impinging on the body may produce inflammation, coagulation, charring and incineration at all body levels (i.e., first-, second- and third-degree burns), with the specific result depending on the location and manner in which the energy is dissipated. The energy which impinges on the body is delivered by various means, usually by inanimate objects. These correspond to the "carriers" and "vectors" of disease. Wires carry electricity, moving objects carry mechanical or kinetic energy and poisonous plants are vectors of their toxins. Thus, the modification of the vehicles or vectors of injurious energy is an important means of preventing injury (Haddon, 1967).

Also, the variation in natural or acquired resistance to injury corresponds to resistance to infection. Increased susceptibility to mechanical insults characterizes such conditions as osteogenesis imperfecta and hemophilia. Shifts in resistance with age and sex also occur. Lower death rates from falls are found in areas having water with naturally high fluoride content (Iskrant and Joliet, 1968). Physical conditioning and training in contact sports increase resistance to injury. Repeated or continuous exposures to moderately high altitudes produces some tolerance for anoxia (McFarland, 1953).

Prevention of Harmful Exchanges of Energy

The prevention of abnormal exchanges of energy between the body and the environment can be done through interference in the early stages leading to the transfer event, or by directly blocking or attenuating the exchange. Four initial levels of prevention are (1) to eliminate the source of hazardous energy (e.g., prohibit the manufacture of fireworks, of flammable blankets and clothing, of lead-based paints), (2) to prevent or modify the release of hazardous energy (e.g., replace wooden handles in lollipops with paper ones, use scissors with blunt ends which will cut only paper), (3) to separate the energy and the persons in time or space (e.g., prohibit traffic on streets reserved for play, provide pedestrian overpasses) and (4) to interpose between the energy source and the person a barrier which blocks or attenuates the energy transfer (e.g., use fences around swimming pools, electrical insulation, child-proof tops for containers of medicine or toxic household products, helmets and pads for football players.

Pediatricians have long recognized the need for improved control over the agents of injury in children's accidents, and have been active in efforts to bring this about, for example, in relation to the flammability of fabrics used in children's clothing. From 40 to 60 per cent of burn injuries seen in various clinics have resulted from burning clothing (McFarland and Moore, 1965; Haddon, 1967). Loose garments, such as girls' dresses and nightgowns, have been particularly implicated, ignited from contact with open flame or elements of electrical heaters (Colebrook and Colebrook, 1949; Wheatley, 1956; Bleck, 1955; Jensen, 1959; Iskrant, 1967).

Consequently, pediatricians have played an especially important role in attempts to prevent children's injuries through the control of injurious agents: The American Standards Association, at the request of the American Academy of Pediatrics, established a committee to consider safety standards for the flammability of children's clothing, the proper labeling of toxic paints and coatings, the design of harnesses and sleeping garments and the design and manufacture of furniture, carriages and toys (McFarland, 1955).

Another important step for the control of injuries was the passage of the Flammable Fabrics Act of 1954 by the U.S. Congress. The purpose of this Act was to reduce the danger of injury and loss of life by providing national standards for testing and rating the flammability of textile products used in clothing. Originally, the provisions of the Act were restricted to fabrics coming in contact with the body. In 1967 it was amended to include all articles of wearing apparel, and fabrics used in interior furnishings (Oglesbay, 1969).

Other developments with far-reaching implications for control of injurious exchanges of energy through the safe design of vectors relate to the concept of product liability. Under this, manufacturers may be held financially responsible for the results of unsafe features of their products. Also, there have been significant recent legislative activities in the field of consumer protection, culminating in the Child Protection Act of 1966,[2] and the establishment in 1968 of the National Commission of Product Safety.

These developments should result in increased attention to potentially unsafe features of products at the stage of their design, and in more extensive evaluation of possible unsafe uses subsequent to purchase. The economic pressure of the threat of expensive lawsuits or of removal of profitable items from the market through governmental action is likely to provide an incentive for greater awareness of safety implications. Indeed, there have recently been notable instances where manufacturers or distributors have voluntarily recalled or removed from the market items called to their attention as defective from a safety standpoint, or as potentially dangerous. For example, in the area of children's acci-

[2]This Act dealt only with certain hazardous substances. A recommendation was made in 1969 by the Commission on Product Safety to extend the provisions to include electrical, mechanical and thermal hazards found in toys and other products used by children.

dents, a surveillance team of the Public Health Service monitoring thermal injuries found that numerous scaldings resulted when electric coffee percolators were upset by children pulling on cords. One manufacturer, when presented with this information, recalled his product and replaced it with a percolator redesigned with a lower center of gravity, a retractable cord and a top that would remain closed in case of upset. Another example is the decision by the Association of Home Appliance Manufacturers to require its members to conform not only to the requirements of the U.S. Public Law 930 for refrigerator doors which may be opened from the inside, but to extend this provision to the design of freezer doors.[3]

Human Factors in the Design of Children's Equipment

The elimination of recognized hazards in the design stage of products accessible to children and of equipment for children is of great importance for the prevention of injury, as is the prevention of the interactions between child and injurious agents. Securing the sides of cribs, using restraining straps on infant's dressing tables and storing poisonous materials in places inaccessible to toddlers are obvious examples of the latter. Accidents may also be reduced if equipment intended for children (e.g., furniture, toys, recreational devices) is designed in terms of the size, physical and psychological capabilities, and limitations, of the children (McFarland, 1955). This approach, known in the United States as human engineering and as ergonomics in Great Britain, was developed in relation to the design of machinery, military devices, aircraft and various types of transport vehicles. The basic principles, however, are applicable in many other fields—the design of children's furniture, play and recreational equipment and household appliances, and in architectural arrangements of dwellings. There are numerous instances where a difference in the size or design of children's furniture, toys or clothing would have prevented an accident, or resulted in less severe injury. When human engineering data are incorporated in the original design of equipment, fewer accidents should result. Advance analysis of children's equipment can be carried out, so that features increasing the likelihood of accidents due to incompatibility between child and his equipment can be eliminated at the design-board stage.

Infant furniture provides some examples of design deficiencies. The magazine *Good Housekeeping* conducted a survey of accidents resulting from design shortcomings of infant furniture. There were many reports in which injuries and near-accidents were related to design features that reflected inadequate consideration of the physical and behavioral characteristics of infants. The National Safety Council has reported details of the survey (1970b), some of which follow:

Crib design was especially implicated. In some models, strangulation accidents occurred because of spacing of the slats of the sides, allowing an infant to wriggle legs, soft buttocks and body through the opening, only to be caught by the relatively large and unyielding head. The height of crib sides relative to the "low" position of the mattress was the subject of frequent complaint based on the fre-

[3] An interesting experimental study relating to the highly publicized problem of entrapment of children in refrigerators has been carried out to analyze the behavior of children when so entrapped and to evaluate their ability to find and use various escape mechanisms (Bain et al., 1958).

quency that active children pulled themselves or bounced over the top rail. Another common complaint involved designs with horizontal cross members onto which the child could hook his toes and climb over the top.

A study of injuries to infants from falls has indicated that the most common accident involves an infant climbing over the sides of a crib (Kravitz et al., 1969). Design recommendations from this study included lower mattresses and netting over the top of the crib from the time an infant can pull himself to a standing position, as well as elimination of features conducive to climbing. Attention was also called to the practice of placing in cribs large toy animals or other playthings which can be used as steps for climbing, and accidents.

In *Good Housekeeping*'s survey there were frequent references to problems of balance and stability of infant seats, plastic baby carriers and strollers, particularly in relation to changes in size, weight and center of gravity in the growing child. Tipovers with consequent spills and falls were often reported. More adequate restraining straps were also urged, to secure active children on the tops of dressing tables and in "bounce" seats and highchairs.

There is a great deal of information relating to height, weight and body dimensions of children. Also, much is known about child growth and the behavioral and developmental capabilities at different ages. Such data, however, are to be found chiefly in reports from the field of anthropometry and in the literature of pediatrics and child development. They are seldom easily available in a form useful to the designer. In regard to design of equipment for adult use, a considerable amount of human engineering data has been developed. In the case of children, however, there is a great need to develop, integrate and augment the existing information for application in design.

INJURIES AND DEATHS FROM MOTOR VEHICLE ACCIDENTS

Considerable publicity attends the accidental deaths of children from house fires, falls from windows, drowning in backyard pools, play in unattended construction projects and the like. However, a fact not always appreciated is that except among infants under one year of age, accidents involving motor vehicles result in far more child deaths than does any other type of accident (see Table 8–2). This phenomenon has perhaps also been obscured by the attention given to the excessive motor vehicle deaths and death rates in the adolescent and young adult years. National estimates on the frequency of nonfatal injury from accidents involving motor vehicles and children suggest that some 290,000 children under the age of 15 years were injured in 1968 (National Safety Council, 1969a). Further, the National Health Survey estimates that in 1967 among children under 6, there were 2.74 million days of restricted activity from injuries received in moving motor vehicle accidents; and in children between 6 and 16, there were 4.65 million days of restricted activity (National Center for Health Statistics, 1969). It should be noted, however, that the types of accidents with highest fatality rates are not necessarily those with the greatest injury rates. In general, fatality rates for motor vehicle injuries are high compared to those for other major types of accidents, and the numbers of persons suffering injury from accidents in the home, for example, far exceed those incurring injuries in motor vehicle accidents.

In regard to motor vehicle deaths among children, further analysis reveals a significant pattern, according to whether the victims were pedestrians or the occupants of vehicles, or were involved in accidents which were not on the highway. This pattern is shown in Figures 8–2 and 8–3. Two aspects of these figures are especially noteworthy. One is the shift with age in the numbers of children killed as pedestrians, in comparison to the other classes in both absolute and relative terms. The ages at which children are more likely to be involved as pedestrians are clearly evident. Beyond the ages shown, pedestrians form but a small proportion of the fatalities in comparison with occupants of vehicles until about middle age, when the proportions of pedestrian deaths begin to increase rapidly.

One implication of childhood fatalities in motor vehicles is the need for improvement, and use, of restraining devices specifically designed to accommodate children of different ages. While in general there is some evidence to suggest that child occupants of vehicles in crashes tend to be less severely injured than adults (Moore et al., 1960), it is also clear that much remains to be done to provide adequate protection against crash injury specifically in the case of children (Snyder, 1969).

The second observation from Figure 8–2 relates to the nontraffic deaths. These are of greatest magnitude in the years one through four, and especially at the crawling and toddler ages. These deaths represent mostly accidents that occur in private driveways and in other nonhighway locations.

Although not shown separately, deaths to bicycle riders from collisions with motor vehicles are greatest

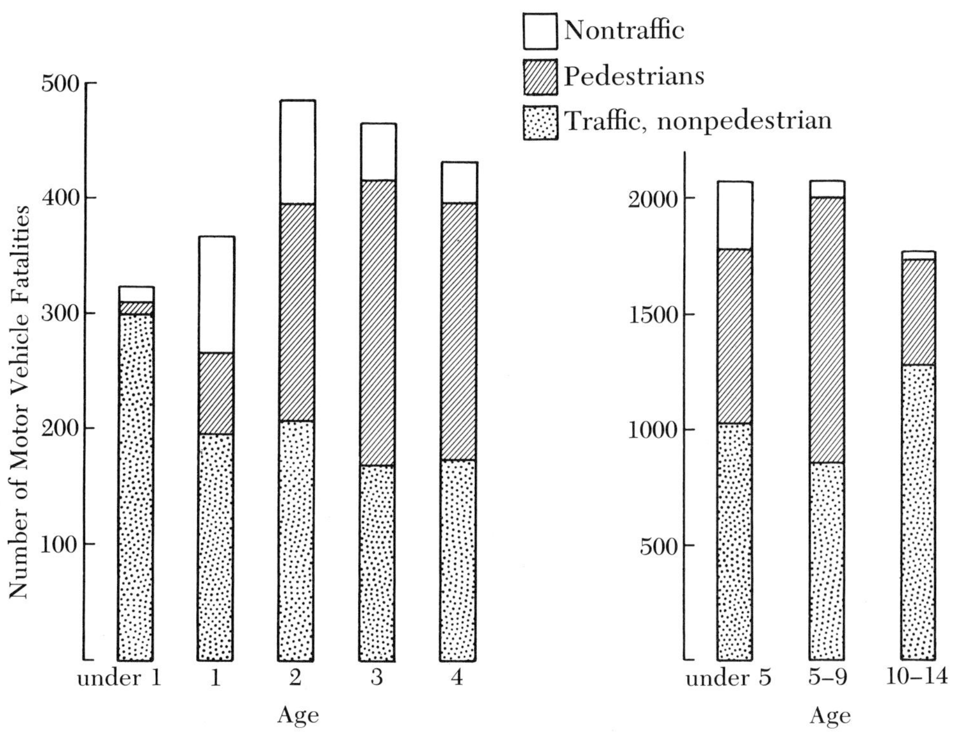

Figure 8–2 The number of children fatally injured in motor vehicle accidents in the U. S. in 1967, classified by age of child and type of accident.

The fatalities are divided into those accidents occurring in nonpublic places (i.e., private driveways, yards and other nonhighway sites), those occurring in motor vehicle–pedestrian collisions on roads and public ways, and those occurring in traffic, nonpedestrian accidents (i.e., involving mostly occupants of motor vehicles). (Based on data from *Vital Statistics of the U.S., 1967.*)

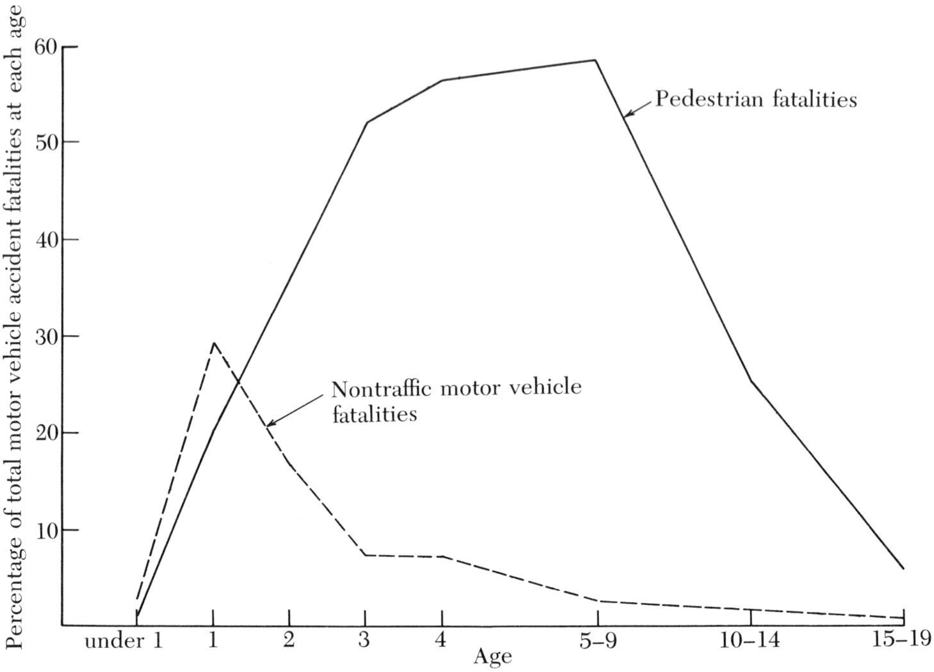

Figure 8–3 The relative frequency of fatalities among children from nontraffic motor vehicle accidents (i.e., those occurring in private driveways and yards) and from highway pedestrian accidents, in relation to age of the victims.

Note the concentration of the nontraffic cases at the earlier ages. Pedestrian fatalities comprise more than half of the total fatalities from age 2 through the 5-to-9-year-old group. These then sharply decrease among the older children.

In the 10 to 14 year range, the relative contribution of these two classes of accidents to the total number of fatalities is markedly less, and in the 15 to 19 year range almost all the fatalities were occupants of motor vehicles. (Based on data from *Vital Statistics of the U.S., 1967.*)

in number in the 5 to 14 age range, accounting for approximately 500 of the deaths shown for ages 5 to 9 and 10 to 14. They are chiefly included in the "traffic-nonpedestrian" class, with a few in the "nontraffic" category. Consideration of this category of motor vehicle accident will be given in a subsequent section on bicycle safety.

Studies of Child Pedestrian Accidents

As already noted, the numbers of fatalities among child pedestrians in traffic accidents are especially high from age 2 through 9, and, more specifically, from age 3 into the 5 to 9 year range, accounting for more than half of the deaths from motor vehicle accidents at these ages. Boys consistently outnumber girls in these deaths by about 2 to 1. Above age 10, fewer children are killed as pedestrians, and the fatalities in motor vehicle accidents are predominantly the occupants of vehicles.

In general, injuries to pedestrians are likely to be fatal about twice as often per case as are injuries to vehicle occupants. However, this does not hold for children, even though far more children are struck by motor vehicles than pedestrians in other age ranges. In a study covering all reported pedestrian accidents occurring in a recent one-year period in a Michigan county (including the city of Detroit), 53 per cent of the 7853 victims were under 15 years of age. The fatalities among these children, however, constituted only 19 per cent of the total pedestrian deaths in the series (Huelke and Davis, 1969). The high rate of involvement among children may be a function of their more frequent exposure as pedestrians. The lower fatality rates may depend on such factors as an impact area of body exposure different from that of adults, or more resistance to trauma in comparison to that of elderly victims.

Medico-engineering investigations of pedestrian accidents (Ryan, 1969) and studies of experimental crashes involving "dummy" pedestrians (Severy and Brink, 1966) have indicated that pedestrians are not usually "run over" and that injuries are sustained both from impact with the vehicle and from striking the road. The size of the pedestrian relative to the height and configuration of the front of the car has an effect on the distribution of injuries sustained. If the center of gravity of the body is higher than the front of the hood, as in many adults, the lower part of the body is thrown upward and rotates, so that the head hits the hood or windshield, and the pedestrian falls off the car onto the road. Children, however, having less height, are projected forward in the direction of car travel or to the side, to strike the road or ground with considerable force. Injuries tend to be multiple, with head and thoracic injuries frequent in the fatalities. One difference between adult and child pedestrian injuries is the relative infrequency of pelvic injuries in children.

Among school-age children, the peak numbers of pedestrian accidents correspond with times of movement to and from school. However, those which have a fatal result are more frequent from 5 to 7 P.M., and in warm weather and summer months (Huelke and Davis, 1969).

Studies of the circumstances under which children are struck by cars indicate three basic action patterns of behavior on the part of the youngsters. In order of frequency these involve (1) running from behind or between parked cars, (2) playing in the street and (3) crossing at an intersection or crosswalk. Analysis of the cases occurring in Vancouver, B.C., revealed that about 20 per cent of the involved drivers did not see the child before the impact, and in about another 40 per cent, drivers first saw the child at a distance too short to avoid the collision. Environmental conditions related to high accident frequencies included (1) areas traversed by busy thoroughfares, (2) congested populations, (3) areas of crowded and conventional housing, (4) high industrialization and (5) limited play facilities (Read, 1969).

In the Canadian series, the accidents were most frequent in the 3 to 7 age group, with boys far outnumbering girls and with accidents more frequently the result of running from between parked cars or playing in the street, rather than of crossing at intersections or crosswalks. Within this age range, as age increased there was a reduction in the frequency of accidents involving running from between cars and playing in the street, compared to intersection and crosswalk accidents. Above age 8 the accidents were more likely to occur at crosswalks.

In recent years an extensive series of observations has been carried out in Sweden on the behavior of child pedestrians, aged 4 to 10, in relation to vehicular traffic, and on their ability to cope with traffic situations. Some of the findings suggest that adults overestimate the ability of children as pedestrians and frequently expose them to traffic conditions before they have the physical maturity necessary to deal with them. For example, distinction between right and left is difficult for 6-year-olds, and even 9-year-olds confuse this about 10 per cent of the time. Also, children do not perceive and interpret moving objects by peripheral vision as do adults, and they are limited in their localization of sounds which come from the side. Preschool and beginning school children cannot be expected to understand traffic signs nor the complex abstract words of traffic safety or its rules and regulations. Thus, teaching children pedestrian safety must be structured in terms of their characteristic degree of comprehension and behavior at various ages, and their interpretations (Sandel, cited in National Safety Council, 1970a).

While some attention has been paid to the characteristics of childhood pedestrian victims in terms of age, sex and gross behavioral tendencies, only limited work has involved the psychosocial environment as a predisposing element. One investigator has raised the question whether it might not be more accurate to think in terms of families vulnerable to accidents rather than children as vulnerable individuals. In Scotland a comparison was made between families in which children had been injured as pedestrians and families in which child pedestrians had not been injured. Children so injured tended to come from families in which there was stress of illness, maternal preoccupation with pregnancy or work outside the home and less opportunity for protected play (Backett and Johnston, 1959). In the Vancouver study previously mentioned, it was noted that the mothers of those children involved in pedestrian accidents tended to be younger and more often worked outside the home. Also, the families tended to relax supervision of the children's play areas early in the child's life. Fathers tended to be unskilled workers, and the families resided in multiple-dwelling housing in the more densely populated areas (Read, 1969).

POISONING ACCIDENTS INVOLVING CHILDREN

One of the problems accentuated by advances made in science and technology is that of accidental poisoning. The proliferation of pharmacological preparations and of time- and labor-saving household substances has greatly increased possibilities for inadvertent ingestion of hazardous or toxic materials.

Death rates from poisoning in children under 5 have improved in the last 15 years by about 14 per cent, but the death rates for those over age 15 have increased. Deaths from poisoning are relatively fewer in school-age children. Estimates as to the annual frequency of nonfatal poisoning among children run from 500,000 to 2 million (Verhulst and Crotty, 1968). Recent studies suggest that as many as 37 per cent of families with young children experience child poisoning incidents (Manheimer and Mellinger, 1967; Baltimore and Meyer, 1969).

Poison Control Centers

It is believed that the decrease in deaths and death rates (Fig. 8–4) among children may be related to the establishment and activities of Poisoning Control Centers across the nation. The first center was formally established in Chicago in 1953. There are now more than 550 of these centers in the United States, usually associated with a medical school or large hospital. Some of those with the most varied facilities act as master centers, offering information on poisons and treatment on a 24-hour basis. Others act as treatment subcenters, contacting master centers for information. In 1956, a National Clearinghouse for Poison Control Centers was established in the U.S. Public Health Service to provide a bank of informa-

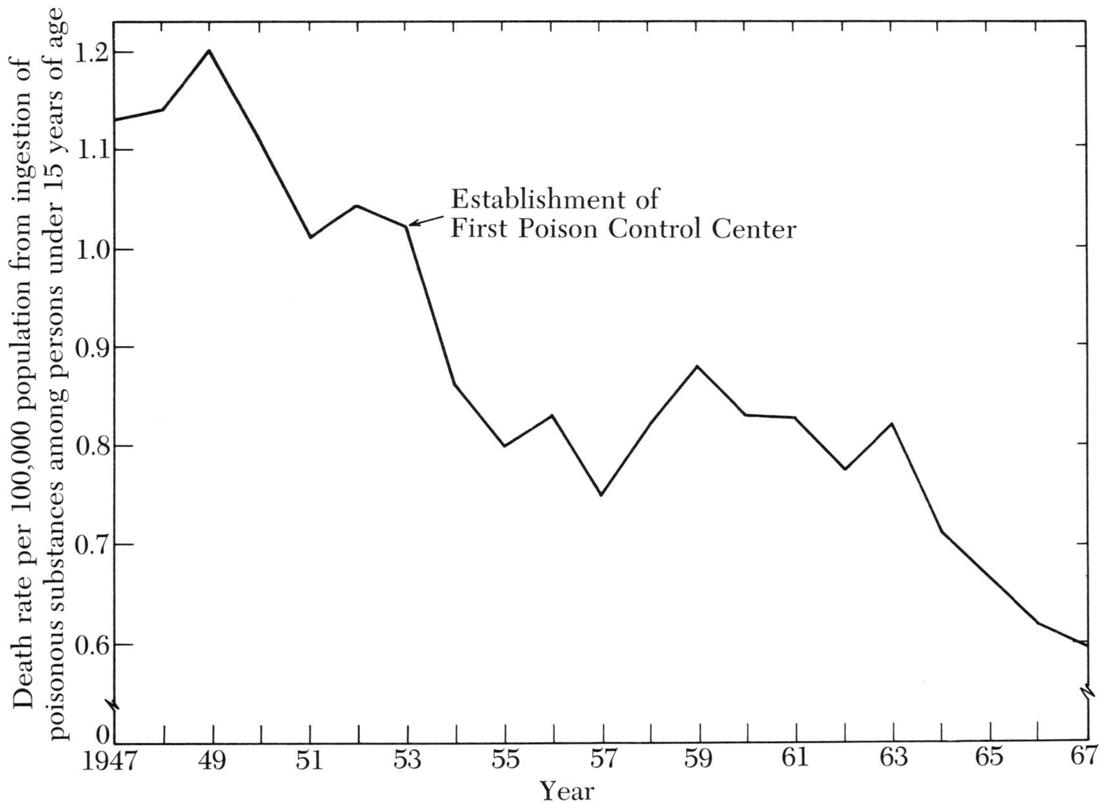

Figure 8–4 Death rates from the ingestion of poisonous substances among children under 15 years of age in the U.S., 1947 to 1967.

The rates shown are per 100,000 persons of this age group. The general decline in the rates over the past 20 years is clearly evident, despite the great increases which have occurred in the numbers and variety of potentially noxious substances. (Based on data from *Vital Statistics of the U.S.*, various years.)

tion on poisons or potential poisons, to disseminate information on new products and on changes in composition of existing products and to collect and analyze data on poisonings reported from the Control Centers (Cann et al., 1958).

A number of findings with important implications for prevention have emerged from analyses of the thousands of cases reported to the National Clearinghouse, as well as from numerous smaller-scale studies in specific areas (Iskrant and Joliet, 1968; Verhulst and Crotty, 1968). Among these are the following:

1. Approximately 90 per cent of the accidental poisonings reported to the Clearinghouse involve children under 5 years of age. The age at which poisoning among children is most frequent is 18 to 24 months. About one-fourth of the incidents in children under 5 occur in this six-month period; about three-fourths are within the age span of 12 to 36 months.

2. There are differences in the types of products ingested by children in different age groups. Household cleaning and polishing agents, pesticides, petroleum products and paint and paint solvents are ingested most frequently by one-year-olds. Two-year-olds ingest medications more frequently than children in other age groups: 39 per cent of external-medication ingestions and 46 per cent of internal-medication ingestions occur at this age. However, with increasing age, the pattern changes from external to internal medications. There is also a reduction in the frequency of poisoning by the various types of household products (see Table 8–6).

3. Among children ingesting internal medications, aspirin is involved in about 50 per cent of the cases; ingestion of "baby" aspirin constitutes about 80 per cent of these cases. (Among older persons, barbiturates are the most frequent type of medication ingested.)

4. The type of product ingested is related to socioeconomic status, cultural patterns, geography and other factors. Poisonings by medicines, for example, are found more frequently in well-to-do homes than in poorer homes. In general, medicines are ingested more frequently in the Northeast and Great Lakes areas. In southern states, petroleum distillates and pesticides form a high proportion of the substances ingested. Within the home, the kitchen is the most frequent site of ingestion. Lead is most often ingested by children eating paint in old, substandard housing areas. Often the paint flakes or peels off walls, ceilings and window sills, and is ingested. Thus, a recognition of the predisposing environmental conditions in the child's home and

*Table 8–6 Type of Product Ingested as Percentage of the Accidental Poisonings at Each Age in Children Under 5 Years**

	Internal Medicine	External Medicine	Cleaning and Polishing Products	Petroleum Products	Cosmetics	Pesticides	Paint Solvents	Other
Under 1 Year	16%	13%	21%	4%	6%	15%	5%	20%
1 Year	23%	8%	27%	8%	7%	11%	7%	9%
2 Years	51%	5%	16%	4%	5%	6%	4%	9%
3 Years	62%	3%	10%	3%	3%	6%	3%	10%
4 Years	55%	5%	12%	2%	2%	8%	3%	13%

*Based on data from Iskrant, A., and Joliet, P.: *Accidents and Homicide*. Cambridge, Massachusetts, Harvard University Press, 1968.

neighborhood is important for the recognition and prevention of poisoning.

5. In about two-thirds of the instances of poisoning by household substances, the toxic materials are not in their customary place of storage, and an important contributing factor is the transfer of products from the original container to vessels often associated with edible substances, such as soft drink bottles, cups or glasses.

The concentration of accidental poisonings in children between one and three years of age has led to the prevalent view that these accidents are a direct result of the developmental and behavioral patterns characteristic of this age range. As stated by Wheatley (1956, p. 204):

> The grasping functions and the drinking function are well developed. The child's most naturally developed method of learning about the physical properties of this world is to put the object or material in his mouth. This method of satisfying curiosity has full play during the runabout, exploring stage. This is the hand-to-mouth stage. This is the period of susceptibility to accidental poisoning.

Consequently, the emphasis in preventive measures has been on the education of parents in the toxicity of potentially hazardous substances and the necessity for the storage of medicines and toxic household preparations in ways to prevent their accessibility to young children. One pilot project, for example, carried out in Charleston County, South Carolina, was an informational and educational program aimed at overcoming adult carelessness or lack of awareness in placing within reach of small children common household products and medicines that can poison. Within one year after the start of the project there was a 27 per cent decrease in the number of hospitalized cases of accidental poisoning in that county (Joliet et al., 1965).

Labeling and Packaging Poisonous Substances

A related aspect of prevention is the proper precautionary labeling of products used in the home; this is now under increased surveillance in the activities of the Food and Drug Administration and in the field of consumer protection. Another aspect is an accelerated attempt to develop child-proof methods of packaging medicine dispensers, medicine containers and containers of toxic household products. The design of such features is based on the inability of young children to perform various manipulative actions simultaneously, such as push-down-and-twist at the same time, or to take advantage of such child characteristics as lack of manual dexterity and short attention span—e.g., as in extracting tablets individually contained in "strip" or "blister" packs (National Safety Council, 1969b). Such devices are currently the subject of legislative activity for the establishment of standards for child-resistant packaging for many products such as medicines, detergents, bleaches, cleaners, polishes and insecticides.

Lead Poisoning

One type of childhood poisoning that is heavily dependent on environmental conditions—and preventable through environmental means—is lead poisoning, or plumbism. This problem poses particular diagnostic difficulties to physicians and pediatricians because of the commonplace and nonspecific nature of the early signs and symptoms. Also, definite clinical manifestations may not be apparent until a child has ingested lead for a period of two or three months as a result of chewing on such substances as painted objects, plaster, wallpaper or putty (Smith, 1964; Zavon, 1964).

The incidence of lead poisoning among children is not known with any certainty. In New York City in a recent two-year period, about 3 per cent of poisonings known to the Department of Health were of this type. There was a substantial increase in the number of cases reported during the last decade. This, however, is believed to reflect improved surveillance and case-finding methods rather than increased incidence. During the same period the fatality rates for plumbism decreased sharply. Encephalopathies and mental disturbances were reported as sequelae in about 25 per cent of cases (Jacobziner, 1959).

Various studies on the epidemiology of lead poisoning have indicated that children one to five years of age are the chief victims, and the existence of pica has been indicated in from 40 to 90 per cent of the poisoned children in different studies (Jacobziner, 1966; Moncrieff et al., 1964; Griggs et al., 1964).

Lead poisonings are considerably more frequent in the summer months than in the winter months. The reason for this is unclear. Two hypotheses suggested are increased absorption resulting from metabolic changes induced by the actinic rays of the summer sun, and greater opportunity during summer months for children to ingest exterior surface paints.

While some cases of lead poisoning may result from ingestions of water or food, inhalation of lead in air or absorption through the skin, almost all cases in children have been traced to the ingestion of lead-bearing paint. Old housing in dilapidated condition, usually in run-down, urban slum areas, is primarily implicated. This consistency has led public health workers to designate the specific housing areas in which the vast majority of such poisoning incidents occur as "lead belts."

Social and economic variables are also associated with lead poisoning. Poverty, crowded living, disruption of families, racial differences and inadequate child supervision have been implicated. With the possible exception of inadequate child supervision, these obviously interrelated factors seem to influence lead poisoning primarily as determinants of the quality of the neighborhood and the housing.

Technical developments in recent years have made possible the evaluation of the incidence of plumbism by mass screening programs for the level of lead in the blood. For example, using techniques of atomic absorption spectroscopy, a survey was carried out in Chicago on nearly 70,000 slum area children aged one to six. Some 5.7 per cent of the children showed elevated lead levels. The purposes of this survey were (1) to detect children with incipient intoxication for treatment prior to the development of encephalopathy, (2) to identify children who were mild or temporary ingesters and (3) to reduce the incidence of lead poisoning through educational aspects of participation in mass screening procedures (Blanksma et al., 1969).

While urban redevelopment and current mass housing programs may reduce exposure to the risk of lead poisoning, large segments of our urban populations still reside under circumstances of great exposure to lead-bearing paints that have been accumulated layer over layer through the years. An example of ameliorative steps taken in this area is the program in New York City, where inspectors take samples of paint and plaster for analysis of lead content, and landlords or owners of housing can be required to remove paints found toxic (Jacobziner, 1966). It has recently been reported in the press that the task of locating and evaluating dwellings for lead exposures in the New York program is now being facilitated by the development of a sophisticated portable analyzer for rapid on-the-spot detection and measurement of lead.

Implications of Recent Studies on Child Poisoning

While no one can deny the accessibility of hazardous substances as a necessary condition for childhood poisonings, some recent studies have suggested that the hand-to-mouth-availability formula may be an oversimplification of the problem of child poisonings. The traditional concepts of prevention assume that children are not at all selective about what they put into their mouths. There is some experimental evidence to suggest that this may not be entirely true. For example, in one experiment some 600 children between the ages of one and eight were offered free access to a collection of 10 colored tablets. The children tended to take those which were brightly colored and to reject those of dark color (with the exception of brown, possibly on the basis of resemblance to chocolate). The age of the child did not affect this order of preference (Jolly and Forrest, 1958). White ranked among those colors of tablets less frequently taken. This might appear paradoxical in view of the prevalence of aspirin poisonings. However, the relative universality of the availability of white aspirin compared to tablets of other colors is probably an important factor.

Two recent studies also have raised the question of whether the degree of availability of noxious substances in the toddler's environment is as important a predisposing factor as is generally believed. In these, the availability, toxicity and storage of medicines and household preparations, and the mothers' awareness of the potential hazards were studied in families in which children aged 2 to 3 had ingested such materials, and in families having children of comparable age but who were free from poisoning incidents. The "poisoning" and "nonpoisoning" families did not differ in regard to the above factors. In view of this, and on the basis of investigations concerning the circumstances of poisoning incidents, it has been suggested that children of this age may often be neither innocent nor ignorant when they consume a bottle of aspirin or drink kerosene. While they do not know the unhealthy consequences of their actions, they may often be well aware that they are doing something wrong or forbidden. Cited as supporting this view are the typically stealthy manner in which the child acquires the substances and the ingenuity and tenacity of his methods to achieve access to materials barred to him. Thus, at this age, factors of self-control in the face of negativistic impulses, and the interpersonal relationships within the psychological climate of the family may be important (Baltimore and Meyer, 1969; Sobel, 1969).

BURNS AND OTHER THERMAL INJURIES

In the age group under 5 years, death rates involving fires, conflagrations and explosions are second only to those involving motor vehicles. They decrease sharply between ages 5 and 14 to about half that at the younger period. The rates for males and females are approximately equal until about age 14, after which males are more frequently involved. Rates are consistently higher among nonwhites than whites. By far, most of these incidents occur in dwellings and frequently involve entrapment (Iskrant and Joliet, 1968). The National Safety Council estimates that in 1967 there were 530,500 fires in one- and two-family dwellings, and 87,900 in apartment buildings. From a medical standpoint, many of these deaths result from asphyxia as well as from thermal effects.

House fires usually result from (1) cooking and heating sources, (2) smoking and the misuse of matches, (3) defective or misused electrical sources, (4) fires in rubbish or trash or (5) flammable liquids or gases. The death rates are highest in the East South Central, West South Central, and South Atlantic areas of the country. The variation probably is related to social and economic conditions. For example, the use of petroleum products and flammable liquids in stoves and heating devices is more common in the southern states, and central heating is less usual. In nonmetropolitan areas, fire protection services may often be less adequate and emergency medical services less available. Prevention of these deaths is obviously complex, involving as it does such factors as housing construction, equipment for cooking and heating and poor safety habits in the use of electrical equipment, wiring systems and flammable liquids. The problems of cause and control of these and some other types of burn injuries cannot be separated from the social and economic problems of the family and therefore require consideration of factors of a broad social nature beyond the traditional scope of medical control (Smith, 1969).

Thermal injuries, apart from those associated with fires and explosions of combustible materials, may also be acquired through contact of a part of the body with a hot object or liquid, an electrical source or flames. Injuries of these kinds are less often fatal but are far more numerous than the nonfatal injuries resulting from conflagration or explosions. For example, of 548 burn admissions in one year to one large hospital for children, only 12 received their injuries from housefires, and 11 from explosions (Munro et al., 1967). Thermal injuries, however, can be permanently disfiguring and often require prolonged hospitalization and specialized treatment, particularly if infection sets in or if skin grafts are necessary. A high frequency of psychological disturbances has been noted in children undergoing extensive treatment for burns, and no one can doubt the emotional complications of residual deformities and permanent cosmetic sequelae (Long and Cope, 1961; Woodward and Jackson, 1961).

Epidemiological surveys and reports from various specialized burn treatment centers established in recent years have indicated the variety of sources giving rise to burn injuries and the various associated circumstances. An early study in Britain called attention to the disproportionately high involvement of young children, and especially of instances where nightgowns and girls' dresses were ignited by flame from an open grate or from contact with the element of unguarded electric heaters (Colebrook and Colebrook, 1949). This resulted in requirements for providing guards on heaters and initiated activity toward standards for nonflammable children's clothing.

Subsequent studies have confirmed the concentration of burns in young children. Highest incidence appears to be in the range from 12 to 17 months, an age when a child is "unsteady on his feet, inquisitive, and irresponsible" (Munro, et al., 1967). Scalds from hot liquids are the most frequent type of injury, usually accounting for somewhat over half in the various reports. Most of these involve hot water spilled when containers are pulled or knocked over. Hot fat or grease, hot soup and the steam and water from vaporizers are less frequent causes. A common pattern is for a child to pull a vessel off the stove or a table. Coffee and tea also account for a large number of scalds; a pot is tipped over or cups are pulled off table edges when an adult's attention is diverted. Some scaldings involve immersion in the bath when water is too hot or are caused by a hot water tap that has been left running (Williams et al., 1958; Smith, 1969).

Contact with hot metal objects is another major source of burns, as when children touch or fall against hot stoves or open oven doors, or crawl onto a hot floor register. While this type of accident may not result in burns as extensive in terms of body surface as those from scalds and flame, many are quite serious and leave permanent scars.

In areas of the United States where winters are less rigorous, there has been wide adoption of the gas-fired floor furnace to provide heat when needed. The metal registers of these cause a typical burn in infants and young children of crawling and toddling age. Because of the characteristic grid pattern in the resulting burns, these have been termed "tic-tac-toe" burns (Waller, 1961; Waller and Mannheimer, 1964). As noted elsewhere, this type of heating device has come under consideration by the National Commission of Product Safety. One city (Denver) has outlawed the installation of floor furnaces; also being explored are methods to protect against burns from the exposed floor grills without impairing the usefulness of the furnaces for heating purposes (National Commission of Product Safety, 1970).

Burns from contact with flame form another major category. These frequently also involve clothing set afire from the original source of flame. Fireplaces, open gas heaters and back-flash from petroleum products used as fire starters, both indoors and out, are prominent sources of the flames. Playing with matches is a not infrequent cause. Bonfires and burning rubbish are also a source of burns acquired outside the home, more frequently among older than younger children.

In recent years there has been a great deal of activity by committees of the American Academy of Pediatrics concerning the flammability of children's clothing, resulting in legislation at the federal level. These have great promise for reducing the frequency and severity of burns by offering protection to extensive areas of the body surface when contact is made with flame or another source capable of igniting clothing. Until national standards are uniformly developed and enforced, until further progress is made in the permanent flame-proofing of fabrics, and until the backlog of outgrown but not outworn hand-me-down clothing is exhausted, parents must consider differences in the ease with which different fabrics may ignite and in the speed of the spread of flame. Wool, for example, is quite safe, while untreated cotton has high flammability. Certain synthetics will not catch fire but instead melt to deposit a hot residue that burns the flesh beneath. Pajamas are very much to be preferred to nightgowns and dressing robes. Little girls' dresses have been a particular hazard as are, among older children, tight-fitting cotton jeans (Oglesbay, 1969; National Commission of Product Safety, 1970).

Statistics from burn treatment centers show a very low frequency of electrical burns in small children. This is surprising in view of the emphasis in safety literature on the dangers electric cords and outlets pose for children. Whether this low frequency indicates a public that is well educated in the problem, successful elimination of hazards by equipment manufacturers or less frequent involvement of children in such incidents than has been supposed is not known (Williams et al., 1958; Blocker et al., 1961; Munro et al., 1967; Smith, 1969).

In children under 5, almost all burn injuries occur within the home and predominantly in the kitchen. Both burns and scalds decrease through ages 5 to 9 and 10 to 14 but increase in proportion to the presence of garages, sheds, yards and other outside areas.

As noted before, death rates from household fires and explosions show variations between geographical areas and socioeconomic levels. These variations are far less apparent in the distribution of burn injuries from other sources (Williams et al., 1958). One study has indicated an excess of such deaths in the families of laborers, as compared to those of skilled workers (Jensen, 1959). Also, one writer has concluded that disease problems of the child, chronic and acute family stresses and accident repeatedness among family members appear to be independent variables associated with thermal injuries (Borland, 1966). Pre-existing disease or emotional problems have also been mentioned as factors contributing to thermal injuries (Williams et al., 1958; Monro et al., 1967; Smith, 1969). An interesting finding in this connection is from a British survey, which reported that epileptic children less frequently are burned from falls against hot objects or into flames than are adult epileptics. This suggests greater protection on the part of those responsible for the children (Bull et al., 1964).

For those interested in the general problem of burn injuries, Strause and Westaby (1968) provide an extensive annotated bibliography that contains more than 800 references relating to the epidemiology, mortality, specific causes, treatment and prevention of burn injuries; studies on flammability of materials; and research on fire and other thermal phenomena.

INJURIES INCURRED DURING RECREATIONAL ACTIVITIES

Activities described as play or recreation occupy a large proportion of children's waking hours. Hence, a consideration of safety in play has great importance. The nature of play and recreational activities varies, of course, with age and sex, with physical, mental and social development and with the environmental resources. So also do the hazards and nature of injury. Studies on accidents in children frequently cite "playing with," "playing near," "playing on," "playing (particular games)," as activities associated with injury, but definitive knowledge in the field of playtime safety is quite fragmentary and incomplete. Attention will be given here to areas in which at least some information has been developed. These include safety in the use of bicycles, in general play and playground activities (the use of toys and other play equipment) and in relation to home swimming and wading pools.

The Problem of Bicycle Safety Among Children

Industry sales figures indicate that some 50 million bicycles are currently in use in the United States, and projections suggest a one-third increase between 1967 and 1980. It has been estimated that some 125,000 to 150,000 persons are injured each year in various kinds of bicycle mishaps, and the largest proportion of these involve child riders.

Collisions Between Motor Vehicles and Bicycles. In addition to pedestrian accidents, another type of accident in which children are overrepresented in comparison with other age groups is the collision between a motor vehicle and a bicycle. The number of bicyclists killed in these accidents has been rising slightly each year, and the National Safety Council states that there were 800 such fatalities in the United States in 1968. These occurred predominantly in the 5 to 10 year age range. Persons receiving nonfatal injuries also were most often in this age group, with 28,800 children between 5 and 14 years injured, in a total of 38,000 children of all ages who were disabled for a day or more after the day of the accident (National Safety Council, 1969a). The above data, while giving an indication of the extent of this problem, also illustrate the limited amount and kinds of information previously available in this area.

An analysis has recently been made of the 2455 motor vehicle–bicycle collisions in the motor vehicle department records in North Carolina for a three-year period through June of 1968 (Waller and Reinfurt, 1969). Four per cent of the bicycle riders in this series were fatalities, and Class A and B injuries were reported for 84 per cent.[4] Class C injuries were reported for 11.5 per cent. The small remainder of instances (probably under-reported) were "property damage only" accidents.

Approximately half of both the fatal and nonfatal accidents involved bicyclists between 10 and 14 years of age. Those aged 5 to 9 were next in order of frequency, and older children 15 to 19 years of age formed the third greatest portion. Exposure factors undoubtedly are reflected in this distribution. Statistical analysis of the data in the series suggested that nonfatal accidents are more likely to involve the younger riders and occur in residential areas. It seems likely that younger bicyclists tend to ride nearer home, and motor vehicle speeds tend to be lower in residential areas than on other streets and highways. The younger riders may also be riding during daylight hours, when accidents, though more frequent, are proportionately less often fatal. The typical daytime, residential area occurrence of bicycle accidents is probably also related to the fact that while more car drivers in accidents are males, female drivers are proportionately more frequently involved in collisions with bicycles than they are in all other accidents. The higher fatality rates for bicycle riders during periods of darkness underscore the importance of having adequate reflectors and lights on bicycles, and wearing high-visibility clothing.

In both fatal and nonfatal accidents, boy cyclists outnumbered girls by about nine to one. Possibly boy cyclists tend to ride more adventurously, or to ride bicycles more than girls. This ratio is close to that reported in an earlier study of bicycle fatalities described below.

In relation to the circumstances of motor vehicle–bicycle accidents, the National Safety Council conducted a nationwide survey in 1957. In addition to the concentration of accidents among males and those under 16 years of age, it was noted that (1) riding on the left of the road carried more risk than riding on the right, (2) about three-fourths of the accidents occurred in the five-month period of April to September, (3) accidents were most frequent on Saturdays and least frequent on Sundays, (4) 70 per cent occurred during daylight, but 80 per cent occurred in the P.M., (5) in about one-third of the cases the bicycle struck the motor vehicle and (6) the bicycle rider was violating a traffic rule in about 80 per cent of the accidents—rules such as right of way, improper turning, disregard of signal or riding against traffic. These data have formed the basis for most of the programs of bicycle safety carried out by a variety of organizations.

---

[4]Under a current system, injuries are reported by police as Class A (visible injury such as bleeding wound, distorted member, or had to be carried from scene), Class B (visible injury such as bruises, abrasions, swellings, limping) or Class C (no visible injury but complains of pain or momentary unconsciousness).

More recent analyses of the circumstances of collisions between motor vehicle and bicycles have revealed that most involve a bicyclist turning across the path of a car proceeding straight ahead, or riding into a car's path or side when emerging from a driveway, alley or intersection of some sort. Those in which the bicycle strikes the side or rear of the car are less likely to be fatal. Also, it has been observed that the distribution of injuries sustained by bicycle riders in collision with motor vehicles tends to be similar to that of pedestrians in terms of severity and parts of the body affected (Ryan, 1969; Waller and Reinfurt, 1969).

Bicycle Injuries in Nonmotor-Vehicle Accidents. The epidemiology of child bicyclist injuries incurred other than in collisions with motor vehicles has received little study.[5] Many organizations have been involved in bicycle safety activities, but the emphasis seems to have been directed mainly to the problem of bicycles in traffic. Information on the prevalence, severity and circumstances of injuries in spills from bicycles or collisions between bicycles and various environmental objects has been scanty.

Consideration of the relative magnitude of the forces involved in motor vehicle and nonmotor-vehicle accidents might suggest that many of the injuries from the latter type of accident would be of a minor nature. Some indirect evidence of the prevalence of the more incapacitating injuries comes from data on 85,000 school jurisdiction accidents reported to the National Safety Council for the 1965–1966 school year (1967a). These are given in terms of the number of accidents per 100,000 student days, an accident being defined as one requiring a doctor's attention or causing absence of a half day or more from school. The rates for such accidents among boys and girls while traveling to or from school on bicycles are shown in Table 8–7, in contrast to the rates for the accidents which involve collision with motor vehicles.

It may be noted in Table 8–7 that for both boys and girls, the frequency rates for injuries in bicycle accidents which do *not* involve motor vehicles are in general considerably higher than those which do, although the average time lost from school (i.e., severity of injury) is greater in the case of the motor vehicle–bicycle collisions. Also to be noted is the considerably elevated rate for boys in grades 4 through 9, corresponding roughly to the age range 10 to 15. The data in the table cannot reliably be

[5]One such study has been carried out under the direction of Dr. Julian Waller at the University of Vermont Medical School (1971).

*Table 8–7 Rate of Accidents per 100,000 School Days Among Children While Riding Bicycles To or From School**

Pupils Injured	Type of Accident	All Grades	Kindergarten	Grades 1 to 3	Grades 4 to 6	Grades 7 to 9	Grades 10 to 12	Average Number of Days Lost per Injury
Boys	Nonmotor-Vehicle	0.06	0.02	0.04	0.11	0.11	0.02	1.59
	Motor Vehicle	0.03	0.00	0.01	0.04	0.05	0.03	2.95
Girls	Nonmotor-Vehicle	0.02	0.01	0.02	0.05	0.01	0.00	1.10
	Motor Vehicle	0.01	0.01	**	0.01	**	0.01	2.25

*Based on data from National Safety Council: *Accident Facts, 1967*, Chicago, 1967a.
**Less than 0.005.

reduced to absolute numbers of accidents. In general, however, in extrapolation to the national scene, a rate of 0.1 in the "All Grades" column would correspond to about 4000 accidents.

Additional data, though not directly comparable to that in Table 8–7, have also been reported concerning children's bicycle injuries causing lost time from school which occur at times other than traveling to or from school. While forming only a small part of the total injuries from all kinds of accidents, the proportion of injuries among boys in all grades from *non*motor-vehicle–bicycle accidents was three times that from motor vehicle–bicycle collisions, and the ratio was more than four to one in grades 4 to 6. A similar pattern was found for girls. For girls as well as boys the injuries in nonmotor-vehicle accidents, though more frequent, were less severe, as shown by average time lost from school (National Safety Council, 1967a).

Unfortunately the foregoing relates only to the school year. It is known that fatalities and injuries in motor vehicle–bicycle collisions are more frequent during the summer period, when there is an increase both in vehicular traffic and in bicycle riding (Waller and Reinfurt, 1969). There is some evidence that other types of bicycle accidents also increase in the period between May and September (Vilardo and Anderson, 1969).

The nature of injuries received in bicycle mishaps has received only limited attention in the medical literature. In one series of 42 boys and 19 girls who were hospitalized because of head injuries, 20 of the boys and 2 of the girls had been injured in falls from bicycles (Burkinshaw, 1960). Falls from bicycles have also been noted as causing injuries involving the teeth and jaws in young children (MacLennan, 1957). One particular type of injury which occurs is the "bicycle spoke" injury, so called because it results from the foot being caught between the spokes of the wheel and the fork or fender braces. The full severity of this injury may not be appreciated on initial inspection, since damage to underlying structures is not readily apparent. These injuries almost always involve a passenger being carried on the handlebars or riding on the crossbar, where there is no support for the feet (Strauch, 1966; Izant, et al., 1969).

An approximate distribution of injuries received by children in bicycle accidents can be drawn from a recent analysis of bicycle accidents among school-age children carried out by the National Safety Council (Vilardo and Anderson, 1969). This was based on questionnaires completed by the parents of children in grades 2 to 8 in various parts of the country. Injury data were reported for more than 4000 children in various types of bicycle accidents. The types of accident are shown in Table 8–8.

The injury data relating to the accidents listed in the table unfortunately do not distinguish between the motor vehicle and nonmotor-vehicle incidents. However, those involving motor vehicles comprised less than 12 per cent of the total, and the series involved only two fatalities. Also, the data are not completely representative because of limitations inherent

Table 8–8 Distribution of Types of Bicycle Accidents Among School-Age Children*

Type of Accident	Per Cent of Total Accidents (N=4151)
Bicycle hit car	7.08
Car hit bicycle	4.83
Bicycle hit bicycle	15.81
Bicycle hit fixed object	13.04
Spills and falls	45.44
Other, and not stated	12.60

*Adapted from Vilardo, F., and Anderson, J.: *Bicycle Accidents to School Age Children.* Report No. 169. Research Department, National Safety Council, Chicago, September, 1969, p. 18.

in the questionnaire approach, and in the nature of the information requested. The data are, however, the most extensive known to the present authors and are at least indicative of the wide variety of injuries. The percentage distribution of the major categories of injuries, as reported in lay terms by the parents, are shown in Table 8–9, arranged in decreasing order of frequency.

Other injuries reported, each accounting for less than 1 per cent of the total, included fractured facial bones, fractured collarbones, fractured ribs, sprained wrists or ankles and "black eyes."

The Background of Children's Bicycle Injuries. As noted before, bicycle safety programs have been based to a great extent on the traffic violations of bicycle riders in collisions with motor vehicles. The development of more effective and more comprehensive preventive measures, however, requires additional information on the population "at risk"—and on their exposure. One needs to know which children ride bicycles and what kinds of bicycles, and how, when, where, why and how much the children use them. Only recently has there been an attempt to develop this kind of information on a systematic basis and to relate it to accidents.

*Table 8–9 Distribution of Injuries Among School-Age Children in Bicycle Accidents**

Body Part and Type of Injury	Per Cent of Total Injuries
Skinned knee	27.03
Abrasion, head or face	14.21
Abrasion, leg	9.76
Abrasion, arm/hand	9.57
Skinned elbow	7.94
Abrasion, body	4.21
Teeth, lost or chipped	3.73
Hand, broken and other	3.11
Cut foot, ankle	2.82
Fractured skull or concussion	1.70
Fractured arm or elbow	1.63
Nose injury	1.46
Fractured leg or ankle	1.44

*Adapted from Vilardo, F., and Anderson, J.: *Bicycle Accidents to School-Age Children.* Report No. 169. Research Department, National Safety Council, Chicago, September, 1969, p. 44.

A preliminary survey during 1968 on bicycle usage by school-age children was carried out through questionnaires administered to 4321 school pupils in four communities: Nassau County, New York; Atlanta, Georgia; Arlington Heights, Illinois; and Sacramento, California (Vilardo et al., 1968). This was followed by a second survey, which yielded some 27,000 questionnaires on usage completed by pupils in grades 2 through 8 in schools from five different geographic areas of the country, including schools in urban, suburban and rural settings. Information was also collected to relate usage to accident frequencies and type (Vilardo and Anderson, 1969). While there were certain limitations to the accident data, some suggestive trends emerged.

According to these surveys, about 93 per cent of pupils in grades 2 through 8 ride bicycles; there are about as many girl as boy bicyclists. With some geographic and seasonal variations, it appears that less than 10 per cent usually ride to and from school by bicycle. More riding is done on Saturdays, at least during the school year, than on any other day of the week, with Sundays second. During the daytime the bicycles are used most frequently for going to see friends and for playing games. At night "just riding around," going to see friends and running "errands" are the largest categories. About twice as many boys as girls ride after dark (22 per cent *versus* 10 per cent), and while about 75 per cent had either a reflector or a taillight on their bicycles, whether the bicycle was so equipped did not seem to affect the practice of riding after dark. The boys rode the newer "high-rise" type of bicycle (with smaller front wheel and higher **V** handlebars) about twice as often as the conventional "middleweight" type, and about 5 times as often as the "lightweight" type. "Middleweights" comprised the bicycles ridden by girls about two-and-one-half times as frequently as the "high-rise," and about eight times as frequently as the "lightweights."

One of the most interesting features of the data on bicycle usage suggests that a child considers his bicycle as a plaything as well as a means of transportation. This is revealed by the high frequency of their use in games, and in the variety of games played. In all, some 93 different titles of bicycle games were listed by the pupils in these surveys, with a high consistency in both the types of games and the order of their frequency across the different geographic areas. Some of the major classes into which these games fall, and examples of names, are shown in Table 8–10.

In general, "Racing" games are the type most often played, with "Pretend" and "Tag" types next. Overall, about 10 per cent of the children mentioned participation in the games classed "Violent," and about 7 per cent in "Daredevil" games. Each class of games listed in Table 8–10 was indicated by some boys and some girls, at each age from 7 to 14 years. There were some variations, however, in terms of the proportions at each age, and by sex. In general, game participation tended to drop off in the older children aged 13 to 14. Among 7-year-olds, game participation tended to be relatively low except for "Pretend," "Wheelies," "Tag" and "General" games. "Pretend" games were also more characteristically played by girls, and by the younger boys. Boys participated more frequently than girls in "Violent" and "Sports" games, and to an older age.

Bicycle Usage in Relation to Accidents. Some of the findings from the National Safety Council study which relate the ways children use bicycles and children's accidents are briefly summarized in the following paragraphs.

Younger children, those under 10, have significantly more falls and fewer accidents involving motor vehicles than is to be expected by chance. This tendency reverses between ages 10 and 12. One suggested

*Table 8–10 Bicycle Games Played by Children**

Class of Game	Number of Game Titles in Class	Examples of Games
Violent	14	Chicken, Murderbike, Wipeout, Terror, Kill, Demolition
Pretend	23	Cops and Robbers, Police, Cars and Traffic, Batman, Rat Patrol
Daredevil	8	Tailgating, Over Ramps, No Hands, Swerve in Traffic
Racing	8	Drag Racing, Beat the Car, Speed around Corners, Time Races
Chasing	5	Chase, Catch, Wolf and Fox
Wheelies	3	Wheelies, Stand on Back Wheels, Drag Wheelies
Sports	8	Frisbee, Hockey, Basketball, Soccer, Kick the Can
Skill	5	Circle, Figure 8's, Slalom, Obstacle Course
General and miscellaneous	19	Tag, Hide and Seek, Hiking, Skid and Spin, Squirt Gun Fight

*Adapted from Vilardo, F., and Anderson, J.: *Bicycle Accidents to School-Age Children.* Report No. 169. Research Department, National Safety Council, Chicago, September, 1969.

explanation is that children under 10 report more riding on the sidewalk only, and less riding in the street. Lack of experience and skill also seems to be a factor in the higher rate of falls and other nonmotor-vehicle accidents in younger children.

While boys are clearly over-represented in various studies of accidents involving motor vehicles, no such differences were found in regard to involvement in other bicycle accidents, which are proportionate to exposure, except that girls more frequently are injured in accidents involving falls.

A frequent question is whether it is safer to ride a bicycle facing oncoming traffic, on the left side of the road—as recommended for pedestrians—or on the right, with traffic. Present evidence seems to indicate no clear safety advantage for either method, though there may be situations involving the relative maneuvers of the bicycle and motor vehicle (i.e., left turns), where the side of the street may be an important factor.

Collisions with motor vehicles occur more frequently when the bicycles are being used for transportation than when being used in play, falls being significantly more frequent in the latter case. However, direct data are lacking on whether injuries are incurred more frequently in some types of games than in others.

As new bicycle styles have been introduced, questions have been raised about their accident potentials. The National Safety Council, for example, called attention to the additional demands on skill and experience required in the safe operation of "lightweight" bicycles (Licht, 1965). More recently there has been controversy over the relative safety of the new style "high-rise" bicycle. A chief consideration relates to the acrobatics possible when the rider shifts his weight to the rear on the long narrow seat and rides with the front wheel off the ground, making steering entirely dependent on balance (National Safety Council, 1967b). Present evidence does not clearly indicate whether there is a difference in accident potential among bicycle styles. One study suggests that accidents to users of "high-rise," "lightweight" and "middleweight" cycles, in both girls' and boys' models, are distributed in close correspondence to the percentages in use (Vilardo and Anderson, 1969). One physician, however, reports an increased incidence of maxillofacial and nasal injuries in accidents involving the newer styles. These are sustained when forward rotation of the small front wheel is suddenly stopped by a curb or rough terrain and the child is catapulted forward through the open handlebars.

The size of the bicycle relative to the size of the child does seem to be a factor in the frequency of accidents and injuries. Smaller children riding bicycles too large for them are involved in more accidents than would be statistically expected. This holds true when pedals are augmented by blocks. Also, there are significant differences in the injuries sustained by small children riding larger bikes and those of taller children on the same-sized vehicle; the smaller children experience more facial injuries and fewer injuries to arms and hands as compared to the taller children in the same type of accident (Howell, 1968).

Safety of the Child at Play

Some tentative estimates have been offered by the U.S. Public Health Service of the numbers of injuries involving various environmental factors or agencies. One of the categories relates to injuries sustained in recreational activities, or in the use of recreational equipment. Unfortunately, no breakdown by age is included. In some instances, however, the category titles suggest an exposure in which juveniles predominate. The most obvious ones are shown in Table 8–11. (Injuries included are those resulting in a day of restricted activity or those requiring medical attention, or both.)

Toys and Playthings. An attempt to measure the frequency of injuries involving toys and playthings was made some years ago in a survey in Florida. Details were reported by pediatricians, general practitioners and hospital emergency wards across the state on 748 accidents to children under 15 years of age which involved "any object which child was using for recreation, play, or amusement purposes," during three separate months in 1960 and 1961 (Dykstra, 1962). Though extrapolation of the data to other states would not be justified because of climatic and perhaps other characteristics of the Florida locale, the findings are nevertheless of interest.

In agreement with most studies of various types of accidents in children, boys' injuries were found to outnumber girls' injuries by about two to one. The differences were slight at the younger ages but showed increasing divergence in the older children.

Small commercial toys were involved in only 7 per cent of the cases, and about three-fourths of these accidents occurred to children under 6 years. They were most frequent among 3-year-olds. Misuse of the toys was more often implicated than defective toys. Bicycles and tricycles were the most frequently involved specific types of plaything, bicycles particularly at ages 5 to 8. Playground equipment accounted for most of the injuries to the 2 to 7 year group. An unexpected finding was the high incidence of injuries associated with play with items which are not usually considered toys or playthings by adults—broken glass, rusty cans, lawn mowers, household tools and a wide variety of other objects. More than 25 per cent of all the injuries involved this type of play.

Falls were the mechanism of injury in nearly half the cases. About one-quarter of the children were injured when hit by playthings thrown, swung or ridden by others. Heads and faces were injured in about a third of the cases, with the other accidents mostly involving the extremities. About twice as many of the accidents occurred in the yard as in the house; 17 per cent were sustained while playing in school yards or in public parks and playgrounds. Lacerations were the most frequent type

Table 8–11 Injuries in Recreational Activities Presumed to Involve Chiefly Children*

Recreational Activity or Equipment	Estimate of Numbers Injured Annually	
Playing, general (e.g., tag)	*2,000,000*	
Playing on stationary equipment	*1,000,000*	
Swings	500,000	
Slides	200,000	
Seesaws	50,000	
Other	250,000	
Playing on mobile equipment	*1,300,000*	
Bicycles	1,000,000	(including 120,000 fractures and 60,000 concussions)
Tricycles	100,000	
Other	200,000	
Playing with toys	700,000	

*Based on data from Public Health Service: *Estimates of Injuries Involving Various Environmental Factors,* 1970.

of injury, followed, respectively, by fractures, abrasions, contusions and punctures as the chief classes. These medically attended injuries were severe enough to require hospitalization in only 5 per cent of the cases; this included two cases that resulted in death. One fatality involved a bicycle-automobile collision; the other was the strangulation of an infant playing with a "stretch toy" placed across the top of a crib.

Absent or inadequate adult supervision of play activities or play areas was a prominent contributing circumstance, especially in the homes and yards. Lack of instruction of children in the proper use of play equipment was also noted. Although in this series toys of unsafe construction did not play a prominent role, the high number of injuries involving playground equipment among the 2 to 7-year-olds raised the question of the suitability of the existing equipment for this age group and the possible need for improved and safer designs as well as improved supervision.

Pediatricians, through the Committee on Accident Prevention of the American Academy of Pediatrics, have long been active in bringing attention to unsafe features of children's toys and playthings. This has resulted in improved designs on the part of toy manufacturers in certain instances, but much remains to be done in the further identification and elimination of specific hazards. Increased attention to this area of safety has also been noted among the general public and at governmental levels in connection with product liability and the use of hazardous substances and products.

It is often difficult for parents contemplating purchase of play equipment to evaluate the item for possible unsafe features of construction or design, or for features conducive to misuse. Price has not always been an effective gauge of quality. To obtain information which might provide some guidelines, a feature column writer in a national woman's magazine requested letters from parents telling of incidents in which children received injuries while playing on backyard gym sets (Montgomery, 1967). Replies were received concerning 174 accidents from 37 of the 50 states. The information was tabulated by the National Safety Council but was inadequate for valid epidemiological analysis. Some items that parents specifically related to these kinds of injuries were the following: protruding bolts and screws, some which loosened or broke; uncapped ends of pipes and tubes; chain links and "S" hooks; the hinge on sky gliders; "pinch points" in the mechanism of lawn gliders; and edges and ladders of slides. There were also several instances reported of sets toppling over and falling on children when clothing caught on the handrail of a slide or a protruding bolt.

In the work of the National Commission on Product Safety, some 350 categories of consumer products have been listed for eventual consideration, and a surveillance system of injuries associated with the use of consumer products has been developed. Thus far, this has included data developed by the Public Health Service, a touch-tone telephone reporting system from emergency rooms of selected hospitals, reports solicited from physicians and surveys of product liability litigation. Also, in hearings before the Commission, testimony has been presented on injuries attributed to unsafe features of numerous specific products. So far, only a limited number of product categories have been explored by the Commission. The age distribution obtained indicates a high proportional involvement of children under 15 in several of these – i.e., architectural glass (50 per cent of 501 cases reported were under age 15), floor furnaces (31 per cent under 5), glass bottles and containers (36 per cent under 15), household cleaning agents and compounds (54 per cent under 5), bleaches and dyes (70 per cent under 5), wringer-washers (57 per cent under 15) and infant furniture (84 per cent under 5). In the context of children's play equipment were toys (75 per cent of cases were under age 15), bicycles (75 per cent under 15) and fireworks (age not specifically stated).

To some extent, the preceding age-injury data reflect essentially the age composition of the populations chiefly exposed to the product categories (e.g., infant furniture). The identification of "unreasonable hazards" involves specific features of categories and of individual makes and models where items are not manufactured according to a uniform standard.

No voluntary industry-wide safety standards exist concerning children's recreational products such as swings, slides, seesaws, tricycles and sports and hobby equipment. In regard to toys, the only voluntary safety standard has been that of the Underwriter Laboratory approval for protection against electric shock in electric toys. Some standards exist for the manufacture of bicycles, but these are not directed at primary injury hazards.

A few examples of unsafe, injury-producing features in toys identified by the Commission are as follows: One electric toy oven for young girls produced temperatures of about 300 degrees Fahrenhe t on the outer surface and about 600 degrees inside.[6] A metal-casting set produced temperatures of 800 degrees on the cooking surface and 600 degrees on the sides, and was packaged without a warning label. A design-sketching set was made with frangible glass panels, and injuries from the broken glass have resulted in at least 22 suits against the manufacturer. The noisemaker of one infant's rattle consisted of sharp spike points under a thin cardboard and plastic cover. Predictable misuse was also involved in some cases. For example, children put the wrong end of a blow gun for darts in their mouths and were injured from inhaling the small darts into their lungs.[7]

As a result of such findings, the Child Protection and Toy Safety Act of 1969 was passed by Congress. This amended the earlier Hazardous Safety Act to cover electrical, mechanical and thermal hazards from toys or other articles intended for children.

Playground Safety. The need to provide public places for children to play in urban and populous communities is generally recognized. Whether existing facilities have been usually located with safety (other than segregation from motor vehicle traffic) in mind or adequately designed, equipped, maintained and supervised to keep injuries to a minimum may be open to question. For example, in a study on pedestrian accidents among city children, it was observed that if a playground was more than about five blocks distant from their homes, they tended not to use it (Read, 1969). Recognition of the frequency of injuries from falls from swings and other equipment has prompted the provision of a soft landing surface, such as sand, underneath such equipment in many playgrounds, but this practice is by no means universal.

Only scant information on the prevalence of injuries to children on playgrounds is available, illustrated by the findings of the limited study in

[6]In reference to burns from floor furnace gratings, it was noted in the Commission hearings that a one-second contact between skin and surface of 155°F. will produce second degree burns; surfaces of 300 to 350° will produce instantaneous burns, often permanently disfiguring.

[7]Subsequently, some corrective action was taken in regard to all of these specific items. These included redesign by the manufacturers to eliminate hazards, cessation of manufacture, inclusion of instructions and warnings against misuse and cessation of sales by retailers.

Florida already mentioned. The Public Health Service estimate of 1 million play equipment injuries includes both playground and home installations, and provides no information on age and sex. There are a few additional data from the National Safety Council based on reports from school jurisdictions. These, however, refer only to the school year. The report for the school year 1965–66 indicates that frequency rates for injuries among children in grades 1 to 6 were higher in unorganized activities on school grounds and outdoor play areas than in regard to any other part of the school plant. Accidents involving playground equipment were more frequent among the younger pupils, decreasing through succeeding grade levels. Injuries while playing ball games and in activities involving running increased in frequency with grade level, peaking at grades 4 to 6. Less extensive data are available on injuries causing loss of school time from accidents occurring away from school. Those injuries due to sports activities formed a rising proportion of the totals for successive grade levels. Among boys in grades 1 to 3, almost 10 per cent had been hurt in activities such as baseball, football, winter sports, water sports and miscellaneous sports. The proportions were 21 per cent at grades 4 to 6 and 34 per cent in grades 7 to 9. For girls, the corresponding percentages of injuries due to sports were, respectively, 6, 13 and 18 per cent.

Currently there is much activity in the fields of urban renewal, construction of housing projects for low and middle income families, residential development and model town planning. These afford both an opportunity and a challenge to the designers and sponsors. In their planning, consideration should be given not only to safety in the architectural arrangements of the homes and buildings, but also to safety in the recreational and play facilities provided for the children of the families concerned.

Children and Backyard Pools

One feature of modern suburban life which has important implications for child safety is the advent and proliferation of private residential swimming pools. Pools of all types have vastly increased in number during the past 25 years and include those sponsored by communities, institutions and private clubs, and those classified as residential at motels, apartments and private homes. The greatest growth has taken place in the number of home pools. Permanent, in-ground, backyard pools totaled about 2500 in 1946. By 1966 these had increased to more than half a million, and the number has grown by about 50,000 a year. Portable, on-surface swimming pools are believed to number about 4 million at present, and plastic wading pools far outnumber these (Webster, 1967). Thus, a new dimension of growing proportions has been added to the risks of submersion accidents, beyond the traditional dangers associated with open natural bodies of water, thin ice and such artifacts as open wells and cisterns.

A comparison of deaths from accidental drowning among children under 15 years of age for two five-year periods within the growth period of home pools, 1954 to 1958 and 1963 to 1967, indicates that at each age there has been an increase in the number of children drowned (U.S. Vital Statistics). When these are related to population changes in the two periods, it is evident that the death rates from drowning increased appreciably for children under 5, and especially for those aged 3 and younger. They decreased somewhat among those aged 5 to 9 and 10 to 14.

The lack of detailed information on

the places where these drownings occurred prevents an accurate appraisal of the role of the increase in backyard pools. There is some evidence, however, that children of preschool age comprise the group most frequently affected. This comes from a survey carried out on the basis of a nationwide coverage of newspaper reports of drownings in various types of pools during the year 1965 (Webster, 1967).

In all, 484 cases of pool drownings were identified, of which 343 were children under 15 years of age, and 207 were under age 5. Home swimming or wading pools were involved in 54 per cent of the drownings under age 15, and 155 or three-quarters of those cases were under age 5. Of these, children aged 2 were most often involved, followed in frequency by children 1, 3 and 4 years of age. An additional 30 children under age 5 were drowned in other residential pools (i.e., motel and apartment house pools), 10 in decorative or fish pools and 3 in public pools.

Play adjacent to the edges of pools —ball tossing, sailing floating toys, riding tricycles and the gamut of other juvenile recreations—was the chief precursor of the accidents among the younger children. The most frequently found contributing cause at the preschool age was the lack of adequate adult supervision, considered even more important than the lack of swimming ability. A frequent circumstance involved a child left unattended while a parent or other adult went to answer the telephone or was occupied in some other temporary distraction. In numerous cases only children, if anyone at all, were present. Among older children, trespass into the pool area over fences or through unlocked gates, in addition to inability to swim, was a frequent factor. These findings highlight the importance of constant and close supervision when children are in pool areas, and of thorough indoctrination in the safe use of swimming and wading pools for the families possessing them.

Inadequate environmental controls were also prominent among the factors contributing to the home pool accidents, and especially in reference to protection against trespassers. The design and construction of fences, often of inadequate height, frequently provided hand and foot holds and consequent access to the pool for even very small children. Many gates did not have self-locking features. In some cases, where a wall of the house formed a side of the pool area, easy access was provided by sliding doors or windows. A variety of unsafe features relating to pool design and construction were also implicated, including slippery decks around pools, pool bottoms affording abrupt changes in depth and lack of float lines. Some of the fatalities involved head injuries from striking the sides or bottoms of pools while diving or jumping.

In the context of accidents involving persons of adolescent and young adult age, attention has been called to the frequency of upper cervical fractures in diving accidents, resulting in quadriplegia (Guttmann, 1964). It is estimated that diving accidents now cause about 500 cases of quadriplegia annually in the United States, and the question has been raised concerning the prevalence of unrecognized injury of this type in deaths attributed to drowning (Rado, 1964). Adequate protection is needed against diving into empty or shallow pools at night, and adequate depth is required for diving into pools from the newer plastic springboards. Also, many accidents have occurred in seaside swimming areas when a child has dived into water lowered by changes in tide.

The development of local ordinances concerning the design, construction, protection and accessory safety equipment of home pools has varied greatly from area to area. In this connection, guidelines have been offered by the American Public Health Association in a "model" ordinance, and by the National Swimming Pool Institute.

It is evident that increased efforts to indoctrinate the owners and other guardians of home pools in the various aspects of pool safety—including resuscitation—should be made. Health workers and physicians can play an important role in directing community activities in this direction. Also, in reference to water safety both in private pools and at the sites of the drownings of older children, which more frequently involve a wide variety of other types of exposure, encouragement should be given to expand opportunities for instruction in learning to swim and play in water. Programs of the American Red Cross, YMCA and other organizations have demonstrated that children of even preschool age can be taught to float and swim and to master rudimentary procedures of water survival. The view that water safety and swimming instruction should more uniformly form a part of the physical education programs in our public schools deserves consideration. While programs of this kind are available in some systems at the high school level, much could be accomplished at the lower grade levels. It is apparent, however, that among younger children there can be no substitute for supervision of play in or near bodies of water of any type.

THE QUESTION OF EXCESSIVE SUSCEPTIBILITY TO ACCIDENTS

It has been proposed that some children are unusually susceptible to accidents and that accidents may be reduced by identifying and treating such individuals. In general, there are three approaches used to deal with this question: (1) the psychiatric approach, which postulates that accidents may be psychologically motivated, (2) the statistical demonstration of differences in individual liability to accidents and (3) the behavioral theory, involving personality traits and behavior in accident-potential situations. The statistical approach has been confined largely to adult populations, chiefly in industrial settings, and the results have been quite negative. There is no evidence of an appreciable effect on accident frequencies due to a "proneness" factor in the statistical sense (McFarland and Moore, 1961; Suchman, 1961). Only one application of the statistical approach to the distributions of accident frequencies among children has been located. This was interpreted to demonstrate individual differences in accident liability (Mellinger et al., 1965; Manheimer et al., 1966).

The Concept of Psychologically Motivated Accidents

The psychiatric study of injured adults resulted in the concept of the "motivated" accident; i.e., that accidental injuries may resolve emotional tensions, especially those involving unexpressed hostility and guilt (Dunbar, 1943). Some studies of children who have had repeated accidents have been undertaken using this viewpoint. In one, about half of a series of 65 children with head injuries were found to have histories of two or more serious injuries. The investigators concluded that the combination of a sadistic father and a passive, masochistic mother was a significant factor, and the children's accidents represented aggressive reactions to frustration (Fabian and Bender, 1947). Other studies have compared children having a history of accidents or repeated accidents, with children having none. Questions have been raised concerning how prevalent "motivated" accidents may be, and whether conflicts about hostility and authority are as important in predisposing children to accidents as may be the case in adults. For example, in one study of accident-repeater children, only a limited number of the accidents appeared to be satisfying emotional needs, such as resolving tensions or gaining parental attention. More often they seemed associated with such factors as poor control when children extended themselves in competition for status among other children, or in undertaking hazardous activities with which their older companions could cope safely. In general, the accident repeaters were characterized as bolder and more daring (Langford et al., 1953).

Children in nursery school have been observed in play situations in an attempt to relate the frequency and kinds of injuries to their basic patterns of behavior. A common feature in those having had the greatest number of accidents was difficulty in adjusting to the group situation. In general, the accident group was characterized by exceptional physical strength, daredevil attitudes, emotional instability and impulsivity. The highest rate was found among those who were "insistent and obstinate" and "rude" (Fuller, 1948; Fuller and Baune, 1951).

In one study, accident-repeater and accident-free children aged 5 to 8 were compared in their behavior in play with dolls. The repeaters were characterized by more aggressive actions in the doll play (Krall, 1953).

Tests were used in another study comparing accident-repeater and accident-free boys in a junior high school. The accident-free subjects were superior on tests of safety knowledge and of personal adjustment. The repeaters were superior in gymnastic skills and on strength tests, but gave more indication of emotional maladjustments. They were also observed to be more aggressive, to dominate social relationships by physical means and to be show-offs and poor losers (Birnbach, 1947). Poor social adjustment as a characteristic of accident repeaters has also been cited in other studies (Krall, 1953, Marcus et al., 1960).

Behavioral Theory in Accident Causation

A more recent approach to the question of the propensity of some children to accidents relates to (1) the extent to which a child possesses personality and behavioral traits which might result in relatively high exposure to hazards and (2) the extent to which a child has psychological or physical traits which, in the presence of exposure to hazard, may impair his abiliy to cope with them (Mellinger and Manheimer, 1967).

Traits which may *impair* coping ability include motivations which compete with those to avoid injury (e.g., the need to satisfy aggressive impulses, a degree of competitiveness which may interfere with perception of hazards); lack of self-control, impairing ability to make rational decisions (e.g., impulsivity, or anger when frustrated); and other impairing traits such as inattentiveness, carelessness or day-dreaming tendencies.

An extensive study was carried out on the foregoing basis in California, using a study population of 453 boys and 231 girls aged 4 to 18 (Manheimer and Mellinger, 1967). These represented groups of approximately equal numbers of children of high, intermediate or low accident liability, selected on the basis of records of medically attended injuries among the children of families enrolled in a large medical service plan. The children were matched for age and social class. In addition to the accident frequency data from the records, ratings on various traits and behavioral characteristics were obtained from interviews with the children's mothers and from their teachers and school records. The ratings were made in relation to traits associated with exposure, to attitudes presumed to influence coping behavior and to adjustment factors.

The results of this investigation indicated that children are more likely to sustain accidental injuries if they are daring, active, exploring and extraverted, and if they engage in activities such as "rough-housing." Also, boys with more accidents tended to have characteristics which impair coping ability—the greater the accident frequency, the greater the tendency to hostility toward parents and peers, to be competitive and to show-off, to be impulsive and angry when frustrated and to be careless and inattentive. They also tended to show more social maladjustment. Girls showed in general a similar though less marked pattern; there was not as strong a relationship between over-rebellion and accidents, but there was a stronger relation between accident frequency and the need for attention.

The investigators stressed the large variety of characteristics related to accident frequency, and the relatively small number of children who comprise the extreme group of repeaters. Certain characteristics should not be taken to imply that a child will have accidents, but they do affect the *probability* that he will. Children of different accident liability differ in degree but not in kind. Thus, the question of what characteristics increase the *probability* of accident is one which applies to all children, and not only to the repeater.

SOCIAL INFLUENCES IN THE OCCURRENCE OF INJURY AMONG CHILDREN

The emphasis of environmental factors as determinants of accidental injuries among children has to a large extent focused on a taxonomy of physical hazards in relation to the age, sex and developmental characteristics of children. Attention to the social environment in the earlier studies related chiefly to socioeconomic influences in the distribution of different classes of accidents, with the chief implications relating to variations in the quantity and quality of exposure to various types of hazard. However, other social factors are important as well. For example, cultural and social norms influence participation in activities which are characteristically different for boys and girls, and for different ages. These involve different exposures to hazard and are reflected in the age-sex variations in the injury statistics. Cultural variations in child-rearing practices and in family knowledge—or ignorance—of safety practices also have a bearing on the occurrence of children's accidents (Dietrich, 1952; McFarland, 1955). As mentioned previously, the quality of parent-child relationships has been cited in studies of the accident-repeater (Dunbar, 1943; Bakwin and Bakwin, 1948) and in relation to children suffering head injuries (Fabian and Bender, 1947). The factor of acceptance among other children in the group is important (Fuller, 1948; Fuller and Baune, 1951). Effort to maintain status among playmates has been noted as a factor increasing accident frequency (Langford et al., 1953). With such exceptions, however, the social behavior and social-influence aspects of accidents have received little systematic attention until recent years.

A survey of research and activities in accident prevention during the late 1950's revealed that there was a relative dearth of information in relation to such factors as the influence of the emotional climate of the family, the social forces at work in the community and the general social values of society. This led to a conference in 1960 for the exploration of the potential contributions to accident research of the behavioral and social sciences. Participating were representatives of such disciplines as child and developmental psychology, social psychiatry, sociology, cultural anthropology, preventive medicine and biostatistics, among other professions more traditionally concerned with the field of accidents (Association for the Aid of Crippled Children, 1961). Attempts to implement some of the concepts and theories presented at this conference can be discerned in subsequent research and development of viewpoints concerning accident causation and control, as exemplified in the variety of approaches included in presentations at two national symposia on childhood injury (Meyer et al., 1966; Meyer and Klein, 1969).

One of the early large-scale studies in which patterns of family life and the emotional climate within the family were specifically investigated as distinct from the more usual socioeconomic considerations has already been mentioned in the context of child pedestrian accidents (Backett and Johnston, 1959). From this came the concept of the "vulnerable family": a set of influences within certain families which increase children's vulnerability to accidents. Families which included children aged 5 to 14 who had been injured as pedestrians were compared with families in which children had not been so injured; the children were matched according to age, sex, school grade and geographic area of residence. Significantly more of the injured children came from families where there was one or more of the following: (1) illness in the mother or other household member, especially a more serious illness, (2) maternal preoccupation with other children, pregnancy or work outside the home, (3) more dependents per earner in the family and (4) lack of supervised, protected play areas.

Another investigation of accident circumstances in relation to family attitudes and patterns of behavior was carried out with regard to a series of 168 children hospitalized for injuries at the Children's Medical Center in Boston in one 12-month period. Though no comparison was made to a control group, it was observed that immediately preceding the accidents there was frequently an impairment in the quality of child supervision. Also, the quality and amount of supervision and protection available often were associated with maternal or other illness in the family or with significant episodes of life stress impinging on the family (Meyer et al., 1963). Subsequently, the same investigator has proposed that an emphasis on alteration of the physical environment and dependence on health and safety education have not proven very effective in achieving control over children's accidents, and that greatest promise for control lies in the areas of the child development aspects and the subsystem of family attitudes, beliefs and practices concerning health and safety (Meyer, 1969).

A final example may be given to illustrate further the trends in the current concepts and research concerning children's accidents. An interesting approach to the analysis of children's interactions with the physical and social environment in the production of injury is found in a study based on 250 infants who were referred for x-ray following accidents involving a physical blow of some kind. In this study, 164 families participated in social interviews, pediatric examinations and psychosocial tests and ratings. Observations were also made of parent-child interactions in the hospital and at home. The purpose of the study was to determine whether particular types of accident situations could be differentiated on the basis of child characteristics, home environments and family interaction patterns. The results reported thus far are based on an analysis of 77 of the cases, which were followed for one year (Wight, 1969). (The series included 16 cases of suspected child abuse.[8])

The accidents were classified in two main categories—child-active and child-passive—on the basis of whether activity of the child in the environment led to the mechanical insult or whether the injury resulted from the activity of persons or movement of objects in the environment. The assumption was that variability of the child in the environment affects the risk of dangerous exchange of energy. Secondly, it was assumed that the probability of accidents is also influenced by a complex set of variables, represented by the role of the mother and by family background factors. "Child-active" cases were subdivided as "open-field" (e.g., child crawling, walking, colliding with furniture) and "fall" cases (e.g., falls from dressing table). Three kinds of "child-passive" accidents were discerned: (1) those where the child was dropped, (2) those where children were struck by another person and (3) "unusual" cases (e.g., struck by baseball, peculiar collapse of baby equipment, knocked out of mother's arms by a dog).

A number of factors were found to differentiate between the child-active and child-passive accidents, and to some extent, in regard to the subclassifications. From the standpoint of child characteristics, the "open-field" children were more motoric, more negativistic and more frequently were characterized by atypical sleeping and eating patterns. The "child-passive" cases were considered easier to manage, showed moderate activity levels and less deviation in behavioral patterns. Children in the "struck" and "unusual" groups tended to be described as bland and apathetic (as were their mothers). Developmentally, children in the "open-field" were relatively accelerated. Those in the "struck" and "unusual" groups tended to be developmentally retarded and appeared to become more so during the year of follow-up.

In terms of general background, "struck" children were predominantly from families of low socioeconomic status, with frequent family disruptions and family stress. The opposite picture prevailed in the "open-field" cases.

Special emphasis was given to child-parent interactions and relationships, with emphasis on the mother: how she cared for the baby, how she perceived and reacted to the child's behavior and her general coping behavior. Various kinds of mothers' failures appeared in all the groups (e.g., mother disabled and no adequate substitute available; mother placed child in unsafe place, failed to protect child from dangerous objects or failed to control behavior of others potentially dangerous to child). Some differences in the mothers between the various groups were, however, apparent. Mothers in the "open-field" cases tended to seek medical assistance for the injuries early. Long delays were frequently found in the "struck" and "unusual" groups. Hostility and guilt feelings as mothers' reactions to the accidents were prominent in the "struck" group but were not apparent in the "open-field" cases. Mothers of the "open-field" cases did not emphasize any particular kind of behavior on the part of the child as meriting punishment. The mothers of children in the "fall" and "dropped" cases tended to punish for exploratory behavior

[8]Consideration of the "abused child," or the "battered child syndrome" is beyond the scope of this chapter. For a discussion of this area, see Chapter 1; for additional references, see Gil, 1969.

considered dangerous, while the focus for punishment of children in the "struck" and "unusual" groups related to demanding and disobedient behavior.

The mothers showing the greatest verbal responsiveness to their children's behavior were those of the "open-field" cases. This was considerably less characteristic of the mothers in all three of the "child-passive" groups, and the investigators suggested a possible relationship to the finding of more and persistent developmental retardation in the "struck" and "unusual" groups mentioned earlier.

While the findings in the study just described are based on relatively small numbers of cases in the various groupings, they suggest promising areas for further investigation. Thus far, a relatively high degree of subjectivity has been apparent in data from studies in the area of family climate and social inter-relationships as influences in accidents. Measurement and scaling techniques in regard to quantifying some of the quantitative aspects of social behavior are constantly being improved, however, and more precise definition of the inter-relationships resulting in accidents should result. Developing ways of applying such findings in effective preventive activities will constitute a considerable challenge to physicians and pediatricians, as well as to social workers, health educators and others representing community health resources.

It is important to note that public attitudes can be developed to influence safety among children. An example can be taken from the field of motor vehicle accidents, to which, until recently, the public as a whole has remained relatively apathetic. Bus transportation of school children, however, is an exception. The public has been made aware of the dangers in passing school buses, especially when they are stopped to load and unload children. The response of the driving public to this danger has been in general one of caution and conformity to the traffic regulations concerning this situation. The fact that only 50 pupils were killed in 1968 from being struck by vehicles while leaving or approaching loading zones suggests a public awareness of this problem, especially in view of the magnitude and extent of school bus transportation operations. Some 18 million pupils are transported each day of the school year, usually both to and from school, by about 260,000 buses (National Safety Council, 1969a).

SUMMARY

Advances in curative medicine and particularly in the prevention of communicable diseases have markedly reduced mortality among children. As a result, deaths and injuries from accidents have moved prominently into the foregound as the major threat to the health and well-being of the young (and other) members of our population. Advances in the treatment and handling of injuries have played a significant role in reducing fatality rates in cases of trauma. However, progress in the prevention of childhood injuries from accidents has lagged behind that in regard to disease. Among children above age one—in fact, among persons between ages 1 and 37—there are more deaths from accidents than from any disease entity.

Nonfatal injuries are far more numerous than fatal ones. With the technological advances and changes in ways of living in our modern society, there are increasing opportunities for injuries to occur. Increased exposure to hazards of poisoning and chemical burns is a result of the proliferation of products designed to assist the housewife. More automobiles, more trucks, more travel—

more overall traffic—have multiplied risks for child pedestrians and bicyclists as well as for those who ride in motor vehicles. Also, new forms of playthings and recreational activities have added to or altered the earlier parameters in the cases of children's injuries.

Information that can be used to prevent injuries has been developed through epidemiological methods of analyzing the causes of accidents and injury. Among children especially, it is clear that inter-relationships between multiple factors are involved in the production of injury. Rather than a single cause, an intricate web of causation is usual. This complex involves the individual characteristics of the child; the environmental setting, including both physical and social influences; and exposure to agencies, in these circumstances, that are capable of producing injury. However, much remains to be accomplished in the proper use of biostatistics and the newer epidemiological concepts to define these problems more specifically. Before effective control can be instituted, parameters of age, sex, developmental level, time, place, specific categories of injurious agencies, and environmental circumstances must be further clarified. Childhood injuries involve a wide variety of threats and hazards to a wide variety of individual children who differ only grossly from one another as the babe-in-arms, the toddler, the preschooler, the school-age child and the adolescent.

Many injuries may be prevented if one considers that all injuries result from an exchange of some form of energy between the environment and the human body. Control of injury may be accomplished through the elimination of hazardous energy sources, through barrier measures to prevent the impingement of hazardous energy upon the body or through measures to attenuate, to levels below tissue thresholds of injury, energy reaching the body. The form of energy against which control measures have been most effectively devised is electricity. The control of thermal energy that causes burns, and of mechanical energy that produces most of the injuries from motor vehicle accidents, recreation and sports as yet leaves much to be desired. The activities of the American Academy of Pediatrics and the National Commission on Product Safety are hopeful harbingers of progress in these areas.

Poison control centers have undoubtedly saved the lives of many children and have contributed greatly to our knowledge of the circumstances of children's ingestions of toxic and poisonous substances. The problem of preventing instances of ingestion still lacks a solution. At the very least, the education of families regarding the safe handling, use and storage of toxic household materials and medicinal preparations is a continuing necessity. It will probably remain so, even in addition to recent national legislative activity pertaining to improved warning labeling, and construction of child-proof containers for medicine and toxic substances. The problem of lead poisoning, for example, will be eliminated not when all new paint is lead-free, but when the many coats of paint present in countless older homes and apartments have also been scraped away or safely covered.

Considerable attention has been given to the question of the child who is involved in frequent accidents. While some behavioral characteristics have been outlined as favoring accident frequency, this area requires further investigation. At present, emphasis on parental education, child supervision, safety in the design of children's equipment and modification of hazardous energy sources in the home seem to be the areas of emphasis more likely to achieve a significant reduction in the total frequency of accidents.

Accidents among children cannot be controlled effectively without consideration of the influence of parent-child relationships, the influence of the emotional climate of the family and the psychological and socioeconomic factors which influence the way the family copes and lives. Parent-child relationships, family tensions and maternal preoccupations with various problems are important factors. Parental ignorance, inadequate substitutes for parent supervision, substandard housing and lack of adequate play areas also contribute.

The foregoing areas seem to lie outside the role of traditional medicine. But such influences are becoming increasingly recognized in an attempt to supply adequate medical and health services to inhabitants of the less privileged areas of our cities and rural areas. Moreover, these problems cannot be solved separately from some of the other products facing contemporary society.

Almost all injuries to young children occur within the home, or in its immediate environs. The first line of prevention is obviously in regard to the knowledge, attitudes and practices of the parents and other immediate family. Parents not only need to recognize and control hazards in the home, yards and play areas. They must also be aware of the changing possibilities for injury as children progress through successive levels of maturation and development, in respect to both physical and social spheres. In infancy, complete protection against hazards is the only way to prevent injury. Complete and constant supervision is required as the child acquires locomotive and rudimentary psychomotor abilities. At some point, depending on both parent and child, a balance between supervision and permissive encouragement of activity must be achieved.

The high incidence of injuries on school playgrounds and other play areas away from home attests to the importance of supervision being extended beyond the home and continued until there are indications of safe independence on the part of the child. Parents and the medical representatives of our communities have the responsibility for seeing that properly supervised and safely equipped play areas are available in the community, as well as insuring that school boards and school administrators are aware of their responsibilities to provide safety not only in the corridors and classrooms but also in the playground and physical education programs of the public schools.

The prevention of accidents in childhood thus involves the cooperation and combined efforts of parents, schools and educators, physicians and health services of communities, engineers and designers of equipment, architects of housing developments, town and city planners, and public administrators.

ACKNOWLEDGMENTS

The authors are indebted to a number of colleagues and other persons for assistance of various kinds in the preparation of this chapter. Among these many, Mr. Richard Manuell and Mr. Richard Fowler of the Home Accident Department of the National Safety Council have been especially helpful in directing us to relevant studies and statistical materials relating to children's accidents, and in allowing us access to certain unpublished data on play equipment accidents. Mr. Jack Morrison, of the Injury Control Program of the Public Health Service has provided us with the most recent national estimates on various aspects of children's injuries. In the typing of the manuscript, the very able assistance of Miss Mary Ann Van Bleek, secretary in the Children's Service of the Massachusetts General Hospital, has been invaluable. Finally, the authors are particularly grateful to Dr. Nathan B.

Talbot for his encouragement and many helpful suggestions throughout the preparation of this chapter.

REFERENCES

Armstrong, D. B., and Cole, W. G.: Can child accidents be prevented in your community? *Amer. J. Public Health, 39*:585, 1949.

Association for the Aid of Crippled Children: *Behavioral Approaches to Accident Research.* New York, 1961.

Backett, E. M., and Johnston, A. M.: Social patterns of road accidents to children. Some characteristics of vulnerable families. *Brit. Med. J., 1*:409, 1959.

Bain, K., Faegre, M. L., and Wylie, B. S.: Behavior of young children under conditions simulating entrapment in refrigerators. *Pediatrics, 22*(Pt. I):628, 1958.

Bakwin, R. M., and Bakwin, H.: Accident proneness. *J. Pediat., 32*:749, 1948.

Baltimore, C., Jr., and Meyer, R. J.: A study of storage, child behavioral traits, and mother's knowledge of toxicology in 52 poisoned families and 52 comparison families. *Pediatrics, 44*(Pt. II. Suppl.):816, 1969.

Birnbach, S. B.: Comparative study of accident free and accident repeater pupils. Doctoral dissertation. New York, School of Education, New York University, 1947.

Blanksma, L. A., Sachs, H. K., Murray, E. F., and O'Connell, M. J.: Incidence of high blood lead levels in Chicago children. *Pediatrics, 44*(Part I. Suppl.):661, 1969.

Bleck, E. C.: Causes of burns in children. *J.A.M.A., 158*:100, 1955.

Blocker, T. G., Washburn, W. W., Lewis, S. P., and Blocker, V.: A statistical study of 1000 burn patients admitted to the plastic surgery service of the University of Texas medical branch, 1950–1959. *J. Trauma, 1*:409, 1961.

Borland, B.: The burned child: An epidemiological survey. Paper presented at the Childhood Accident Symposium, University of Virginia, Charlottesville, Virginia, April 22–29, 1966.

Bull, J. P., Jackson, D. M., and Walton, C.: Causes and prevention of domestic burning accidents. *Brit. Med. J., 2*:1421, 1964.

Burkinshaw, J.: Head injuries in children: Observations on their incidence and causes with an inquiry into the value of routine x-rays. *Arch. Dis. Child., 35*:205–214, 1960.

California State Department of Public Health. *Home Safety Project, Final Report, 1953–1957.* Berkeley, California, October, 1957.

Cann, H. M., Neyman, D. S., and Verhulst, H. L.: Control of accidental poisoning. *J.A.M.A., 168*:717, 1958.

Colebrook, L., and Colebrook, V.: Prevention of burns and scalds; Review of 1000 cases. *Lancet, 2*:181, 1949.

Dietrich, H. F.: Clinical application of the theory of accident prevention in childhood. *Amer. J. Public Health, 42*:849, 1952.

Dunbar, F.: *Psychosomatic Diagnosis.* New York, Hoeber Medical Division, Harper & Row, Publishers, 1943.

Dykstra, P.: *Survey of Injuries Involving Toys and Playthings Sustained by Children in Florida.* Chicago, National Safety Council, 1962.

Fabian, A. A., and Bender, L.: Head injury in children; predisposing factors. *Amer. J. Orthopsychiat., 17*:68, 1947.

Fowler, R. G.: Accidents in childhood. A survey of 150 cases in private pediatric practice. *Canad. Med. Ass. J., 79*:241, 1958.

Fuller, E. M.: Injury prone children. *Amer. J. Orthopsychiat., 18*:708, 1948.

Fuller, E. M., and Baune, H. B.: Injury-proneness and adjustment in second grade: Sociometric study. *Sociometry, 14*:210, 1951.

Gibson, J. J.: The contribution of experimental psychology to the formulation of the problem of safety—A brief for basic research. In *Behavioral Approaches to Accident Research.* New York, Association for the Aid of Crippled Children, 1961, pp. 77–87.

Gil, D. G.: Physical abuse of children. Findings and implications of a nationwide survey. *Pediatrics, 44*(Pt. II, Suppl.):856, 1969.

Gordon, J.: The epidemiology of accidents. *Amer. J. Public Health., 39*:505, 1949.

Griggs, R. C., Sunshine, P., Nevill, V. A., Newton, B. W., Buchanan, S., and Rasch, C. A.: Environmental factors in childhood lead poisoning. *J.A.M.A., 187*:703, 1964.

Guttmann, L.: Neurological injuries sustained through diving. *Brit. Assn. Sport Med. Bull. 1*:32, 1964.

Haddon, W., Jr.: The prevention of accidents. *In* Clark, D. W., and MacMahon, B. (Eds.): *Preventive Medicine.* Boston, Little, Brown and Company, 1967.

Haddon, W., Jr., Suchman, E. A., and Klein, D.: *Accident Research Methods and Approaches.* New York, Harper and Row Publishers, Inc., 1964.

Hemphill, F. M.: A sample survey of home injuries. *Public Health Rep., 67*:1026, 1952.

Hemphill, F. M., and Velz, C. J.: *Investigation and Application of Home Injury Survey Data in Development of Prevention Procedures* (February 1, 1952 to January 31, 1953). School of Public Health, University of Michigan, Ann Arbor, 1953.

Howell, T. R.: Accidents and those bizarre bicycles. *Pediatrics, 42*:214, 1968.

Huelke, D. F., and Davis, R. A.: *A Study of Pedestrian Fatalities in Wayne County, Michigan.* Highway Safety Research Institute Report Bio-9, University of Michigan, Ann Arbor, Michigan, 1969.

Iskrant, A. P.: Statistics and epidemiology of burns. *Bull. N.Y. Acad. Med., 43*:636, 1967.

Iskrant, A. P., and Joliet, P. V.: *Accidents and*

Homicide. Cambridge, Massachusetts, Harvard University Press, 1968.

Izant, R. J., Jr., Rothmann, B. F., and Frankel, V. H.: Bicycle Spoke Injuries of the Foot and Ankle in Children: An underestimated "minor" injury. *J. Pediat. Surg.*, *4*:654, 1969.

Jacobziner, H.: Causation, prevention, and control of accidental poisoning. *J.A.M.A.*, *171*:1769, 1959.

Jacobziner, H.: Lead poisoning in childhood; epidemiology, manifestation, and prevention. *Clin. Pediat.*, *5*:277, 1966.

Jensen, G. D.: Preventive implications of a study of 100 children treated for serious burns. *Pediatrics*, *24*:623, 1959.

Joliet, P. V., Schaplowsky, A. F., and Huyck, E. E.: Accidents and the nation's health. *H.E.W. Indicators*, December, 1964 to January, 1965.

Jolly, H., and Forrest, T. R. W.: Accidental poisoning in childhood. An experimental approach to the prevention of poisoning by tablets. *Lancet*, *1*:1308, 1958.

King, B. G.: Accident prevention research. *Public Health Rep.*, *64*:373, 1949.

Krall, V.: Personality characteristics of accident repeating children. *J. Abnorm. Soc. Psychol.*, *48*:99, 1953.

Kravitz, H., Driessen, G., Gomberg, R., and Korach, A.: Accidental falls in infancy. *Pediatrics*, *44*(Pt. II, Suppl.):869, 1969.

Langford, W. S., Gilder, R. J., Jr., Wilking, V. N., Genn, M. M., and Sherrill, H. H.: Pilot study of childhood accidents, preliminary report. *Pediatrics*, *11*:405, 1953.

Licht, K.: Once upon a light-weight. *Safety Education*, 1965.

Long, R. T., and Cope, O.: Emotional problems of burned children. *New Eng. J. Med.*, *264*:1121, 1961.

McFarland, E. F.: *Community Health Educat on for Child Safety.* Harvard School of Public Health, Boston, Massachusetts, 1956.

McFarland, R. A.: *Human Factors in Air Transportation—Occupational Health and Safety.* New York, McGraw-Hill Book Company, 1953.

McFarland, R. A.: Epidemiological principles applicable to the study and prevention of child accidents. *Amer. J. Public Health*, *45*:1302, 1955.

McFarland, R. A.: A critique of accident research. *Ann. N.Y. Acad. Sci.*, *107*:686, 1963.

McFarland, R. A., and Moore, R. C.: The epidemiology of accidents. *In* Halsey, M. N. (Ed.): *Accident Prevention: The Role of Physicians and Public Health Workers.* New York, McGraw-Hill Book Company, 1961, pp. 17–45.

McFarland, R. A., and Moore, R. C.: The prevention of accidental injury and death. *In* Leavell, H. R., and Clark, E. G. (Eds.): *Preventive Medicine for the Doctor in His Community.* New York, McGraw-Hill Book Company, 1965, pp. 284–299.

MacLennan, W. D.: Injuries involving the teeth and jaws in young children. *Arch. Dis. Child.*, *32*:492, 1957.

MacMahon, B., Pugh, T. F., and Ipsen, J.: *Epidemiological Methods.* Boston, Little, Brown and Company, 1960.

MacQueen, I. A. G.: *A Study of Home Accidents in Aberdeen.* London, E. & S. Livingstone Ltd., 1960.

Manheimer, D. I., Dewey, J., Mellinger, G. D., and Corsa, L.: 50,000 child-years of accidental injuries. *Public Health Rep.*, *81*:519, 1966.

Manheimer, D. I., and Mellinger, G. D.: Personality characteristics of the child accident repeater. *Child Develop.*, *38*:491, 1967.

Marcus, I. M., Wilson, W., Kraft, I., Swander, D., Southerland, F., and Schulhafer, E.: An interdisciplinary approach to accident patterns in children. *Monogr. Soc. Res. Child Develop.*, *25*, No. 2, 1960.

Marland, R. E., and Burg, F. D.: The injury control program of the U.S. Public Health Service. *Pediatrics* *44*(Pt. II, Suppl.):858, 1969.

Mellinger, G. D., and Manheimer, D. I.: An exposure-coping model of accident liability among children. *J. Health Soc. Behav.*, *8*:96, 1967.

Mellinger, G. D., Sylvester, D. L., Gaffey, W. R., and Manheimer, D. I.: A mathematical model with applications to a study of accident repeatedness among children. *J. Amer. Stat. Assoc.*, *60*:1046, 1965.

Meyer, R. J.: Introduction: The Horizons of Childhood Injury. *Pediatrics*, *44*(Part II, Suppl.):793, 1969.

Meyer, R. J., Austin, R. H., and Symmers, A. T., (eds.): *Childhood Accidental Injury Proceedings.* Charlottesville, Virginia, University of Virginia, 1966.

Meyer, R. J., and Klein, D. (Eds.): Childhood injuries: Approaches and perspectives. A report of the Second National Childhood Injury Symposium, June 28 to 30, 1968, Charlottesville, Virginia. *Pediatrics*, *44* (Part II, Suppl.):791, 1969.

Meyer, R. J., Roelofs, H., Bluestone, J., and Redmond, S.: Accidental injury to the preschool child. A study of some child, family, and environmental associations with injuries requiring hospitalization. *J. Pediat.*, *63*:95, 1963.

Moncrieff, A. A., Koremides, O. P., Clayton, B. E., Patrick, A. D., Renwick, A. G. C., and Roberts, G. E.: Lead poisoning in children. *Arch. Dis. Child.*, *39*:1, 1964.

Montgomery, C.: Speaker for the house. *Good Housekeeping*, March, 1967.

Moore, J. O., Tourin, B., and Garrett, J. W.: Child injuries in automobile accidents. *Traffic Safety Res. Rev.*, *4*:16, 1960.

Munro, I. R., Farmer, A. W., Csima, A., and Lindsay, W. K.: An analysis of burns in children. *Canad. Med. Ass. J.*, *97*:459, 1967.

National Center for Health Statistics: *Current Estimates from the Health Interview Survey, United States, 1967.* U.S. Dept. of Health, Education and Welfare, Public Health Service. Vital and Health Statistics, Series 10, Number 52, May, 1967.

National Center for Health Statistics: *Types of Injuries, Incidence, and Associated Disability, United States, 1965–1967.* U. S. Dept. of Health, Education and Welfare, Pub ic Health Service. Vital and Health Statistics, Series 10, Number 57, 1969.

National Commission of Product Safety: *Final Report.* Washington, D.C., U.S. Government Printing Office, June, 1970.

National Safety Council, *Accident Facts, 1967.* Chicago, 1967a.

National Safety Council: Look what's happening to bikes. *Family Safety, 26*:13, 1967b.

National Safety Council: *Accident Facts, 1969.* Chicago, 1969a.

National Safety Council: Child-proof caps are coming. *Family Safety, 28*:28, 1969b.

National Safety Council: The child pedestrian. *Family Safety* 5:4, 1970a.

National Safety Council: Do we want better baby beds? *Family Safety, 29*:8, 1970b.

Oglesbay, F. B.: The flammable fabrics problem. *Pediatrics, 44*(Pt. II, Suppl.):827, 1969.

Public Health Service: *Estimates of Injuries Involving Various Environmental Factors.* Unpublished report, Bureau of Environmental Management, Cincinnati, Ohio, 1970.

Rado, R. W.: Immediate handling of diving injuries, a rational approach. *Bull. Amer. Coll. Surg., 49*:105, 1964.

Read, J. H.: Traffic accidents involving child pedestrians: A program for their prevention. *Pediatrics, 44*(Pt. II, Suppl.):838, 1969.

Rice, R. G., Starbuck, G. W., and Reed, R. B.: Accidental injuries to children. *New Eng. J. Med., 255*:1212, 1956.

Rowntree, G.: Accidents among children under two years of age in Great Britain. *J. Hyg., 48*:323, 1950.

Ryan, G. A.: Children in traffic accidents. *Pediatrics, 44*(Pt. II, Suppl.):847, 1969.

Severy, D., and Brink, H.: *Auto-Pedestrian Collision Experiments.* SAE Report No. 660080, New York, Society of Automotive Engineers, 1966.

Smith, E. I.: The epidemiology of burns. The cause and control of burns in children. *Pediatrics 44*(Pt. II, Suppl.):821, 1969.

Smith, H. D.: Pediatric lead poisoning. *Arch. Environ. Health,* 8:256, 1964.

Snyder, R. G.: *A Survey of Automotive Restraint Systems: Where We've Been, Where We Are, and Our Current Problems.* SAE Report No. 690243, New York, Society of Automotive Engineers, 1969.

Sobel, R.: Traditional safety measures and accidental poisoning in childhood, *Pediatrics, 44*(Pt. II. Suppl.):811, 1969.

Stallones, R. A., and Corsa, L., Jr.: Epidemiology of childhood accidents in two California counties. *Public Health Rep., 76*:25, 1961.

Strauch, B.: Bicycle spoke injuries in children. *J. Trauma,* 6:61, 1966.

Strause, D. F., and Westaby, J. R.: *Accident Research Bibliographical Series, Vol. I, Fire and Burn Injury, 1960–1967.* Department of Public Health Administration, School of Public Health, University of North Carolina, Chapel Hill, North Carolina, 1968.

Suchman, E. A.: A conceptual analysis of the accident phenomenon. In *Behavioral Approaches to Accident Research.* New York, Association for the Aid of Crippled Children, 1961, pp. 26–47.

Verhulst, H. L., and Crotty, J. J.: Childhood poisoning accidents. *J.A.M.A., 203*:1049, 1968.

Vilardo, F. J., and Anderson, J. H.: *Bicycle Accidents to School Age Children.* Report No. 169. Research Department, National Safety Council, Chicago, September, 1969.

Vilardo, F. J., Nicol, M. J., and Heldreth, H. E.: *An Investigation into Bicycle Usage.* Report No. 268, Research Department, National Safety Council, Chicago, September, 1968.

Waller, J. A.: Tic-tac toe burns. The hazard of exposed floor type heaters. *New Eng. J. Med., 265*:1256, 1961.

Waller, J. A.: Bicyc e ownership, use, and injury patterns among elementary school children. *Pediatrics, 47*:1042, 1971.

Waller, J. A., and Manheimer, D. I.: Non-fatal burns of children in a well-defined urban population. *J. Pediat., 65*:869, 1964.

Waller, P. F., and Reinfurt, D. W.: Bicycles: *An Analysis of Accidents in North Carolina.* Highway Safety Research Center, University of North Carolina, Chapel Hill, North Carolina, February, 1969.

Webster, D. P.: Pool drownings and their prevention. *Public Health Rep., 82*:587, 1967.

Wheatley, G. M.: Accident prevention and the general practitioner. *Postgrad. Med., 10*:442, 1951.

Wheatley, G. M.: Prevention of accidents in childhood. *Advances Pediat.,* 8:191, 1956.

Wheatley, G. M., and Richardson, S. A.: Some approaches to research in childhood accidents. *Pediatrics, 25*:343, 1960.

Wight, B. W.: The control of child-environment interaction: A conceptual approach to accident occurrence. *Pediatrics, 44*(Pt. II, Suppl.):799, 1969.

Williams, H., Bowman, N., and Malare, G.: A social study of burns and scalds in children. *Med. J. Aust., 2*:599, 1958.

Woodward, J., and Jackson, D. M.: Emotional reactions in burned children and their mothers. *Brit. J. Plast. Surg., 13*:316, 1961.

Zavon, M. R.: Problems in the recognition of lead intoxications. *Arch. Environ. Health,* 8:262, 1964.

9 PSYCHO-PHARMACOLOGY IN CHILDHOOD

Leon Eisenberg, and C. K. Conners

Drugs are prescribed for the treatment of behavioral disorders in children at a remarkably high rate, a rate which seems extraordinary in contrast to the paucity of evidence for the effectiveness of most of the agents which are used. The frequency of prescription makes it clear that complaints about disturbing behavior are common in medical practice. The ready resort to drugs suggests that alternative modes of treatment are either unfamiliar to physicians, too time consuming for them or too unsatisfactory in outcome. One can guess that all three factors obtain, given the limited psychiatric training most medical students receive, the uneconomic nature of most psychological treatment methods and the difficulty in obtaining substantive evidence of their efficacy (Levitt, 1959; Eisenberg, 1962). Moreover, the continuing use of drugs, despite the frequently negative outcome of controlled studies, indicates that behavioral disorders in children are placebo responsive.

Alternatively, it might be argued that children's behavioral disorders themselves are subject to such high rates of spontaneous remission that any "treatment" will bring about good results; i.e., no treatment is really required. But that the latter alternative is not correct has been demonstrated by the longterm follow-up studies of Robins (1966), which clearly indicate that children with diagnosed psychiatric disorders are at high risk for continued disability into adulthood. Nonetheless, many *do* improve, and if improvement is subsequent to some intervention, the physician is all too ready to credit the result to the particular intervention.

Given the scientific evidence, the frequency with which psychopharmacological agents are prescribed points to a failure in medical education. Practitioners are given insufficient grounding in the nature, course and treatment of psychiatric disorders. Moreover, in this as in other fields of therapeutics our educational efforts fail to meet our professed goals of preparing physicians to evaluate critically the reports of new agents. It is not medical education alone that is at fault, however. The organization of medical practice, with its insufficiency of manpower and its inability to provide systematic opportunities for educational "renewal" through postgraduate training, leaves the practitioner at the mercy of the detail man and the drug house. But perhaps both the educator and the physician are openly reflecting our general culture, which is drug oriented (Lennard et al., 1970). Though it has become fashionable for adults to bemoan the hedonistic use of drugs by adolescents and college students, it should be remembered that ours is a society that uses tobacco, alcohol, sedatives and stimulants at a rate without parallel. Documentation of the dire consequences of this injudicious use of chemical aids to control the anxiety of existence has unfortunately had little effect in deterring their use. It may be asking a great deal of the physician to transcend the culture which shapes him.

Our objective is not to suggest that drugs which affect behavior should never be used, but rather that they should be used only when a condition exists that requires treatment, when the agent prescribed is likely to be effective in treating that condition, when the likelihood of benefit outweighs the risk of toxicity and then only for the shortest period possible. Indeed, it is an error of equal magnitude to deny a patient an agent which can help relieve his symptoms and hasten his recovery. If pediatricians are to be faulted for the overprescription of drugs in an effort to avoid the burdens of dealing with the troubled child in a troubled family, the child psychiatrist all too frequently errs in the opposite direction and disdains the use of drugs because of an unsubstantiated faith in the superiority of psychological over pharmacological treatment methods (Eisenberg, 1969).

DEVELOPMENTAL PHARMACOLOGY

The authors lack the competence to treat the subject of developmental pharmacology in depth, and the reader is referred to the succinct discussion and pertinent bibliography supplied by Nyhan (1968). Unfortunately, medical knowledge of the pharmacology of infancy and childhood is sparse in comparison to its importance. Among the factors that influence the response of the young organism to drugs are the following. The size of the patient, as reflected either by weight or by surface area, is a significant determinant of the concentration of the drug in body fluids, which is the most immediate parameter controlling its effects. Absorption and distribution differ from the adult because of differences in binding to serum proteins, differences in circulation and the immaturity of the blood-brain barrier (differential permeability). The metabolism of drugs in children is influenced by the rate at which enzyme systems develop, particularly in the liver and kidney. Finally, there are peculiarities of receptor response, best exemplified by the sensitivity of the retina of the premature infant to high concentrations of oxygen, which results in the production of retrolental fibroplasia. The well-established but still perplexing paradoxical response of infants and young children to sedatives and stimulants (described later in this chapter) as yet defies adequate explanation.

Only recently have pharmacologists studied genetically controlled individual differences in the metabolic responses to drug action. This, as with many other areas of pharmacology in childhood, is difficult to study systematically because of the ethical barriers to the experimental administration of drugs to "volunteers," a technique available with an adult population who can give informed consent. Clearly, the child is incapable of informed consent, and it is dubious that a physician has the right to ask or that parents have the right to give consent for the use of children in experimental drug trials, except when those drugs are being given in the effort to treat an existing disorder. The inability to use the normal control makes difficult the distinction between an age-related "normal" difference in response to a drug, and a difference in response that is attributable to a difference in the responsiveness of the disorder itself in the child as opposed to the adult.

A few documented clinical examples may serve to alert the reader to some of the complexities of drug effects on the growing oganism; this listing is partial and for illustrative purposes only. The tragic production of phocomelia following thalidomide ingestion by pregnant women brought to public attention the teratogenic potential of drugs administered during pregnancy. A recent study (Berlin and Jacobson, 1970) has indicated that lysergic acid ingested during pregnancy is associated with the production of midline central nervous system defects in the fetus and newborn. The syndrome of fetal feminization (Money et al., 1968), caused by cellular insensitivity to androgen at a crucial point in early development, results in female external genitalia despite a male chromosomal pattern and abdominal testes. Progesterone, given to sustain pregnancy in cases of threatened abortion, may result in induced masculinization of the infant and a tendency toward masculine behavioral traits (Money et al., 1968).

Narcotic withdrawal symptoms have been observed in the infants of mothers addicted to heroin or morphine (Cobrinik et al., 1959) and require appropriate treatment (paregoric or chlorpromazine) if serious illness or even death is to be avoided. Diagnosis depends on alertness to the addictive state in the mother; present indications are that complete recovery of the infant ensues if treatment is adequate; the ultimate prognosis depends upon effective help for the mother in order to provide a suitable environment for the child. Indeed, acute alcohol withdrawal symptoms have been reported in the infant of an alcoholic mother (Nichols, 1967).

It has long been recognized that the use of narcotics to diminish maternal discomfort during delivery can have an effect on the behavior of the neonate, an effect maximized by the immaturity of the newborn's liver and kidney, which are unable to detoxify the drugs received through the maternal circulation (Baker, 1960). Brazelton (1970) has noted a lag in adaptation to breast feeding, and an effect on the relationship between the infant and the mother during the first week of life has been noted by Brazelton and Robey (1965).

It should be clear from the data just cited that drug use should be avoided during pregnancy except in the presence of major indications in behalf of the mother; when drugs are employed, the infant should be closely monitored for the consequences of their use.

DESIGN OF THERAPEUTIC TRIALS

The cautions expressed in the introductory paragraphs to this chapter will have prepared the reader for the fact that the great majority of reports on the use of psychopharmacological agents with children are difficult to accept with confidence because of the inadequacy of study design. Clearly, when a new agent has gone through the preliminary animal studies that render it fit for use with human subjects, the initial clinical studies should maximize the likelihood of detecting drug effects in humans. This can be accomplished by having a clinician who is alert to what he may find study carefully selected patients in great detail. Once such clinical trials have suggested that the new agent may be useful, more elaborate investigations designed to rule out placebo effects and investigator bias are essential. Variability in course and susceptibility to psychological influence are the hallmarks of psychiatric disorders. Thus, careful attention to methodology is necessary if we are to discriminate true drug effects, to learn how to produce them reliably and to maximize their benefit by employing appropriate adjunctive psychological methods.

However elaborate the design necessary to attain it, the basic element in a therapeutic drug trial is nothing more than a contrast of the results obtained with and without the agent in question. Complexities arise in efforts to control the many variables, other than the drug under study, that can influence outcome, either independently of or in interaction with the drug. Thus, a generalized design for such a study would include the following features: the division of the patient population into subsamples so chosen as to be approximately equivalent in variables relevant to outcome; the administration of contrasting treatment schedules to the subsamples, one maintained (where possible) as an untreated group; the measurement of change (improvement) in the patients by reliable and valid methods; and the assessment of the confidence to be placed in the obtained results by the use of appropriate statistical techniques.

Patient-related variables

Patient-related variables that must be taken into account are those associated with demographic characteristics, with the disease process itself and with "idiosyncratic" factors.

Demographic factors of importance include age, sex and social class, all of which have been shown to influence course and outcome. School phobia provides an example of an age effect. In our own experience (Rodriquez et al., 1959), as well as in that of others (Coolidge et al., 1960; Warren, 1960), school phobia in children of elementary school age has proven to have a much better prognosis than the same presenting syndrome in children of high school age. A study of drug "x" in the treatment of this disorder could result in quite misleading conclusions if the drug-treated group were either younger or older than the control group. The high ratio of boys to girls having psychiatric disorders of childhood (Bahn et al., 1962) suggests that sex is potentially a variable of importance, though its precise meaning in this context is not clear. Moreover, as in adults (Hollingshead and Redlich, 1958), social class interacts significantly with the assignment of diagnosis, the choice of treatment, the likelihood of remaining in treatment and the outcome of illness (Eisenberg, 1962).

Whereas the characteristics of age, sex and social class can be specified (with an appreciable margin of error in the methods of assigning social class), the problems related to diagnosis have thus far defied consensus. Not only is there no common and completely satisfactory terminology, there is also considerable disagreement between clinicians of the same theoretical persuasion on the diagnosis to be assigned a given patient (Fish, 1969). As a result, some investigators have abandoned serious concern with diagnoses and rely instead upon symptoms; others employ a therapeutic procedure against a heterogeneous group of patients and report overall outcome without relationship to diagnostic subgroups.

No serious investigator elsewhere in medicine would propose such a course. Even when his target is the relief of a nonspecific symptom such as headache, he is careful to deal separately with the headaches of migraine, cerebral neoplasm, tension and so forth. Obviously an agent efficacious for one may be completely ineffectual against another and harm the patient by delaying his access to appropriate treatment. These considerations apply with equal force to the psychiatric disorders of children (Eisenberg, 1957). The thorough follow-up studies of O'Neal and Robins (1958a and b) have demonstrated that the longterm prognosis of psychiatric disorders in children bears a significant relationship to the nature of the presenting syndrome. The relevance of diagnosis to outcome in psychopharmacologic studies has been clearly illustrated in several of our own studies (Cytryn et al., 1960; Eisenberg et al., 1961).

Table 9–1 contrasts the outcome for children classified as neurotic with that for children classified as hyperkinetics; in the latter category we include overactive, impulsive, distractible children with behavior distressing to others but associated with no apparent distress to the child (except for its secondary consequences: reprimands, school exclusion and so forth). Excluded from both groups were children with IQ's of less than 80, gross neurologic impairment, psychosis or adjudicated delinquents. Noteworthy in Table 9–1 is the significantly greater likelihood (p. 0.01) of a favorable outcome for the neurotic children. Comparison of treatment effects within diagnostic categories revealed that none of the three drugs employed (meprobamate, prochlorperazine or perphenazine) yielded a result better than that obtained with placebo or brief psychotherapy, or both. (If anything, children on active medication did less well than the comparison groups when toxic effects were taken into account.) Yet, the differences between the diagnostic groups is so great that, *had diagnosis been ignored*, uneven allocation of cases to the several "therapeutic" regimens could have produced an entirely spurious impression of a therapeutic difference.

These results have led us to deal with the two diagnostic groups as different patient populations. So high is the improvement rate among neurotic children treated by brief psychotherapy, a regime well within the practicalities of ordinary office practice, that we have abandoned further psychopharmacologic investigations with such patients; an agent would have to be spectacularly effective (given the limited sensitivity of clinical measures of improvement) to meet the statistical criteria for superiority over this baseline therapeutic regime. For these patients, the relevant question becomes: Is the apparent improvement a simple function of the "natural history" of neurotic syndromes in children, or a conse-

Table 9–1 Relevance of Diagnosis to Outcome in Neurotic* versus *Hyperkinetic Children

Diagnosis	Outcome			Total
	Much Improved	Somewhat Improved	No Change	
Neurotic	48	17	6	71
Hyperkinetic	24	22	25	71
Total	72	39	31	142

quence of the brief psychotherapy? Recent results (Conners et al., 1965) suggest that the psychotherapy is indeed efficacious.

The "idiosyncratic" (perhaps better termed "unknown") variables include those factors which can lead to differences in outcome between untreated patients who are apparently equivalent on all specifiable variables. That is, two schizophrenics (or neurotics or sociopaths) adjudged clinically to have similar prognoses may nonetheless show quite divergent courses in the hospital. There is always the possibility that the clinical investigator may be intuitively sensitive to subtle prognostic factors despite his inability to specify them explicitly. To control such unwitting bias in assigning patients to treatment regimes, it becomes necessary to insist upon the principle of random allocation of treatment conditions within the major diagnostic groups. Furthermore, in view of the possibility of variation in severity or course of illness—or in the skill of the therapist as he accumulates experience—in relation to time of year, contrasting treatment programs should be carried out synchronously. For example, the "complaint value" of the child is likely to be less, with the same behavioral traits, when good weather comes and he is out of the home for more of the day, or when the school term ends and, with it, vexing calls from the teacher. Had drug "x" been given to the first 30 patients seen from September to February, and drug "y" to the next 30 seen from March to July, the study could well be biased in favor of "y" by this time-of-year factor. Cases coming to attention early in the school year may well be more severe than those surviving without major complaint through the greater part of the term; the later cases, in addition, may show an apparent remission as school ends.

TREATMENT SCHEDULES

The two basic design strategies for teasing out the treatment effect from the other intertwined variables are (1) the patient as his own control and (2) the untreated or standard treatment control.

The first procedure economizes on the size of the clinical population needed and offers the further advantage of providing, at least nominally, complete matching of patient variables. However, the sequential nature of the "own control" design (i.e., a period without medication, followed by one on drug x, followed by a period on placebo, followed by one on drug y—or some variant thereof) makes two special precautions essential. Unless one is dealing with a static disorder from which no one recovers without therapy, we know in advance that more and more patients will be registered as recovered the greater the lapse of time (i.e., fewer and fewer schizophrenics in the hospital the longer the interval after admission). To take this into account, drug and placebo must be given in counterbalanced order, so that half the patients receive the drug first and half receive the placebo first. Secondly, the investigator must be alert for position effects. The impact of placebo after drug may be different from that of placebo before drug (rebound effect). In "own control" designs, the requirement that the patients remain under observation for a considerably longer period of time (at least twice as long) than in the standard treatment control design makes the problem of patients dropping out of treatment a particular hazard.

The practical problems encountered with the use of this design in outpatient studies can be illustrated by the study of Whitehouse et al. (1964). The purpose of the study was to contrast the effectiveness of phenobarbital, methylphenidate, and placebo in the treatment of hyperkinetic retarded children. Each patient was to receive each medication for four weeks, the order being counterbalanced and the administration double blind. However, four patients dropped out after the first drug, and nine dropped out after the second; it is of interest that only two of the thirteen drop-outs were on methylphenidate at the time of drop-out as compared with five on placebo and six on phenobarbital. Analysis of responses to the first and second drug trials separately, and of 19 cases treated by all three drugs, revealed consistent evidence of the superiority of methylphenidate (p 0.05) over phenobarbital, with some evidence of its superiority over placebo (on two of the three analyses). A final analysis based on change in condition in passing from one medication to another demonstrated that both methylphenidate (p 0.0002) and placebo (p 0.01) were superior to phenobarbital, but that there was only a trend (p 0.20) for methylphenidate to be better than placebo. Although the separate analyses tend to complement each other, the asymmetry and decrease in sample size resulting from the sequential and differential drop-outs make interpretation of the findings less clear-cut than we had hoped for.

The alternate research strategy, the one more commonly employed, is a division of the total patient group into two or more matched samples, each of which is then placed in a different treatment condition. Clearly, the preferred design includes a patient group maintained in an untreated condition. This, however, is not always attainable. Patients have, as they clearly should, freedom of movement, and those who are maintained on a waiting list or deliberately denied treatment may well seek help elsewhere. "Defectors" from a waiting list may differ significantly in discomfort or initiative from those who accept delay; the fraction left in the untreated "control" may no longer be representative of the initial patient population. When the patients are in an institution and thus willy-nilly in the "control" condition, the very fact of denial of treatment may influence their course. This seemed clearly to be the case in a study of the effectiveness of perphenazine in the treatment of institutionalized delinquents (Molling et al., 1962). Whereas the youngsters given either placebo or perphenazine displayed improved behavior (as rated by house parents on symptom charts), those who were in a cottage and whom we naively designated as an "untreated control" showed significant worsening of behavior instead of the random fluctuations that we had expected to serve as a check on the stability of our measurement techniques. In the institutional environment, the grapevine among the boys had it that getting the medicine offered the prospect of an earlier discharge, since length of stay was known to depend on adjustment. Those who learned that they were being denied the magic elixir appeared to respond to this condition by increasing dissatisfaction and consequent behavioral disturbance. Clearly, this was a major flaw in the design of the experiment; in such a setting, an undisguised control condition vitiates its intended features. However, serendipity had called our attention to the fact that *not* giving something to patients can be as meaningful to them as giving something, when they know that such a decision has been made.

The customary control is the use of the placebo: a pharmacologically inert substance which resembles the active medication in external form. The ideal placebo would be one which would mimic all of the properties of the active preparation except those relevant to its therapeutic action. The customary use of a pharmacodynamically inert substance suffers from the deficit that the subjective awareness of the physiologic change in state produced by the active drug is missing. Yet, these nonspecific effects of medication may have a significant psychological impact on behavior (that is, if the patient experiences flush or tachycardia after taking medication, this may convince him of its potency and thus lead him to anticipate and experience benefit, even though no direct drug action on the basic disorder has occurred.)

Placebo effects in pediatric drug studies can include effects upon the child, his parents and the physician. A very considerable literature has grown up demonstrating the power of expectancy. If the patient or his family, on the basis of prior experience, of confidence in their physician or of a general conviction about the potency of drugs, anticipates consequences from taking medication, this expectation can lead to a marked alteration in the subjective state. These expected consequences may be either positive or negative. Thus, there are placebo responders who regularly report improvement after taking drugs, and others who report increased distress. The physician is no less vulnerable to anticipations of the value of his treatment. His expectations can influence the outcome of the experiment, either by the attitude he conveys to his patient or by an unwitting bias that skews his judgment of outcome (even in so "objective" a problem as measuring the behavior of laboratory rats—Rosenthal and Lawson, 1964).

The standard method for dealing with the unpredictable and ubiquitous placebo effect is to employ a double-blind design: active drug and placebo are made up to appear identical, coded and administered in a way that neither the patient nor the physician is aware of whether drug or placebo is being given. While it would be absurd to conduct the initial clinical trial with a hitherto untried medication using the double-blind method and thus lose the advantage of increased sensitivity to possible effects, it is equally clear that precise delineation of the role of a new drug requires double-blind studies if the initial clinical trial suggests utility. Medical annals are replete with instances of enthusiastic appraisals of new treatments (from blood letting to tranquilizers) which were finally abandoned after extensive experience. Moreover, so universal are placebo effects in the treatment of psychiatric disorders that a critical reader should be highly suspicious of any study that includes a placebo group and alleges that no or inconsiderable effects were found.

A final consideration anent the role of expectation is alertness to the possibility of interaction between expectation and drug effects. It is customary to assume that placebo effects and drug effects are simply additive; that is, that the amount of improvement in the group receiving placebo provides a baseline to be subtracted from the improvement reported in the group receiving the drug. However, the expectancy or set of the patient can interact differentially with medication, so as either to enhance or to inhibit the drug effect. The response of a patient who anticipates sedation but who receives a stimulant may be different from the response of a patient who anticipates stimulation. A drug may produce effects that depend upon the attitude of the physician administering it, and upon the physician's relationship to the patient. Experimental efforts to investigate drug-set interactions are currently under way by means of strategies that involve deliberate manipulation of set variables (Fisher, 1962b; Uhlenhuth and Park, 1964).

METHODS OF ASSESSING IMPROVEMENT

For the clinician, the essential question is whether the patient improves under the treatment. In office or hospital practice he judges outcome with his clinical skills, integrating into an overall judgment his observations of the behavior of the patient, the patient's subjective account and the reports from the parents and others. Properly enough, this is the method most commonly used in therapeutic studies. Outcome is scored in categories such as "much improved," "somewhat improved," "no change" or "worse." Unfortunately, clinical estimation of change is subject to a considerable margin of uncertainty (reducible by pretraining of raters and by narrowing the focus of the rating from the overall to the specific); this "noise" in the measurement system magnifies apparent within-group differences and hence makes it more difficult, on statistical analysis, to detect potentially significant between-group differences.

More fundamental than even the issue of the reliability of a measuring system is that of its validity: with what precision does the score the system yields correspond to the magnitude of the "real" phenomenon? To determine this we must agree upon the salient characteristics of the phenomenon itself, as well as upon a standard system for the measurement of these characteristics. Much of the bitter controversy over therapeutic outcome studies in psychiatry stems from implicit differences in the criteria of improvement which becloud technical arguments over measurement. What is to be the touchstone of clinical success: reduction in symptoms, reduction in signs, personality change, customer satisfaction, more effective work performance or some or all of these and, if combined, in what proportion?

Discussion of the theoretical issues underlying criterion choice would require a chapter in itself; the problem is stated here only to call attention to the necessity for choice and full realization of the implications of that choice. If the focus is on symptom relief, there is some burden on the investigator to demonstrate that the symptoms are nontrivial, and that the relief of symptoms "a" and "b" is not attained at the cost of substituting "x" and "y" (or at least that "x" and "y" are less disabling than the original set). If "personality change" is taken to be crucial, this requirement must be matched by methods of measurement that fulfill scientific canons; it is simply to negate the possibility of investigation if the stance is taken that only the psychotherapist himself can assess personality "in depth" (the very nature of his involvement precludes a role as both plaintiff and judge).

In our outpatient studies we have made use of clinical appraisal as the central criterion measure, with recognition of its limited reliability but in acknowledgment of its correspondence with daily medical practice. However, at the same time we have sought other independent methods of assessment as cross-checks. A valuable source of information for school-age children is the teacher's report. She is assigned the role of judge of the child's academic progress, as well as of peer interactions and response to institutional rules. She employs, by virtue of her training and her task, a universe of discourse that may not readily be translatable into psychiatric phraseology. If her estimate of change differs from that of the mother or of the clinician, this is not necessarily a reflection of unreliability, since she is judging behavior in a setting substantially different from home or clinic (and it is precisely this that gives her judgment value as an equally important sounding on the performance of the child). In our experience, teachers have tended to anticipate that children will benefit from psychiatric intervention. However, when teachers are asked to rate children on several different treatment programs—and do not know which child is on which regime—then the bias in favor of "treatment" should be distributed among children on all regimes; under this circumstance, differences in outcome can be related to type of treatment.

The mother is an important, although highly involved, observer of her child's behavior. Her satisfaction or dissatisfaction with his initial behavior and with the course of treatment is a key element to be taken into account in rating outcome. Her report of improvement is of course subject to the restriction that it may reflect a change in her response to his behavior, or an actual change in his behavior, or both. Again, with the use of control groups, differences in mothers' reports add valuable data.

The treating physician, though the most expert observer, has an investment in the outcome of the experiment. His assessment of change in the child, while in part based upon what he can see for himself in the clinic, is also (and should be) influenced by what the teacher and the mother report. Indeed, the mother herself is influenced by the comment she receives from the teacher. Thus, although it may be useful to treat the three ratings as separate sources of information, they are not to be considered independent sources.

A clinical method frequently used in therapeutic drug studies is the symptom list. The rater (mother, school teacher, ward attendant or another) is asked to estimate change in each of a list of symptoms chosen to cover the spectrum of aberrant behavior. Symptom lists may ask for a simple "present" or "absent" judgment or they may require a semiquantitative statement of severity. The total score is employed as a measure of overall severity. The advantage of the symptom list lies in requiring the observer to give relatively specific estimates of the level of particular behaviors rather than a single global estimate. The separate judgments, however, are subject to a "halo" effect; marked change in a particularly troublesome symptom may lead to a report of improvement in other symptoms, even though they have not changed. The most serious deficit of the total count of the symptom list is its assumption of an equivalence in the significance of symptoms, an assumption contrary to clinical reality. Cessation in enuresis or headache is clearly not the same as the disappearance of hallucinations or stealing. Yet for all its limitations, the symptom score has yielded useful results. Moreover, it permits detailed study of those symptoms which have changed as contrasted with those that have not (Conners and Eisenberg, 1963).

A method of considerable utility for groups of children who share a common setting is the sociogram. The children are asked to rate each other by a scheme which gives a measure of "social standing." In the class play of Bower and Larsen (1960), children in the same classroom (or cottage) are asked to cast their classmates in roles in a play; both positive and negative roles are available. By assessing the number of times a given child is assigned positive and negative parts in the play, one can estimate his position in the social structure of the classroom. In a study at an institution for delinquents (Eisenberg et al., 1963), a before and after analysis of the sociogram revealed significant gains in peer estimates for the child receiving dextroamphetamine, gains paralleling the improvement independently recorded by school teachers and house parents on symptom rating charts.

The uncertainties associated with clinical ratings suggest the importance of psychological test measures that can be objectively scored and assessed for reliability and validity. Whatever the utility of projective tests as diagnostic instruments, they have not been designed to measure change over the short run. It would appear more fruitful to center on tests sensitive to those psychological dimensions central to the treatment effort. The Porteus Maze Tests, scored as they are to penalize the subject for lack of planning in the search for the exit from the labyrinth, provide a screen to detect impulsivity, a key problem in the hyperkinetic and distractible child.

The examples cited serve only to indicate the possibility of documenting impressions of clinical change by objective tests. A note of caution should be added. Performance measures offer advantages in quantitation and precision, but the investigator must still deal with the ultimate problem of their relevance to the clinical state of the patient. Demonstration of change or lack of change in any given test bears on the question of therapeutic efficacy only if the test performance can be demonstrated to relate directly to the disorder from which the patient suffers.

Statistical Analysis

Except in those rare instances in which diseases have a regular, predictable and documented course, the decision as to whether the improvement following treatment is to be ascribed to the treatment must be based on a statistical analysis of the results from an appropriately designed experiment. The choice of statistical procedures bears an intimate relationship to the design of the experiment and to the methods employed in it. The biostatistician can suggest the most efficient design, once the clinical questions have been posed, and should be a participant at the planning stage rather than a consultant called in out of desperation after the investigator has been inundated by obscure data. Fisher (1962a), using a hypothetical experiment, has demonstrated the relationship between the method of analysis of the data and the conclusions reached.

Statistics are invested with no magic. No statistical manipulations can compensate for failures in design and methodology. The patient sample must be representative of the patient population from which it is drawn if the conclusions from the experiment are to be generalizable. Statistical analysis then enables the investigator to make a statement of the probability that chance alone produced the observed difference; but however improbable, chance remains a finite possibility. The more unreliable the methods used in the experiment, the greater the likelihood of failing to detect a significant difference when it exists. The bedrock of the experiment remains the accuracy of its methodology; biostatistical elegance cannot transmute dross into gold.

SYNOPSIS OF CURRENT VIEWS ON DRUG EFFECTIVENESS

The drugs used to modify behavior may be classified into stimulants, tranquilizers, antidepressants and anticonvulsants. Major emphasis will be placed on the stimulant drugs, for which the greatest documentation of effectiveness exists, and which serve to exemplify general principles. The remaining categories will be dealt with in summary fashion, and the reader will be referred to the appended bibliography.

Stimulant Drug Treatment of Behavioral Disorders in Children

Effects on General Behavior and Symptomatology. Charles Bradley's earliest report of the use of Benzedrine (amphetamine) for treatment of behavioral disorders in children (1937) described the effects of the drug on 30 children of normal intelligence between 5 and 14 years of age. He noted a "striking change" in school activities of many of the patients during the week of Benzedrine therapy. A great increase of interest in school material was noted immediately, with a "definite drive to accomplish as much as possible during the school period." He also noted an increased sense of well-being, decrease of mood swings, mild euphoria and less self-preoccupation. Arithmetic performance was the school subject most strikingly improved.

Bradley's later report of observations on 100 children from the same residential inpatient setting noted that 54 children became subdued, 21 showed no change in behavior, 19 appeared generally stimulated and 6 showed improved school behavior without other changes (1941). Only children with demonstrable neurologic deficits failed to show improvement. Bradley's (1950) summary of 275 children, reflecting more than a decade of observations with Benzedrine and Dexedrine (dexamphetamine) indicated that 60 per cent to 75 per cent were clinically improved, 10 per cent to 15 per cent showed no change and 10 per cent to 15 per cent showed unfavorable effects. School adjustment, academic performance, readiness for testing, enuresis, subdued behavior, stimulation of shy and seclusive children, increased drive for achievement and increase in attention span were described as effects of these stimulants.

These early studies merit careful consideration, since they were carried out in a well-controlled environment in which detailed observation by staff members was possible over a long period of time. The children were under intensive observation by people who knew them well, and the reports show a conservative, critical approach that gives the reader confidence in the final results despite the limitations in experimental design. These findings are in accord with most subsequent work, and they anticipate most of the effects described in rather different settings and with different methods in later research. To be sure, placebo controls and double-blind conditions were not usually established, but the findings are in many respects superior to those from studies done on patients in less controlled settings.

Bender and Cottington (1942) reported the effects of Benzedrine on 40 children with psychoneuroses, neurotic behavioral disorders, psychopathic personality, organic brain disease and schizophrenia. Among the changes observed were "feeling of well-being," stimulation of drive in learning, relief of fear, decrease of sexual tension, integration of activity, more sociability and the ability to relate in therapy. The authors attempted to explain results in individual children by taking into account the dynamics of the child in relation to the effects of the drug. For example, psychopathic personalities were adversely affected, and this was presumed to occur because the "personalities became overwhelmed by the sudden awareness of affects which led to a breakdown of a superficial integration overlying the disorganization in the emotional sphere." The authors noted that although the aggression in these children decreased, sensitivity to criticism increased, and they retired into corners to sit and cry for prolonged periods. While this study uses small samples and is impressionistic and uncontrolled, the observations just cited are noteworthy; in particular, the negative mood changes which occurred are of interest and will be discussed more fully later.

The paucity of systematic investigation of the type of effects described in these clinical studies is partially a function of the difficulty of making the clinical concept operational, but it is also undoubtedly due to a tendency among researchers to focus on easily observable symptom changes without regard to more complex aspects of personality function. It seems reasonable to expect that if given in adequate dosages, most drugs will have *some* effects on behavior; but the more interesting question of why certain effects appear in one child and not in another has seldom been attacked except in clinical studies, such as the ones mentioned here. Other clinicians have also reported observations indicating that the personality of the child may be importantly related to the type of outcome with stimulant drugs. Fish (1960) found that amphetamine "was markedly effective only in children with behavior disorders. In this group it was most effective in the more mature, better organized children with more neurotic features. Some of the most dramatic responses occurred in children with school phobias and sexual preoccupations."

A number of clinical reports and controlled studies have reported changes in a variety of behaviors through the use of rating scales or checklists of behavior. In general, these reports show that it is disruptive behavior that is most noticeably affected by the stimulants. Knobel et al. (1959) used a checklist of behavioral traits (such as temper tantrums, fighting, irritability) and also developed a Guttman scale of hyperkinesis. The effect of methylphenidate in one study with 20 children was felt to be unrelated to whether the child was hyper- or hypokinetic. Burks' rating scale of symptoms showed a 35 per cent overall reduction in symptom score, but again no details of individual symptom change are given. Knobel (1962) reported on 150 patients treated over a period of eight months. The symptoms most modified in this uncontrolled study were a decrease in hyperactivity, an increase in frustration tolerance, less agressiveness and destructiveness, diminished impulsivity, classroom performance improvement, better peer relationships and a marked decrease in hostility and resentment to authority figures.

Eisenberg et al. (1963), in a controlled study, found a significant decrease in disruptive symptoms in juvenile delinquents treated with dextroamphetamine, and Conners and Eisenberg (1963) found the following symptoms significantly reduced in a group of severely disturbed and deprived children treated with methylphenidate: the leading of others into trouble, demanding, disobedience, lying, listlessness, apathy, childlishness or immaturity, and quarrelsomeness. Interestingly, nail-biting was significantly *increased*. This might appear to be an isolated and chance phenomenon, although recently Knights and Hinton (1968) found an increase in "fiddling" behavior at meals as reported by parents of children treated with methylphenidate. They also found a reduction in symptoms of laziness, distractibility, restlessness, disobedience, fluctuating performance, restlessness while shopping, wiggling during homework, and periods of quiet play.

Conners and Rothschild (1968) found an overall reduction in ratings of activity level in specific situations using the Werry-Weiss-Peters scale as rated by parents of children treated with Dexedrine (see Fig. 9–1). A factor analysis of a 93-item symptom scale used by these parents produced two factors which Conners et al. (1970) employed in a double-blind study with Dexedrine. One cluster of symptoms consisted of symptoms of restlessness, disruptive behavior, short attention span and the like, and these showed marked reduction in the Dexedrine group. On the other

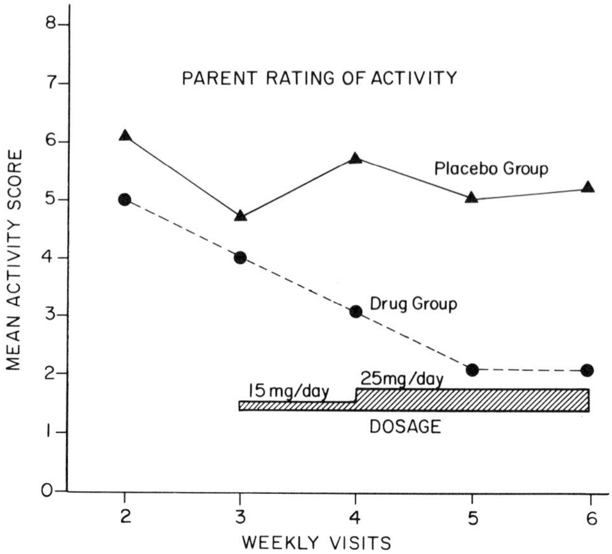

Figure 9–1 Effects of dextroamphetamine on parent ratings of activity level at home. The rating scale consists of seven items regarding the child's activity during common household activities such as eating, watching television and so forth. The score is the sum of ratings for all items. The scale was devised by Werry, Weiss and Peters (Werry, 1968b).

hand, the symptoms of seclusiveness, anxiety and inhibited behavior failed to improve significantly more than those in the placebo group (see Fig. 9–2).

Two studies, by Conners et al. (1967) and Conners (1970), employed ratings by teachers. A factor analysis of the scale produced five factors, all of which showed significant reduction with dextroamphetamine treatment over a one-month period. Factor I consisted of items reflecting disturbing, disruptive behavior (selfishness, disturbance of others, quarrelsomeness, defiance, impudence and so forth. Factor II included poor concentration, poor motor coordination, daydreaming, inattentiveness, and being easily led by others. Factor III consisted of oversensitivity, overly seriousness or sadness, fearfulness, shyness and anxiety to please. Factor IV included restless and overactive behavior, but unlike Factor I it lacked the aggressive content (excitability, making odd noises, fiddling with small objects, excessive demands for the teacher's attention and so forth). Factor V appeared to reflect sociable, cooperative behavior. These ratings were highly reliable as separate scales over a one-month period, with the test-retest reliability for subjects receiving placebo being between 0.72 and 0.91 for the five scales.

However, the difficulty with such rating studies is the possibility that raters may experience a strong "halo" effect, rating a child who shows *any* improvement as improved across all areas. The presumed specific changes may therefore be spurious. Other studies, however, tend to support these general findings of the effects of stimulants. Moreover, in perhaps the best study of its kind, Werry (1968a) used time sampling of specific individual behaviors and showed that certain deviant classroom behaviors, attention to work, nontask-related activity and points earned for "good" behavior were improved by methylphenidate as compared with placebo.

In summary, there are many clinical reports which support the view that stimulant drugs have positive effects on symptoms of a disturbing, uncontrolled, impulsive nature. For the most part these reports are based on children in whom such symptoms represent the basis of the original sample selection; that is, these are children that have been seen in clinical settings precisely because of presenting complaints of a disturbing nature at home or in school. Therefore, the degree of severity of these symptoms is probably in general above that of a normal sample, and more apparent than for other types of disturbance of development. The occasional reports of stimulation of the shy, seclusive child to more active, outgoing behavior are seen less frequently in the literature, possibly because such behavior is less likely to come to the attention of adults. In careful studies such as those by Bradley and coworkers, where this type of improvement was noted, the children were sufficient problems to warrant residential treatment. It may be the case, then, that the action of these drugs is not as paradoxical as it is usually assumed to be. Rather, they *may* produce behavioral changes in either overcontrolled or undercontrolled children, depending on which symptoms are of sufficient severity to show detectable changes.

Effects on Activity Level and Motor Performance. Perhaps because of the disruptive behavioral patterns which are frequently seen by clinicians as responding to stimulant drugs, and because of the similarity, in many respects, of these behavioral patterns to those of the organically driven, hyperkinetic syndrome described by Kahn and Cohen (1934), a good deal of attention has been focused on the effects of drugs on activity level. It has already been noted that Bradley found that many children became quieter and calmer when treated with stimulants. Molitch and Eccles (1937) found improvement in form-board tasks, with strength of grip and a form-board test being among those showing improvement after Benzedrine treatment. Blum et al. (1964) found no effects on tapping speed and reaction time, though performance was improved if the task required concentrated attention.

Conners (1966) found no effects

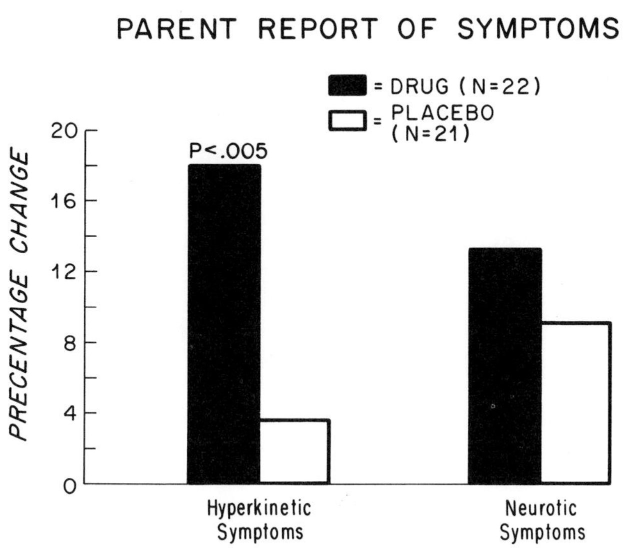

Figure 9–2 Changes in symptoms reported by parents following treatment with dextroamphetamine.

of amphetamine on a Luria-type tremorgram, though visual discriminations performed during the motor task showed significant improvement. Another study from the same laboratory (Epstein et al., 1968) found that motor steadiness was significantly improved by Dexedrine. In a more complete study, Knights and Hinton (1968) also found improvement of steadiness using a similar apparatus requiring the holding of a stylus in progressively smaller holes, and a maze tracing task.

Millichap and Boldrey (1967) reported a significant *increase* in activity measured by an actometer (an activity-watch that tabulates as a function of locomotion in the horizontal plane); and at the same time teachers and parents reported impressions of more motor coordination and less impulsivity. In a subsequent study, Millichap and coworkers (1968) measured actometer changes and keytapping speed, and found significant improvement (less actometer activity and faster keytapping) in a group treated with Ritalin (methylphenidate) as compared with control levels, but neither test improved more than those taken by the placebo-treated group.

In the best study dealing specifically with motor behavior and stimulants, Sprague et al. (1970) found that Ritalin reduced reaction times, improved accuracy, lower seat activity, (measured with an activity cushion) and reduced troublesome behavior in the classroom. Interestingly, dosage level did not influence the results, suggesting either an all-or-none type of effect or a too narrow range of dosage.

Werry (1968a), using a time-sampling observational method, found that noisy behavior and nontask-oriented activity were reduced by Ritalin in a classroom setting. This study is particularly valuable inasmuch as it is one of the few that attempts to use a molecular analysis of activity, rather than global judgments. Such measurements are both more meaningful in terms of relevance to molar behavior, and less likely to be confounded with "halo" or attitudinal variables that impinge on ratings of a more global type.

The effects of the stimulants on motor activity in children are, in general, contradictory—at least from a superficial point of view. A similar apparent divergence of findings may be found in the literature on amphetamine and activity level in animals (Dews and Morse, 1961). Part of the difficulty lies in inexact terminology. As Werry (1968a) and others have remarked, it is important to distinguish between modal activity level, and situationally appropriate motor behavior. Lytton and Knobel (1958) noted that "the administration of methylphenidate . . . resulted [not only] in a decrease in the absolute amount of motor activity but in an increase in the amount of motoric activity devoted to goal-directed behavior." Knobel et al. (1959) also make a useful distinction between a *related* type of hyperactivity; "that is, the child even though disorganized shows an interpersonal relatedness which can be easily differentiated from the *unrelated* type of hyperactivity, which is seen in some schizophrenic children who show the autistic, apparently meaningless, personally uninvolved type of hyperactivity."

Clinical reports on stimulant effects frequently point to *a better integrated or more controlled performance,* not simple alteration of activity level *per se.* Moreover, it appears that with both animals and humans the starting level of activity is an important factor in determining whether a drug will alter the level. In the rat, cortical lesions do not alter activity level itself but rather sensitize the animals to amphetamine-induced hyperkinesis (Adler, 1961), and in general, animal studies show that the animals with the most active predrug condition display the greatest response to drugs (Irwin, 1961).

Some of the divergent findings with children are almost certainly due to varying levels within a heterogeneous population of activity level and degree of motor control.

The best indication derived from the literature suggests that in the child (within the dose ranges used therapeutically), the stimulants facilitate motor performance either by increasing speed or by giving more selective control over motor response. This type of effect is well illustrated by findings reported by Conners and Rothschild (1968) for a continuous performance test: the drug-treated group showed a decreased latency of response on trials in which no signal occurred, but they showed an *increased* latency when a target signal appeared; the placebo-treated group had significantly shorter latency periods on trials in which errors occurred. These data suggest that the drug group becomes slower when it is more appropriate to do so in terms of the demands of the particular task.

Effects on Mood and Personality. Very little systematic work is available on the effects of any kind of psychotropic drugs on mood and personality in children. It has already been noted that Bradley remarked on a generalized euphoria and positive attitude in his patients, and Bender and Cottington described some improvements in mood. The zestful, energetic approach to tasks described by Bradley was confirmed in a study by Conners et al. (1967) using a very large battery of objective personality tests devised by Cattell and coworkers. The factor showing the largest effect of Dexedrine consisted of a number of tests reflecting a vigorous and energetic approach to the tasks. The results were interpreted in terms of an enhanced need for achievement, in the sense described by McClelland (1953). A study specifically designed to test this effect of amphetamine in adults also showed enhanced "n ach" (Evans and Smith, 1964).

Another study by Conners et al. (1965) used Clyde Mood Scale descriptions by parents of their children, who were being treated with Dexedrine. Two factors, termed "friendliness" and "concentration," showed significant improvements in this group over children given placebo. An examination of the items involved in these factors suggests that the children were judged as being happier and more cooperative and as showing enhanced concentration and attention span. A similar effect on sociability was reported by Eisenberg et al. (1963) in a study of delinquent boys using a sociometric device.

A less frequently reported effect of the stimulants is the production of sadness and depression. Ounstead (1955), in a study of hyperkinetic children with epilepsy, found that two-thirds responded with a depressive reaction, including crying and withdrawn and motionless behavior, while only 9 per cent showed the more frequently described positive responses of decreased hypermotility, reduced aggression and improved attention. This is no doubt a somewhat different sample of behavioral disorders in children from that used in most other reports; the hyperkinesis, poor impulse control, destructive behavior and labile moods and attention fit a syndrome of behavior frequently noted, even in the absence of demonstrable neuropathology.

Conners (1965) used the Holtzman Inkblot Test and found no effect of Dexedrine on scoring factors usually associated with mood and affect, such as the color responses and shading responses frequently presumed in clinical literature to reflect emotionality and responsiveness to the blots.

Effects on Cognition, Attention and

Perception. A number of studies have shown that stimulants have facilitatory effects on complex intellectual performances. These effects are frequently difficult to interpret, however, because they can represent either direct changes in the higher cognitive functioning of the individual, or more limited changes in specific aspects of the information-processing sequence. For example, there is good reason to suppose that stimulants alter the child's ability to attend to the task at hand; and given such alterations, almost any task will show enhanced performance unless the specific attending component has been controlled. The process of attending is itself complex, involving aspects of arousal, orienting reaction, cessation of distracting motor movements and internal processes such as filtering or sensory rating; any or all of these processes are conceivably altered by psychoactive agents.

Bradley and Bowen (1941) secured data on school performance over a one-month period prior to and after Benzedrine Sulfate (amphetamine sulfate) administration. Before medication only 6 of 19 children were making normal progress. Seventeen of the 19 produced more work while on drug than before taking the drug. Spelling was not noticeably improved. In another study, Bradley and Green (1940) found that "in general there was no striking change in intelligence quotient when amphetamine sulfate was used." That study also found no noticeable change on psychomotor tasks. These results led Bradley to conclude that positive effects to be found in testing of this type are mainly due to a change in the emotional attitude of the child rather than to any intrinsic elevation of intellectual capability.

In a pilot study, Sprague et al. (1967) found decreased latencies of response in a two-choice discrimination learning task, but no changes in levels of correct performances, possibly due to a low performance ceiling of the test. The subjects treated with Dexedrine also showed decreases over the levels of activity of subjects given placebo, but the designs of the study did not permit a separation of effects of practice and drug. In a more carefully designed study, Sprague et al. (1970) treated 12 underachieving boys in a special classroom with Ritalin, Mellaril and placebo. Ritalin significantly increased correct responding, it decreased reaction times and hyperactivity and it significantly increased attention and cooperative behavior in the classroom.

Knights and Hinton (1968) found a significant positive effect on performance IQ with Ritalin, as did Epstein et al. (1968) with Dexedrine. Conners and Rothschild (1968) found no significant effects of Dexedrine on the WISC IQ scores, though performance IQ's after treatment were consistently higher than those of the group given placebo. Millichap and coworkers (1968) found improvements in the Draw-A-Man IQ and a figure-ground subtest from the Frostig Developmental Test of Visual Perception in a study of 30 children with learning disorders treated with Ritalin. The latter result was obtained by Conners and Rothschild, as well as significant effects on the Spatial Relations subtest and the overall Perceptual Quotient of the Frostig test. Significant improvement was also found on tests of continuous attention, reading and arithmetic, auditory synthesis and paired-associate learning.

In a series of studies, we have found consistently significant drug-induced improvements in children with learning problems or behavioral problems, or both, in the Porteus Maze Test (1968). This test requires the subject to trace his way through a pencil maze at his own rate and penalizes impulsive darting into blind alleys, thus placing a premium on planned, controlled responding. The improvements have often been striking, being as much as 16 to 25 IQ points over the placebo controls. It is our belief that much of the change seen in many intellectual and performance tests is due to this change in the more basic capacity to selectively inhibit, plan and control response (see Fig. 9–3).

In a well-controlled study, Creager and Van Riper (1967) documented an oft-noted clinical response to stimulants: they found that the total number of words spoken and the number of verbal responses were significantly increased by Ritalin in a group of 30 children. It seems plausible that an increase in available verbal production together with more controlled or selective responding should lead to enhanced performance of children in a number of situations.

Potential for Abuse. In 1970, public attention focused on the potential for the abuse of stimulant drugs in children (Eisenberg, 1971). Two issues have been paramount: addiction and misuse. Amphetamines have long been known to be addictive in adolescents and adults (Connell, 1958; Ellenwood and Cohen, 1971); by extrapolation, they have been assumed to have such effects in children.

Furthermore, their demonstrated effectiveness in decreasing activity in hyperkinetic children has led to charges that they are being misused by teachers (and parents) as chemical strait jackets for normal but "active," "exuberant" and "creative" children whose behavior challenges authority. These two concerns, addiction and

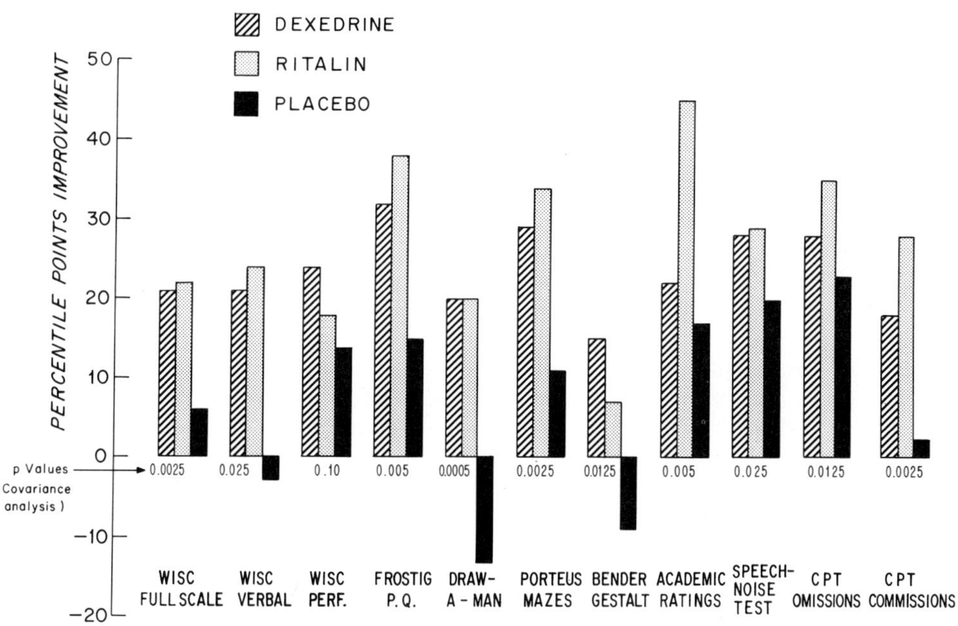

Figure 9–3 Changes in psychological tests following treatment with Dexedrine, Ritalin or placebo. Changes are displayed in terms of percentile changes based on the normal curve. Probability differences between treatments are based on analysis of covariance. Tests are as follows: WISC = Wechsler Intelligence Scale for Children; Frostig P.Q. = perceptual quotient from the Frostig Developmental Test of Visual Perception. Draw-A-Man scores are based on the Goodenough-Harris scoring system. The speech-noise test is a measure of word-discrimination in background noise; CPT refers to a continuous performance test, with errors of omission and errors of commission. All scores are displayed to show improvement (e.g., reduction in errors, gain in performance).

misuse, raise quite different pharmacologic and policy questions and require separate analysis.

ADDICTION. Extensive clinical experience since the 1940's has not led to recognized and recorded instances of addiction to amphetamines in children. Amphetamine can be discontinued totally, even after several years of daily use, with no deleterious effects and no necessity for graduated withdrawal, unlike the situation with anticonvulsants or steroids. If the patient is still hyperkinetic when the drug is withdrawn, his symptoms will return; if the underlying disorder has diminished with maturation, the patient is able to function normally without further requirement for medication. Such a child has no craving for the drug because it does not produce euphoria (as it does with adolescents); thus, it is not sought after by the patient. The reasons for these differences remain unknown, but the fact of the difference is another illustration of the importance of developmental psychopharmacology.

Nonetheless, it has been contended that the experience of drug use might predispose to the risk of indiscriminate use of drugs later in life. Until recently, there has been no systematic data by which to assess this theoretical possibility. In a study undertaken by members of our staff, no evidence of subsequent drug abuse was found in a series of patients who had been treated during childhood for hyperkinesis and who were followed into adolescence and young adulthood (Laufer et al., 1971). Further, Klein (1970), in a survey of adolescent drug addicts at Hillside Hospital, found a group who, by history, had been hyperkinetic children but who had been *untreated.* Thus, the available data suggest that effective treatment of this disorder, probably by enhancing the adaptive capacities of hyperkinetic children, diminishes their vulnerability to adolescent drug addiction.

MISUSE. Regarding the misuse of stimulant drugs, potential must be distinguished from actuality. The ethical barriers to experimentation with normal children leaves us with no information on the effects of amphetamines on normal levels of activity. If we assume that there may be a "sedative" effect, then it remains possible for the drugs to be misused in the effort to suppress troublesome behavior. This serves to reinforce the importance of a thorough medical evaluation of children thought to be candidates for treatment (Eisenberg, 1971). The subject of misuse has been thoroughly reviewed by a panel convened for this purpose by the Office of Child Development (1971). In essence, this expert report emphasizes the usefulness of pharmacologic treatment for hyperkinetic children under medical supervision and stresses the necessity for adequate safeguards to protect against indiscriminate and inappropriate use of these agents.

Summary. It has been found that stimulant drugs such as dextroamphetamine and methylphenidate are a useful clinical tool for the management of disruptive symptoms and for some psychoneurotic complaints. Effects on activity level and motor performance are generally in the direction of more controlled, skilled performances, particularly where goal-directed striving is an important component of the tasks. Various perceptual, intellective and performance tasks have been enhanced by the stimulants in children with a variety of behavioral disturbances, most notably in those with poor impulse control and impulsivity. These changes are most likely a function of enhanced attention to the tasks or control over response, or both. Effects on mood and personality are less well understood, though often the drugs appear to produce a sense of well-being and a more vigorous, zestful approach to the environment. Well-controlled studies on other stimulant drugs such as deanol have not been performed.

Effects of Tranquilizers and Sedatives

A rather large literature on the tranquilizers and their use with children exists, but most of this literature is uncontrolled and contradictory in its findings. Carefully controlled studies usually show small effects (Molling et al., 1962). Little is to be gained by a detailed review of the extensive literature in view of the paucity of experimental findings. The best survey of findings on these drugs is to be found in a chapter by Karen Veazie Davis in a report compiled by Sprague and Werry (1968).

In brief, the following conclusions seem to be warranted from the existing literature:

1. Mellaril (thioridazine) appears to be the most effective of the phenothiazine derivatives which have been tried, particularly in retarded-hyperactive, brain-injured or highly excitable patients. Thorazine (chlorpromazine) has been most widely used, with one or two well-controlled studies showing positive clinical benefits, again in those children with *severe* hypermotility.

2. While the tranquilizers may be useful for symptom control, most evidence indicates that they have deleterious effects on cognitive functions and learning, and they are therefore contraindicated for children of normal intellectual endowment (Garfield et al., 1962). The conclusion which is sometimes drawn that these drugs are desirable for children of low intelligence, however, seems unwarranted, since it is precisely those children who would stand to lose most from reduced intellectual capability.

3. In the opinion of Fish (1967), one of the most experienced clinicians in the field, many of the studies have utilized dosages too small for maximum clinical benefit.

4. Sedatives, such as phenobarbital, are generally contraindicated because of a tendency, except in very high doses, to produce hyperexcitement in many children, though many clinicians attest to the calmative effects of the antihistamine drug, Benadryl (diphenhydramine) (Effron and Freedman, 1953).

Antidepressant Drugs

A number of recent studies have suggested that antidepressant drugs may be useful in certain disorders (Mariuz and Walter, 1963; Treffert, 1964). The use of the tri-cyclic amines (imipramine, nortriptyline, amitriptyline) with children is relatively recent but deserves mention because of promising reports on enuresis and behavioral disorders. Two studies using hospitalized patients (Abrams, 1963; Fisher et al., 1963) found no effects of imipramine on enuresis, while a number of studies have reported quite striking diminution of wetting in a variety of children in both inpatient and outpatient settings. The relapse rate when the drug is withdrawn is high, though apparently this may be reduced by gradual drug withdrawal (Poussaint and Ditman, 1965). The possible mechanism for this specific action is not known, though it may be a direct action on diuretic hormones or the sleep cycle. It is of interest, however, to note that other drugs such as Dexedrine and Ritalin, which are essentially central nervous system stimulants, have occasionally been noted to reduce enuresis. Whether this occurs because of a change in the sleep pattern, by direct autonomic effects or otherwise, is not known.

Krakowski (1965) studied 122 children in various diagnostic categories and ranging in age from 2 to 18 years. He found sufficient benefits from amitriptyline to warrant a controlled study of this agent. Fifty hyperkinetic children, with a mean age of approximately 10 years, were followed over a six-month period or until symptoms disappeared. In general, improvement was excellent or good in 72 per cent to 87 per cent of the cases, with 8 out of 10 enuretics showing complete remission of symptoms. Seventy-two per cent showed excellent or good response when switched from placebo to drug. This study is methodologically unsound in many respects, but it suggests that more work with this drug might be worthwhile in children with hyperkinesis.

Anticonvulsant Drug Therapy

Few well-controlled studies of the use of anticonvulsants in behavioral disorders of children have been carried out, though many clinicians use such drugs for these disorders, often being quite convinced of dramatic benefits in certain cases, regardless of whether the child also has accompanying EEG abnormalities. Undoubtedly the most serious neglect in the published studies is the use of very heterogeneous samples, which is bound to obscure any meaningful changes in smaller subgroups, and the absence of placebo controls.

The most widely used and longest tested drug of this class is diphenylhydantoin (DPH). Pasamanick (1951) treated 21 boys, 6 to 13 years old, with behavioral patterns "not acceptable in the community or home;" some had abnormal EEG records. No improvement attributable to DPH was found. Cohn and Nardini (1958) treated children with unruly, violent behavior and abnormal slowing on EEG, with no change in either behavior or EEG pattern. Green (1961) found DPH ineffective for behavioral disorders in children with an EEG focus. On the other hand, Walker and Kirkpatrick (1947) gave DPH to behavioral problem children with abnormal EEG records, and they "appeared" improved. Brown and Solomon (1942) found that three of seven boys with serious behavioral difficulties in a training school setting and with grossly abnormal EEG's of the psychomotor type showed definite decrease in hyperactivity, inattention, excitability and temper tantrums. Putnam and Hood (1964) found the drug useful in a study of delinquents. Chao et al. (1964) studied the effect of DPH on the convulsive equivalent syndrome (paroxysmal cerebral disorder characterized by autonomic disturbances and dysfunction in behavior and communication), with good overall clinical results that were often of a dramatic quality. Resnick (1967) carried out a double-blind controlled study that included delinquents ranging in age from 12 to 15 years. This study carefully selected the subjects on the basis of symptoms thought by some to be particularly suitable for DPH treatment: overthinking, sleep difficulties, depression, anger and hostility, with chronic impatience and irritability being prominent features. Significant positive benefits were reported, although the study has serious flaws in the manner the data were obtained.

Two studies by Conners and coworkers (1971), in which double-blind placebo control, random group assignments, objective performance measures, behavioral ratings by trained observers and naturalistic observations were used, failed to show any benefit for children in a training school for delinquents or for children with severe temper outbursts. However, these studies also suffer from heterogeneity of the subject population and from the necessity to use subjects who were only mildly disturbed.

SUMMARY

The bulk of this chapter is devoted to studies with stimulant drugs (specifically Dexedrine and Ritalin), which partially reflects the longer use of these agents, the larger number of controlled studies and positive findings and the authors' own predilections. The large numbers of reports on other agents that have been tried with children are so poorly documented or restricted to limited populations or symptom conditions that they are not yet of sufficient generalizability to warrant extensive discussion.

Apart from clinical considerations of treatment and management of behavior, there is the profoundly important contribution that drugs can make in the understanding of the mechanisms of behavior, of personality and of development in children. The effect of the stimulants, for example, in altering attentional behavior and drive level while at the same time also altering the behavioral disorder (hyperkinetic or impulsive behavior in particular), has important implications for the genesis of the behavioral disorder in neurophysiologic disturbances of arousal and inhibitory mechanisms. Whether these occur because of delayed maturation of the cortices, because of diencephalic disorders or because of imbalance in corticoreticular regulation of afferent input remains to be decided by much further work. This work must involve cooperative efforts of scientists and clinicians and must be carried out with due attention to clinical obligations to the child and his family. These obligations can be formulated as follows:

1. No drug should be employed without firm indication for its use, without careful control of the patient to be treated and without due precautions for toxicity. With any potent drug, toxicity is inevitable; to justify its use, the severity of the presenting condition and the likelihood of benefit must outweigh the risk of toxicity. Toxicity studies on adults cannot be safely extrapolated to children because of differences in the immature organism. Clinical decisions must be based upon data from pediatric studies.

2. An old and familiar drug is to be preferred to a new one unless evidence for superiority for the new drug is preponderant. This principle of pharmacologic conservatism is based on the fact that unexpected toxicity from a new agent may be apparent only after prolonged experience with its use. This is not a statement of pharmacologic nihilism. Drugs can make a decisive difference in treatment, but their very potency commends us not to use them lightly.

3. Despite these cautions, drugs can be useful agents in the management of pediatric psychiatric disorders when chosen appropriately and applied with discrimination. They can be effective in controlling symptoms not readily managed by other means and can facilitate other methods of psychiatric treatment by allaying symptoms that disrupt learning. If they are not the panaceas portrayed in advertisements, neither are they the poisons claimed by those wedded to exclusively psychological methods of treatment.

4. Every drug study reveals the potency of placebo effects; that is, benefits occurring from the relationship between physician and patient and from positive expectations in the patient. Skill in the use of drugs requires, in addition to knowledge of their pharmacologic properties, sensitivity to their psychologic implications.

5. Drugs should be used no longer than necessary. Dosage should be reduced periodically with the goal of cessation of treatment if symptoms do not return on lower dosage. Dosage must be individualized. Undertreatment as well as overtreatment can result in incorrect judgments about the appropriateness of particular drugs for the patient.

6. The use of drugs does not relieve the physician of the responsibility for seeking to identify and eliminate the factors causing or aggravating the psychiatric disorder. All of the currently

available psychopharmacologic agents treat symptoms, not diseases. Clearly, symptomatic relief is not be disparaged; indeed, it will remain a major part of medicine so long as causes are unknown and cures unattainable in many diseases. However, symptom suppression may also delay diagnosis and hence effective treatment. To prescribe drugs for a child whose symptoms stem from correctable social, familial, biological or intrapersonal disturbances without attempting to alter the factors causing the symptoms is poor medicine.

ACKNOWLEDGMENTS

The work by the authors that is reported in this chapter has been supported by research grant MH-02583 and Research Scientist Development Award MH-07839 from the National Institute of Mental Health, as well as by grant support from the Dreyfus Medical Foundation.

REFERENCES

Abrams, A. L.: Imipramine in enuresis. *Amer. J. Psychiat., 120*:177–178, 1963.

Adler, M. W.: Changes in sensitivity to amphetamine in rats with chronic brain lesions. *J. Pharmacol. Exp. Ther., 134*:214–221, 1961.

Alexandris, A., and Lundell, F.: Effect of thioridazine, amphetamine and placebo on the hyperkinetic syndrome and cognitive area in mentally deficient children. *Canad. Med. Ass. J., 98*:92–96, 1968.

Apgar, V.: A Proposal for a new method of evaluation of the newborn infant. *Current Research in Anesthesia and Analgesia, 32*: 260–268, 1960.

Bahn, A., Chandler, C., and Eisenberg, L.: Diagnostic characteristics related to services in psychiatric clinics for children. *Milbank Mem. Fund Quart., 40*:289–318, 1962.

Baker, J. B. E.: The effects of drugs on the fetus. *Pharmacol. Rev., 12*:37–90, 1960.

Baker, R. R.: The effects of psychotropic drugs on psychological testing. *Psychol. Bull., 69*:377–387, 1968.

Bender, L., and Cottington, F.: The use of amphetamine sulfate (Benzedrine) in child psychiatry. *Amer. J. Psychiat., 99*:116–121, 1942.

Berlin, C. M., and Jacobson, C. B.: Congenital anomalies associated with LSD ingestion. *Society for Pediatric Research Abstracts*, 1970, p. 13.

Blum, B., Stern, M., and Melville, K.: A comparative evaluation of the action of depressant and stimulant drugs on human performance. *Psychopharmacologia, 6*:173–177, 1964.

Bower, E. M., and Larson, C. A.: A class play. *In* Bower, E. M.: *Early Identification of Emotionally Handicapped Children in School.* Springfield, Illinois, Charles C Thomas, Publisher, 1960.

Bradley, C.: The behavior of children receiving Benzedrine. *Am J. Psychiat. 94*:577–585, 1937–1938.

Bradley, C.: Benzedrine and Dexedrine in the treatment of children's behavior disorders. *Pediatrics, 5*:24–36, 1950.

Bradley, C., and Bowen, M.: School performance of children receiving amphetamine (Benzedrine) sulfate. *Amer. J. Orthopsychiat., 10*:782–788, 1940.

Bradley, C., and Bowen, M.: Amphetamine (Benzedrine) therapy of children's behavior disorders. *Amer. J. Orthopsychiat., 11*:92–103, 1941.

Bradley, C., and Green, E.: Psychometric performance of children receiving amphetamine (Benzedrine) sulfate. *Am. J. Psychiat., 97*:388–394, 1940–1941.

Brazelton, T. B.: Effect of prenatal drugs on the behavior of the neonate. *Amer. J. Psychiat., 126*:1261–1266, 1970.

Brazelton, T. B., and Robey, J. S.: Observations of neonatal behavior. The effect of perinatal variables, in particular that of maternal medication. *J. Amer. Acad. Child Psychiat., 4*:613–637, 1965.

Brown, W. T., and Solomon, C. I.: Delinquency and the electroencephalograph. *Amer. J. Psychiat., 98*:499–503, 1942.

Cattell, R. B.: *Personality and Motivation Structure and Measurement.* New York, Harcourt Brace Jovanovich, Inc., 1957.

Chao, D., Sexton, J., and Davis, S.: Convulsive equivalent syndrome of childhood. *J. Pediat., 64*:499–508, 1964.

Cobrinik, P. W., Hood, R. T., and Chusis, E.: The effect of maternal narcotic addiction on the newborn infant. *Pediatrics, 24*:288–290, 1959.

Cohn, R., and Nardini, J. E.: Bilateral occipital slow activity in the EEG. *Amer. J. Psychiat., 115*:44–48, 1958.

Connell, P. H.: *Amphetamine Psychosis.* London, Chapman & Hall Ltd., 1958.

Conners, C. K.: Effects of brief psychotherapy, drugs, and type of disturbance on Holtzman inkblot scores in children. *Proceedings of American Psychological Association*, 1965.

Conners, C. K.: A teacher rating scale for use in drug studies with children. *Amer. J. Psychiat., 126*:152–156, 1969.

Conners, C. K., and Eisenberg, L.: The effects of methylphenidate on symptomatology and learning in disturbed children. *Amer. J. Psychiat., 120*:458–464, 1963.

Conners, C. K., Eisenberg, L., and Barcai, A.: Effect of dextro-amphetamine in children. *Arch. Gen. Psychiat., 17*:478–485, 1967.

Conners, C. K., Eisenberg, L., and Sharpe. L.: Effects of methylphenidate (Ritalin) on paired-associate learning and Porteus Maze performance in emotionally disturbed children. *J. Consult. Psychol., 28*:14–22, 1964.

Conners, C. K., Eisenberg, L., and Sharpe, L.: A controlled study of the differential application of outpatient psychiatric treatment for children. *Japanese Journal of Child Psychiatry, 6*:125–132, 1965.

Conners, C. K., and Greenfeld, D.: Habituation of motor startle in anxious and restless children. *J. Child Psychol. Psychiat., 7*:125–132, 1966.

Conners, C. K., Kramer, R., Rothschild, G. H., Schwartz, L., and Stone, A.: Treatment of young delinquent boys with diphenylhydantoin sodium and methylphenidate. *Arch. Gen. Psychiat., 24*:156–160, 1971.

Conners, C. K., and Rothschild, G. H.: Drugs and learning in children. *In Learning Disorders.* Seattle, Washington, Special Child Publications, 1968, Vol. III, 191–224.

Conners, C. K., Rothschild, G. H., Eisenberg, L., Schwartz, L., and Robinson, E.: Dextroamphetamine Sulfate in children with learning disorders: Effects on perception, learning and achievement. *Arch. Gen. Psychiat., 21*:182–190, 1969.

Coolidge, J. C., Willer, M. L., Tessman, E., and Waldfogel, S.: School phobia in adolescence. *Amer. J. Orthopsychiat., 30*:599–607, 1960.

Creager, R. O., and Van Riper, C.: The effect of methylphenidate on the verbal productivity of children with cerebral dysfunction. *J. Speech Hearing Res., 10*:623–628, 1967.

Cytryn, L., Gilbert, A., and Eisenberg, L.: The effectiveness of tranquilizing drugs plus supportive psychotherapy in treating behavior disorders of children: A double-blind study of eighty outpatients. *Amer. J. Orthopsychiat., 30*:113–129, 1960.

Davis, K. V.: The use of phenothiazine derivatives with children. *In* Sprague, R., and Werry, J.: *Survey of Research on Psychopharmacology of Children.* Urbana, University of Illinois Press, 1967–1968, pp. 87–135.

Dews, P. B., and Morse, W. H.: Behavioral pharmacology. *Ann. Rev. Pharmacol., 1*: 145–174, 1961.

Effron, A., and Freedman, A.: The treatment of behavior disorders in children with Benadryl. *J. Pediat., 42*:261–266, 1953.

Eisenberg, L.: The course of childhood schizophrenia. *Arch. Neurol., Psychiat., 78*:69–83, 1957.

Eisenberg, L.: If not now, when? *Amer. J. Orthopsychiat., 32*:781–793, 1962.

Eisenberg, L.: Child psychiatry: The past quarter century. *Amer. J. Orthopsychiat., 39*:389–401, 1969.

Eisenberg, L.: Principles of drug therapy in child psychiatry with special reference to stimulant drugs. *Amer. J. Orthopsychiat., 41*:371–379, 1971.

Eisenberg, L., Gilbert, A., Cytryn, L., and Molling, P. A.: The effectiveness of psychotherapy alone and in conjunction with perphenazine or placebo in the treatment of neurotic and hyperkinetic children. *Amer. J. Psychiat., 117*:1088–1093, 1961.

Eisenberg, L., Lachman, R., Molling, P., Lockner, A., Mizelle, J., and Conners, C. K.: A psychopharmacologic experiment in a training school for delinquent boys. *Amer. J. Orthopsychiat., 33*:431–447, 1963.

Ellenwood, E. H., and Cohen, S.: Amphetamine abuse. Science, *171*:420–421, 1971.

Epstein, L. C., Lasagna, L., Conners, C. K., and Rodriguez, A.: Correlation of dextroamphetamine excretion and drug response in hyperkinetic children. *J. Nerv. Ment. Dis., 146*: 136–146, 1968.

Evans, W. O., and Smith, R. P.: Some effects of morphine and amphetamine on intellectual functions and mood. *Psychopharmacologia, 6*:49–56, 1964.

Fish, B.: Drug therapy in child psychiatry: Pharmacological aspects. *Compr. Psychiat., 1*:212–227, 1960.

Fish, B.: Methodology in child psychopharmacology. Presented at the meeting of the American College of Neuropsychopharmacology, San Juan, December, 1967.

Fish, B.: Drug use in psychiatric disorders of children. *Amer. J. Psychiat.,* Supplement, 124, 31–36, 1969.

Fish, B., Shapiro, T., and Campbell, M.: Long-term prognosis and the response of schizophrenic children to drug therapy: A controlled study of trifluoperazine. *Amer. J. Psychiat., 123*:32–39, 1966.

Fisher, G. W., Murray, F., Walley, M. R., and Kiloh, L. G.: A controlled trial of imipramine in the treatment of nocturnal enuresis in mentally subnormal patients. *Amer. J. Ment. Defic., 67*:536–538, 1963.

Fisher, S.: Use of chi-square in simple cross-over designs. *J. New Drugs, 2*:84–87, 1962a.

Fisher, S.: On the relationship between expectations and drug responses. *Clinical Pharmacological Therapy, 3*:125, 1962b.

Freedman, A. M.: Drug therapy in behavior disorders. *Pediat. Clin. N. Amer., 5*:573–594, 1958.

Freedman, A. M., Effron, A. S., and Bender, L.: Pharmacotherapy in children with psychiatric illness. J. Nerv. Ment. Dis., *122*:479–486, 1955.

Freeman, R. D.: Drug effects on learning in children: A selective review of the past thirty years. *Journal of Special Education, 1*:17–44, 1966.

Frommer, E. A.: Treatment of childhood depression with antidepressant drugs. *Brit. Med. J., 1*:729–732, 1967.

Garfield, S. L., Helper, M. M., Wilcott, R. C., and Muffly, R.: Effects of chlorpromazine on behavior in emotionally disturbed children. *J. Nerv. Ment. Dis., 135*:147–154, 1962.

Green, J. B.: Association of behavior disorder with EEG focus in children without seizure. *Neurology, 11*:337–344, 1961.

Helper, M., Wilcott, R. C., and Garfield, S. L.: Effects of chlorpromazine on learning and related processes in emotionally disturbed children. *J. Consult. Psychol., 27*:1–9, 1963.

Hollingshead, A. B., and Redlich, F. C.: *Social Class and Mental Illness.* New York, John Wiley & Sons, Inc., 1958.

Hunt, B. R., Frank, T., and Krush, T. P.: Chlorpromazine in the treatment of severe emotional disorders of children. *A.M.A. J. Dis. Child., 91*:268–277, 1956.

Hutt, C., Jackson, P. M., and Level, M.: Behavioral parameters and drug effects: A study of a hyperkinetic epileptic child. *Epilepsia, 7*:250–259, 1961.

Irwin, S.: The actions of drugs on psychomotor activity. *Rev. Canad. Biol., 20*:239–250, 1961.

Irwin, S.: A rational framework for the development, evaluation, and use of psychoactive drugs. *Amer. J. Psychiat., 124(Suppl.)*: 1–19, 1968.

Jonas, A.: *Ictal and Subictal Neurosis: Diagnosis and Treatment.* Springfield, Illinois, Charles C Thomas, Publisher, 1965.

Kahn, E., and Cohen, L.: Organic driveness: A brain stem syndrome and an experience. *New Eng. J. Med., 210*:748–756, 1934.

Klein, D.: Personal Communication, 1970.

Knights, R. M., and Hinton, G.: The effects of methylphenidate (Ritalin) on the motor skills and behavior of children with learning problems. Research Bulletin No. 102, University of Western Ontario, October, 1968.

Knobel, M.: Psychopharmacology for the hyperkinetic child – Dynamic considerations. *Arch. Gen. Psychiat., 6*:198–202, 1962.

Knobel, M., Wolman, M. B., and Mason, E.: Hyperkinesis and organicity in children. *Arch. Gen. Psychiat., 1*:310–321, 1959.

Krakowski, A. J.: Amitriptyline and the treatment of hyperkinetic children. *Psychosomatics, 6*:355–360, 1965.

Lane, G. G., Huber, W. G., and Smith, F. L.: The effect of chlorpromazine on the behavior of disturbed children. *Amer. J. Psychiat., 114*:937–938, 1958.

Laties, V. G., and Weiss, B.: A critical review of the efficacy of meprobamate in the treatment of anxiety. *J. Chronic Dis., 7*:500–519, 1958.

Laufer, M. H., Conners, C. K., and McCarthy, P. D.: Unpublished Manuscript, 1971.

Lennard, H., Epstein, L. J., Bernstein, A., and Ransom, D. C.: Hazards implicit in prescribing psychoactive drugs. *Science, 169*:438–441, 1970.

Levitt, E.: A followup evaluation of cases treated at a community child guidance clinic. *Amer. J. Orthopsychiat., 29*:337–349, 1959.

Lytton, G. J., and Knobel, M.: Diagnosis and treatment of behavior disorders in children. *Dis. Nerv. Syst., 20*:596–599, 1958.

Mariuz, M. J., and Walter, C. J.: Enuresis in non-psychotic boys treated with imipramine. *Amer. J. Psychiat., 120*:596–599, 1963.

McClelland, D. C., Atkinson, J. W., Clark, R. A., and Lowell, E. L.: *The Achievement Motive.* New York, Appleton-Century-Crofts, 1953.

McConnel, T. R., Cromwell, R. L., Bialer, I., and Son, C. D.: Studies in activity level VII. Effects of amphetamine drug administration on the activity level of retarded children. *Amer. J. Ment. Defic., 68*:647–651, 1964.

Millichap, J. G., Aymat, F., Sturgis, L. H., Larsen, K., and Whittle, R.: Hyperkinetic behavior and learning disorders. III. Battery of neuropsychological tests in controlled trial of methylphenidate. *Amer. J. Dis. Child., 116*:235–244, 1968.

Millichap, J. G., and Boldrey, E. E.: Studies in hyperkinetic behavior. *Neurology, 17*:467–471, 1967.

Millichap, J. G., and Fowler, G.: Treatment of minimal brain dysfunction syndrome. *In* Millichap, J. G. (Ed.): *The Pediatric Clinics of North America: Pediatric Neurology.* Philadelphia, W. B. Saunders Company, 1967, Vol. XIV, pp. 767–777.

Molitch, M., and Eccles, A. K.: The effect of Benzedrine sulfate on the intelligence scores of children. *Amer. J. Psychiat., 94*: 587–590, 1937.

Molling, P. A., Lockner, A., Sauls, R. J., and Eisenberg, L.: The impact of perphenazine and placebo in committed delinquent boys. *Arch. Gen. Psychiat., 7*:70–76, 1962.

Money, J., Ehrdardt, A. A., and Masica, D. N.: Fetal feminization induced by androgen insensitivity in the testicular feminizing syndrome: Effect on marriage and maternalism. *Johns Hopkins Med. J., 123*:105–114, 1968.

Nichols, M. M.: Acute withdrawal syndrome in a newborn. *Amer. J. Dis. Child., 133*:714–715, 1967.

Nyhan, W. L.: Developmental pharmacology. *In* Cooke, R. E. (Ed.): *Biological Basis of Pediatric Practice,* New York, McGraw-Hill Book Company, 1968.

Office of Child Development: Report of the Conference on the use of stimulant drugs in the treatment of behaviorally disturbed young school children. Washington, D. C., January 11–12, 1971.

O'Neal, P., and Robins, L. N.: The relation of childhood behavior disorders to adult psychiatric status. *Amer. J. Psychiat., 114*:961–968, 1958a.

O'Neal, P., and Robins, L. N.: Childhood patterns predictive of adult schizophrenia. *Amer. J. Psychiat., 115*:385–391, 1958b.

Ounstead, C.: The hyperkinetic syndrome in epileptic children. *Lancet, 2*:303–311, 1955.

Pasamanick, B.: Anticonvulsant drug therapy of behavior problem children with abnormal EEG. *Arch. Neurol. Psychiat., 65*:752–766, 1951.

Pauig, P., Deluca, M. A., and Ostenheld, R. G.: Thioridazine hydrochloride in the treatment of behavior disorders in epileptics. *Amer. J. Psychiat., 117*:832–833, 1961.

Porteus, S. D.: New application of the Porteus Maze Test. *Percept. Motor Skills, 26*:787–798, 1968.

Poussaint, A. F., and Ditman, K. S.: A controlled study of imipramine (Tofranil) in the treatment of childhood enuresis. *J. Pediat., 67*:283–290, 1965.

Putnam, T. J., and Hood, O. E.: Project Illinois: A study of therapy in juvenile behavior problems. *Western Med., 5*:231–233, 1964.

Resnick, O.: Appendix to: The psychoactive properties of diphenylhydantoin: Experiences with prisoners and juvenile delinquents. *Int. J. Neuropsychiat.* 3 Suppl.2: 37–48, 1967.

Robins, L.: *Deviant Children Grown Up.* Baltimore, The Williams & Wilkins Co., 1966.

Rodriguez, A., Rodriguez, M., and Eisenberg, L.: The outcome of school phobia. *Amer. J. Psychiat., 116*:540–544, 1959.

Rosenthal, R., and Lawson, R.: A longitudinal study of the effects of experimenter bias on the operant learning of laboratory rats. *J. Psychiat. Res., 2*:61–72, 1964.

Shaw, C. R., Lockett, H. J., Lucas, A. R., Lamontagne, C. H., and Grim, F.: Tranquilizer drugs in the treatment of emotionally disturbed children. I. Inpatients in a residential treatment center. *J. Amer. Acad. Child Psychiat., 2*:725–741, 1963.

Smith, S. W.: Trifluoperazine in children and adolescents with marked behavior problems. *Amer. J. Psychiat., 122*:702–703, 1965.

Sprague, R., Barnes, K., and Werry, J.: Methylphenidate and thioridazine: Learning, reaction time, activity, and classroom behavior in disturbed children. *Amer. J. Orthopsychiat., 40*:615–628, 1970.

Sprague, R., et al.: Effects of dextroamphetamine on activity level and learning in retarded children. Presented at Midwestern Psychological Association, Chicago, May 5, 1967.

Tec, L.: Efficacy of diphenylhydantoin in childhood psychiatric disorders. *Amer. J. Psychiat., 124*:1138–1139, 1968.

Treffert, D. A.: Evaluation of imipramine in enuresis. *Amer. J. Psychiat., 121*:178–179, 1964.

Uhlenhuth, E. H., and Park, L. C.: The influence of medication (imipramine) and doctor in relieving depressed psychoneurotic outpatients. *J. Psychiat. Res., 2*:101–122, 1964.

Walker, C. F., and Kirkpatrick, B. B.: Dilantin treatment for behavior problem children with abnormal electroencephalograms. *Amer. J. Psychiat., 103*:484–492, 1947.

Warren, W.: Some relationship between the psychiatry of children and adults. *J. Ment. Sci., 106*:815–826, 1960.

Weiss, G., Werry, J., Minde, K., Douglas, V., and Sykes, D.: Studies on the hyperactive child. V. The effects of dextroamphetamine and chlorpromazine on behavior and intellectual functioning. *J. Child Psychol. Psychiat., 9*:145–156, 1968.

Werry, J.: The effects of methylphenidate and phenobarbital on the behavior of hyperactive and aggressive children. Unpublished manuscript. University of Illinois, 1968a.

Werry, J.: Developmental hyperactivity. *Pediat. Clin. N. Amer., 15*:581–599, 1968b.

Werry, J. S., Weiss, C., Douglas, V., and Martin, J.: Studies on the hyperactive child. III. The effect of chlorpromazine upon behavior and learning ability. *J. Amer. Acad. Child Psychiat., 5*:292–312, 1966.

Whitehouse, D., Conners, C. K., and Eisenberg, L.: A double-blind study of phenobarbital methylphenidate and placebo in defective hyperkinetic children. Unpublished manuscript. Johns Hopkins University, 1964.

Wilcott, R. C., Helper, M. M., and Garfield, S. L.: Some psychological effects of chlorpromazine on emotionally disturbed children. *J. Nerv. Ment. Dis., 135*:233–238, 1962.

Zrull, J. P., Westman, J. C., Arthur, B., and Bell, W. A.: A comparison of chlordiazepoxide, D-amphetamine, and placebo in the treatment of the hyperkinetic syndrome in children. *Amer. J. Psychiat., 120*:590–591, 1963.

Zrull, J. P., Westman, J. C., Arthur, B., and Rice, D. L.: An evaluation of methodology used in the study of psychoactive drugs for children. *J. Amer. Acad. Child Psychiat., 5*:284–291, 1961.

Zrull, J. P., Westman, J. C., Arthur, B., and Rice, D. L.: A comparison of diazepam, D-amphetamine, and placebo in the treatment of the hyperkinetic syndrome in childhood. *Amer. J. Psychiat., 121*:388–389, 1964.

INDEX

Page numbers in *italics* refer to illustrations.
Page numbers followed by *t* refer to tables.